I0478736

Atherosclerosis: Risks, Mechanisms and Management

Atherosclerosis: Risks, Mechanisms and Management

Editor: Grace Flynn

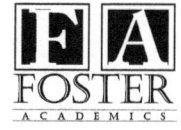

FOSTER
ACADEMICS

www.fosteracademics.com

www.fosteracademics.com

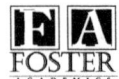

Cataloging-in-Publication Data

Atherosclerosis : risks, mechanisms and management / edited by Grace Flynn.
    p. cm.
Includes bibliographical references and index.
ISBN 978-1-63242-968-1
1. Atherosclerosis. 2. Atherosclerosis--Complications. 3. Atherosclerosis--Diagnosis.
4. Atherosclerosis--Treatment. I. Flynn, Grace.

RC692 .A84 2020

616.136--dc23

© Foster Academics, 2020

Foster Academics,
118-35 Queens Blvd., Suite 400,
Forest Hills, NY 11375, USA

ISBN 978-1-63242-968-1 (Hardback)

This book contains information obtained from authentic and highly regarded sources. Copyright for all individual chapters remain with the respective authors as indicated. All chapters are published with permission under the Creative Commons Attribution License or equivalent. A wide variety of references are listed. Permission and sources are indicated; for detailed attributions, please refer to the permissions page and list of contributors. Reasonable efforts have been made to publish reliable data and information, but the authors, editors and publisher cannot assume any responsibility for the validity of all materials or the consequences of their use.

Trademark Notice: Registered trademark of products or corporate names are used only for explanation and identification without intent to infringe.

Contents

Preface

The main aim of this book is to educate learners and enhance their research focus by presenting diverse topics covering this vast field. This is an advanced book which compiles significant studies by distinguished experts in the area of analysis. This book addresses successive solutions to the challenges arising in the area of application, along with it; the book provides scope for future developments.

Atherosclerosis is a clinical condition characterized by the narrowing of an artery due to the build-up of plaque. The arterial narrowing limits the flow of oxygen and blood to different parts of the body. The disease does not usually show symptoms at the outset, but starts exhibiting signs around middle age. Several factors can play a contributing role to the development of atherosclerosis, such as high blood pressure, obesity, high cholesterol, smoking, diabetes, etc. It can be prevented by following a healthy diet, refraining from smoking, exercising regularly and maintaining a normal weight. By conducting a physical examination, and performing exercise stress tests and electrocardiograms, this condition can be diagnosed. Its management typically consists of medications for lowering cholesterol such as blood pressure medication, statins and drugs that decrease clotting. Various procedures can also effectively treat this condition, such as coronary artery bypass graft, percutaneous coronary intervention or carotid endarterectomy. The topics included in this book on atherosclerosis are of utmost significance and bound to provide incredible insights to readers. It presents researches and studies performed by experts across the globe on the risks, mechanisms and management of atherosclerosis. This book is an essential guide for both academicians and those who wish to study this disease further.

It was a great honour to edit this book, though there were challenges, as it involved a lot of communication and networking between me and the editorial team. However, the end result was this all-inclusive book covering diverse themes in the field.

Finally, it is important to acknowledge the efforts of the contributors for their excellent chapters, through which a wide variety of issues have been addressed. I would also like to thank my colleagues for their valuable feedback during the making of this book.

Editor

Differential associations of central and brachial blood pressure with carotid atherosclerosis and microvascular complications in patients with type 2 diabetes

Chan-Hee Jung[1†], Sang-Hee Jung[2†], Kyu-Jin Kim[1], Bo-Yeon Kim[1], Chul-Hee Kim[1], Sung-Koo Kang[1] and Ji-Oh Mok[1*]

Abstract

Background: We examined the relationship between central blood pressure (BP), brachial BP with carotid atherosclerosis and microvascular complications in type 2 diabetes mellitus (T2DM).

Methods: We recruited 201 patients who were evaluated for central BP, brachial BP, carotid ultrasonography, brachial-ankle pulse wave velocity (baPWV), ankle-brachial index (ABI) and microvascular complications. Central BP were calculated using a radial automated tonometric system.

Results: Agreement between central BP and brachial BP was very strong (concordance correlation coefficient between central and brachial SBP = 0.889, between central and brachial PP = 0.816). Central pulse pressure (PP) was correlated with mean carotid intima-media thickness (CIMT), baPWV and ABI, whereas brachial PP was borderline significantly correlated with CIMT. The prevalence of nephropathy(DN) and retinopathy(DR) according to the brachial PP tertiles increased, the prevalences of microvascular complications were not different across central PP tertiles. In multivariate analysis, the relative risks (RRs) for the presence of DR were 1.2 and 4.6 for the brachial PP tertiles 2 and 3 when compared with the first tertile. Also, the RRs for the presence of DN were 1.02 and 3 for the brachial PP tertiles 2 and 3 when compared with the first tertile.

Conclusions: Agreement of central BP and brachial BP was very strong. Nonetheless, this study showed that higher brachial PP levels are associated with increased probability for the presence of microvascular complications such as DR/DN. However, there are no associations with central SBP and central PP with microvascular complications. Central BP levels than brachial BP are correlated with surrogate marker of macrovascular complications.

Keywords: Central blood pressure, Brachial blood pressure, Microvascular complications, Carotid atherosclerosis, Type 2 diabetes

Background

Blood pressure (BP) management is important for the prevention and management of cardiovascular disease (CVD) and microvascular complications in T2DM [1]. Brachial BP remains the standard of reference for the evaluation and management of BP, and has been a key element in predicting target organ damage (TOD) and CVD [2]. However, there is increasing evidence that central BP may be a more sensitive indicator of CV risk than brachial BP in specific groups [3-5]. In a study of American Indians, central BP more strongly related to the extent of carotid atherosclerosis, vascular hypertrophy and CV events than brachial BP [4]. The Conduit Artery Function Evaluation study demonstrated the superiority of central BP to brachial BP as a CV predictor in hypertensive patients [5]. In patients with T2DM, a few studies have documented that increased augmentation of central BP is associated with increases in CIMT [6,7]. However, to our knowledge, no study has compared central BP

* Correspondence: hanna@schmc.ac.kr
†Equal contributors
[1]Division of Endocrinology and Metabolism, Department of Internal Medicine, Soonchunhyang University College of Medicine, #170 Jomaru-ro, Wonmi-gu, Bucheon-si, Gyeonggi-do 420-767, South Korea
Full list of author information is available at the end of the article

with brachial BP regarding to association with both micro-and macrovascular complications in patients with T2DM.

Pulse pressure (PP) is traditionally thought of as a marker of arterial stiffness and has been suggested as an independent CV risk factor [8,9]. Recent several studies reported that brachial PP may be significantly associated with CIMT [10,11]. Brachial PP is reportedly a better predictor of coronary heart disease events than other BP components in patients with T2DM [9]. However, the significance of central PP versus brachial PP regarding macrovascular complications in patients with diabetes remains to be clarified. In addition, some authors suggested that brachial PP is associated with microvascular complications, although some authors disagree [12-14].

Central BP is most accurately measured by an invasive method. It has been evaluated noninvasively by mathematically transforming the radial artery pulse waveform to the aortic pulse waveform recently [15,16]. Although a few studies evaluated the relations of brachial and central pressures to carotid atherosclerosis, no studies have reported the relative importance of central and brachial BP into microvascular complications in patients with T2DM.

Therefore, the aim of this study was to evaluate the value of central BP and brachial BP components in relation to microvascular complications and surrogate markers of macrovascular diseases (CIMT, baPWV and ABI), in patients with T2DM.

Methods

Patients

We recruited 201 patients with T2DM who were evaluated for central BP, carotid ultrasonography and standard brachial BP measurement at the diabetes clinic of Soonchunhyang University Bucheon Hospital, from June 2012 to July 2012. We reviewed detailed demographic data, biochemical data and clinical history using medical records. Participants provided written informed consent for the use of their data for research. This study was reviewed and approved by the Institutional Review Board of Soonchunhyang University College Medicine, Bucheon Hospital.

Measurement of central BP

Central BP was evaluated noninvasively by mathematically transforming the radial artery pulse waveform to the aortic pulse waveform with an automated tonometric system, HEM-9000AI (Omron Healthcare, Kyoto, Japan) in a sitting position after at least 5 min of rest. The radial artery pressure waveform was recorded for 10 sec with the HEM-9000AI system. The radial pulse wave was calibrated to brachial BP, measured with an automated oscillometric device. From the average radial pulse wave form, the corresponding ascending aortic pulse wave form was derived, using a validated generalized transfer function incorporated in the software (Omron Healthcare), which also provided the calculated central BP and the calculated central Aix. The measurements of blood pressure were performed twice by the same trained observer in same day at intervals of at least one minute.

Carotid atherosclerosis

Carotid atherosclerosis was assessed by the use of a model SSA-660A high-resolution B-mode ultrasonograph device (Toshiba, Tokyo, Japan) performed with an ultrasound scanner equipped with a 12-MHz linear-array transducer. IMT measurements were performed on the right and left common carotid arteries 1.0 cm proximal to the origin of the bulb and the mean IMT values were calculated. Carotid IMT thickening was defined as mean CIMT ≥ 1.0 mm [17,18].

Microvascular complications

Diabetic nephropathy (DN) was defined using albuminuria, which was measured by radioimmunoassay (Immunotech, Prague, Czech Republic). Albumin excretion rate (AER) in the range of 20-200 µg/min or urine albumin 30-300 mg/g creatinine was defined as microalbuminuria, and AER > 200 µg/min or urine albumin ≥ 300 mg/g creatinine as overt proteinuria. Patients were considered to have nephropathy if they displayed microalbuminuria or overt proteinuria.

Diabetic retinopathy (DR) was evaluated by experienced ophthalmologists while the patients' pupils were dilated. If needed, fluorescein angiography was performed. DR was classified as normal, nonproliferative and proliferative retinopathy [19]. Patients were considered to have retinopathy if they displayed the nonproliferative or proliferative stage.

Diabetic peripheral neuropathy (DPN) was diagnosed with recommendation by the Expert Committee of Korean Diabetes Neuropathy Study Group, as: the presence of typical symptoms using the Michigan Neuropathy Screening Instrument (MNSI) and compatible findings on neurologic screening examinations or electrophysiologic studies [20,21]. Although electrophysiological studies are not essential, current perception threshold (CPT) test was performed in all patients using a Neurometer CPT/C (Neurotron, Baltimore, MD).

Cardiac autonomic neuropathy (CAN) was assessed by autonominc function test (AFT). CAN was assessed by the five standard cardiovascular reflex tests according to the Ewing's protocol [22]. The severity of CAN was quantitated by summation of points obtained from each of the five tests, where each test was given a point of 0, 0.5, or 1 if it yielded a normal, borderline, or abnormal value, respectively. CAN was defined as the presence of at least two abnormal tests or an autonomic neuropathy points ≥ 2 [23,24].

An automated device (VP-1000; Colin, Komaki, Japan) was used to measure arterial baPWV and ABI. The insulin resistance status was evaluated by the HOMA-IR index, which was calculated by the formula: [fasting insulin (uIU/mL) × fasting blood glucose (mmol/L)]/22.5. The HOMA-IR score was available only in 164 patients not receiving exogenous insulin.

Statistical analyses

Data are presented as mean ± standard deviation (SD) for variables normally distributed or as median (interquartile range) for variables not normally distributed or as number of participants (percentages). Non-normally distributed variables of, triglyceride, high-sensitivity C-reactive proein (hsCRP) and HOMA-IR were transformed as natural logarithm before analysis. The concordance correlation coefficient between central BP and brachial BP was measured to evaluate the agreement between two variables. The categorical variables of the groups were compared by Chi-square test. Correlation between BP and other clinical parameters were analyzed by Spearman's correlation analysis. The significance of the mean differences including several parameters of BP between patients with and those without microvascular complications was evaluated with Student's t-test. Patients were divided into theree groups by the tertiles of central or brachial PP levels, respectively. One-way ANOVA was used to evaluate differences of means among tertiles of central or brachial PP groups. The prevalence of microvascular complications and carotid atherosclerosis according to the tertile of brachial PP, central SBP and central PP were analyzed using Chi-square test. Relationships of central BP and brachial BP with microvascular complications were determined in multivariate logistic regression analyses. Two-tailed p < 0.05 was considered significant. Statistical analyses were performed with SPSS, version 18 (SPSS, Chicago, IL).

Results

General characteristics of the study populations

A total of 201 patients with T2DM (115 males) participated in this cross-sectional study. Clinical and biochemical characteristics of the study subjects are presented in Table 1. The mean age was 55.8 years and duration of DM was 8.5 years. Ninety-six (47.8% of total, 57% of men and 43% of women) were treated for hypertension. Eighty-three (86.5%) were treated with angiotensin converting enzyme inhibitor (ACEI) or/and angiotensin receptor blocker (ARB), 41 (47.2%) were treated with calcium channel blocker, 14 (14.6%) with beta blockers and 15 (15.6%) with diuretics. Central and brachial blood pressures and parameters of carotid atherosclerosis are presented in

Table 1 General characteristics of the study populations

Age (year)	55.8 ± 11.3
Men/Women (%)	115/86 (57.2/42.8)
Duration of DM(year)	8.5 ± 7.5
Hypertension, n (%)	96 (47.8%)
Body mass index (kg/m^2)	24.9 ± 3.1
Central SBP (mmHg)	121.7 ± 17
Central PP (mmHg)	49.4 ± 13.3
Brachial PP (mmHg)	49 ± 12
Systolic BP (mmHg)	121.4 ± 15.6
Diastolic BP (mmHg)	72.3 ± 10
Total Cholesterol (mg/dL)	162.7 ± 36.2
Triglyceride (mg/dL)*	121 (88, 169)
HDL-cholesterol (mg/dL)	48 ± 13
LDL-cholesterol (mg/dL)	94.7 ± 33
hsCRP (mg/dL)*	0.09 (0.05, 0.18)
HbA1$_C$ (%)	7.6 ± 1.6
eGFR (mL/min/1.73 m^2)	76 ± 18
Mean CIMT (mm)	0.62 ± 0.14
Mean ABI	1.14 ± 0.07
Mean baPWV (cm/sec)	1555 ± 405
HOMA-IR*	2.81 (1.89, 4.5)
DPN, n(%)	56 (28%)
CAN, n (%)	65 (32.6%)
Diabetic nephropathy, n (%)	47 (23.4%)
Diabetic retinopathy, n (%)	39 (19.4%)

Data are reported as mean ± standard deviation (SD) for variables which are normally distributed or as median (interquartile range) for variables which are not normally distributed or as number of participants (percentages). DM: diabetes mellitus; SBP: systolic blood pressure; PP: pulse pressure; HDL: high density lipoprotein; LDL: low density lipoprotein; hsCRP: high-sensitivity C-reactive protein; HbA1c: hemoglobin A1c; eGFR: estimated glomerular filtration rate; CIMT: carotid intima-media thickness; ABI: ankle-brachial index; baPWV: brachial-ankle pulse wave velocity; HOMA-IR: homeostasis model assessment-insulin resistance; DPN: diabetic peripheral neuropathy; CAN: cardiac autonomic neuropathy.
*Natural logarithmic transformation were performed before analysis.

Table 1. The prevalence of DN, DR, DPN and CAN was 23.4%, 19.4%, 28% and 32.6%, respectively.

Bivariate correlations between central and brachial BP with carotid atherosclerosis, vascular stiffness and clinical CV risk factors

The concordance correlation coefficient between central SBP and brachial SBP was 0.889 and between central PP and brachial PP was 0.816 (Figure 1).

The correlations of central BP components (central SBP, central PP) and brachial BP components (brachial SBP, brachial PP) to carotid atherosclerosis, vascular stiffness and other clinical variables are presented in Table 2. Central SBP showed significant positive correlation with mean ABI and baPWV (r = 0.162, p = 0.04,

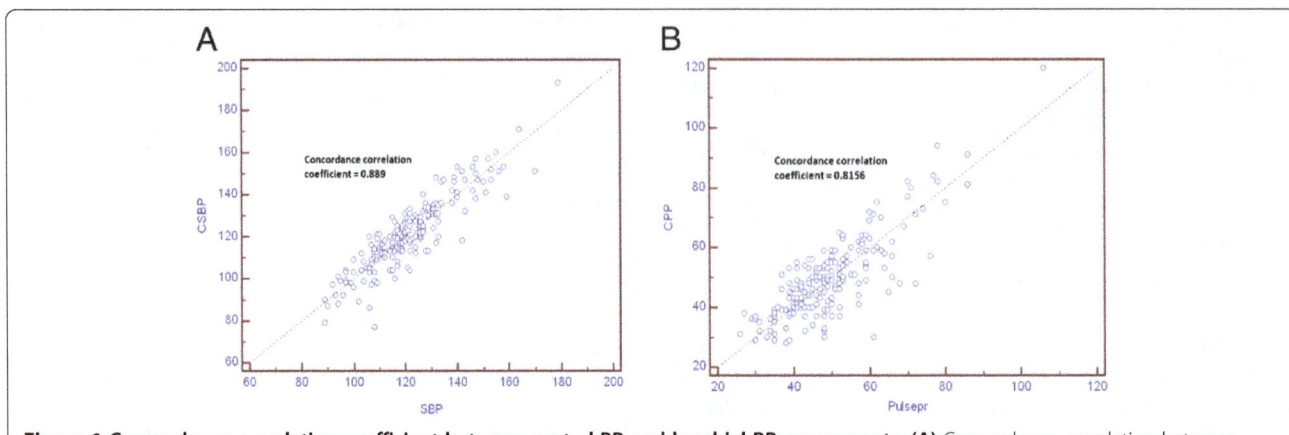

Figure 1 Concordance correlation coefficient between central BP and brachial BP components. (A) Concordance correlation between central SBP and brachial SBP. **(B)** Concordance correlation between central PP and brachial PP.

r = 0.449, p < 0.01, respectively). Brachial SBP levels were correlated positively with total cholesterol, triglyceride and baPWV and were not correlated ABI. Brachial DBP showed negative correlations with age and duration of DM and positive correlations with eGFR and triglyceride (data not shown). Central PP was correlated positively with age, ABI and baPWV and negatively with eGFR.

Brachial PP was not correlated with ABI and was correlated positively with duration of DM, age, eGFR, and baPWV. (r = 0.234, p < 0.01 for duration of DM; r = 0.473, p < 0.01 for age; r = –0.349, p < 0.01 for eGFR; r = 0.576, p < 0.01 for baPWV). Univariate analysis revealed that central PP is significantly correlated with CIMT (r = 0.235, p = 0.01) and brachial PP values also showed positive

Table 2 Bivariate correlations between central and brachial blood pressure with clinical variables

	Central SBP		Central PP		Brachial SBP		Brachial PP	
	r	p	r	p	r	p	r	p
Age (years)	0.131	0.06	0.431	<0.001	0.119	0.091	0.473	<0.01
Duration of DM (years)	0.019	0.78	0.126	0.083	0.082	0.26	0.234	<0.01
BMI (kg/m²)	0.049	0.49	−0.015	0.834	0.091	0.2	0.04	0.56
Central SBP (mmHg)	-	-	0.767	<0.001	0.875	<0.001	0.544	<0.01
Central PP (mmHg)	0.767	<0.001	-	-	0.596	<0.001	0.748	<0.001
Brachial SBP (mmHg)	0.875	<0.01	0.596	<0.001	-	-	0.692	<0.01
Brachial DBP (mmHg)	0.643	<0.01	0.077	0.274	0.66	<0.001	0.005	0.94
Brachial PP (mmHg)	0.643	<0.01	0.748	<0.001	0.692	<0.001	-	-
HbA1$_C$ (%)	0.06	0.4	−0.039	0.5	0.042	0.561	−0.034	0.64
eGFR (mL/min/1.73 m²)	−0.083	0.29	−0.217	0.006	−0.152	0.459	−0.349	<0.01
Total cholesterol (mg/dL)	0.143	0.06	0.068	0.376	0.194	0.011	0.139	0.07
Triglyceride (mg/dL)	0.108	0.15	−0.057	0.451	0.164	0.029	0.016	0.84
HDL-C (mg/dL)	0.051	0.504	0.035	0.647	0.08	0.293	0.035	0.65
LDL-C (mg/dL)	0.121	0.16	0.049	0.565	0.127	0.138	0.066	0.44
HsCRP (mg/dL)	0.1	0.31	0.072	0.469	0.072	0.466	0.037	0.44
HOMA-IR	0.05	0.62	0.02	0.844	0.071	0.481	0.068	0.5
Mean CIMT (mm)	0.082	0.38	0.235	0.01	0.068	0.467	0.197	0.047
Mean ABI	0.162	0.04	0.185	<0.019	0.083	0.297	0.069	0.38
Mean baPWV (cm/sec)	0.449	<0.01	0.531	<0.001	0.477	<0.001	0.576	<0.01

DM: diabetes mellitus; BMI: body mass index; SBP: systolic blood pressure; PP: pulse pressure; HbA1c: hemoglobin A1c; eGFR: estimated glomerular filtration rate; HDL: high density lipoprotein; LDL: low density lipoprotein; hsCRP: high-sensitivity C-reactive protein; HOMA-IR: homeostasis model assessment-insulin resistance; CIMT: carotid intima-media thickness; ABI: ankle-brachial index; baPWV: brachial-ankle pulse wave velocity.
Spearman's correlation analysis was used for the statistical analyses.

correlation but weaker correlation than central PP (r = 0.197, p = 0.047).

Carotid atherosclerosis, vascular stiffness and other clinical variables according to the tertile of central PP and brachial PP

Comparison of carotid atherosclerosis, vascular stiffness and clinical variables among tertile groups of central PP or brachial PP is shown in Tables 3 and 4. The mean CIMT, baPWV and ABI was significantly increased progressively across central PP tertiles (p = 0.04, p < 0.001, and p = 0.023, respectively). In addition, the age and duration of DM were significantly increased progressively across central PP tertiles (Table 3). Stage of DN (normoalbuminuria, microalbuminuria, overt proteinuria) among tertile groups of central PP was not different (p = 0.69). Whereas stage of DN among tertile groups of brachial PP was significantly different (p = 0.02). The age and duration of DM were significantly increased progressively, eGFR were decreased progressively across brachial PP tertiles

(Table 4). Mean CIMT and baPWV in the third tertile group of a brachial PP were significantly higher than those levels in the first and second tertile group (p = 0.03, p < 0.01). Mean carotid IMT levels among tertile groups of central SBP and brachial SBP were not different (data not shown).

Prevalence of diabetic microvascular complications according to the tertile levels of central PP or brachial PP

Comparisons of the prevalence of diabetic microvascular complications according to the tertile levels of central PP or brachial PP are shown in Figure 2. The prevalence of nephropathy and retinopathy according to the brachial PP tertiles significantly increased (21% vs 20% vs 44%, p = 0.006; 19% vs 22% vs 51%, p = 0.002, respectively). The prevalence of DPN and CAN did not show significant differences according to the brachial PP tertiles. The prevalence of diabetic microvascular complications did not differ across central PP tertiles.

Table 3 Difference of mean values of the clinical variables according to the tertile levels of central PP

	1st tertile	2nd tertile	3rd tertile	P for trend
Central PP (mmHg)	37.1 ± 4.2	48.6 ± 2.8	63.7 ± 10	0.001
Central SBP (mmHg)	108.2 ± 11.8	122.1 ± 10.4	135.9 ± 13.8	<0.01
Brachial SBP (mmHg)	111.4 ± 11.9	121.7 ± 11.4	132.0 ± 15.1	<0.01
Brachial DBP (mmHg)	71.1 ± 10	73.4 ± 9.8	72.2 ± 10.2	0.53
Brachial PP (mmHg)	40.3 ± 7.2	48.2 ± 7.3	59.7 ± 10.6	<0.01
Age (years)	51.2 ± 11	54.2 ± 10.3	59.7 ± 10.6	<0.01
BMI (kg/m²)	24.9 ± 3.4	25.1 ± 2.7	24.7 ± 3.2	0.67
Duration of DM (years)	7.5 ± 5.4	7.3 ± 6.4	10.5 ± 9.2	0.02
HbA1c (%)	7.7 ± 1.6	7.5 ± 1.5	7.6 ± 1.9	0.75
Total cholesterol (mg/dL)	158.3 ± 34.6	164.6 ± 37.6	166 ± 36.7	0.27
Triglycerides (mg/dL)	112 (91, 169)	133 (88, 185)	114 (77, 144)	0.35
HDL-C (mg/dL)	47.5 ± 11.9	47.6 ± 13.2	48.5 ± 13.7	0.67
LDL-C (mg/dL)	93.5 ± 32.6	93.4 ± 34.8	98.9 ± 31.4	0.45
eGFR (mL/min/1.73 m²)	79.5 ± 16.1	78.5 ± 19	69.5 ± 16	0.01
Diabetic nephropathy, n (%)				0.69
No albuminuria	55 (36.9)	52 (34.8)	42 (28.2)	
Microalbuminuria	13 (35)	12 (31.6)	13 (44.4)	
Overt proteinuria	2 (26.8)	4 (34.2)	3 (33.3)	
HOMA-IR	2.6 (1.8, 4.5)	2.9 (2.0, 4.1)	2.9 (1.9, 5.0)	0.92
hsCRP (mg/dL)	0.09 (0.05, 0.13)	0.08 (0.04, 0.18)	0.1 (0.05,0.25)	0.35
Mean CIMT (mm)	0.58 ± 0.14	0.62 ± 0.13	0.66 ± 0.15	0.014
Mean baPWV (cm/sec)	1385 ± 253	1581 ± 495	1751 ± 359	<0.01
Mean ABI	1.13 ± 0.06	1.15 ± 0.06	1.15 ± 0.06	0.02

Data are shown as mean ± SD, median (interquartile range) or number (percentages).
PP: pulse pressure; SBP: systolic blood pressure; SBP: systolic blood pressure; DBP: diastolic blood pressure; BMI: body mass index; DM: diabetes mellitus; HbA1c: hemoglobin A1c; HDL: high density lipoprotein; LDL: low density lipoprotein; eGFR: estimated glomerular filtration rate; HOMA-IR: homeostasis model assessment-insulin resistance; hsCRP: high-sensitivity C-reactive protein; CIMT: carotid intima-media thickness; baPWV: brachial-ankle pulse wave velocity; ABI: ankle-brachial index.

Table 4 Difference of mean values of the clinical variables according to the tertile levels of brachial PP

	1ST tertile	2nd tertile	3rd tertile	P for trend
Central PP (mmHg)	40.1 ± 6.6	47.5 ± 7.0	60.6 ± 14.6	<0.01
Central SBP (mmHg)	113.2 ± 13	119.9 ± 12.3	132 ± 19.1	<0.01
Brachial SBP (mmHg)	110.9 ± 11.6	120 ± 9.8	133.5 ± 15.5	<0.01
Brachial DBP (mmHg)	73.1 ± 9.6	72.4 ± 9.4	71.3 ± 10.9	0.3
Brachial PP (mmHg)	37.8 ± 4.3	47.6 ± 2.1	62.1 ± 10.2	<0.01
Age (years)	50.5 ± 9	54.6 ± 10.7	62.4 ± 10.8	<0.01
BMI (kg/m^2)	24.5 ± 3.2	25.5 ± 3	24.7 ± 3	0.82
Duration of DM (years)	6.1 ± 5.1	7.7 ± 5.7	11.8 ± 9.9	<0.01
HbA1$_C$ (%)	7.8 ± 1.6	7.6 ± 1.8	7.5 ± 1.5	0.3
Total cholesterol (mg/dL)	159 ± 35.7	159.3 ± 36.4	170.6 ± 35.8	0.09
Triglycerides (mg/dL)	123 (80, 162)	121 (91, 181)	117 (81, 153)	0.69
HDL-C (mg/dL)	47.4 ± 11	46.6 ± 12.1	50.2 ± 15.9	0.26
LDL-C (mg/dL)	93.6 ± 32.9	90.5 ± 32.7	101.4 ± 33.4	0.28
eGFR (mL/min/1.73 m^2)	82.2 ± 16	78.1 ± 14.9	67.2 ± 19.8	<0.01
Diabetic nephropathy, n (%)				0.02
No albuminuria	56 (37.6)	53 (35.6)	40 (26.8)	
Microalbuminuria	11 (28.9)	10 (26.3)	17 (44.7)	
Overt proteinuria	2 (22.2)	1 (11.1)	6 (66.7)	
HOMA-IR	2.4 (1.7, 4.5)	2.9 (2.2, 4.8)	2.7 (1.9, 3.9)	0.97
hsCRP (mg/dL)	0.08 (0.05, 0.18)	0.09 (0.04, 0.16)	0.09 (0.05, 0.22)	0.68
Mean CIMT (mm)	0.58 ± 0.11	0.63 ± 0.16	0.75 ± 0.14	0.03
Mean PWV (cm/sec)	1370 ± 205	1587 ± 537	1752 ± 341	<0.01
Mean ABI	1.14 ± 0.05	1.14 ± 0.07	1.14 ± 0.08	0.74

Data are shown as mean ± SD, median (interquartile range) or number (percentages).
PP: pulse pressure; SBP: systolic blood pressure; SBP: systolic blood pressure; DBP: diastolic blood pressure; BMI: body mass index; DM: diabetes mellitus; HbA1c: hemoglobin A1c; HDL: high density lipoprotein; LDL: low density lipoprotein; eGFR: estimated glomerular filtration rate; HOMA-IR: homeostasis model assessment-insulin resistance; hsCRP: high-sensitivity C-reactive protein; CIMT: carotid intima-media thickness; baPWV: brachial-ankle pulse wave velocity; ABI: ankle-brachial index.

Differences of parameters of BP according to the presence of each diabetic microvascular complications

Differences of several parameters of BP according to the presence or absence of microvascular complications are presented in Table 5. Significantly increased levels of brachial SBP and brachial PP were detected in patients with DN compared to those without DN (p = 0.02 and p = 0.01, respectively). In patients with DR, brachial SBP and brachial PP were significantly higher than in those without DR (p = 0.02 and p = 0.03, respectively).

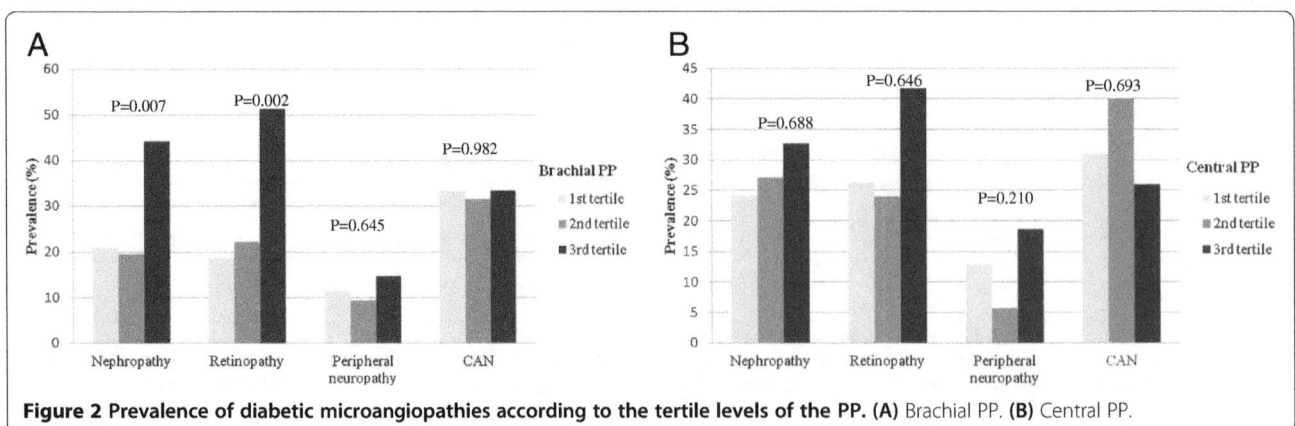

Figure 2 Prevalence of diabetic microangiopathies according to the tertile levels of the PP. (A) Brachial PP. **(B)** Central PP.

Table 5 Blood pressure according to the presence of each microangiopathies

	DR			DN			DPN		
	(−)	(+)	p	(−)	(+)	p	(−)	(+)	p
Central SBP	119.5 ± 15.7	123.6 ± 20	0.22	120.4 ± 14.6	123.9 ± 17.8	0.20	123.2 ± 13.6	121.5 ± 21.3	0.73
Central PP	47.7 ± 11.4	53 ± 17.4	0.08	47.8 ± 11.8	51.5 ± 13.9	0.09	49.8 ± 11.4	52 ± 15.3	0.53
Brachial SBP	117.8 ± 13.6	124.7 ± 17	0.02	119.2 ± 13.9	125 ± 15.7	0.02	121.6 ± 13	122 ± 20.6	0.93
Brachial PP	46 ± 8.9	54.2 ± 15	0.03	46.6 ± 10.1	52.6 ± 13.1	0.01	48.3 ± 10.2	52.5 ± 15.1	0.21

Data are shown as mean ± SD.
DR: diabetic retinopathy; DN: diabetic nephropathy; DPN: diabetic peripheral neuropathy.

The levels of central BP were not different between in patients with DN or DR and those without DN or DR.

Multivariate logistic regression analysis for the relationship of central or brachial blood pressure with presence of diabetic retinopathy/nephropathy

Clinical variables showing significantly different values between the presence or absence of DR/DN were examined by t-test (data not shown). Total cholesterol, LDL-cholesterol, eGFR and mean baPWV levels were significantly different according to the presence or absence of DN. HbA1$_C$, duration of DM and mean baPWV levels were significantly different according to the presence or absence of DR. After adjustment for these variables, age and gender, multivariate logistic regression analysis was done to examine the relationship of central or brachial BP with the presence of DR/DN (Table 6). In multivariate analysis, only brachial PP among all BP components was significantly associated with the presence of DR/DN. An increased brachial PP independently increased the odds for the presence of diabetic nephropathy and retinopathy. The relative risks for the presence of DR were 1.2 and 4.6 for the brachial PP tertiles 2 and 3 when compared with the first tertile (p = 0.003). Also, the relative risks for the presence of DN were 1.02 and 3.0 for the brachial PP 2nd, 3rd tertiles when compared with first tertile (p = 0.01). Higher HbA1$_C$ and longer duration of DM independently increased the odds for the presence of DR (Table 6).

Discussion

To the best of our knowledge, our study is the first to report associations between central versus brachial BP with all diabetic microvascular complications as well as carotid atherosclerosis.

The main finding of this study is that central BP and brachial BP show very strong agreement. Nevertheless, the higher brachial PP levels are associated with increased probability for the presence of diabetic microvascular complications and are more powerful than central BP in relation to DR and DN. But, to the contrary, central BP levels rather than brachial BP are correlated with surrogate marker of macrovascular complications.

Peripheral (brachial) BP is an essential parameter for the evaluation and management of BP and remains the standard reference. On the other hand, there is increasing evidence that measurement of central BP, reflecting ascending aortic BP, is more strongly correlated to CVD or TOD than brachial BP levels [4,25]. Although superiority of central BP than brachial BP in relation to CVD or TOD has been suggested in several studies, measurement of central BP in real practice is not easy. Therefore, it is meaningful to examine the relationship or concordance between central BP and brachial BP. In this study, agreement between central BP and brachial BP was very strong as evidenced by the concordance correlation coefficient > 0.8. High concordance values may indicate little difference between two BP components is present and these two can be interchangeable.

Few studies have evaluated whether central and brachial BP are associated differently with carotid atherosclerosis and microvascular complications in patients with T2DM. The Strong Heart Study revealed that central PP was more strongly related to CIMT and plaque score than was brachial PP in 3520 population (including diabetes in 46.5% of women and 38.1% of men) [4]. Central pressure augmentation and aortic SBP, but not brachial SBP, were age-independent determinants of CIMT in another study [7]. To the contrary, whereas the superiority of central BP relative to brachial BP in terms of its association with TOD such as cardiac hypertrophy has been reported, central and brachial BP levels are not reportedly different in relation with cardiac hypertrophy [26]. In a recent meta-analysis of 11 longitudinal studies, the relative risk of any CV event was 1.088 ([1.040-1.139], n = 3285) for an increase of central SBP by 10 mmHg and 1.137 ([1.063-1.215], n = 4778) for an increase of central PP by 10 mmHg, but neither the RR associated with higher central SBP nor the RR associated with higher central PP differed significantly from the relative risks associated with its brachial counterparts, respectively [27].

The present study revealed that central PP is significantly correlated with CIMT and brachial PP values also showed positive, but weaker, correlation than central PP. The levels of mean CIMT demonstrated an increasing trend as the levels of central PP or brachial PP increased.

Table 6 Multivariate logistic regression analysis with presence or absence of diabetic nephropathy/retinopathy as the dependent variable

(1) diabetic retinopathy as dependent variable

Independent variable	Odds ratio (95% CI)	P-value
Central SBP		0.65
1st tertile	1	
2nd tertile	1.50 (0.60-3.77)	0.39
3rd tertile	1.44 (0.56-3.73)	0.45
Central PP		0.18
1st tertile	1	
2nd tertile	0.89 (0.35-2.29)	0.81
3rd tertile	2.02 (0.80-5.15)	0.14
Brachial PP		0.003
1st tertile	1	
2nd tertile	1.21 (0.44-3.54)	0.67
3rd tertile	4.59 (1.72-12.27)	0.002
Gender (Male)	1.85 (0.85-4.03)	0.12
Age	1.03 (0.99-1.07)	0.12
mean baPWV	1.01 (0.99-1.01)	0.91
HbA1C	1.85 (1.27-2.71)	0.002
Duration of DM	1.19 (1.09-1.30)	0.001

(2) diabetic nephropathy as dependent variable

Independent variable	Odds ratio (95% CI)	P-value
Central SBP		0.69
1st tertile	1	
2nd tertile	1.28 (0.50-3.0)	0.57
3rd tertile	1.45 (0.60-3.40)	0.39
Central PP		0.61
1st tertile	1	
2nd tertile	1.17 (0.52-2.64)	0.71
3rd tertile	1.52 (0.66-3.50)	0.33
Brachial PP		0.01
1st tertile	1	
2nd tertile	1.02 (0.38-2.26)	0.86
3rd tertile	3.0 (1.32-6.80)	0.01
Age	1.02 (0.99-1.05)	0.25
Gender (Male)	1.11 (0.56-2.22)	0.76
mean baPWV	1.01 (0.99-1.01)	0.14
Total cholesterol	1.03 (0.99-1.06)	0.18
LDL-cholesterol	0.98 (0.94-1.02)	0.35

SBP: systolic blood pressure; PP: pulse pressure; baPWV: brachial-ankle pulse wave velocity; LDL: low density lipoprotein; HbA1c: hemoglobin A1c.

However, measures of central or brachial SBP/DBP were not correlated with carotid atherosclerosis. In contrast to this our study, Westerbacka et al. reported measures of central SBP correlate with CIMT [7]. One report showed

that central SBP predicted CV mortality independently of brachial SBP and traditional cardiovascular risk factors (Hazard ratio per 10 mmHg increase in central SBP: 1.34 [1.107-1.612], whereas central PP did not predict CV mortality independently of brachial PP and traditional CV risk factors in 1272 Chinese people recruited from the community [28].

PP, the arithmetic difference between systolic and diastolic BP, has been reported as a potent predictor for CVD [29]. Several studies pointed out that a CV risk in subjects with wide PP increased with the presence of diabetes [9]. In addition, PP is increased in patients with intima-media thickening [11]. In our study, brachial PP was significantly correlated with age, duration of diabetes, baPWV and CIMT. Also, central PP was correlated with age, estimated glomerular filtration ratio (eGFR), ABI, baPWV and CIMT. Especially, central or brachial PP, but not central or brachial SBP/DBP, was presently associated with carotid atherosclerosis. However, the majority of previous studies did not compare the brachial PP and central PP in relation to CV risk factors. Associations and clinical values of several components of BP such as SBP, DBP, mean BP and PP with CVD have been studied extensively. However, it is not definitively identified whether one of these measures is more strongly associated with CVD than the other. Moreover, the answer to the question of whether central BP provides value over and above peripheral BP in relation to CVD is still open.

Central BP can be directly measured only using a pressure sensor or catheter inserted into the aorta. This procedure is invasive and can lead to complications. Recently, central BP has been evaluated noninvasively by mathematically transforming the radial artery pulse waveform to the aortic pulse waveform [15,16]. However, the clinical significance of central BP, which can be measured easily by automated applanation tonometry, has not been fully elucidated. More data are needed to establish and differentiate the clinical utility of central BP using automated applanation tonometry or brachial BP as a surrogate marker in predicting CV events in T2DM.

To our knowledge, no study has examined the relative importance of central and brachial BP in their relations to microvascular complications in patients with T2DM. This present study examined the relationship between central BP, brachial BP and all microvascular complications. We established good association higher brachial PP levels and increased probability for the presence of diabetic nephropathy and retinopathy. However, our study showed that no associations of any central BP components or brachial BP components with CAN and DPN. In agreement of our study, Knudsen et al. reported that in 80 patients with T2DM, brachial PP is associated with DR and DN [12]. Also, in another study, brachial PP was reported as an important risk factor for eGFR decline and incident chronic kidney disease over a 5-year period, especially in patients with T2DM [13]. In contrast to our study, brachial PP was not a risk factor for DN in T1DM [14]. One of the possible explanation for association PP and microvascular complications such as DN and DR is that elevated PP is associated with endothelial activation and pertubation in patients with T2DM. Endothelial dysfunction could represent a pathophysiological link between these wide PP and the development of microvascular complications in T2DM [30]. However, the reasons are not clear why central PP is not associated with any diabetic microvascular complications. Prospective data on the predictive value of central BP for microvascular complications, such as renal outcome and retinal vascular impairment in diabetic patients, are currently lacking. The ongoing LOD-DIABETES study is expected to answer this question [31]. Also, it is not clear the reason why brachial PP is not associated with DPN and CAN. A possible explanation can be suggested. Regarding to the pathogenesis of DPN, several important mechanisms, such as glycemic control and duration of diabetes, have been related. Although roles of CV risk factors such as hypertension have been proposed, the effect of BP on pathogenesis of DPN may be not more prominent than other traditional risk factors of DPN [32].

Several limitations of our study should be addressed. First, due to the cross-sectional design, we cannot determine the causative relationship between brachial PP and diabetic microvascular complications, DN or DR. Prospective studies are required to address this important question. Second, because our study population included individuals who received the examination for diabetic complications, some characteristics of the present study population may be substantially different from other populations that did not perform complication study. Therefore, the generalizability of our study may be limited. Third, the present study included a small numbers of subjects. A larger number of patients should be analyzed for the confirmation of our results. Fourth, information for central BP is that derived from automated radial artery tonometry. Although the clinical significance of central BP by automated applanation tonometry, has not been fully elucidated, many studies revealed that central BP from radial artery automated tonometry showed excellent correlation with direct measured central BP [33]. However, our study is meaningful in that this is the first study for the evaluation of relationships between central versus brachial BP with all diabetic microvascular complications as well as vascular stiffness and carotid atherosclerosis in patients with T2DM.

Conclusions

In conclusion, this study showed that agreement of central BP and brachial BP was very strong. Brachial BP

are associated with presence of microvascular complications such as DR/DN than central BP. On the other hand, central BP levels rather than brachial BP are correlated with surrogate marker of macrovascular complication. However, further prospective studies are needed to evaluate the superiority or difference of central BP versus brachial BP in respective of associations with development of micro-and macrovascular complications in T2DM.

Competing interests
The authors declare that they have no competing interests.

Authors' contributions
Study design: CHJ, JOM. Data collection: CHJ, SHJ, BYK. Data analysis: CHJ, SHJ, JOM. Writing the first draft: CHJ, KJK, BYK, JOM. Data interpretation, discussion and preparation of the final manuscript: CHJ, SHJ, KJK, BYK, CHK, SKK, JOM. All authors read and approved the final manuscript.

Authors' information
Chan-Hee Jung and Sang-Hee Jung both should be considered as first authors.

Acknowledgements
We would like to thank Jee-Sung Lee for review of the manuscript for its statistical content.

Author details
[1]Division of Endocrinology and Metabolism, Department of Internal Medicine, Soonchunhyang University College of Medicine, #170 Jomaru-ro, Wonmi-gu, Bucheon-si, Gyeonggi-do 420-767, South Korea. [2]Department of Obstetrics and Gynecology, Cha University School of Medicine, Bundang, Korea.

References
1. Reaven GM, Lithell H, Landsberg L: **Hypertension and associated metabolic abnormalities: the role of insulin resistance and the sympatho-adrenal system.** *N Engl J Med* 1996, **334**:374–381.
2. Messerli FH, Grossman E, Goldbourt U: **Antihypertensive therapy in diabetic hypertensive patients.** *Am J Hypertens* 2001, **14**:12S–16S.
3. McEniery CM, Yasmin, McDonnell B, Munnery M, Wallace SM, Rowe CV, Cockcroft JR, Wilkinson IB: **Central pressure: variability and impact of cardiovascular risk factors: the Anglo-Cardiff Collaborative Trial II.** *Hypertension* 2008, **51**:1476–1482.
4. Roman MJ, Devereux RB, Kizer JR, Lee ET, Galloway JM, Ali T, Umans JG, Howard BV: **Central pressure more strongly relates to vascular disease and outcome than does brachial pressure: the strong heart study.** *Hypertension* 2007, **50**:197–203.
5. Williams B, Lacy PS, Thom SM, Cruickshank K, Stanton A, Collier D, Hughes AD, Thurston H, O'Rourke M: **CAFÉ Steering Committee and Writing Committee: differential impact of blood pressure-lowering drugs on central aortic pressure and clinical outcomes: principal results of the Conduit Artery Function Evaluation (CAFÉ) study.** *Circulation* 2006, **113**:1213–1225.
6. Fukui M, Kitagawa Y, Nakamura N, Mogami S, Ohnishi M, Hirata C, Ichio N, Wada K, Kamiuchi K, Shigeta M, Sawada M, Hasegawa G, Yoshikawa T: **Augmentation of central arterial pressure as a marker of atherosclerosis in patients with type 2 diabetes.** *Diabetes Res Clin Pract* 2003, **59**:153–161.
7. Westerbacka J, Leinonen E, Salonen JT, Salonen R, Hiukka A, Yki-Jarvinen H, Taskinen MR: **Increased augmentation of central blood pressure is associated with increases in carotid intima-media thickness in type 2 diabetic patients.** *Diabetologia* 2005, **48**:1654–1662.
8. Franklin SS, Khan SA, Wong ND, Larson MG, Levy D: **Is pulse pressure useful in predicting risk for coronary heart disease? The Framingham Heart Study.** *Circulation* 1999, **100**:354–360.

9. Cockcroft JR, Wilkinson IB, Evans M, McEwan P, Peters JR, Davies S, Scanlon MF, Currie CJ: **Pulse pressure predicts cardiovascular risk in patients with type 2 diabetes mellitus.** *Am J Hypertens* 2005, **18**:1463–1467.

10. Zureik M, Touboul PJ, Bonithon-Kopp C, Courbon D, Berr C, Leroux C, Ducimetiere P: **Cross-sectional and 4-year longitudinal associations between brachial pulse pressure and common carotid intima-media thickness in a general population: the EVA study.** *Stroke* 1999, **30**:550–555.

11. Wakabayashi I, Masuda H: **Association of pulse pressure with carotid atherosclerosis in patients with type 2 diabetes mellitus.** *Blood Press* 2007, **16**:56–62.

12. Knudsen ST, Poulsen PL, Hansen KW, Ebbehoj E, Bek T, Mogensen CE: **Pulse pressure and diurnal blood pressure variation: association with micro-and macrovascular complications in type 2 diabetes.** *Am J Hypertens* 2002, **15**:244–250.

13. van den Hurk K, Magliano DJ, Alssema M, Schlaich MP, Atkins RC, Reutens AT, Nijpels G, Dekker JM, Shaw JE: **Type 2 diabetes strengthens the association between pulse pressure and chronic kidney disease: the AusDiab Study.** *J Hypertens* 2011, **29**:953–960.

14. Gordin D, Waden J, Forsblom C, Thorn L, Rosengard-Barlund M, Tolonen N, Saraheimo M, Harjutsalo V, Groop PH: **Pulse pressure predicts incident cardiovascular disease but not diabetic nephropathy in patients with type 1 diabetes (The FinnDiane Study).** *Diabetes Care* 2011, **34**:886–891.

15. Takazawa K, Kobayashi H, Shindo N, Tanaka N, Yamashina A: **Relationship between radial and central arterial pulse wave and evaluation of central aortic pressure using the radial arterial pulse wave.** *Hypertens Res* 2007, **30**:219–228.

16. O'Rourke MF, Adji A: **Noninvasive studies of central aortic pressure.** *Curr Hypertens Rep* 2012, **14**:8–20.

17. Chambless LE, Folsom AR, Clegg LX, Sharrett AR, Shahar E, Nieto FJ, Rosamond WD, Evans G: **Carotid wall thickness is predictive of incident clinical stroke: the Atherosclerosis Risk in Communities (ARIC) study.** *Am J Epidemiol* 2000, **151**:478–487.

18. Chambless LE, Heiss G, Folsom AR, Rosamond W, Szklo M, Sharrett AR, Clegg LX: **Association of coronary heart disease incidence with carotid arterial wall thickness and major risk factors: the Atherosclerosis Risk in Communities (ARIC) study.** *Am J Epidemiol* 1997, **146**:483–494.

19. Watkins PJ: **ABC of diabetes; retinopathy.** *Bri Med J* 2003, **326**:924–926.

20. Expert Committee of Korean Diabetes Neuropathy Study Group: *Diabetic neuropathy management guidebook.* 3rd edition. Korean: Gold Planning and Development; 2010.

21. Feldman EL, Stevens MJ, Thomas PK, Brown MB, Canal N, Greene DA: **A practical two-step quantitative clinical and electrophysiological assessment for the diagnosis and staging of diabetic neuropathy.** *Diabetes Care* 1994, **17**:1281–1289.

22. Ewing DJ, Martyn CN, Young RJ, Clarke BF: **The value of cardiovascular autonomic function test: 10 years experience in diabetes.** *Diabetes Care* 1985, **8**:491–498.

23. Bellavere F, Bosello G, Fedele D, Cardone C, Ferri M: **Diagnosis and management of diabetic autonomic neuropathy.** *BMJ (Clin Res Ed)* 1983, **287**:61.

24. O'brien IAD, O'hare JP, Lewin IG, Corrall RJM: **The prevalence of autonomic neuropathy in insulin-dependent diabetes mellitus: a controlled study based on heart rate variability.** *QJM* 1986, **61**:957–967.

25. Sharman JE, Fang ZY, Haluska B, Stowasser M, Prins JB, Marwick TH: **Left ventricular mass in patients with type 2 diabetes is independently associated with central but not peripheral pulse pressure.** *Diabetes Care* 2005, **28**:937–939.

26. Zhang Y, Li Y, Ding FH, Sheng CS, Huang QF, Wang JG: **Cardiac structure and function in relation to central blood pressure components in Chinese.** *J Hypertens* 2011, **29**:2462–2468.

27. Vlachopoulos C, Aznaouridis K, O'Rourke MF, Safar ME, Baou K, Stefanadis C: **Prediction of cardiovascular events and all-cause mortality with central haemodynamics: a systematic review and meta-analysis.** *Eur Heart J* 2010, **31**:1865–1871.

28. Wang KL, Cheng HM, Chuang SY, Spurgeon HA, Ting CT, Lakatta EG, Yin FC, Chou P, Chen CH: **Central or peripheral systolic or pulse pressure: which best relates to target organs and future mortality?** *J Hypertens* 2009, **27**:461–467.

29. Thomas F, Blacher J, Benetos A, Safar ME, Pannier B: **Cardiovascular risk as defined in the 2003 European blood pressure classification: the assessment of an additional predictive value of pulse pressure on mortality.** *J Hypertens* 2008, **26**:1072–1077.

30. Knudsen ST, Jeppesen P, Frederiksen CA, Andersen NH, Bek T, Ingerslev J, Mogensen CE, Poulsen PL: **Endothelial dysfunction, ambulatory pulse pressure and albuminuria are associated in type 2 diabetic subjects.** *Diabetic Med* 2007, **24**:911–915.

31. Gomez-Marcos MA, Recio-Rodriguez JI, Rodriguez-Sanchez E, Castano-Sanchez Y, de Cabo-Laso A, Sanche-Salgado B, Rodriguez-Martin C, Castano-Sanchez C, Gomez-Sanchez L, Garcia-Ortiz L: **Central blood pressure and pulse wave velocity: relationship to target organ damage and cardiovascular morbidity-mortality in diabetic patients or metabolic syndrome: an observational prospective study: LOD-DIABETES study protocol.** *BMC Public Health* 2010, **10**:143–150.

32. Forrest KY, Maser RE, Pambianco G, Becker DJ, Orchard TJ: **Hypertension as a risk factor for diabetic neuropathy: a prospective study.** *Diabetes* 1997, **46**:665–670.

33. Ding FH, Fan WX, Zhang RY, Zhang Q, Li Y, Wang JG: **Validation of the noninvasive assessment of central blood pressure by the SphygmoCor and Omron devices against the invasive catheter measurement.** *Am J Hypertens* 2011, **24**:1306–1311.

2

Impact of clinical input variable uncertainties on ten-year atherosclerotic cardiovascular disease risk using new pooled cohort equations

Himanshu Gupta[1,2]*, Chun G. Schiros[1], Oleg F. Sharifov[1], Apurva Jain[3] and Thomas S. Denney Jr[4]

Abstract

Background: Recently released American College of Cardiology/American Heart Association (ACC/AHA) guideline recommends the Pooled Cohort equations for evaluating atherosclerotic cardiovascular risk of individuals. The impact of the clinical input variable uncertainties on the estimates of ten-year cardiovascular risk based on ACC/AHA guidelines is not known.

Methods: Using a publicly available the National Health and Nutrition Examination Survey dataset (2005–2010), we computed maximum and minimum ten-year cardiovascular risks by assuming clinically relevant variations/uncertainties in input of age (0–1 year) and ±10 % variation in total-cholesterol, high density lipoprotein- cholesterol, and systolic blood pressure and by assuming uniform distribution of the variance of each variable. We analyzed the changes in risk category compared to the actual inputs at 5 % and 7.5 % risk limits as these limits define the thresholds for consideration of drug therapy in the new guidelines. The new-pooled cohort equations for risk estimation were implemented in a custom software package.

Results: Based on our input variances, changes in risk category were possible in up to 24 % of the population cohort at both 5 % and 7.5 % risk boundary limits. This trend was consistently noted across all subgroups except in African American males where most of the cohort had ≥7.5 % baseline risk regardless of the variation in the variables.

Conclusions: The uncertainties in the input variables can alter the risk categorization. The impact of these variances on the ten-year risk needs to be incorporated into the patient/clinician discussion and clinical decision making. Incorporating good clinical practices for the measurement of critical clinical variables and robust standardization of laboratory parameters to more stringent reference standards is extremely important for successful implementation of the new guidelines. Furthermore, ability to customize the risk calculator inputs to better represent unique clinical circumstances specific to individual needs would be highly desirable in the future versions of the risk calculator.

Keywords: Cholesterol, Statins, Cardiovascular disease, Atherosclerosis, Primary prevention, Computer simulations

Abbreviations: AA, African-American; ACC/AHA, American College of Cardiology/American Heart Association; ARIC, Atherosclerosis risk in communities study; ASCVD, Atherosclerotic cardiovascular disease; BP, Blood pressure; c, Cholesterol; CARDIA, Coronary artery risk development in young adults; CHS, Cardiovascular health study; CLIA, Clinical laboratory improvement amendment; DM, Diabetes mellitus; FHS, Framingham heart study; HDL, High density lipoprotein; MESA, Multi-ethnic study of atherosclerosis; NCEP, National cholesterol education program; NHANES, National health and nutrition examination survey; REGARDS, Reasons for geographic and racial differences in stroke

* Correspondence: hgupta@uab.edu
[1]Department of Medicine, Cardiovascular Disease, University of Alabama at Birmingham, 1808 7th Ave South, BDB 101, Birmingham, AL 35294, USA
[2]VA Medical Center, Birmingham, AL, USA
Full list of author information is available at the end of the article

Background

The recent American College of Cardiology/American Heart Association (ACC/AHA) guideline on the treatment of blood cholesterol to reduce atherosclerotic cardiovascular disease (ASCVD) risk in adults recommends the use of the new pooled cohort equations to calculate ten-year risk to help define the population cohorts that are likely to benefit from either the initiation of statin therapy in non-diabetics or define the intensity of statin therapy in patients with diabetes for the primary prevention of ASCVD [1, 2]. These equations were derived from analyzing five major longitudinal studies that include the Framingham Heart Study (FHS and offspring cohort) [3–5], the Coronary Artery Risk Development in Young Adults (CARDIA) [6], the Cardiovascular Health Study (CHS) [7], and the Atherosclerosis Risk in Communities Study (ARIC) [8]. The equations incorporate sex- and race-specific proportional hazards models consisting of covariates of objectively measured values of systolic blood pressure (BP), total-cholesterol (c) and HDL-c with other clinical and demographic features to calculate ten-year risk of ASCVD. A risk calculator is available for download [http://my.americanheart.org/cvriskcalculator].

The ten- year risk assessment has profound implications for clinical decision-making for an individual patient and for formulating health policies for primary prevention [9, 10]. Application of the pooled cohort equations to the National Health and Nutrition Examination Survey (NHANES) dataset from 2007 to 2010 reveals that approximately 20 % of the US population (about 20 million people) have predicted ten- year risk between 5 and 9.9 % and are therefore potential candidates for statin therapy [11]. Despite multiple recent analyses that suggest good calibration in general population based cohorts [12–14], there is a considerable ongoing debate about the value of the new pooled cohort equations as a tool to define thresholds for drug therapy including the major impact of advanced age on calculated risk [15]. When the risk equations are applied to a distinct population cohort different from original studied cohorts, there has been conflicting data. Application of these risk equations to the Reasons for Geographic and Racial Differences in Stroke (REGARDS) cohort demonstrated that observed and predicted CVD risks at 5 years were similar suggesting that these equations are well calibrated with moderate to good discrimination [14]. In contrast when the risk equations are applied to the Multi-Ethnic Study of Atherosclerosis (MESA) cohort, there appears to be an overestimation of risk and a lack of superior calibration or discrimination compared with the older risk scores [16]. We have recently published in-depth analysis of the ten-year risk equations [17] and also described a modified treatment approach based on ten year risk assessment [18].

Because risk equations represent mathematical best fit based on the results of prospective cohort studies, certain inherent uncertainties (i.e., predictive intervals) always exist when applying group equation to the individual. This aspect has been highlighted in the ten-year risk guidelines and discussed elsewhere [1, 2, 19]. Another important aspect of the new pooled cohort equations that has not been well described is the influence of the uncertainties in clinical input measurements of the discrete variables that are needed for risk calculation on ten-year risk. Age in the longitudinal studies is usually expressed in years corresponding to the last birthday which would indicate that there can be a variance of up to 1 year compared to actual age (for example 60.75 years = 60 years, indicating difference of 0.75 years). BP measurement is prone to a number of errors and uncertainties [15]. Furthermore, in CARDIA, ARIC and CHS, a random zero sphygmomanometer was used that produces readings 2–3 mmHg lower than manual sphygmomanometer [20, 21]. In contrast, in FHS, BP measurements were made with a mercury-column sphygmomanometer and the average of two physician-obtained measures constituted the examination BP. This approach is markedly different from routine clinical practice. Similarly for total-c and HDL-c, the measurement results in longitudinal studies were generally standardized to those of a reference laboratory. The National Cholesterol Education Program (NCEP) guidelines recommend total analytical error in clinical models for the measurement of total-c of ≤ 9.6 % and HDL-c of ≤ 13.3 % [22]. These operating characteristics may not hold true for many commercial assays [23]. Moreover the clinical labs are certified to Clinical Laboratory Improvement Amendment (CLIA) standards where the acceptable total error for total-c is ±10 %, and for HDL-c is ±25 % [24].

Based on the hazard ratio of each variable to the ten-year risk [1, 2], the variations/uncertainties in age, systolic BP, HDL-c and total-c may have a significant influence on the ten-year ASCVD risk. It is therefore conceivable that due to the uncertainties in the input values of these variables in routine clinical practice, there is variable categorization of individuals into a high or low risk grouping, which in turn may cause erroneous management decisions based on the guidelines. Therefore it is important to define the effects of the input uncertainties to the risk calculation. Here, we evaluate the influence of these uncertainties on the ten-year risk and hence on the proposed treatment algorithms.

Methods

Study dataset

We used the publicly available NHANES dataset (2005–2010). Participants with all the variable values required for ten- year risk calculation between ages 40–75 years were included ($n = 2355$, Table 1 describes the

Table 1 Baseline characteristics

Variable	Entire cohort (N = 2355)	Without Hispanic Ethnicity (N = 1805)
AA/White/Hispanic, %	29/48/23	38/62/0
Male/Female, %	45/55	46/54
Age, yrs	60 ± 10	60 ± 10
Total Cholesterol, mg/dl	200 ± 41	199 ± 41
HDL Cholesterol, mg/dl	53 ± 17	54 ± 17
Blood Pressure, mmHg	133 ± 20	133 ± 20
Diabetes, %	32	28
Smoker, %	16	17
Hypertension, %	89	90

Values are n, % or mean ± standard deviation
AA African-American

baseline characteristics). Age was reported based on last birthday (i.e., age in completed years) calculated by subtracting the date of birth from the reference date, with the reference date being the date of contact with an individual. Gender and treatment for hypertension was self-reported. Diabetes mellitus (DM) included self-reported physician diagnosis or fasting plasma glucose of ≥126 mg/dL or a hemoglobin A1c ≥ 6.5 %. Current smokers were persons who smoked 100 cigarettes and who currently smoked every day or some days. Race was self-reported based on 1997 Revisions to the Standards for the Classification of

Federal Data on Race and Ethnicity [25]. Total-c and HDL-c measurements were using standard methods as described [26]. Individuals with self-reported coronary artery disease, heart attack (or myocardial infarction), angina and stroke were excluded.

Pooled cohort equations analysis
The new pooled cohort equations were implemented in a custom software package (MATLAB, Natick, MA). Our version of the risk calculator is available online [18]. Predicted ten-year risk for a given set of parameters for the NHANES database (called 'base calculated' risk in this paper) along with possible maximum and minimum risks were computed by assuming a variation in age of 0–1 year, and a ± 10 % variation in total-c, HDL-c, and systolic BP. The change in risk category at 5 % and/or 7.5 % risk boundary limits were analyzed. These boundary limits were chosen as these define thresholds for discussion of drug therapies in the new guidelines. For the patient cohort with base calculated risk < (less than) the boundary limits, the percentage of the designated patient cohort that had maximum possible risk ≥ (greater or equal to) the boundary limits indicated the potentially re-categorized population that may be eligible for more intensive therapy but were deemed lower risk based on base calculated measurement (Fig. 1). On the other hand, for the patient cohort with base calculated

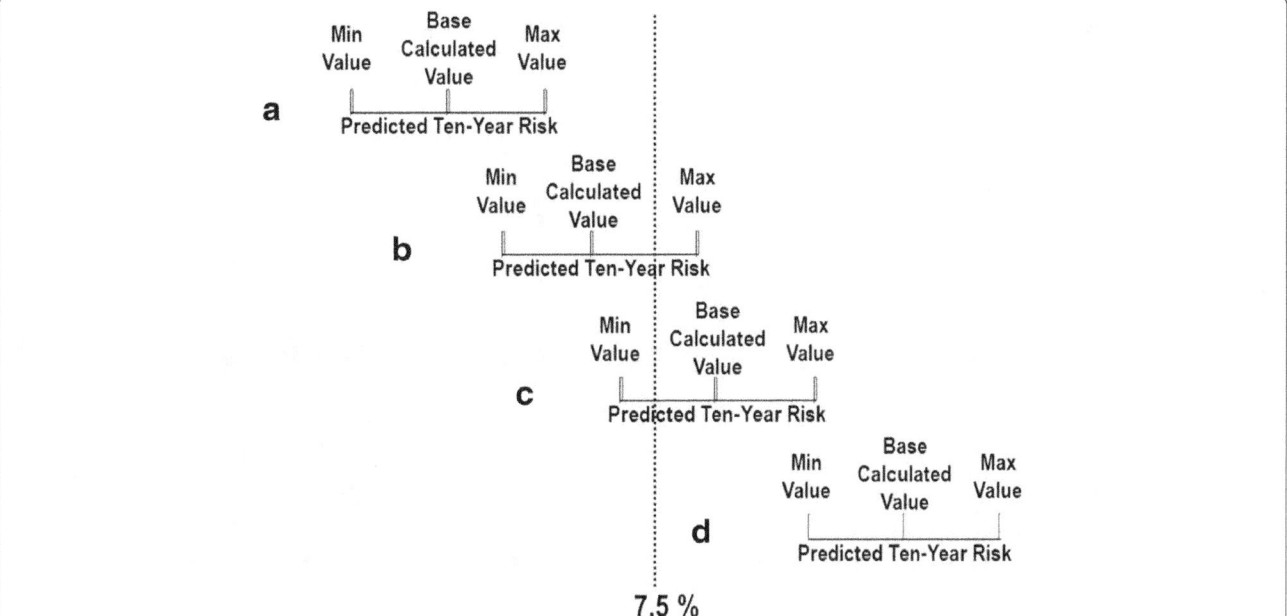

Fig. 1 Illustration of four classification scenarios according to boundary limit of 7.5 % due to the uncertainty of clinical measurements on predicted ten-year atherosclerotic cardiovascular disease risk using the new pooled cohort equations. Scenario **a**, the base calculated ten-year risk is well below the boundary limit, the variation in clinical measurements does not result in the change in risk category; For scenario **b** when the base calculated ten-year risk is below or close to the boundary limit, and scenario **c** when the base calculated ten-year risk is equal to or slightly beyond the boundary limit, the variation in clinical measurements may result in the change in risk category; Scenario **d**, the base calculated ten-year risk is well beyond the boundary limit, the variation in clinical measurements does not result in the change in risk category

risk ≥ the boundary limits, the percentage of the designated population that had minimum possible risk < the boundary limits indicated the re-categorized population that may be eligible for more conservative therapy but were deemed higher risk based on baseline calculated measurement (Fig. 1). For the primary analysis, we analyzed white and African American (AA) ethnicity (combined whites and AA $N = 1805$) because the ACC/AHA risk guidelines were primarily based on the white/AA population. We also performed secondary analysis for all participants that includes Hispanic ethnicity ($n = 2355$) (Data Supplement).

Statistical analysis

The change in risk category at 5 % and/or 7.5 % risk boundary limits were assessed by the Fisher's exact test (SAS 9.4). A $P < 0.05$ was considered statistically significant. Total number of cohort with possible risk category changes was defined as the total number of differences in base calculated risk and maximum risk in the patient cohort with base calculated ten-year risk < the boundary limits (i.e., for 7.5 % boundary limit, $N_{[Base\ Calculated\ Risk}$ $_{<7.5\%]}$ $-N_{[no\ change\ in\ risk\ categorization\ compared\ to\ base\ risk}$ $_{<7.5\%]})$ and differences in base calculated risk and minimum risk in the patient cohort with baseline calculated ten-year risk ≥ the boundary limits (i.e., for 7.5 % boundary limit, $N_{[Base\ Calculated\ Risk\ \geq7.5\%]}$ $-N_{[no\ change\ in\ risk}$ $_{categorization\ compared\ to\ base\ risk\ \geq7.5\%]})$. Percentage of total risk categorization changes was defined as the percent total number of cohort with possible risk category changes to the total patient cohort.

Results

In Figs. 2, 3 and 4, we provide the examples of application of the modified calculator [18] with customizable uncertainty limits for the realistic case scenarios. For these case scenarios, the calculated maximum and minimum risk based on the variations/ uncertainties of rounding of age and measurements of total-c, HDL-c and systolic BP reveals that the upper and lower boundary limits of ten-year risk crosses the 5 % and 7.5 % boundary limits (Figs. 2, 3 and 4). Thus, due to effect of input variable uncertainties, base-calculated risk category could be potentially increased from <5 % to ≥5 %

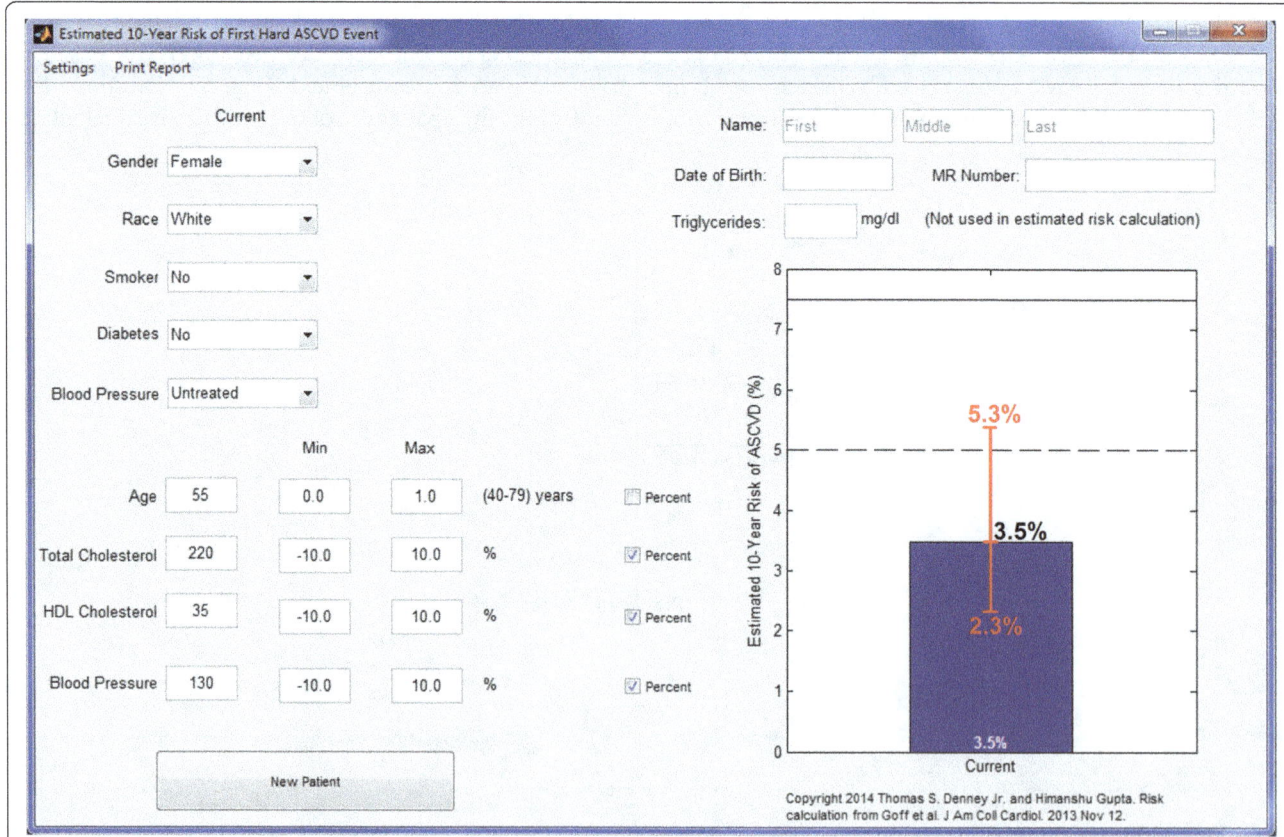

Fig. 2 Example illustrating the modified calculator with customizable uncertainty limits for a white female with baseline calculated ten-year risk of 3.5 %. The uncertainty in the measurement values of age, total-c, HDL-c and BP can be input using this customizable tool. The blue bar depicts the calculated baseline ten-year risk, and the red bar represents the maximum and minimum risk. In the depicted example, maximum and minimum risks were computed by assuming variations in input of age (0–1 year) and ± 10 % variation in total-cholesterol (c), HDL-c, and systolic blood pressure. Boundary limits of 5 % and 7.5 % are marked by dashed and solid line, respectively. Our version of the risk calculator is available online [18]

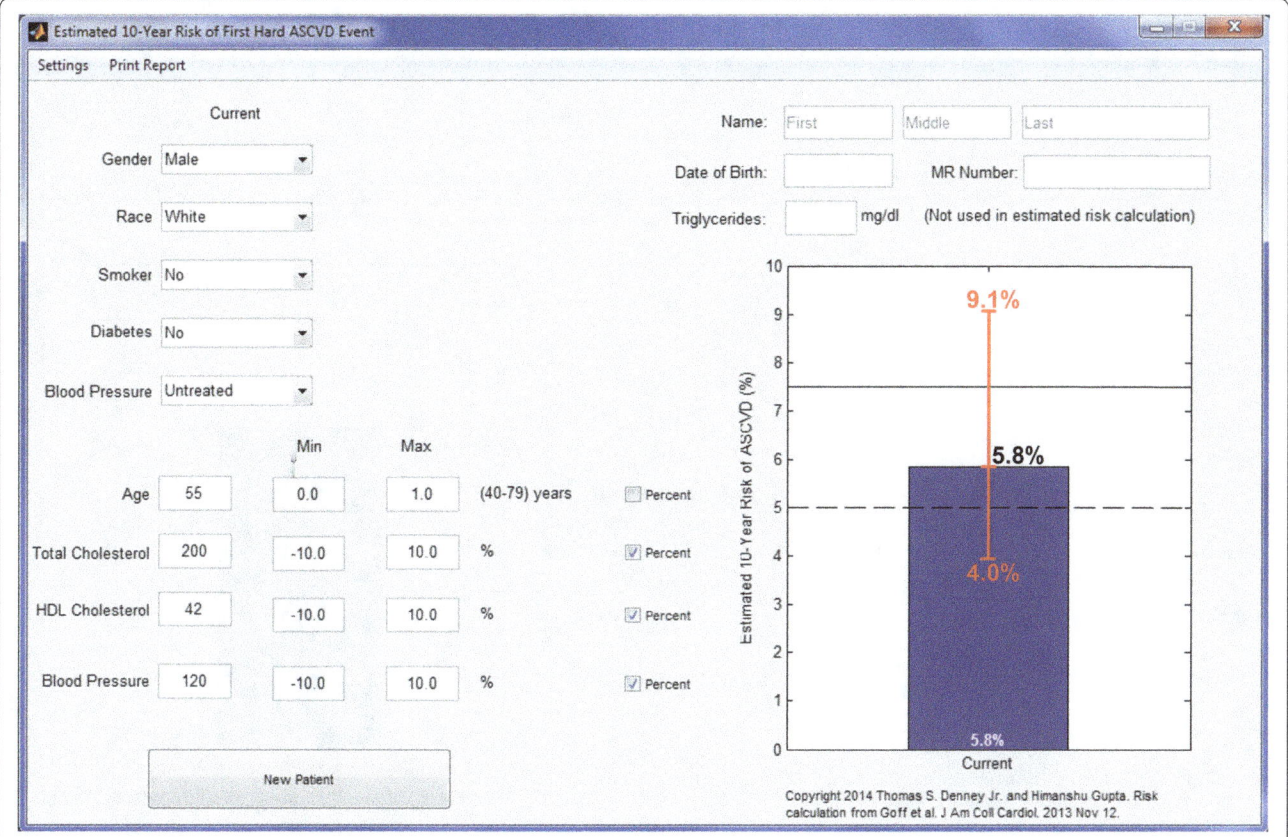

Fig. 3 Example illustrating the modified calculator with customizable uncertainty limits for a white male with baseline calculated ten-year risk of 5.8 %. Explanations and abbreviations as in Fig. 2

for patient in Fig. 2 or decreased from ≥7.5 % to <7.5 % in patient in Fig. 4. For example depicted in Fig. 3 with base-calculated risk of 5.8 %, risk category could potentially range from low risk (<5 % boundary limit) to a higher risk (≥7.5 % boundary limit).

Using modified calculator [18], we determined the base and the upper and lower boundary limits of ten-year risk for our study cohort. Baseline characteristics of the participant cohort are described in Table 1. Our detailed analysis dataset of NHANES data is attached as Additional file 1.

For the primary analysis, we analyzed white and AA ethnicity (combined $N = 1805$). We find that around 33 % of the total cohort had base calculated risk of < 7.5 % while the other 67 % had base calculated risk ≥7.5 %. On evaluating the possible risk category changes, up to 38 % of the cohort with base calculated risk <7.5 % (12.57 % of total cohort) may have ≥7.5 % risk based on possible risk. These may therefore need to be treated more aggressively. Furthermore, up to 17 % of the cohort with base calculated risk ≥7.5 % (12.36 % of total cohort) may be re-categorized based on their possible minimum risk, indicating that these individuals may not be treated appropriately. This trend was

consistently noted across all subgroups except for African American males where most of the cohort had ≥ 7.5 % baseline risk regardless of the variation in the variables (Table 2).

We also calculated possible changes in risk category based on the variation described at 5 % boundary limit for non-diabetics (Table 3).

We find similar trends and results for possible risk re-categorization as for 7.5 % boundary limit for the total cohort and the subgroups except for African American males for <5 % risk where the number of possible change in risk category did not reach statistical significance as most of the cohort had ≥5 % baseline risk regardless of the variation in the variables. When we incorporated Hispanics and calculated the risk based on white cohort (as per the guideline recommendations), we find that the results remained consistent (Additional file 2: Table S1 and Additional file 3: Table S2).

Discussion

Our analysis of the new-pooled cohort equations for ten-year ASCVD risk quantification provides important caveats that need to be considered: a) The variations/ uncertainties in the input values of continuous variables

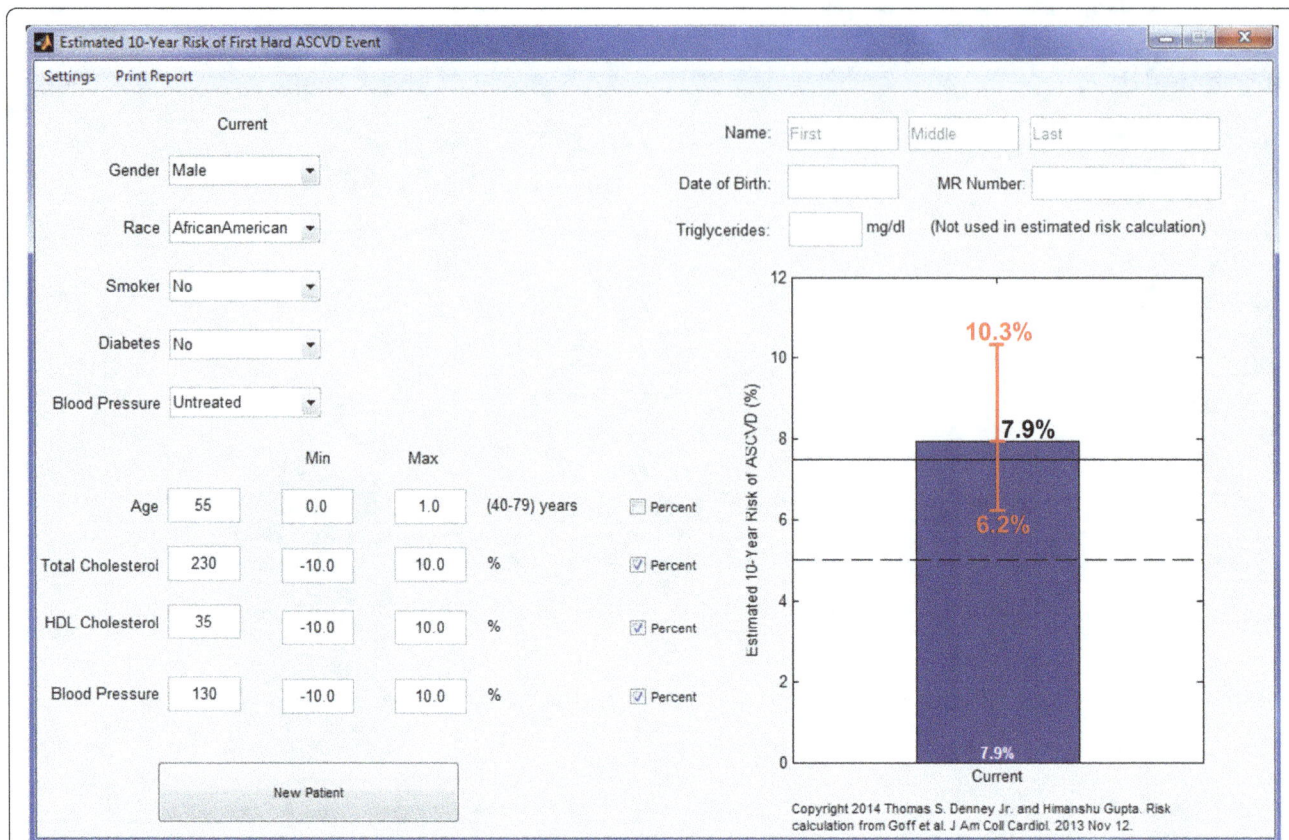

Fig. 4 Example illustrating the modified calculator with customizable uncertainty limits for African American male with baseline calculated ten-year risk of 7.9 %. Explanations and abbreviations as in Fig. 2

(age, systolic BP, total-c and HDL-c) used for ten-year risk calculation have an important effect on the calculated ten-year risk; b) At the proposed important decision nodes of 5 % and 7.5 % ten-year risk, we find that these variations/ uncertainties in the input values can influence the categorization into a high or low risk grouping in a substantial number of people. This therefore may have important effects on treatment planning and preventive policies. Uncertainty is a quantification of the doubt about the measurement results [27]. Any parameter which influences the risk calculation, and whose value we do not know precisely, is a source of uncertainty [1]. We report our results based on 0–1 year uncertainty, assuming that the age of individual is typically rounded or truncated based on how his date of birth compared to the date of encounter. The ACC/AHA risk calculator allows for inputting precise age in years (using decimal numbers) which is likely to reduce the uncertainty in the absolute calculated risk and should therefore be taken into account when calculating ten-year risk. Defining uncertainties in routine clinical practice of systolic BP, total-c and HDL-c for calculating 10-year risk is more challenging. The measurements uncertainty

(coefficient of variance) of a particular assay is generally reported by the manufactures and similar test characteristics should therefore be replicated wherever the test is performed in a clinical setting. In clinical reports these known uncertainty/variability due to known test characteristics are not generally reported. There are additional parameters that can affect the certainty of the measurements, which may be due to biological factors and/environmental factors or other undefined reasons, and are therefore difficult to quantify. This latter aspect is likely more important for BP measurements. Guidelines have been proposed regarding optimal techniques for BP measurement including instrumentation [15]. Adhering to these guidelines may reduce some of the well described uncertainties in the clinical BP measurements [15, 28]. Although CLIA standards are frequently used for clinical labs, NCEP standards for total and HDL-c are more stringent. The use of repeated measures has been previously shown to improve risk prediction by reducing regression dilution bias and providing more stable risk factor values [29]. Therefore, in patients with borderline risk (e.g. between 5-7.5 %), it may be prudent to perform repeat measurements (at a certain time apart, preferably triplicate

Table 2 Analysis of the impact of input variable variations in categorizing subjects based on ten-year risk threshold of 7.5 %

Patient groups	Base Calculated Ten Year Risk <7.5 % (% of total)			Base Calculated Ten Year Risk ≥7.5 % (% of total)			Total Change of Risk Categorization (% of total)
	Base Calculated Risk <7.5 %	No change of risk categorization (Maximal calculated risk <7.5 %)	Change of risk categorization (Maximal calculated risk ≥7.5 %)	Base Calculated Risk ≥7.5 %	No change of risk categorization (Minimal calculated risk ≥7.5 %)	Change of risk categorization (Minimal calculated Risk <7.5 %)	
All (n = 1805)	32.96	20.39***	12.57	67.04	55.68***	11.36	23.93
Non-DM (n = 1292)	41.80	26.55***	15.25	58.20	46.90***	11.3	26.55
AA (n = 426)	36.15	20.42***	15.73	63.85	52.11***	11.74	27.46
AA Male (n = 196)	14.29	6.63*	7.66	85.71	78.57	7.14	14.80
AA Female (n = 230)	54.78	32.17***	22.61	45.22	29.57***	15.65	38.26
White (n = 866)	44.57	29.56***	15.01	55.43	44.34***	11.09	26.10
White Male (n = 404)	34.90	19.31***	15.59	65.10	52.72***	12.38	27.97
White Female (n = 462)	53.03	38.53***	14.5	46.97	37.01***	9.96	24.46
DM (n = 513)	10.72	4.87***	5.85	89.28	77.78***	11.5	17.35
AA (n = 255)	5.88	2.35	3.53	94.12	84.71***	9.41	12.94
AA Male (n = 107)	0.00	0.00	0	100.00	98.13	1.87	1.87
AA Female (n = 148)	10.14	4.05	6.09	89.86	75.00**	14.86	20.95
White (n = 258)	15.50	7.36***	8.14	84.50	70.93***	13.57	21.71
White Male (n = 130)	10.77	3.85	6.92	89.23	81.54	7.69	14.62
White Female (n = 128)	20.31	10.94	9.37	79.69	60.16**	19.53	28.91

Values are % or n. Base calculated: predicted ten-year risk using the raw NHANES data; Minimal Risk: minimum predicted ten-year risk computed by the calculator assuming a variation in age of 0–1 year, and ± 10 % variation in total-cholesterol (c), HDL-c, and systolic blood pressure (BP); Maximal Risk: maximum predicted ten-year risk computed by the calculator assuming a variation in age of 0–1 year, and ± 10 % variation in total-cholesterol (c), HDL-c, and systolic blood pressure (BP); DM: Diabetes mellitus; AA: African-American; Comparisons between Base versus Max/Min Risk were performed using Fisher's Exact Test; * for P < 0.05, ** for P < 0.01, and *** for P < 0.001

Table 3 Analysis of the impact of input variable variations in categorizing subjects based on ten-year risk threshold of 5 %

Patient groups	Base Calculated Ten Year Risk < 5 % (% of total)			Base Calculated Ten Year Risk ≥ 5 % (% of total)			Total Change of Risk Categorization (% of total)
	Base Calculated Risk <5 %	No change of risk categorization (Maximal calculated risk <5 %)	Change of risk categorization (Maximal calculated risk ≥5 %)	Base Calculated Risk ≥5 %	No change of risk categorization (Minimal calculated risk ≥5 %)	Change of risk categorization (Minimal calculated Risk <5 %	
Non-DM (n = 1292)	28.79	16.02***	12.77	71.21	59.83***	11.38	24.15
AA (n = 426)	23.47	10.80***	12.67	76.53	65.49***	11.04	23.71
AA Male (n = 196)	4.08	1.53	2.55	95.92	90.82	5.1	7.65
AA Female (n = 230)	40.00	18.70***	21.3	60.00	43.91***	16.09	37.39
White (n = 866)	31.41	18.59***	12.82	68.59	57.04***	11.55	24.36
White Male (n = 404)	22.77	10.89***	11.88	77.23	66.34***	10.89	22.77
White Female (n = 462)	38.96	25.32***	13.64	61.04	48.92***	12.12	25.76

Values are % or n. Base calculated: predicted ten-year risk using the raw NHANES data; Minimal Risk: minimum predicted ten-year risk computed by the calculator assuming a variation in age of 0–1 year, and ± 10 % variation in total-cholesterol (c), HDL-c, and systolic blood pressure (BP); Maximal Risk: maximum predicted ten-year risk computed by the calculator assuming a variation in age of 0–1 year, and ± 10 % variation in total-cholesterol (c), HDL-c, and systolic blood pressure (BP); DM: Diabetes mellitus; AA: African-American; Comparisons between Base versus Max/Min Risk were performed using Fisher's Exact Test; * for $P < 0.05$, ** for $P < 0.01$, and *** for $P < 0.001$

measurements). A similar approach has been previously proposed in NCEP Adult Treatment Panel III guidelines and in a US Preventive Services Taskforce statement that recommends repeating the lipid profile to confirm abnormal values [http://www.uspreventiveservicestaskforce.org/uspstf08/lipid/lipidrs.htm [30],]. In addition, use of NCEP network laboratories may be prudent in certain situation such as of wide variability in the measurement values.

It should be emphasized that clinical judgement and discussion with the individual patient is important when deciding for optimal treatment approach based on calculated ten-year risk. This aspect has also been highlighted in the ten-year risk guidelines. Risk equations provide important guidance to the clinicians and the patients for such discussion. However since these equations represent mathematical functions/ best fit based on the results of prospective cohort studies, they do have inherent uncertainties and hence cannot supersede the judgement of a clinician. Our analysis does have important limitations. The distribution function of the variance of the continuous variables in actual clinical situations is not well described. We calculated the outermost boundaries of ten-year risk and the net uncertainty assuming uniform distribution and predictable direction in the variance of each variable. This therefore would result in greater net risk re-categorization than in clinical situations. However, we have provided a practical framework for estimating the impact of uncertainties in important clinical variables. Assessment of the whole spectra of intermediate effects due to bidirectional uncertainties in clinical variable measurements as well as the assessment of relative role of specific input variables on the risk re-categorization was not considered in the present study. The relative interaction of clinical input variable uncertainties and model inherent uncertainties (i.e., group risk prediction intervals) in individual risk predictions [19], was also beyond the scope of the present study. Such analysis would require much more sophisticated simulation and incorporating data from large clinical datasets.

Based on our previous publications [17, 18] and present work, we would suggest two additional features for the future iterations of the risk calculator. Firstly, it should allow the customizable input of uncertainty limits for relevant variables based on the local or reference laboratory standards. Further, it should estimate the upper and lower boundaries for ten-year ASCVD risk taking into account various uncertainties including that for individual datasets and model fits.

Conclusions

Our intent in writing this manuscript is to raise awareness about certain aspects of the new pooled cohort equations for ten-year risk calculation that are not immediately apparent. We describe effects of the uncertainty in measurements of important variables for calculating ten-year risk that may have a significant impact in preventive approaches to ASCVD. Incorporating good clinical practices for the measurement of critical clinical variables and robust standardization of laboratory parameters to more stringent reference standards is extremely important for successful implementation of the new guidelines. Furthermore, ability to customize the risk calculator inputs to better represent unique clinical circumstances specific to individual needs would be highly desirable in the future versions of the risk calculator.

Acknowledgements
None.

Funding
This work was partially supported by grant NIH NHLBI R01-HL104018. The funders had no role in study design, data collection and analysis, decision to publish, or preparation of the manuscript.

Authors' contributions
HG conceived of the study, participated in its design and coordination, analysis and interpretation of data, wrote and finalized the manuscript. CGS performed the analysis and interpretation of the data, wrote the manuscript. OFS revised the manuscript critically for important intellectual content, edited and submitted the manuscript. AJ performed acquisition of data. TSD contributed to the analysis and interpretation of the data, writing and finalizing the manuscript. All authors read and approved the final manuscript.

Competing interests
The authors declare that they have no competing interests.

Author details
[1]Department of Medicine, Cardiovascular Disease, University of Alabama at Birmingham, 1808 7th Ave South, BDB 101, Birmingham, AL 35294, USA. [2]VA Medical Center, Birmingham, AL, USA. [3]School of Public Health, The University Of Texas Health Science Centre, Houston, TX, USA. [4]Department of Electrical and Computer Engineering, Auburn University, Auburn, AL, USA.

References
1. Goff Jr DC, Lloyd-Jones DM, Bennett G, Coady S, D'Agostino RB, Gibbons R, Greenland P, Lackland DT, Levy D, O'Donnell CJ, et al. 2013 ACC/AHA guideline on the assessment of cardiovascular risk: a report of the American College of Cardiology/American Heart Association Task Force on Practice Guidelines. Circulation. 2014;129(25 Suppl 2):S49–73.
2. Stone NJ, Robinson JG, Lichtenstein AH, Bairey Merz CN, Blum CB, Eckel RH, Goldberg AC, Gordon D, Levy D, Lloyd-Jones DM, et al. 2013 ACC/AHA guideline on the treatment of blood cholesterol to reduce atherosclerotic cardiovascular risk in adults: a report of the American College of Cardiology/American Heart Association Task Force on Practice Guidelines. Circulation. 2014;129(25 Suppl 2):S1–45.
3. Anderson K, Odell P, Wilson P, Kannel W. Cardiovascular disease risk profiles. Am Heart J. 1991;121:293–8.
4. Lloyd-Jones DM, Leip EP, Larson MG, D'Agostino RB, Beiser A, Wilson PWF, Wolf PA, Levy D. Prediction of Lifetime Risk for Cardiovascular Disease by Risk Factor Burden at 50 Years of Age. Circulation. 2006;113(6):791–8.
5. Wilson PWF, D'Agostino RB, Levy D, Belanger AM, Silbershatz H, Kannel WB. Prediction of Coronary Heart Disease Using Risk Factor Categories. Circulation. 1998;97(18):1837–47.
6. Friedman GD, Cutter GR, Donahue RP, Hughes GH, Hulley SB, Jacobs Jr DR, Liu K, Savage PJ. CARDIA: study design, recruitment, and some characteristics of the examined subjects. J Clin Epidemiol. 1988;41(11):1105–16.
7. Fried L, Borhani N, Enright P, Furberg C, Gardin J, Kronmal R, Kuller L, Manolio R, Mittelmark M, A N, et al. The Cardiovascular Health Study: design and rationale. Ann Epidemiol. 1991;1(3):263–76.
8. The ARIC Investigators. The atherosclerosis risk in community (ARIC) study: design and objectives. Am J Epidemiol. 1989;129(4):687–702.
9. Keaney Jr JF, Curfman GD, Jarcho JA. A pragmatic view of the new cholesterol treatment guidelines. N Engl J Med. 2014;370(3):275–8.
10. Psaty BM, Weiss NS. 2013 ACC/AHA guideline on the treatment of blood cholesterol: A fresh interpretation of old evidence. JAMA. doi:10.1001/jama2013284203.
11. Ridker PM, Cook NR. Statins: new American guidelines for prevention of cardiovascular disease. Lancet. 2013;382(9907):1762–5.
12. Karmali KN, Goff Jr DC, Ning H, Lloyd-Jones DM. A systematic examination of the 2013 ACC/AHA pooled cohort risk assessment tool for atherosclerotic cardiovascular disease. J Am Coll Cardiol. 2014;64(10):959–68.
13. Mortensen MB, Afzal S, Nordestgaard BG, Falk E. Primary Prevention With Statins: ACC/AHA Risk-Based Approach Versus Trial-Based Approaches to Guide Statin Therapy. J Am Coll Cardiol. 2015;66(24):2699–709.
14. Muntner P, Colantonio LD, Cushman M, Goff Jr DC, Howard G, Howard VJ, Kissela B, Levitan EB, Lloyd-Jones DM, Safford MM. Validation of the atherosclerotic cardiovascular disease Pooled Cohort risk equations. JAMA. 2014;311(14):1406–15.
15. Pickering TG, Hall JE, Appel LJ, Falkner BE, Graves J, Hill MN, Jones DW, Kurtz T, Sheps SG, Roccella EJ. Recommendations for Blood Pressure Measurement in Humans and Experimental Animals: Part 1: Blood Pressure Measurement in Humans: A Statement for Professionals From the Subcommittee of Professional and Public Education of the American Heart Association Council on High Blood Pressure Research. Circulation. 2005;111(5):697–716.
16. DeFilippis AP, Young R, Carrubba CJ, McEvoy JW, Budoff MJ, Blumenthal RS, Kronmal RA, McClelland RL, Nasir K, Blaha MJ. An analysis of calibration and discrimination among multiple cardiovascular risk scores in a modern multiethnic cohort. Ann Intern Med. 2015;162(4):266–75.
17. Schiros CG, Denney Jr TS, Gupta H. Interaction analysis of the new pooled cohort equations for 10-year atherosclerotic cardiovascular disease risk estimation: a simulation analysis. BMJ Open. 2015;5(4):e006468.
18. Gupta H, Schiros CG, Denney Jr TS. Modified treatment approach using cardiovascular disease risk calculator for primary prevention. PLoS One. 2014;9(8):e104478.
19. Sniderman AD, D'Agostino Sr RB, Pencina MJ. The Role of Physicians in the Era of Predictive Analytics. JAMA. 2015;314(1):25–6.
20. Conroy R, O'Brien E, O'Malley K, Atkins N. Measurement error in the Hawksley random zero sphygmomanometer: what damage has been done and what can we learn? BMJ. 1993;306:1319–22.
21. McGurk C, Nugent A, McAuley D, Silke B. Sources of inaccuracy in the use of the Hawksley random-zero sphygmomanometer. J Hypertens. 1997;15(12):1379–84.
22. National Cholesterol Education Program. Recommendations on lipoprotein measurement (NIH Publication No. 95-3044). Bethesda: National Heart, Lung, and Blood Institute; 1995.
23. Miller W, Myers G, Sakurabayashi I, Bachmann L, Caudill S, Dziekonski A, Edwards S, Kimberly M, Kozun W, Leary E, et al. Seven direct methods for measuring HDL and LDL cholesterol compared with ultracentrifugation reference measurement procedures. Clin Chem. 2010;56(6):977–86.
24. Warnick G, Kimberly M, Waymack P, Leary E, Myers G. Standardization of Measurements for Cholesterol, Triglycerides, and Major Lipoproteins. Lab Medicine. 2008;39(8):481–90.
25. Federal Register. 1997;62:58781–90
26. https://www.gpo.gov/fdsys/pkg/FR-1997-10-30/pdf/97-28653.pdf. Accessed 22 Jan 2014.
27. Bell S. A Beginner's Guide to Uncertainty of Measurement. Teddington: TW11 0LW: National Physical Laboratory; 1999. available at http://www.wmo.int/pages/prog/gcos/documents/gruanmanuals/UK_NPL/mgpg11.pdf.
28. Campbell N, Chockalingam A, Fodor J, McKay D. Accurate, reproducible measurement of blood pressure. CMAJ. 1990;1(143):19–24.
29. Karp I, Abrahamowicz M, Bartlett G, Pilote L. Updated risk factor values and the ability of the multivariable risk score to predict coronary heart disease. Am J Epidemiol. 2004;160(7):707–16.
30. Executive Summary of The Third Report of The National Cholesterol Education Program (NCEP). Expert Panel on Detection, Evaluation, And Treatment of High Blood Cholesterol In Adults (Adult Treatment Panel III). JAMA. 2001;285(19):2486–97.

3

Serum 25-hydroxyvitamin D levels are associated with carotid atherosclerosis in normotensive and euglycemic Chinese postmenopausal women: the Shanghai Changfeng study

Hui Ma[1], Huandong Lin[2], Yu Hu[1], Xiaoming Li[2], Wanyuan He[3], Xuejuan Jin[4], Jian Gao[5], Naiqing Zhao[6], Zhenqi Liu[7] and Xin Gao[2*]

Abstract

Background: The role of serum 25-hydroxyvitamin D (25 (OH) D) in atherogenesis is unclear. We investigated whether the 25 (OH) D is independently associated with the carotid intima–media thickness (CIMT) and carotid plaques in normotensive and euglycemic postmenopausal women.

Methods: A total of 671 normotensive and euglycemic postmenopausal women (mean age, 58.8 years) were enrolled from the Changfeng Study. A standard interview, anthropometrics measurements and laboratory analyses were performed for each participant. Bilateral CIMTs were measured using ultrasonography, and the presence of carotid plaques was assessed. The serum 25 (OH) D was measured using electrochemiluminescence immunoassay.

Results: Serum 25 (OH) D was 43.6 ± 18.2 nmol/L in the postmenopausal women. Compared with subjects with 25 (OH) D in the first, second and third quartiles, subjects with 25 (OH) D in the fourth quartile had decreased CIMT and prevalence of carotid plaque (0.684 ± 0.009 mm vs 0.719 ± 0.009 mm, 0.708 ± 0.009 mm and 0.709 ± 0.009 mm; 10.8% vs 19.0%, 14.8% and 16.8%, respectively). After adjusting for conventional CVD risk factors, PTH, liver and renal function, postmenopausal women with 25 (OH) D in the fourth quartile still had lower CIMT than those in the first, second and third quartiles ($p = 0.039$) and the subjects in the fourth quartile had a 0.421-fold decreased risk of carotid plaques relative to those in the lowest quartile (95% confidence interval 0.209 to 0.848).

Conclusions: These results suggest serum 25 (OH) D is independently and inversely associated with carotid atherosclerosis in postmenopausal women with normal blood pressure and normal glucose tolerance.

Keywords: 25-hydroxyvitamin D (25 (OH) D), Carotid intima-media thickness (CIMT), Carotid plaque, Carotid atherosclerosis

Background

Vitamin D, a fat-soluble vitamin and steroid hormone, is well known for its pivotal role in calcium homeostasis and bone metabolism. Beyond the role in bone health, vitamin D is receiving increasing attention for its influence on non-skeletal health problems and chronic diseases [1,2]. Serum 25-hydroxyvitamin D (25(OH) D), the major storage form of vitamin D, is formed in the liver, and is a clinical indicator of overall vitamin D3 status [3]. The association of serum 25 (OH) D levels with cardiovascular diseases (CVD) is debated in the literature. The Framingham Offspring Study revealed that low serum 25 (OH) D was independently associated with an increased incidence of CVD in Caucasians during a 5.4-year follow-up period [4]. Additionally, European studies have shown that serum 25 (OH) D levels are inversely associated with the prevalence of CVD and carotid intima-medial thickening in patients with type 2 diabetes mellitus (DM) [5]. More recently, the meta-analysis by Wang et al. [6] of nineteen independent prospective

* Correspondence: zhongshan_endo@126.com
[2]Department of Endocrinology and Metabolism, Zhong Shan Hospital, Fudan University, Shanghai 200032, China
Full list of author information is available at the end of the article

cohort studies reported an inverse association between serum 25 (OH) D concentrations and risk of CVD outcome. However, several other studies observed no significant association between serum 25 (OH) D levels and CVD. For example, Deleskog A et al and Blondon M et al demonstrated that levels of 25 (OH) D showed multiple associations with established and emerging cardiovascular risk factors but were not consistently, independently related to measures of carotid IMT and carotid plaque[7,8]. The Korean National Health and Nutrition Examination Survey (KNHANES-2008-2009) indicates that the prevalence of CVD is not associated with low serum 25 (OH) D levels in the total population [9]. The study by Melamed et al. [10], using the third National Health and Nutrition Examination Survey cohort, while CVD risk was not statistically significant, the all-cause mortality data suggested a U- or reverse J-shaped dose-relationship, with increased total mortality for both the lowest and highest serum 25 (OH) D concentrations (<44.4 and >80.1 nmol/l, respectively) in this cohort followed for 9 years. As noted, the majority of the previous studies were conducted using populations with different proportions of hypertension or diabetes. In addition, 25 (OH) D is associated with hyperglycemia and hypertension [11], which may themselves be linked to CVD. Therefore, the association between 25 (OH) D and atherosclerosis may be confounded by the inclusion of subjects with hypertension, diabetes or pre-diabetes. Moreover, it has been shown that 25 (OH) D values vary between different ethnicities. There are few reports on the relationship between 25 (OH) D and CVD in the Chinese postmenopausal women. Given the high risk of CVD in this population [12], more evidence is needed to evaluate the association between 25 (OH) D and atherosclerosis in the Chinese postmenopausal women.

The use of high-resolution color-coded duplex sonography offers the opportunity to assess the carotid intima-media thickness (CIMT) and carotid plaques as reliable markers of atherosclerosis [13]. Therefore, in the present study, we investigated the relationship between 25 (OH) D and carotid atherosclerosis in a community-based population of normotensive and euglycemic postmenopausal women.

Methods
Study population
The subjects were participants in the Changfeng Study, a community-based study of chronic diseases among middle-aged and elderly individuals which has been described elsewhere [14]. The Changfeng community is a middle-class community in Shanghai [14]. From June 2009 to June 2012, 2717 postmenopausal women were initially enrolled. We excluded 2046 participants for the following reasons: lack of physical examination and laboratory

assessments (n = 51), prevalent CVD (myocardial infarction, stroke, or peripheral arterial disease) (n = 202), prevalent hemodialysis (n = 2), bone fracture within 3 months and use of drugs known to influence bone metabolism including the use of postmenopausal hormone therapy, calcium, diphosphonate, vitamin D and glucocorticoid (n = 384), prevalent hypertension (systolic blood pressure ≥ 140 mmHg, diastolic blood pressure ≥90 mmHg, the use of antihypertensive medications, or diagnosed hypertension) (n = 1076), prevalent diabetes mellitus or pre-diabetes (fasting glucose ≥5.6 mmol/L, OGTT 2 h glucose ≥7.8 mmol/L, the use of hypoglycaemic medications, or diagnosed diabetes; n = 320), or the use of lipid-lowering therapy or use of the antiplatelet agents (n = 11). Finally, 671 subjects were included in the analysis.

The study was approved by the ethical committee of Zhongshan Hospital, Fudan University and was conducted in accordance with the guidelines of the Declaration of Helsinki. All the patients provided consent upon enrolment in the study. Interviews, physical examinations and ultrasound scans were performed at the Changfeng Community Health Service Center.

Clinical measurements
Letters were sent to participants with instructions asking them not to alter their diet or level of physical activity for at least 3 days before the test. A questionnaire was administered by trained nurses to evaluate the medical history and lifestyle of each participant. Weight and height were measured while the participant was clothed in a light gown. The body mass index (BMI) was calculated as the weight divided by the height squared (kg/m^2). The waist circumference was measured midway between the lowest rib margin and the iliac crest in a standing position, and the hip circumference was measured at the widest level over the greater trochanters. The waist-to-hip ratio (WHR) was calculated as the waist circumference divided by the hip circumference. The resting blood pressure was measured three times, and the mean value was used for the analysis. Blood samples were obtained after a fasting period of at least 10 hours. Total cholesterol (TC), high-density lipoprotein cholesterol (HDL-C), triglycerides (TG) and liver enzymes were measured using a model 7600 automated bio-analyser (Hitachi, Tokyo, Japan). The level of low-density lipoprotein cholesterol (LDL-C) was calculated using the Friedewald equation. The fasting blood glucose (FBG) and 2 h glucose levels following a 75-g oral glucose challenge (PPG) for non-diabetics were measured using the glucose oxidase method. The glomerular filtration rate (GFR) was estimated based on the serum creatinine concentration using the Modification of Diet in Renal Disease (MDRD) formula: estimated GFR (eGFR) = 186 × [serum creatinine

(mmol/L) × 0.0113]$^{-1.154}$ × age$^{-0.203}$ × (0.742 for women) [15]. The serum 25(OH)D, parathyroid hormone (PTH) and insulin were measured by electrochemiluminescence immunoassay using an immunoassay analyzer (Roche Cobas-6001, Switzerland; coefficient of variation <4.0%, <5.0% and <5.0%, respectively). Homeostasis model assessment index for insulin resistance (HOMA-IR) and beta cell function (HOMA-%B) were used to estimate insulin sensitivity and insulin secretion [16].

The carotid arteries of the participants were evaluated by an experienced radiologist who was blinded to the participants' details using a GE Logic P5 (GE Healthcare, Milwaukee, USA) scanner with a 10-MHz probe. The CIMTs on both sides were measured in the common carotid artery approximately 1 cm proximal to the bifurcation at the far wall during end diastole. The CIMT was quantified at plaque-free sections of the carotid arteries as the distance between the lumen–intima and media–adventitia interfaces. Three values were measured on each side, and the average CIMT values were used for the analysis. The study procedure involved scanning the near and far walls of both common carotid arteries, the carotid bifurcation, and the internal carotid artery for the presence of plaques, defined as the presence of focal wall thickening resulting in a thickness that is at least 50% greater than that of the surrounding vessel wall or as a focal region with a CIMT greater than 1.5 mm that protrudes into the lumen that is distinct from the adjacent boundary, according to American Society of Echocardiography [17]. Repeated measurements on the same subjects (performed in 104 subjects) for CIMT and carotid plaque yielded an intraclass correlation coefficient (ICC) of 95% (95% confidence interval, 0.91 to 0.97) and 96% (95% confidence interval, 0.92 to 0.97), respectively.

Hypertension was defined according to the Seventh Report of the Joint National Committee [18]. The diagnoses of impaired fasting glucose, impaired glucose tolerance, and DM were based on the American Diabetes Association 2010 criteria [19]. The diagnosis of cardiovascular disease was based on self-reports and confirmed using hospital medical records.

Statistical analyses

The data were expressed as the means ± SD(SE), frequencies or medians with 25th and 75th percentiles. Skewed variables were logarithmically transformed to improve normality prior to analysis. To evaluate the relationship between each parameter and the 25(OH)D, the subjects were stratified according to the 25(OH)D quartiles. The ranges of 25(OH)D in the quartiles were 12.4-30.7, 30.8 -40.5, 40.6-53.0 and 53.2-153.0 nmol/L. Analysis of covariance and logistic regression, with adjustments for CVD risk factors, liver enzymes and the GFR were

conducted to compare means and proportions, respectively, across the 25(OH)D quartiles. We used a general linear model analyses and complete the homogeneity tests, in which the outcome is the CIMT value of comparison among 25(OH)D quartiles. We test the null hypothesis that the error variance of the dependent variable is equal across groups and get the result that p = 0.366. Regression coefficients and odds ratios (ORs) were calculated for a 1-unit increase in 25(OH)D. SPSS 16.0 for Windows (SPSS 16.0 Inc Chicago, IL, USA)) was used to perform the statistical analyses. All statistical tests were two tailed, and p-values less than 0.05 were considered significant.

Results

Characteristics of the subjects according to the 25(OH)D quartiles

A total of 671 postmenopausal women were evaluated. The mean value of CIMT was 0.703 ± 0.123 mm. The prevalence of carotid plaques was 15.4%. The mean value of 25(OH)D was 43.6 ± 9.2 nmol/L. A total of 1.5% of the subjects was current smokers. Table 1 shows the clinical and biochemical parameters according to the quartiles groups for the 25(OH)D. When the traditional CVD risk factors were examined, WHR, DBP, PPG and PTH were significantly associated with the 25(OH)D quartiles. Other parameters were not significantly different among the groups.

Association of the anthropometric and biochemical parameters with serum 25(OH)D levels

Linear regression analysis showed an association between 25(OH)D and BMI, WHR, DBP, PPG and PTH (Table 2). Multivariate linear stepwise regression analysis was performed to evaluate the independent factors of 25 (OH)D. The analysis demonstrated that age (standardized β = 0.082, p = 0.028), PTH (standardized β = -0.334, p < 0.001), BMI (standardized β = -0.141, p = 0.001) and PPG (standardized β = -0.053, p = 0.003) were independently associated with serum 25(OH)D.

Association between carotid atherosclerosis and 25(OH)D

Table 3 presents the CIMT of the subjects according to 25(OH)D quartile groups. Compared with the subjects in the first, second and third 25(OH)D quartiles, those in the fourth quartile had significantly thinner CIMTs (0.684 ± 0.009 mm vs 0.719 ± 0.009 mm, 0.708 ± 0.009 mm and 0.709 ± 0.009 mm, respectively). After adjusting for conventional CVD risk factors, liver enzymes and the GFR, the subjects with 25(OH)D in the fourth quartile still had lower CIMT than those in the first, second and third quartiles (p = 0.039).

Compared with the subjects in the first, second and third 25(OH)D quartiles, those in the fourth quartile had significantly lower prevalence of carotid plaque (10.8%

Table 1 Characteristics of the subjects according to quartiles groups for 25(OH)D in subjects

Variables	All (n = 671)	1st quartile (n = 168)	2nd quartile (n = 169)	3rd quartile (n = 167)	4th quartile (n = 167)	P among groups
25(OH) D range (nmol/L)	12.4-153.0	12.4-30.7	30.8 -40.5	40.6-53.0	53.2-153.0	
Age (ys)	58.8(7.5)	57.9(7.4)	59.5(7.5)a	58.9(7.0)	59.0(8.0)	0.255
BMI (kg/m^2)	22.8(2.9)	22.9(2.9)	22.8(2.8)	23.1(3.1)	22.4(2.8)c	0.238
WHR	0.853(0.063)	0.846(0.052)	0.855(0.061)	0.847 (0.061)	0.863(0.074)a,c	0.042
Current smoker, n (%)	10(1.5%)	4(2.4%)	3(1.8%)	1(0.6%)	2(1.2%)	0.572
SBP (mmHg)	120.0(11.1)	119.7(11.8)	120.8(11.1)	120.8(10.3)	118.7(11.1)	0.253
DBP (mmHg)	70.4(7.5)	71.2(7.6)	70.0(7.2)	71.3(7.3)	69.1(7.8)a,c	0.023
ALT (U/L)	16.9(9.5)	15.6(7.6)	16.4(7.2)	17.6(7.1)	17.8(7.5)a	0.107
AST (U/L)	21.1(6.1)	20.5(6.9)	20.7(5.5)	21.4(5.5)	21.7(6.5)	0.246
TC (mmol/L)	5.2(0.8)	5.2(0.8)	5.3(0.9)	5.4(0.9)	5.2(0.7)c	0.130
LDL-c (mmol/L)	3.0(0.7)	3.0(0.8)	3.0(0.7)	3.1(0.8)	2.9(0.7)c	0.096
HDL-c (mmol/L)	1.6(0.4)	1.6(0.4)	1.6(0.4)	1.6(0.4)	1.6(0.4)	0.605
TG (mmol/L)	1.4(0.7)	1.3(0.6)	1.3(0.6)	1.4(0.8)	1.4(0.7)	0.467
FBG (mmol/L)	4.9(0.3)	4.9(0.3)	4.9(0.4)	4.9(0.3)	4.9(0.3)	0.516
PPG (mmol/L)	5.7(1.1)	5.9(1.1)	5.5(1.0)a	5.4(1.0)a	5.4(0.9)a	<0.001
PTH (pg/mL)	42.2(15.1)	48.6(16.3)	42.9(13.6)a	41.4(14.5)a	35.7(12.9)a,b,c	<0.001
HOMA-IR	1.4(1.0-1.9)	1.3(1.0-2.0)	1.5(1.1-2.0)	1.5(1.0-2.0)	1.4(1.0-1.8)	0.425
HOMA-B %	97.4(72.7-128.6)	92.1(71.4-127.8)	98.6(75.6-131.0)a	102.1(70.8-134.7)	97.5(73.4-122.9)	0.1
GFR (ml/min per 1.73 m^2)	96.9(18.9)	98.3(19.0)	96.2(19.2)	97.4(19.8)	96.0(17.6)	0.647

Data are mean (SD) or percentage of subjects or median (interquartile range).
BMI: body mass index, WHR: waist-hip-ratio, FBG: Fasting blood glucose, PPG: OGTT 2 h blood glucose, PTH: parathyroid hormone, SBP: systolic blood pressure, DBP: diastolic blood pressure, ALT: alanine transaminase, AST: aspartate transaminase, TC: Total cholesterol, TG: triglyceride, HDL-C: high density lipoprotein cholesterol, LDL-C: low density lipoprotein cholesterol, HOMA-IR: homeostasis model assessment index for insulin resistance, HOMA-B: homeostasis model assessment index for beta cell function, GFR: glomerular filtration rate.
a Analysis of variance with LSD post-hoc test or Chi-square statistical analysis: P < 0.05 versus 1st quartile.
b Analysis of variance with LSD post-hoc test or Chi-square statistical analysis: P < 0.05 versus 2nd quartile.
c Analysis of variance with LSD post-hoc test or Chi-square statistical analysis: P < 0.05 versus 3rd quartile.

vs 19.0%, 14.8% and 16.8%, respectively). After adjusting for conventional CVD risk factors, liver enzymes and the GFR, the subjects with 25(OH)D in the fourth quartile had 0.421-fold decreased risks for carotid plaques relative to those in the lowest quartile (95% confidence interval 0.209 to 0.848) (Figure 1).

Discussion

Our study showed that serum 25(OH)D was independently associated with carotid atherosclerosis in normotensive and euglycemic Chinese postmenopausal women. The CIMT and the prevalence of carotid plaques significantly decreased with increasing serum 25(OH)D levels after adjusting for conventional CVD risk factors, PTH, liver enzymes and renal function in the subjects.

Serum 25(OH)D has recently become an interesting topic in cardiovascular researches [1-6]. Although a number of studies have demonstrated that 25(OH)D is associated with the development of cardiovascular events, it is still conflicting whether there is an independent association between 25(OH)D and atherosclerotic CVD. The participants in the Framingham Offspring Study [4]

had 40% patients with hypertension and 8% diabetic patients. European studies [5] were performed in diabetic adults. The studies eligible for inclusion in the meta-analysis by Wang [6], the study by Deleskog A [7], Blondon M [8], Melamed [10] and the Korean National Health and Nutrition Examination Survey [9] enrolled study populations with different proportions of hypertension or diabetes. As noted, recent studies have demonstrated that there was a close association between 25(OH)D and cardiovascular risk factors, such as hyperglycemia and hypertension [11]. Studies suggest vitamin D deficiency may be a contributor to the development of CVD potentially through associations with diabetes or hypertension [20]. In line with previous studies [11], serum 25(OH)D concentrations were inversely associated with blood pressure and blood glucose in the present study. Therefore, the relationship between carotid atherosclerosis and serum 25(OH)D would be affected by the chronic effects of increased blood glucose levels and blood pressure. The impact of residual confounding factors would remain after adjusting for hyperglycemia and hypertension in previous studies. To eliminate the confounding effects

Table 2 Association of the anthropometric and biochemical parameters with serum 25(OH)D levels in postmenopausal women

	β (95% CI)	Standardized β	P
Age (per 1y)	0.154(-0.029-0.338)	0.064	0.1
BMI (per 1 units)	-0.593(-1.063- -0.123)	-0.095	0.013
WHR	25.129(3.130-47.128)	0.086	0.025
Current smoking	-5.456(-16.840-5.928)	-0.036	0.347
SBP (per 1 mmHg)	-0.104(-0.229-0.020)	-0.064	0.1
DBP (per 1 mmHg)	-0.272(-0.455- -0.09)	-0.112	0.004
ALT (1U/L)	0.130(-0.014-0.275)	0.068	0.077
AST (1U/L)	0.161(-0.064-0.386)	0.054	0.161
TC (1 mmol/L)	-0.679(-2.323-0.965)	-0.031	0.418
LDL-C (1 mmol/L)	-1.199(-3.044-0.646)	-0.049	0.202
HDL-C (1 mmol/L)	-1.489(-5.121-2.143)	-0.031	0.421
TG (1 mmol/L)	-1.838(-2.788-0.111)	-0.071	0.065
FBG (1 mmol/L)	-2.853(-6.953-1.247)	-0.053	0.172
PPG (1 mmol/L)	-2.569(-3.862- -1.275)	-0.149	0.001
PTH (1 pg/mL)	-0.408(-0.494- -0.322)	-0.338	<0.001
logHOMA-IR	-4.853(-11.222-1.516)	-0.058	0.135
logHOMA-B %	1.779(-0.079-3.480)	0.025	0.125
GFR (1 ml/min per 1.73 m2)	-0.052(-0.125-0.021)	-0.054	0.161

BMI: body mass index, WHR: waist-hip-ratio, FBG: Fasting blood glucose, PPG: OGTT 2 h blood glucose, PTH: parathyroid hormone, SBP: systolic blood pressure, DBP: diastolic blood pressure, ALT: alanine transaminase, AST: aspartate transaminase, TC: Total cholesterol, TG: triglyceride, HDL-C: high density lipoprotein cholesterol, LDL-C: low density lipoprotein cholesterol, HOMA-IR: homeostasis model assessment index for insulin resistance, HOMA-B: homeostasis model assessment index for beta cell function, GFR: glomerular filtration rate.

of hyperglycemia and hypertension on the relationship between carotid atherosclerosis and serum 25(OH)D, we explored the relationship in the subjects with normal blood pressure and normal glucose tolerance. Thus, the association between 25(OH)D and carotid atherosclerosis was not confounded by hyperglycemia and hypertension.

In the present study there was an independent association between 25(OH)D and CIMT after adjusting for established cardiovascular risk factors. As we known, CIMT may be affected both by atherosclerosis and wall hypertrophy, we

also assessed the association between 25(OH)D and carotid plaque, which may be more representative of atherosclerosis than CIMT and more informative for predicting cardiovascular risk [21]. We demonstrated a negative and independent relationship between 25 (OH)D and carotid plaque, independently from the traditional risk factors. In contrast, Deleskog A et al [7] reported that there were no independent relationships between 25(OH)D and the baseline and progression measures of carotid IMT in 3430 middle-aged and elderly

Table 3 CIMT in the subjects according to quartile groups for 25(OH)D in the subjects

	Quartile groups for 25(OH) D in the subjects				
	1st quartile	2nd quartile	3rd quartile	4th quartile	p
Unadjusted					
CIMT (mm)	0.719(0.009)	0.708(0.009)	0.709(0.009)	0.684(0.009)a,b,c	0.034
Model I					
CIMT (mm)	0.712(0.009)	0.704(0.009)	0.707(0.009)	0.688(0.009)a,b,c	0.039

Data are mean (SE).
a Analysis of variance with LSD (least significant difference) post-hoc test: P < 0.05 versus 1st quartile.
b Analysis of variance with LSD post-hoc test: P < 0.05 versus 2nd quartile.
c Analysis of variance with LSD post-hoc test: P < 0.05 versus 3rd quartile.
Model I: adjusting for age, FBG (fasting blood glucose), PPG (postprandial blood glucose), PTH(parathyroid hormone), BMI (body mass index), WHR (waist-to-hip ratio), current smoking, SBP (systolic blood pressure), DBP (diastolic blood pressure), ALT(alanine transaminase), AST(aspartate transaminase),TG (triglyceride), HDL-C (high-density lipoprotein cholesterol), LDL-C (low-density lipoprotein cholesterol), logHOMA-IR (homeostasis model assessment index for insulin resistance), logHOMA-%B (homeostasis model assessment index for beta cell function) and GFR(glomerular filtration rate).
cIMT: carotid intima-media thickness, 25 (OH) D: 25-hydroxyvitamin D.

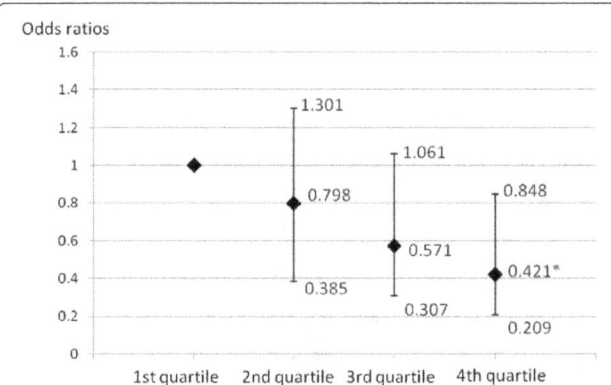

Figure 1 ORs of carotid plaque in the subjects across the 25(OH)D quartile. ORs of carotid plaque in the subjects according to 25(OH)D quartile groups after adjusting for age, BMI, WHR, FBG, PPG, SBP, DBP, TG, HDL-C, LDL-C, smoking, ALT, AST, PTH, logHOMA-IR, logHOMA-B% and the GFR, respectively. * Analysis of variance with logistic regression analysis: P < 0.05 versus 1st quartile ORs and 95% CI are shown.

subjects with high cardiovascular risk but no prevalent CVD. Similarly, Blondon M et al [8] evaluated the associations of 25(OH)D with CIMT and carotid plaques among 3251 participants free of cardiovascular disease in the Multi-Ethnic Study of Atherosclerosis and observed consistent null results for both cross-sectional associations and longitudinal associations evaluating change in IMT and incident plaque during 10 years of follow-up. Several explanations could be involved in the above different results. First, the BMI, blood pressure, blood glucose and lipid profile of the subjects in our study were relatively improved in comparison with those in the above studies. In addition, our subjects had a lower proportion of smoking participants. Thus, the association between 25(OH)D and CVD in subjects with higher cardiovascular risk may be weakened for the greater contribution of traditional atherosclerotic risks to CVD in the studies of Deleskog A [7] and Blondon M [8]. Second, there may be sex-related differences in the association between 25(OH)D and CVD. These sex-related differences might depend on background data. It is known that the life-long risk for CVD is higher for men than women [22]. Third, it is necessary to take ethnic differences into account.

69.9% of subjects have 25(OH)D levels below 50 nmol/L. Similarly, another study in China evaluated vitamin D status of healthy adults living in Guiyang (latitude 26.5° north). The study showed that the average serum 25(OH)D level of 20.4 ng/mL(51 nmol/L) and serum 25(OH)D was below 50 nmol/L in 52.3% [23]. Lu L et al [24] measured plasma 25(OH)D was in a cross-sectional sample of 1,443 men and 1,819 women aged 50-70 years from Beijing (latitude 40° north) and Shanghai (latitude 31° north). The median value of plasma 25(OH)D was 35.6 nmol/l in Beijing and

47.6 nmol/l in Shanghai, and the percentages of vitamin D deficiency, insufficiency, and sufficiency were 69.2, 24.4, and 6.4%, respectively. Indeed, poor vitamin D status in middle and older Chinese individuals was also reported previously in two small bone related studies conducted in Beijing [25] and Shenyang [26]. The above data suggested that vitamin D deficiency was common in middle-aged and elderly Chinese individuals. Another explanation is the exclusion criteria of the intake of the vitamin D supplements in our study. Additionally, unlike in the United States and other western countries, a racial/ethnic difference may be exist in the levels of 25(OH)D concentrations. Although little is known regarding to the high prevalence of vitamin D deficiency in our population, the criteria of vitamin D deficiency in Chinese may differ from that in the western population.

The mechanisms responsible for the independent relationship between 25(OH)D and atherosclerosis have not been well elucidated. In our study, 25(OH)D was negatively associated with BMI, DBP and PPG. These findings were also supported by other studies [27-29]. Therefore, the beneficial effects of 25(OH)D on atherosclerosis might be attributed to its ability to improve the glucose metabolism and blood pressure control. On the other hand, in the present study, we demonstrated an inversely and independent association between 25(OH)D and carotid atherosclerosis after adjustment for established CVD risk factors, PTH, liver and renal function in postmenopausal women with normal blood pressure and normal glucose tolerance. If 25(OH)D and the other risk factors share a common causal pathway, adjusting for these risk factors may attenuate the relationship between 25(OH)D and carotid atherosclerosis. However, 25(OH)D remained a relatively strong predictor after full adjustment in our study, suggesting that there was an independent additive component in the relationship between 25(OH)D and CVD. Thus, other atherogenic mechanisms could conceivably be involved. Because many cell types involved in cardiovascular function like cardiomyocytes, endothelial cells, or vascular smooth muscle cells express vitamin D receptors, a direct influence of vitamin D on the cardiovascular system can be assumed [30]. There are several mechanisms proposed to explain the inverse relationship between vitamin D and CVD. First, activated vitamin D is an inhibitor of the renin-angiotensin system [31]. Vitamin D deficiency predisposes to up-regulation of the renin–angiotensin–aldosterone system and hypertrophy of the vascular smooth muscle cells [20,32]. Second, Vitamin D has effects that may favorably influence cardiovascular system through strengthen in insulin secretion and insulin sensitivity [33], down-regulate coagulation through the up-regulation of thrombomodulin [34], down-regulate vascular calcification [35-37] and modulation of inflammatory processes [38]. Third, long-term vitamin D insufficiency and deficiency cause secondary hyperparathyroidism, which in turn may mediate many of the detrimental CV effects including increasing systemic inflammation, as indicated by increased levels of C-reactive protein, homocysteine, and interleukin-10 [32]. Fourth, vitamin D may play a pivotal role in cardiac function. Cardiac muscle cells possess a vitamin D receptor and a 1,25-dihydroxyvitaminD–dependent calcium-binding protein. Vitamin D has effects on extra- cellular matrix remodeling, myocardial cell hypertrophy, and proliferation [20,39]. Vitamin D deficiency predisposes to lead to hypertrophy of the left ventricle. Fifth, activated vitamin D may also retard atherosclerosis by inhibiting macrophage cholesterol uptake and foam cell formation [40].

Our results suggest that 25(OH)D is a marker or risk factor for atherosclerosis. 25(OH)D could be adopted as an additional marker of the detection of CVD and the implementation of interventions. An early evaluation of the 25(OH)D would be advantageous for the early detection of CVD, and individuals with decreased 25 (OH)D might benefit from more aggressive lifestyle modifications and food-based strategies.

We recognize several limitations of this study: it is cross-sectional, and the 25(OH)D was assessed based on a single morning fasting blood sample. We also acknowledge that in this analysis we do not have data on hours of sunlight per day, albumin and vitamin D binding protein. The cross-sectional nature of this study limits our ability to determine causality. The potential confounding factors remain, particularly in the absence of data for physical activity and socio-economic status. However, the temporal relationship between the 25(OH)D and carotid atherosclerosis has been well established. Our participants were postmenopausal women, and therefore, the results cannot be applied to younger subjects. Hence, the association between 25 (OH)D and carotid atherosclerosis should be confirmed using a larger sample and in prospective studies.

Conclusions

In conclusion, we demonstrated that 25(OH)D has a negatively correlation with carotid atherosclerosis even after adjusting for conventional CVD risk factors, PTH, liver and renal function in postmenopausal women with normal blood glucose levels and normal blood pressure. Our findings suggest that individuals with decreased 25 (OH)D require aggressive management of CVD risk factors. Should causality be affirmed by ongoing and future studies, there are food-based strategies for enhanced vitamin D status in the population which could ultimately lower risk of CVD.

Abbreviations

25(OH)D: 25-hydroxyvitamin D; CIMT: Carotid intima-media thickness; CVD: Cardiovascular disease; BMI: Body mass index; WHR: Waist-hip-ratio; FBG: Fasting blood glucose; PPG: OGTT 2 h blood glucose; PTH: Parathyroid hormone; SBP: Systolic blood pressure; DBP: Diastolic blood pressure; ALT: Alanine transaminase; AST: Aspartate transaminase; TC: Total cholesterol; TG: Triglyceride; HDL-C: High density lipoprotein cholesterol; LDL-C: Low density lipoprotein cholesterol; HOMA-IR: Homeostasis model assessment index for insulin resistance; HOMA-B: Homeostasis model assessment index for beta cell function; GFR: Glomerular filtration rate.

Competing interests
The authors declare that they have no competing interests.

Authors' contributions
Conceived and designed the experiments: HM HDL XML YH XJJ JG NQZ ZQL XG. Performed the experiments: HM HDL XML WYH JG. Analyzed the data: HM NQZ JG. Wrote the paper: HM XG. All authors read and approved the final manuscript.

Acknowledgments
The Shanghai Changfeng Study has also received great support from Changfeng Health Center, the Health Bureau of Putuo District, and the committees of all the sub-communities of Changfeng. The contributions of all the working staffs and inhabitants are greatly acknowledged. This work was supported by grants from the Major State Basic Research Development Program of China (2012CB524906 to X.G.; http://www.973.gov.cn/Default_3.aspx), National Natural Science Foundation of China (81270933 to X.G.), the Major Project of Subject Construction of Shanghai Bureau of Health (Grant No. 2013ZYJB0802 to X. Gao).

Author details
[1]Department of Geriatrics, Zhong Shan Hospital, Fudan University, Shanghai 200032, China. [2]Department of Endocrinology and Metabolism, Zhong Shan Hospital, Fudan University, Shanghai 200032, China. [3]Department of Ultrasonography, Zhongshan Hospital, Fudan University, Shanghai 200032, China. [4]Clinical Epidemiology Center, Zhong Shan Hospital, Fudan University, Shanghai 200032, China. [5]Department of Clinical Nutrition, Zhong Shan Hospital, Fudan University, Shanghai 200032, China. [6]Department of Biostatistics, College of Public Health, Fudan University, Shanghai 200032, China. [7]Division of Endocrinology and Metabolism, Department of Medicine, University of Virginia Health System, Charlottesville, Virginia, USA.

References
1. Zhao G, Ford ES, Li C, Croft JB: **Serum 25-hydroxyvitamin D levels and all-cause and cardiovascular disease mortality among US adults with hypertension: the NHANES linked mortality study.** *J Hypertens* 2012, **30**(2):284–289.
2. Messenger W, Nielson CM, Li H, Beer T, Barrett-Connor E, Stone K, Shannon J: **Serum and dietary vitamin D and cardiovascular disease risk in elderly men: a prospective cohort study.** *Nutr Metab Cardiovasc Dis* 2012, **22**(10):856–863.
3. Holick MF: **Vitamin D deficiency.** *N Engl J Med* 2007, **357**(3):266–281.
4. Wang TJ, Pencina MJ, Booth SL, Jacques PF, Ingelsson E, Lanier K, Benjamin EJ, D'Agostino RB, Wolf M, Vasan RS: **Vitamin D deficiency and risk of cardiovascular disease.** *Circulation* 2008, **117**(4):503–511.
5. Targher G, Bertolini L, Padovani R, Zenari L, Scala L, Cigolini M, Arcaro G: **Serum 25-hydroxyvitamin D3 concentrations and carotid artery intima-media thickness among type 2 diabetic patients.** *Clin Endocrinol (Oxf)* 2006, **65**(5):593–597.
6. Wang L, Song Y, Manson JE, Pilz S, März W, Michaëlsson K, Lundqvist A, Jassal SK, Barrett-Connor E, Zhang C, Eaton CB, May HT, Anderson JL, Sesso HD: **Circulating 25-hydroxy-vitamin D and risk of cardiovascular disease: a meta-analysis of prospective studies.** *Circ Cardiovasc Qual Outcomes* 2012, **5**(6):819–829.
7. Deleskog A, Piksasova O, Silveira A, Gertow K, Baldassarre D, Veglia F, Sennblad B, Strawbridge RJ, Larsson M, Leander K, Gigante B, Kauhanen J, Rauramaa R, Smit AJ, Mannarino E, Giral P, Gustafsson S, Östenson CG, Humphries SE, Tremoli E, de Faire U, Öhrvik J, Hamsten A: **Serum 25-hydroxyvitamin D concentration in subclinical carotid atherosclerosis.** *Arterioscler Thromb Vasc Biol* 2013, **33**(11):2633–2638.

8. Blondon M, Sachs M, Hoofnagle AN, Ix JH, Michos ED, Korcarz C, Gepner AD, Siscovick DS, Kaufman JD, Stein JH, Kestenbaum B, de Boer IH: 25-Hydroxyvitamin D and parathyroid hormone are not associated with carotid intima-media thickness or plaque in the multi-ethnic study of atherosclerosis. *Arterioscler Thromb Vasc Biol* 2013, **33**(11):2639–2645.

9. Park S, Lee BK: Vitamin D deficiency is an independent risk factor for cardiovascular disease in Koreans aged ≥ 50 years: results from the Korean National Health and Nutrition Examination Survey. *Nutr Res Pract* 2012, **6**(2):162–168.

10. Melamed ML, Michos ED, Post W, Astor B: 25-hydroxyvitamin D levels and the risk of mortality in the general population. *Arch Intern Med* 2008, **168**(15):1629–1637.

11. Hypponen E, Berry D, Cortina-Borja M, Power C: 25-Hydroxyvitamin D and pre-clinical alterations in inflammatory and hemostatic markers: a cross sectional analysis in the 1958 British Birth Cohort. *PLoS One* 2010, **5**:e10801.

12. Mosca L, Barrett-Connor E, Wenger NK: Sex/gender differences in cardiovascular disease prevention: what a difference a decade makes. *Circulation* 2011, **124**(19):2145–2154.

13. Ma H, Lin H, Hofman A, Hu Y, Li X, He W, Jeekel J, Jin X, Gao J, Zhao N, Gao X: Low-grade albuminuria is associated with carotid atherosclerosis in normotensive and euglycemic Chinese middle-aged and elderly adults: the Shanghai Changfeng Study. *Atherosclerosis* 2013, **228**(1):237–242.

14. Gao X, Hofman A, Hu Y, Lin H, Zhu C, Jeekel J, Jin X, Wang J, Gao J, Yin Y, Zhao N: The Shanghai Changfeng Study: a communitybased prospective cohort study of chronic diseases among middle-aged and elderly: objectives and design. *Eur J Epidemiol* 2010, **25**(12):885–893.

15. Levey AS, Bosch JP, Lewis JB, Greene T, Rogers N, Roth D: A more accurate method to estimate glomerular filtration rate from serum creatinine: a new prediction equation. Modification of Diet in Renal Disease Study Group. *Ann Intern Med* 1999, **130**(6):461–470.

16. Matthews DR, Hosker JP, Rudenski AS, Naylor BA, Treacher DF, Turner RC: Homeostasis model assessment: insulin resistance and beta-cell function from fasting plasma glucose and insulin concentrations in man. *Diabetologia* 1985, **28**(7):412–419.

17. Stein JH, Korcarz CE, Hurst RT, Lonn E, Kendall CB, Mohler ER, Najjar SS, Rembold CM, Post WS: American Society of Echocardiography Carotid Intima-Media Thickness Task Force: Use of carotid ultrasound to identify subclinical vascular disease and evaluate cardiovascular disease risk: a consensus statement from the American Society of Echocardiography. Carotid intima-media thickness Task Force Endorsed by the Society for vascular Medicine. *J Am Soc Echocardiogr* 2008, **21**(2):93–111.

18. Chobanian AV, Bakris GL, Black HR, Cushman WC, Green LA, Izzo JL Jr, Jones DW, Materson BJ, Oparil S, Wright JT Jr, Roccella EJ; Joint National Committee on Prevention, Detection, Evaluation, and Treatment of High Blood Pressure. National Heart, Lung, and Blood Institute; National High Blood Pressure Education Program Coordinating Committee: Seventh report of the joint national committee on prevention, detection, evaluation, and treatment of high blood pressure. *Hypertension* 2003, **42**(6):1206–1252.

19. American Diabetes Association: Standards of medical care in diabetes—2010. *Diabetes Care* 2010, **33**(suppl 1):S11–S61.

20. Liu L, Chen M, Hankins SR, Nùñez AE, Watson RA, Weinstock PJ, Newschaffer CJ, Eisen HJ: Drexel Cardiovascular Health Collaborative Education, Research, and Evaluation Group: Serum 25-hydroxyvitamin D concentration and mortality from heart failure and cardiovascular disease, and premature mortality from all-cause in United States adults. *Am J Cardiol* 2012, **110**(6):834–839.

21. Simon A, Megnien JL, Chironi G: The value of carotid intima-media thickness for predicting cardiovascular risk. *Arterioscler Thromb Vasc Biol* 2010, **30**(2):182–185.

22. Kim SH, Reaven G: Sex differences in insulin resistance and cardiovascular disease risk. *J Clin Endocrinol Metab* 2013, **98**(11):E1716–E1721.

23. Qiao Z, Li-Xing S, Nian-Chun P, Shu-Jing X, Miao Z, Hong L, Hui-Jun Z, Ming-Xian G, Song Z, Rui W, Ying H, Jing-Lu Z, Shuang C: Serum 25(OH)D Level and Parathyroid Hormone in Chinese Adult Population: A Cross-Sectional Study in Guiyang Urban Community from Southeast of China. *Int J Endocrinol* 2013, **2013**:150461.

24. Lu L, Yu Z, Pan A, Hu FB, Franco OH, Li H, Li X, Yang X, Chen Y, Lin X: Plasma 25-hydroxyvitamin D concentration and metabolic syndrome among middle-aged and elderly Chinese individuals. *Diabetes Care* 2009, **32**(7):1278–1283.

25. Xue Y: Serum levels of 25-hydroxyvitamin D in normal Beijing subjects. *China Prev Med* 1991, **25**(3):177–179.

26. Yan L, Zhou B, Wang X, D'Ath S, Laidlaw A, Laskey MA, Prentice A: Older people in China and the United Kingdom differ in the relationships among parathyroid hormone, vitamin D, and bone mineral status. *Bone* 2003, **33**(4):620–627.

27. Saedisomeolia A, Taheri E, Djalali M, Moghadam AM, Qorbani M: Association between serum level of vitamin D and lipid profiles in type 2 diabetic patients in Iran. *J Diabetes Metab Disord* 2014, **13**(1):7.

28. Mattila C, Knekt P, Männistö S, Rissanen H, Laaksonen MA, Montonen J, Reunanen A: Serum 25-hydroxyvitamin D concentration and subsequent risk of type 2 diabetes. *Diabetes Care* 2007, **30**(10):2569–2570.

29. Grandi NC, Breitling LP, Vossen CY, Hahmann H, Wüsten B, März W, Rothenbacher D, Brenner H: Serum vitamin D and risk of secondary cardiovascular disease events in patients with stable coronary heart disease. *Am Heart J* 2010, **159**(6):1044–1051.

30. Gouni-Berthold I, Krone W, Berthold HK: Vitamin D and cardiovascular disease. *Curr Vasc Pharmacol* 2009, **7**(3):414–422.

31. Li YC, Kong J, Wei M, Chen ZF, Liu SQ, Cao LP: 1,25-Dihydroxyvitamin D(3) is a negative endocrine regulator of the renin-angiotensin system. *J Clin Invest* 2002, **110**(2):229–238.

32. Li YC: Vitamin D regulation of the renin-angiotensin system. *J Cell Biochem* 2003, **88**(2):327–331.

33. Rammos G, Tseke P, Ziakka S: Vitamin D, the renin-angiotensin system, and insulin resistance. *Int Urol Nephrol* 2008, **40**(2):419–426.

34. Ohsawa M, Koyama T, Yamamoto K, Hirosawa S, Kamei S, Kamiyama R: 1alpha,25-dihydroxyvitamin D(3) and its potent synthetic analogs down-regulate tissue factor and up-regulate thrombomodulin expression in monocytic cells, counteracting the effects of tumor necrosis factor and oxidized LDL. *Circulation* 2000, **102**(23):2867–2872.

35. Van der Schueren BJ, Verstuyf A, Mathieu C: Straight from D-Heart: vitamin D status and cardiovascular disease. *Curr Opin Lipidol* 2012, **23**(1):17–23.

36. Schmidt N, Brandsch C, Kühne H, Thiele A, Hirche F, Stangl GI: Vitamin D receptor deficiency and low vitamin D diet stimulate aortic calcification and osteogenic key factor expression in mice. *PLoS One* 2012, **7**(4):e35316.

37. Brandenburg VM, Vervloet MG, Marx N: The role of vitamin D in cardiovascular disease: from present evidence to future perspectives. *Atherosclerosis* 2012, **225**(2):253–263.

38. Deluca HF, Cantorna MT: Vitamin D: Its role and uses in immunology. *Faseb J* 2001, **15**(14):2579–2585.

39. Zittermann A1, Schleithoff SS, Tenderich G, Berthold HK, Körfer R, Stehle P: Low vitamin D status: a contributing factor in the pathogenesis of congestive heart failure? *J Am Coll Cardiol* 2003, **41**(1):105–112.

40. Oh J, Weng S, Felton SK, Bhandare S, Riek A, Butler B, Proctor BM, Petty M, Chen Z, Schechtman KB, Bernal-Mizrachi L, Bernal-Mizrachi C: 1,25(OH)2 vitamin d inhibits foam cell formation and suppresses macrophage cholesterol uptake in patients with type 2 diabetes mellitus. *Circulation* 2009, **120**(8):687–698.

4

Acculturation is associated with left ventricular mass in a multiethnic sample: the Multi-Ethnic Study of Atherosclerosis

Valery S. Effoe[1], Haiying Chen[1], Andrew Moran[2], Alain G. Bertoni[1], David A. Bluemke[3], Teresa Seeman[4], Christine Darwin[5], Karol E. Watson[6] and Carlos J. Rodriguez[1*]

Abstract

Background: Acculturation involves stress-related processes and health behavioral changes, which may have an effect on left ventricular (LV) mass, a risk factor for cardiovascular disease (CVD). We examined the relationship between acculturation and LV mass in a multiethnic cohort of White, African-American, Hispanic and Chinese subjects.

Methods: Cardiac magnetic resonance assessment was available for 5004 men and women, free of clinical CVD at baseline. Left ventricular mass index was evaluated as LV mass indexed by body surface area. Acculturation was characterized based on language spoken at home, place of birth and length of stay in the United States (U.S.), and a summary acculturation score ranging from 0 = least acculturated to 5 = most acculturated. Mean LV mass index adjusted for traditional CVD risk factors was compared across acculturation levels.

Results: Unadjusted mean LV mass index was 78.0 ± 16.3 g/m^2. In adjusted analyses, speaking exclusively English at home compared to non-English language was associated with higher LV mass index (81.3 ± 0.4 g/m^2 vs 79.9 ± 0.5 g/m^2, $p = 0.02$). Among foreign-born participants, having lived in the U.S. for ≥ 20 years compared to < 10 years was associated with greater LV mass index (81.6 ± 0.7 g/m^2 vs 79.5 ± 1.1 g/m^2, $p = 0.02$). Compared to those with the lowest acculturation score, those with the highest score had greater LV mass index (78.9 ± 1.1 g/m^2 vs 81.1 ± 0.4 g/m^2, $p = 0.002$). There was heterogeneity in which measure of acculturation was associated with LV mass index across ethnic groups.

Conclusions: Greater acculturation is associated with increased LV mass index in this multiethnic cohort. Acculturation may involve stress-related processes as well as behavioral changes with a negative effect on cardiovascular health.

Keywords: Acculturation, Left ventricular mass index, Cardiovascular risk, Ethnic disparities

Background

Increased left ventricular (LV) mass, or left ventricular hypertrophy (LVH) is an independent risk factor for cardiovascular disease events, and the prevalence of LVH varies between race/ethnic groups [1]. In a recent analysis of Hispanic, African-American, Chinese, and White participants in the Multi-Ethnic Study of Atherosclerosis (MESA), all Hispanic subgroups had a higher mean LV mass and a higher prevalence of LVH compared with White and Chinese participants at the time of the baseline study examination. Hypertension is strongly associated with the presence of LVH, but the race/ethnic differences in LV mass observed in MESA were not easily explained by a higher prevalence of hypertension among all of the Hispanic subgroups. In fact, Mexican-American participants had a higher mean LV mass and a higher prevalence of LVH compared with White and Chinese participants despite having a similar prevalence of hypertension and similar mean blood pressures [2].

Acculturation is the adoption of the traditions, values, attitudes and cultural practices of another country [3].

* Correspondence: crodrigu@wakehealth.edu
[1]Division of Public Health Sciences, Wake Forest School of Medicine, Medical Center Blvd, Winston Salem, NC 27127, USA
Full list of author information is available at the end of the article

Acculturation may involve stress-related processes as well as behavioral changes. A number of studies have linked higher acculturation to a higher prevalence of hypertension [4–7]. Consistent with most, but not all prior studies, an analysis from MESA found that acculturation was associated with hypertension [5]. However, the association between acculturation parameters and hypertension within race/ethnic groups in this sample was not reported due to lack of statistical power. Given the strong association between hypertension and LVH, a positive association between greater acculturation and LVH would be expected. Acculturation may in part explain the relatively higher LV mass among Hispanic participants, when compared to other race/ethnic groups.

We used data from MESA to examine the associations between acculturation and LV mass. We hypothesized that a higher degree of acculturation, calculated using an acculturation score and acculturation characteristics: i) place of birth in or outside of the U.S.; ii) English vs. non-English language spoken at home; and iii) number of years living in the U.S. (in immigrants), would be associated with a higher mean LV mass, beyond risks accounted for by traditional risk factors for both acculturation and increased LV mass.

Methods
Study participants
Participants were drawn from MESA, a multi-center cohort study of the determinants of subclinical cardiovascular disease in 6814 men and women from four ethnic groups (non-Hispanic whites, Hispanics, African-Americans, and Chinese) aged 45–84 years. MESA cohort participants came from six US communities (Baltimore, MD; Chicago, Il; Forsyth County, NC; Los Angeles County, CA; Northern Manhattan, NY; and St. Paul, MN) and were free of any clinical cardiovascular disease at baseline. Details on the design and objectives of the MESA study have been previously published [8]. This study was approved by the Institutional Review Boards of each study site, and written informed consent was obtained from all participants.

The sample for the present analysis was 5004 men and women with complete baseline data on cardiac MRI assessment.

Data collection and study variables
Measurement of left ventricular mass index
LV mass was measured using cardiac magnetic resonance (CMR) imaging technique. The MESA CMR protocol has been described and published elsewhere [9]. Imaging was performed using 1.5-Tesla MR scanners at each site using a standard protocol and read at a central site (Johns Hopkins University, Baltimore, MD). CMR was performed with a four-element, phased-array surface coil placed anteriorly and posteriorly, electrocardiogram gating, and brachial artery blood pressure monitoring. Cine images of the left ventricle were obtained with a temporal resolution of 50 milliseconds or less. LV mass was determined by the sum of the myocardial area (the difference between endocardial and epicardial contour) times slice thickness plus image gap in the end-diastolic phase multiplied by the specific gravity of myocardium (1.05 g/mL). LV mass was modeled as a continuous measurement, indexed by body surface area and expressed as g/m^2.

Acculturation
Nativity, language spoken at home, and years living in the U.S. were used as proxy measures of acculturation. Nativity was categorized as U.S.-born and foreign-born (including those born in Puerto Rico). Language spoken at home was categorized as English, English and Chinese, English and Spanish, and non-English languages. Among foreign-born participants, number of years lived in the U.S. was categorized as less than 10 years, 10–19 years, and 20 or more years. These proxy measures were chosen for a number of reasons: they show strong correlations with existing acculturation scales, they explain much of the variance of existing scales, [10, 11] and they have also been widely used in other studies examining acculturation [5, 12–17].

For each participant we used the proxy measures of acculturation to compute an acculturation score. A score of 0–2 was assigned to language spoken at home (2 = English only; 1 = English and Chinese or English and Spanish; 0 = non-English languages). A score of 0–3 was assigned for years living in the U.S. combined with nativity (3 = U.S. born; 2 = foreign born and lived in the U.S. for 20 or more years; 1 = foreign born and lived in the U.S. for 10–19 years; 0 = foreign born and lived in the U.S. less than 10 years). For each participant, these individual scores were summed to obtain a summary acculturation score was calculated ranging from 0 (least acculturated) to 5 (most acculturated).

Covariates
Data used in this study were taken from the baseline examination (2000–2002) during which standardized questionnaires (administered in English, Spanish, or Chinese) and calibrated devices were used to obtain demographic data, smoking history, alcohol consumption, medical conditions, current prescription medication use, weight, and height. Three blood pressure readings were obtained with an appropriate-sized cuff at 1-min intervals with subjects seated after 5 min of rest using a Dinamap automated oscillometric sphygmomanometer (model Pro 100; Critikon, Tampa, FL). The average of the last two measurements was used

for analysis. Hypertension was defined as a systolic blood pressure ≥140 mmHg or diastolic blood pressure ≥90 mmHg, use of blood pressure medicine or a self-report of hypertension. Fasting blood glucose was analyzed at a central laboratory. Diabetes was defined as a fasting blood glucose level of ≥126 mg/dl, use of hypoglycemic medications or insulin. Smoking use was defined as never, former, and current smokers. Alcohol consumption was defined as current drinkers or not. Annual income was categorized in 3 levels: participants earning < $20,000, $20,000 - $49,000, and > $49,000. Body mass index was calculated as weight (in kilograms) divided by the square of the height (in meters). Serum creatinine was measured on frozen serum specimens that were stored at −70 °C by rate reflectance spectrophotometry using thin film adaptation of the creatine amidinohydrolase method on the Vitros analyzer (Johnson & Johnson Clinical Diagnostics, Inc.). Physical activity was measured as the number of hours of exercise per week.

Statistical analysis

Sample characteristics by acculturation score or race/ethnicity were summarized using counts and percentages for categorical variables and mean with standard deviation for continuous variables. Linear regression models were used to examine the association between various acculturation factors and LVMI. We started with unadjusted models, and then proceeded to fit models adjusted for age, sex, serum creatinine, smoking status, income level, physical activity, diabetes status, and systolic blood pressure. Least square means (for categorical predictors) and beta coefficients (for continuous predictors) and associated standard errors are reported. A p-value of less than 0.05 was considered statistically significant. All analyses were performed using SAS 9.3 software (SAS Institute; Cary, NC).

Results

Cohort characteristics

The mean age of the sample was 62.1 ± 10.1 years, 39.1 % were white, 25.7 % African-American, 22.1 % were Hispanic, and 13.0 % Chinese. The mean LVMI of the entire cohort was 78.0 ± 16.3 g/m^2. Compared to participants with lower acculturation scores, those with higher scores had higher mean systolic blood pressure and prevalence of hypertension, higher body mass index, tended to be current smokers and drinkers, and were more educated (Table 1). In contrast, a higher acculturation score was associated with a lower prevalence of diabetes. The annual income was $20,000 or less for half of participants who were least acculturated compared to $50,000 or more for half of those who were most acculturated.

LVMI and acculturation factors

In unadjusted analysis, among participants born out of the US, LVMI increased with increasing number of years lived in the US; those who had lived 20 years or more had a higher mean LVMI (78.3 ± 0.5 g/m^2) compared to those who had lived for less than 10 years (LVMI 75.5 ± 1.1 g/m^2, $p = 0.01$) (Table 2). LVMI in participants born in the U.S. and outside the U.S. was not different ($p = 0.2$).

In multivariable analysis, after adjustment for age, sex, serum creatinine, smoking status, income level, physical activity, diabetes status, and systolic blood pressure, exclusively speaking English at home compared to non-English language was associated with higher LVMI (81.3 ± 0.4 g/m^2 versus 79.9 ± 0.5 g/m^2, $p = 0.02$) (Table 2). Among foreign-born participants, after adjustment, having lived in the U.S. for 20 years or more compared to having lived for less than 10 years was associated with greater LVMI (81.6 ± 0.7 g/m^2 versus 79.5 ± 1.1 g/m^2, $p = 0.02$).

LVMI and acculturation score

In unadjusted analysis, increasing acculturation score was associated with greater mean LVMI (75.2 ± 1.2 g/m^2 versus 78.2 ± 0.3 g/m^2 for a score of 0 and 5, respectively, $p < 0.01$). This association persisted after adjustment (78.9 ± 1.1 g/m^2 versus 81.1 ± 0.4 g/m^2 for a score 0 and 5, respectively, $p = 0.002$) (Table 3).

LVMI and acculturation by ethnicity

Blacks had the highest prevalence of hypertension (56.9 %), followed by Hispanics (39.6 %), Chinese (36.6 %), and Whites (36.3 %) (Table 4). Similarly, mean LVMI was highest for Blacks (81.3 ± 18.0 g/m^2), followed by Hispanics (80.4 ± 16.6 g/m^2), Whites (75.8 ± 15.2 g/m^2), and Chinese (73.9 ± 13.6 g/m^2). The majority of Chinese (87.2 %) and about half of Hispanics (51.2 %) had an acculturation score of 2 or less. Among Chinese (96.2 %) and Hispanics (66.4 %) born outside the U.S., a great majority had lived in the U.S. for 10 years or more (79.5 and 88.3 % respectively). Whites and Blacks had higher acculturation scores of 3 or more (99.9 and 99.7 %, respectively).

Associations of acculturation with LVMI varied across ethnic groups. In Table 5, for Blacks, being born outside the U.S. compared to being born in the U.S. (85.8 ± 1.4 g/m^2 versus 82.6 ± 0.7 g/m^2, $p = 0.03$) was associated with higher mean LVMI after adjustment for age, sex, income level, serum creatinine, smoking, physical activity, diabetes, and systolic blood pressure. The association between acculturation score and LVMI also varied across ethnic groups. In Blacks, there appeared to be a significant non-linear association between acculturation score and LVMI. In Chinese participants, however, the results show a graded increase in LVMI across acculturation scores, though not significant.

Table 1 Baseline characteristics of study participants by acculturation score

Characteristic	Acculturation score = 0 N = 188	Acculturation score = 1 N = 260	Acculturation score = 2 N = 547	Acculturation score = 3 N = 169	Acculturation score = 4 N = 311	Acculturation score = 5 N = 3192
Age, years	60.7 ± 10.3	61.5 ± 10.9	62.1 ± 9.7	61.0 ± 10.4	62.2 ± 10.6	62.4 ± 10.0
Females, %	54.3	50.4	51.9	50.9	53.1	52.7
Educational level, %						
< High school	37.8	35.0	48.3	27.8	16.1	6.7
High school or college	55.9	55.0	44.4	55.0	64.6	69.9
> College	6.4	10.0	7.3	17.2	19.3	23.4
Annual income, %						
< $20,000	55.3	47.3	41.9	22.8	22.7	14.3
$20,000–$49,000	32.4	36.3	39.1	41.9	34.1	36.3
> $49,000	12.3	16.4	19.0	35.3	43.2	49.4
Diabetes, %	12.8	12.3	16.5	11.8	10.6	10.8
Hypertension, %	28.7	37.3	42.8	34.9	40.8	44.5
Smoker, %						
Never	68.6	70.4	66.9	58.6	48.2	44.8
Former	22.3	20.4	24.5	26.6	39.6	41.1
Current	9.0	9.2	8.6	14.8	12.2	14.1
Exercise, hrs/week	16.3 ± 26.1	18.3 ± 24.2	15.8 ± 21.9	26.2 ± 32.6	28.1 ± 37.9	30.2 ± 44.1
Current alcohol use, %	58.6	64.0	61.5	67.2	75.8	70.6
Systolic BP, mm Hg	124 ± 22	124 ± 22	127 ± 21	124 ± 21	125 ± 20	126 ± 21
Diastolic BP, mm Hg	71 ± 10	72 ± 10	72 ± 10	71 ± 11	71 ± 11	72 ± 10
Body mass index, kg/m^2	25.3 ± 4.2	25.3 ± 4.3	27.1 ± 4.5	27.9 ± 5.0	28.4 ± 4.9	28.3 ± 5.0
Mean LVMI, g/m^2	75.2 ± 14.3	75.8 ± 13.9	77.4 ± 15.5	78.5 ± 21.3	80.1 ± 16.7	78.2 ± 16.5

Data are mean ± SD for continuous variables or percentages for categorical variables
BP indicates blood pressure, *LVMI* left ventricular mass index

To assess if indexing LV mass to body surface area accounted for the effects of obesity on the association between LV mass and measures of acculturation, we performed sensitivity analyses using LV mass as the outcome variable. The multivariable models were adjusted for the same covariates described above and body mass index. The association between LV mass and the different measures of acculturation (language, nativity, and number of years in the U.S.) were significant and similar to those described above.

Discussion

This study examined the association between acculturation and LVMI in a multi-ethnic cohort of individuals

Table 2 Unadjusted and adjusted mean left ventricular mass index by acculturation characteristic

Acculturation characteristic	Unadjusted analysis			Adjusted analysis[a]		
	Mean LVMI (g/m^2)	SE	p-value	Mean LVMI (g/m^2)	SE	p-value
Language						
Non-English spoken at home	76.8	0.5	0.01	79.9	0.5	0.02
Mixed languages at home	78.6	1.1		81.0	0.9	
English spoken at home	78.4	0.3		81.3	0.4	
Nativity + Years in the US						
Foreign born and in US for < 10 years	75.5	1.1	0.01	79.5	1.1	0.02
Foreign born and in US for 10–19 years	75.9	0.9		79.5	0.9	
Foreign born and in US for ≥ 20 years	78.3	0.5		81.6	0.7	

LVMI indicates left ventricular mass index, *SE* standard error
[a]Models adjusted for age, sex, income, serum creatinine, smoking status, physical activity, diabetes status, and systolic blood pressure

Table 3 Adjusted mean left ventricular mass index by acculturation score

Acculturation score	Adjusted analysis		
	Mean LVMI (g/m^2)	SE	p-value
Least acculturated (score = 0)	78.9	1.1	0.002
Acculturated (score = 1)	78.9	0.9	
Acculturated (score = 2)	80.5	0.7	
Acculturated (score = 3)	81.6	1.1	
Acculturated (score = 4)	83.4	0.8	
Most acculturated (score = 5)	81.1	0.4	

Models adjusted for age, sex, income, serum creatinine, smoking status, physical activity, diabetes status, and systolic blood pressure
LVMI indicates left ventricular mass index, SE standard error

aged 45–84 years at baseline and who had no discernable clinical cardiovascular disease. From the findings, higher levels of acculturation are associated with increased LVMI. Also, LVMI varied by language spoken at home and time spent in the U.S. but not by nativity; different measures of acculturation appeared to have varying effects in differences race/ethnic groups, highlighting the complexity of the acculturation concept.

Among foreign-born participants, having lived in the U.S. for longer periods of time was associated with a higher mean LVMI, even after adjusting for traditional CVD risk factors. In fact mean LVMI increased after 20 or more years of residence in the U.S., compared to those who had lived in the U.S. for less than 20 years. Evidence suggests that the health advantage exhibited by foreign-born individuals over U.S.-born individuals tends to decrease with duration of stay in the U.S. [18, 19]. This decline in the health with increased duration of stay in the U.S. has also been reported for other health measures like obesity [16, 19–21] and heart disease [22]. One explanation could be that some immigrant groups (non-U.S. Whites, Hispanics, and Asians) may be less likely, than U.S.-born individuals, to discuss dietary or physical activity measures with their clinicians, [19] probably in part due to patient-provider characteristics which affect care such as language barriers and cultural sensitivity.

Table 4 Clinical and acculturation characteristics by ethnicity

Characteristic	Non-Hispanic White	Chinese	Black	Hispanic
N	1957	653	1288	1106
Diabetes, n (%)	113 (5.8)	81 (12.4)	215 (16.7)	172 (15.6)
Hypertension, n (%)	710 (36.3)	239 (36.6)	733 (56.9)	438 (39.6)
Systolic BP, mmHg	122 ± 20	123 ± 21	131 ± 21	126 ± 22
Diastolic BP, mmHg	70 ± 10	72 ± 10	75 ± 10	72 ± 10
Current smoker, n (%)	216 (11.1)	35 (5.4)	229 (17.9)	155 (14.0)
Exercise, hrs/week	1707 ± 2248	1145 ± 1472	1879 ± 3049	1361 ± 2009
Body mass index, kg/m^2	27.3 ± 4.7	23.9 ± 3.3	29.4 ± 5.2	28.9 ± 4.5
Mean LVMI, g/m^2	75.8 ± 15.2	73.9 ± 13.6	81.3 ± 18.0	80.4 ± 16.6
Percent life in the US	0.7 ± 0.3	0.3 ± 0.2	0.6 ± 0.3	0.5 ± 0.2
Non-English spoken at Home, n (%)	52 (2.7)	573 (87.8)	34 (2.6)	604 (54.6)
Born out of US, n (%)	136 (7.0)	630 (96.5)	143 (11.2)	764 (69.1)
Nativity + Years in the US, n (%)				
Foreign-born & in US for <10 years	5 (0.3)	120 (19.7)	5 (0.4)	79 (7.8)
Foreign-born & in US for 10–19 years	11 (0.6)	196 (32.2)	21 (1.7)	95 (9.3)
Foreign-born & in US for ≥ 20 years	90 (4.7)	269 (44.2)	84 (6.8)	501 (49.3)
US-born	1817 (94.5)	23 (3.8)	1135 (91.2)	342 (33.6)
Acculturation Score, n (%)				
Least acculturated (0)	0 (0)	115 (21.1)	0 (0)	73 (7.3)
Acculturated (1)	0 (0)	168 (30.8)	1 (0.1)	91 (9.1)
Acculturated (2)	1 (0.1)	192 (35.2)	3 (0.2)	351 (34.9)
Acculturated (3)	12 (0.6)	33 (6.1)	18 (1.5)	106 (10.5)
Acculturated (4)	71 (3.8)	21 (3.9)	77 (6.3)	142 (14.1)
Most Acculturated (5)	1803 (95.6)	16 (2.9)	1130 (91.9)	243 (24.2)

Data are mean ± SD for continuous variables or number (percentages) for categorical variables
BP indicates blood pressure, LVMI left ventricular mass index

Table 5 Adjusted mean left ventricular mass index by acculturation characteristic and by ethnicity

Acculturation characteristic	Race/Ethnicity							
	Non-Hispanic White		Chinese		African-American		Hispanic	
	LVMI, g/m², mean ± SE	p-value	LVMI, g/m², mean ± SE	p-value	LVMI, g/m², mean ± SE	p-value	LVMI, g/m², mean ± SE, p	p-value
Language								
Non-English spoken at home	80.2 ± 1.9	0.56	76.5 ± 0.9	0.24	83.4 ± 3.4	0.69	82.8 ± 0.8	0.075
Mixed languages at home	78.3 ± 4.9		78.2 ± 1.9		78.9 ± 4.7		82.3 ± 1.2	
English spoken at home	78.2 ± 0.7		79.6 ± 2.1		82.9 ± 0.7		84.9 ± 0.9	
Nativity								
US-born	78.2 ± 0.7	0.19	76.0 ± 2.6	0.74	82.6 ± 0.7	0.027*	84.2 ± 0.9	0.24
Foreign-born	79.7 ± 1.3		76.9 ± 0.9		85.8 ± 1.4		83.0 ± 0.8	
Nativity + Years in US								
Foreign born - in US for < 10 years	90.2 ± 6.2	0.92	75.9 ± 1.4	0.37	80.5 ± 10.7	0.73	84.3 ± 1.9	0.61
Foreign born - in US for 10–19 years	87.8 ± 4.7		76.7 ± 1.2		86.7 ± 5.9		82.4 ± 1.7	
Foreign born - in US for ≥ 20 years	87.6 ± 2.7		77.7 ± 1.1		88.5 ± 3.9		82.6 ± 0.9	
Acculturation score								
Least acculturated (0)	-	0.72	75.1 ± 1.5	0.32	-	0.024*	84.3 ± 1.9	0.25
Acculturated (1)	-		76.2 ± 1.2		-		83.1 ± 1.7	
Acculturated (2)	84.5 ± 12.8		76.8 ± 1.2		80.15 ± 8.9		82.9 ± 0.9	
Acculturated (3)	78.9 ± 3.7		77.3 ± 2.3		88.7 ± 3.7		82.7 ± 1.5	
Acculturated (4)	79.4 ± 1.7		81.9 ± 2.8		87.8 ± 1.9		82.5 ± 1.3	
Most Acculturated (5)	77.8 ± 0.7		76.2 ± 3.2		82.8 ± 0.7		85.5 ± 1.0	

Adjusted for age, sex, income, serum creatinine, smoking status, physical activity, diabetes status, and systolic blood pressure

LVMI indicates left ventricular mass index, SE standard error

*$p < 0.05$

Participants who spoke exclusively English at home had higher LVMI compared to those who spoke a language other than English. This finding may be explained by the fact that those who spoke exclusively English may have been either those born in the U.S. or those who had lived in the U.S. for longer periods of time. Ninety-seven percent of Blacks (91 % born in the U.S.) and 97 % of non-Hispanic Whites (94 % born in the U.S.) spoke exclusively English at home. These may have been participants with higher acculturation levels (96 % of non-Hispanic whites and 92 % of Blacks had an acculturation score of 5). This finding corroborates with an analysis using the same cohort which showed a higher prevalence of hypertension, a strong predictor of LVMI, among those who spoke English at home [5]. Other studies have described different associations between language spoken and hypertension. In one study, those who spoke Russian at home reported a higher prevalence of hypertension than those who spoke English [23]. This was attributed to a higher baseline prevalence of self-reported hypertension among those born in Eastern/Central Europe, than US-born whites.

In our study, the association between acculturation and LVMI did not differ when birthplace alone was considered (U.S.-born vs. foreign-born). This finding may be attributed to the fact that among participants born out of the U.S. (33 % of sample), the majority (76 %) had lived in the U.S. for at least 10 years and thus may have had acculturation levels comparable to those born in the U.S.

The race/ethnic stratified analysis demonstrates the complexity and heterogeneity of the associations of acculturation measures and LVMI among the different immigrant groups. Overall, blacks had higher mean LVMI than other race/ethnic groups. This risk was even higher among foreign-born than U.S.-born blacks. The increased risk in blacks may be due to a number of factors including psychosocial stress, chronic adrenergic stimulation [24, 25] and increased sodium retention, [26] both of which are disproportionately increased in blacks. An association between these factors and increased LVMI has been described in other studies [27, 28]. Place of birth, and not language spoken at home, may have been an important dimension of acculturation among blacks in the US (who may be from Haiti, the Caribbean, or Africa) since many countries in the Caribbean and in Africa already have English as the national language. Among Hispanics, preferential English speaking at home (greater acculturation) was associated with increased LVMI. There is strong evidence that points towards a negative effect of greater acculturation and health behaviors, including diet, illicit drug, alcohol and tobacco use, [29] all of which are associated with increased LVMI [30–32].

Despite having higher levels of physical activity, the most acculturated participants had higher mean LVMI. Similarly, blacks with the highest total number of hours of exercise per week had the highest mean LVMI of all ethnicities; Chinese with the least total number of hours of exercise had the least mean LVMI. The fact that the more acculturated participants were more physically active despite having higher LVMI may be explained by a number of factors. First, physical activity may not be an important factor contributing to decreased LVMI in our sample. This is consistent with results from one study which showed that fat mass, rather than inactivity, is an important contributor to disease risk in young Mexican and Mexican–American women [33]. Second, our measure of physical activity (hours of exercise per week) may not be a good correlate of the effects of exercise on LVMI.

To the best of our knowledge, this is the first study investigating the association between acculturation and LVMI. The multiethnic nature of our sample makes it possible to compare the independent associations of measures of acculturation among the different race/ ethnic groups. However, the cross-sectional nature of our analysis makes it impossible to draw any inferences on a causal link between acculturation and LVMI. Another limitation of our study is the scope of our measure of acculturation which may have influenced some of our non-significant findings. Several studies have used different surrogates for acculturation, and our measure may not fully cover the spectrum of acculturation and its related cardiovascular health effects. It is therefore important to consider the measures of acculturation used and outcomes under study when comparing our findings with that of other studies. Also, due to sample size limitations of our race/ethnic stratified analyses, we may have had insufficient power to detect the presence of other associations between measures of acculturation and LVMI among race/ethnic groups. Finally, residual confounding via measurement error may possibly explain some of the associations found, although we would expect significant associations given the results of other studies examining acculturation and other health effects. Our study nevertheless found significant associations between acculturation measures and increased LVMI.

Regardless of the process of acculturation, lifestyle modification (via physical activity, diet, and smoking cessation) provides cardiovascular health benefits. The present study, however, identifies a group a group of individuals (more acculturated) which is at risk of developing increased LVM, and consequently CVD. This reinforces the notion that the immigrant process and making decisions on retaining one's native culture while adapting to a new culture may exert a remarkable stress on cardiovascular health behaviors and subsequent health risks in certain individuals due to factors such as lack of healthcare access and social marginalization which will impede healthy lifestyle modifications.

Conclusion

Given the growing size of the immigrant population in the U.S., it is important to study disease prevalence and associated risks in the different race/ethnic groups, in order to better tailor preventive strategies. Our study showed that different acculturation measures (language spoken at home, nativity, and length of stay in the U.S.) are important determinants of subclinical cardiovascular disease, and the study also highlights the heterogeneity and complexity of studying the acculturation process among different race/ ethnic groups.

Competing interests
The authors have no competing interests.

Authors' contributions
VSE contributed to the study methodology, literature review, interpretation and discussion of findings, and manuscript write-up; HC contributed to study conception, data analysis and interpretation of findings; AM, AGB, and DAB contributed to study conception, study design, and performed a critical review; TS contributed to data interpretation and performed a critical review of manuscript; CD and KEW contributed to data interpretation and performed a critical review of manuscript; CJR contributed to study conception and design, data acquisition, interpretation of findings, and manuscript write-up. All authors read and approved the final manuscript for publication.

Acknowledgements
The authors thank the other investigators, the staff, and the participants of the MESA study for their valuable contributions. A full list of participating MESA investigators and institutions can be found at http://www.mesa-nhlbi.org. This research was supported by contracts N01-HC-95159, N01-HC-95160, N01-HC-95161, N01-HC-95162, N01-HC-95163, N01-HC-95164, N01-HC-95165, N01-HC-95166, N01-HC-95167, N01-HC-95168 and N01-HC-95169 from the National Heart, Lung, and Blood Institute and by grants UL1-TR-000040 and UL1-TR-001079 from NCRR. The research was also partially supported by NHLBI grant R01 HL104199 (Epidemiologic Determinants of Cardiac Structure and Function among Hispanics).

Author details
[1]Division of Public Health Sciences, Wake Forest School of Medicine, Medical Center Blvd, Winston Salem, NC 27127, USA. [2]Department of Medicine, Columbia University College of Physicians & Surgeons, New York, NY, USA. [3]National Institutes of Health/Clinical Center, Bethesda, MD, USA. [4]Division of Geriatrics, University of California at Los Angeles, Los Angeles, CA, USA. [5]University of California at Los Angeles Research Center, Los Angeles, CA, USA. [6]Division of Cardiology, University of California at Los Angeles School of Medicine, Los Angeles, CA, USA.

References

1. Rodriguez CJ, Lin F, Sacco RL, Jin Z, Boden-Albala B, Homma S, et al. Prognostic implications of left ventricular mass among Hispanics: the Northern Manhattan Study. Hypertension. 2006;48(1):87–92.

2. Rodriguez CJ, Diez-Roux AV, Moran A, Jin Z, Kronmal RA, Lima J, et al. Left ventricular mass and ventricular remodeling among Hispanic subgroups compared with non-Hispanic blacks and whites: MESA (Multi-ethnic Study of Atherosclerosis). J Am Coll Cardiol. 2010;55(3):234–42.

3. Marmot MG, Syme SL. Acculturation and coronary heart disease in Japanese-Americans. Am J Epidemiol. 1976;104(3):225–47.

4. Espino DV, Maldonado D. Hypertension and acculturation in elderly Mexican Americans: results from 1982–84 Hispanic HANES. J Gerontol. 1990;45(6):M209–13.

5. Moran A, Diez Roux AV, Jackson SA, Kramer H, Manolio TA, Shrager S, et al. Acculturation is associated with hypertension in a multiethnic sample. Am J Hypertens. 2007;20(4):354–63.

6. Sundquist J, Winkleby MA. Cardiovascular risk factors in Mexican American adults: a transcultural analysis of NHANES III, 1988–1994. Am J Public Health. 1999;89(5):723–30.

7. Vaeth PA, Willett DL. Level of acculturation and hypertension among Dallas County Hispanics: findings from the Dallas Heart Study. Ann Epidemiol. 2005;15(5):373–80.

8. Bild DE, Bluemke DA, Burke GL, Detrano R, Diez Roux AV, Folsom AR, et al. Multi-ethnic study of atherosclerosis: objectives and design. Am J Epidemiol. 2002;156(9):871–81.

9. Natori S, Lai S, Finn JP, Gomes AS, Hundley WG, Jerosch-Herold M, et al. Cardiovascular function in multi-ethnic study of atherosclerosis: normal values by age, sex, and ethnicity. AJR Am J Roentgenol. 2006;186(6 Suppl 2):S357–65.

10. Coronado GD, Thompson B, McLerran D, Schwartz SM, Koepsell TD. A short acculturation scale for Mexican-American populations. Ethn Dis. 2005;15(1):53–62.

11. Deyo RA, Diehl AK, Hazuda H, Stern MP. A simple language-based acculturation scale for Mexican Americans: validation and application to health care research. Am J Public Health. 1985;75(1):51–5.

12. Choi S, Rankin S, Stewart A, Oka R. Effects of acculturation on smoking behavior in Asian Americans: a meta-analysis. J Cardiovasc Nurs. 2008;23(1):67–73.

13. Diez Roux AV, Detrano R, Jackson S, Jacobs Jr DR, Schreiner PJ, Shea S, et al. Acculturation and socioeconomic position as predictors of coronary calcification in a multiethnic sample. Circulation. 2005;112(11):1557–65.

14. Gomez SL, Kelsey JL, Glaser SL, Lee MM, Sidney S. Immigration and acculturation in relation to health and health-related risk factors among specific Asian subgroups in a health maintenance organization. Am J Public Health. 2004;94(11):1977–84.

15. Kandula NR, Diez-Roux AV, Chan C, Daviglus ML, Jackson SA, Ni H, et al. Association of acculturation levels and prevalence of diabetes in the multi-ethnic study of atherosclerosis (MESA). Diabetes Care. 2008;31(8):1621–8.

16. Lauderdale DS, Rathouz PJ. Body mass index in a US national sample of Asian Americans: effects of nativity, years since immigration and socioeconomic status. Int J Obes Relat Metab Disord. 2000;24(9):1188–94.

17. Salant T, Lauderdale DS. Measuring culture: a critical review of acculturation and health in Asian immigrant populations. Soc Sci Med. 2003;57(1):71–90.

18. Frisbie WP, Cho Y, Hummer RA. Immigration and the health of Asian and Pacific Islander adults in the United States. Am J Epidemiol. 2001;153(4):372–80.

19. Goel MS, McCarthy EP, Phillips RS, Wee CC. Obesity among US immigrant subgroups by duration of residence. JAMA. 2004;292(23):2860–7.

20. Gordon-Larsen P, Harris KM, Ward DS, Popkin BM. Acculturation and overweight-related behaviors among Hispanic immigrants to the US: the National Longitudinal Study of Adolescent Health. Soc Sci Med. 2003;57(11):2023–34.

21. Kaplan MS, Huguet N, Newsom JT, McFarland BH. The association between length of residence and obesity among Hispanic immigrants. Am J Prev Med. 2004;27(4):323–6.

22. Mooteri SN, Petersen F, Dagubati R, Pai RG. Duration of residence in the United States as a new risk factor for coronary artery disease (The Konkani Heart Study). Am J Cardiol. 2004;93(3):359–61.

23. Yi S, Elfassy T, Gupta L, Myers C, Kerker B. Nativity, Language Spoken at Home, Length of Time in the United States, and Race/Ethnicity: Associations with Self-Reported Hypertension. Am J Hypertens. 2014;27(2):237–44.

24. Rapaport E. Pathophysiological basis of ventricular hypertrophy. Eur Heart J. 1982;3 Suppl A:29–33.

25. Post WS, Larson MG, Levy D. Impact of left ventricular structure on the incidence of hypertension. The Framingham Heart Study Circulation. 1994;90(1):179–85.

26. Pratt JH, Rebhun JF, Zhou L, Ambrosius WT, Newman SA, Gomez-Sanchez CE, et al. Levels of mineralocorticoids in whites and blacks. Hypertension. 1999;34(2):315–9.

27. de Simone G, Devereux RB, Roman MJ, Schlussel Y, Alderman MH, Laragh JH. Echocardiographic left ventricular mass and electrolyte intake predict arterial hypertension. Ann Intern Med. 1991;114(3):202–9.

28. Rodriguez CJ, Sciacca RR, Diez-Roux AV, Boden-Albala B, Sacco RL, Homma S, et al. Relation between socioeconomic status, race-ethnicity, and left ventricular mass: the Northern Manhattan study. Hypertension. 2004;43(4):775–9.

29. Lara M, Gamboa C, Kahramanian MI, Morales LS, Bautista DE. Acculturation and Latino health in the United States: a review of the literature and its sociopolitical context. Annu Rev Public Health. 2005;26:367–97.

30. Brickner ME, Willard JE, Eichhorn EJ, Black J, Grayburn PA. Left ventricular hypertrophy associated with chronic cocaine abuse. Circulation. 1991;84(3):1130–5.

31. Manolio TA, Levy D, Garrison RJ, Castelli WP, Kannel WB. Relation of alcohol intake to left ventricular mass: the Framingham Study. J Am Coll Cardiol. 1991;17(3):717–21.

32. Markus MR, Stritzke J, Baumeister SE, Siewert U, Baulmann J, Hannemann A, et al. Effects of smoking on arterial distensibility, central aortic pressures and left ventricular mass. Int J Cardiol. 2013;168(3):2593–601.

33. Vella CA, Ontiveros D, Zubia RY, Bader JO. Acculturation and metabolic syndrome risk factors in young Mexican and Mexican-American women. J Immigr Minor Health. 2011;13(1):119–26.

5

Adipo/cytokines in atherosclerotic secretomes: increased visfatin levels in unstable carotid plaque

Teresa Auguet[1,2], Gemma Aragonès[1], Esther Guiu-Jurado[1], Alba Berlanga[1], Marta Curriu[1], Salomé Martinez[3], Ajla Alibalic[2], Carmen Aguilar[1], María-Luisa Camara[5], Esteban Hernández[4], Xavier Ruyra[5], Vicente Martín-Paredero[4] and Cristóbal Richart[1,2]*

Abstract

Background: Novel pro-inflammatory and anti-inflammatory derivatives from adipose tissue, known as adipokines, act as metabolic factors. The aim of this study was to analyse the secreted expression of different adipo/cytokines in secretomes of unstable carotid atherosclerotic plaque versus non-atherosclerotic mammary artery.

Methods: We evaluated the secretion levels of adiponectin, visfatin, lipocalin-2, resistin, IL-6 and TNFR2 by ELISA in human secretomes from cultured unstable carotid atherosclerotic plaque ($n = 18$) and non-atherosclerotic mammary artery ($n = 13$). We also measured visfatin serum levels in patients suffering from atherosclerosis and in a serum cohort of healthy subjects ($n = 16$).

Results: We found that visfatin levels were significantly increased in unstable carotid atherosclerotic plaque secretome than in non-atherosclerotic mammary artery secretome. No differences were found with regard the other adipo/cytokines studied. Regarding visfatin circulating levels, there were no differences between unstable carotid atherosclerotic plaque and non-atherosclerotic mammary artery group. However, these visfatin levels were increased in comparison to serum cohort of healthy subjects.

Conclusions: Of all the adipo/cytokines analysed, only visfatin showed increased levels in secretomes of unstable carotid atherosclerotic plaque. Additional human studies are needed to clarify the possible role of visfatin as prognostic factor of unstable carotid atherosclerotic plaque.

Keywords: Atheroma plaque, Secretome, Visfatin, Atherosclerosis, Adipo/cytokines

Background

Carotid artery stenosis as a causative factor of ischemic strokes or transient ischemic attacks constitutes a major therapeutic target. Since obesity is considered a risk factor associated to atherosclerosis, a lot of research over recent years has tried to gain greater insights into the link between atherosclerosis and adipose tissue that has been described as an endocrine organ that secretes a wide variety of proteins called adipokines [1–3]. Currently, it is well known that adipokines play a relevant role in the pathophysiology of cardiovascular diseases (CVDs) [4–6]. These molecules can act as enzymes, hormones or growth factors in the modulation of insulin resistance and the metabolism of fats and glucose, and, therefore, have an indirect effect on atherosclerosis [7]. To note, visceral fat accumulation associated with adipokine dysregulation affects on both atherosclerotic plaque development and plaque disruption. When the advanced plaque becomes unstable, rupture can occur and may be provided by the adipokine-induced prothrombotic and inflammatory state [8, 9]. During the last century, the epidemic of obesity and CVDs has lead to intense research into the role of adipokines in obesity and atherosclerosis [6]. However, further research is necessary to elucidate more thoroughly the

---

* Correspondence: crichart.hj23.ics@gencat.cat
[1]Grup de Recerca GEMMAIR - Medicina Aplicada. Departament de Medicina i Cirurgia, Universitat Rovira i Virgili (URV), Institut Investigació Sanitària Pere Virgili (IISPV), 43007 Tarragona, Spain
[2]Servei Medicina Interna, Hospital Universitari Joan XXIII, 43007 Tarragona, Spain
Full list of author information is available at the end of the article

pathophysiological pathways that underlie the association between adipokines and atherosclerosis, and their potential role as new therapeutic approaches and biomarkers.

Recently, the study of the secretome has emerged as a new strategy for analysing the formation of atherosclerotic plaques in humans [10]. The secretome is the sub-set of proteins released by a cell or tissue under certain conditions and shows a narrower dynamic range of proteins than serum or plasma, which means less complexity. Furthermore, studies on tissue secretome more closely resemble the in vivo situation than cell culture workflows.

The aim of this study was to analyse the presence of several adipo/cytokines with different profiles, pro- and anti-inflammatory: adiponectin, visfatin, lipocalin-2, resistin, IL-6 and TNFR2, and compare their differential expression in the secretome of an unstable carotid atherosclerotic plaque with the secretome in a non-atherosclerotic mammary artery. Moreover, in order to study whether the differences observed in adipo/cytokine levels were only a local effect or if they were also reflected in serum, we measured circulating levels in the group of patients suffering from atherosclerosis and in a serum group of healthy subjects.

Methods
Subjects/Samples
The study was approved by the institutional review board "Comitè d'Ètica d'Investigació Clínica, Hospital Universitari de Sant Joan de Reus" (10-04-29/4proj3). All participants gave written informed consent for participation in medical research.

Human unstable carotid atherosclerotic plaques were obtained from patients (men, $n = 18$) who underwent carotid endarterectomy at the Angiology and Vascular Surgery Unit of the Hospital Universitari Joan XXIII (Tarragona, Spain). Patients with cerebrovascular ischemia and internal carotid artery stenosis >75 % were included, diagnosed by colour Doppler assisted duplex investigation and arteriography. The diagnosis of unstable carotid atherosclerotic plaques was made by an experienced pathologist following the American Heart Association (AHA) guidelines [11].

Mammary arteries were used as non-atherosclerotic control arteries. Segments of mammary arteries (men, $n = 13$) were obtained during coronary revascularisation surgery at the Cardiovascular Surgery Department of the Hospital Germans Trias i Pujol (Badalona, Spain). Patients who had an acute illness, acute or chronic inflammatory or infective diseases, or malignant neoplastic disease were excluded.

We also recruited serum cohort of healthy men ($n = 16$), whose medical history included no cardiovascular event. Subjects who had an acute illness, acute or chronic inflammatory or infective diseases, or malignant neoplastic disease were excluded.

All subjects recruited were male. Blood samples were obtained from each individual immediately before surgery and after overnight fasting. Serum was obtained by standard protocols and preserved at −80 °C until use.

Clinical and biochemical assessments
A complete anthropometric, biochemical, and physical examination was carried out on each patient. Body height and weight were measured with the patient standing in light clothes and shoeless. Body mass index (BMI) was calculated as body weight divided by height squared (kg/m^2). Laboratory studies included glucose, insulin, glycated haemoglobin (HbA1c), total cholesterol, high-density lipoprotein cholesterol (HDL-C), low-density lipoprotein cholesterol (LDL-C) and triglycerides, all of which were analysed using a conventional automated analyser. Insulin resistance (IR) was estimated using the homeostatic model assessment of IR (HOMA2-IR) [12].

Arterial tissue culture – obtaining the secretome
Tissue samples were transported from the surgery to the laboratory in phosphate buffered saline (PBS) at room temperature. Immediately upon arrival, the tissue was transferred to a Petri dish and washed with PBS. For mammary arteries, we removed the adventitia before incubation of the intima-media. All samples were then cut into similar-sized pieces about 3–5 mm in length and transferred to a 12-well tissue culture plate containing 2 ml/well of protein-free Roswell Park Memorial Institute medium (RPMI) (RPMI-1640, Gibco, Invitrogen, N.Y, USA) supplemented with penicillin (100 U/ml), streptomycin (100 μg/ml) and 50 mM HEPES. These procedures were all carried out under a laminar flow hood using sterile equipment. After 24 h of incubation at 37 °C and 5 % of CO_2, the media containing the secreted proteins, the so-called secretome, were collected, aliquoted and stored at −80 °C until used for analysis.

Additionally, a section of each atherosclerotic plaque was placed in phormol 10 % and further studied by an experienced pathologist from the Hospital Universitari Joan XXIII (Tarragona) following the AHA guidelines [11].

Measurements of adipo/cytokines levels
Defrosted secretome samples were centrifuged at 1200 rpm and 4 °C for 15 min. Then, they were analysed by enzyme-linked immunosorbent assays (ELISA) following the manufacturer's instructions. Adiponectin (EMD Millipore, St. Charles, MI, USA), visfatin (AdipoGen, San Diego, CA, USA), lipocalin-2 (R&D Systems Inc, Minneapolis, USA), resistin (Biovendor, Modrice, Czech Republic), IL-6 (R&D Systems Inc, Minneapolis, USA) and TNFR2 (BioSource Europe, Nivelles, Belgium) were

determined in secretome samples. Only visfatin was determined in both secretome and serum samples. The adiponectin assay sensitivity was 0.2 ng/ml, and intra-assay and inter-assay coefficients of variation (CV) were 3.4 and 5.7, respectively. The visfatin assay sensitivity was 30 pg/ml, and intra-assay and inter-assay CV were 5.63 and 5.92, respectively. The lipocalin-2 assay sensitivity was 0.012 ng/ml, and intra-assay and inter-assay CV were 3.7 and 6.5, respectively. The resistin assay sensitivity was 0.012 ng/ml, and intra-assay and inter-assay CV were 5.9 and 7.6, respectively. The IL-6 assay sensitivity was 0.039 pg/mL, and intra-assay and inter-assay CV were 7.4 and 7.8, respectively. Finally, sTNF-RII assay sensitivity was 0.1 ng/ml, and intra-assay and inter-assay CV were 4.9 and 7.9, respectively. In order to normalize adipo/cytokine measurements, total protein concentration was assessed using the Pierce BCA protein assay kit (Thermo Scientific, Waltham, MA, USA) following the manufacturer's instructions.

Statistical analysis

All the values reported are expressed as mean ± standard deviation (SD) and were analysed using the Windows SPSS/PC+ statistical package (version 22.0; SPSS, Chicago, IL, USA). Differences between groups were calculated using Student's t test or one-way ANOVA analysis. The strength of association between variables was calculated using Pearson's method for parametric variables and the Spearman Rho correlation test for non-parametric contrasts. P values <0.05 were considered to be statistically significant.

Results

Characteristics of the population studied

The general characteristics and biochemical measurements of the population studied are shown in Table 1. Subjects were classified according to the samples obtained: serum group of healthy subjects ($n = 16$), non-atherosclerotic mammary artery samples from patients undergoing coronary artery bypass ($n = 13$) and unstable carotid atherosclerotic plaque samples from patients undergoing endarterectomy ($n = 18$). The three groups studied had similar BMIs and they were all men. Anthropometrical and biochemical parameters showed no significant differences between non-atherosclerotic mammary artery and unstable carotid atherosclerotic plaque groups. As expected, carotid atherosclerotic plaque and mammary artery patients showed significant lower lipid profile because these subjects were taking lipid-lowering drugs. Table 1 also shows that the levels of glucose and HbA1c were significantly higher in the carotid atherosclerotic plaque and mammary artery group than in serum group of healthy subjects.

Table 1 Anthropometric measurements and metabolic analysis of the population studied

	Serum group of healthy subjects	Coronary patients with non-atherosclerotic mammary artery	Unstable carotid atherosclerotic plaque group
	($n = 16$)	($n = 13$)	($n = 18$)
	Mean ± SD	Mean ± SD	Mean ± SD
Age (years)	52.47 ± 13.25	65.08 ± 10.48	69.17 ± 7.44[b]
BMI (kg/m^2)	32.19 ± 11.76	29.39 ± 3.36	27.74 ± 3.13
Glucose (mg/dl)	91.31 ± 14.24	129.19 ± 55.44[a]	123.56 ± 45.37[b]
HbA1c (%)	4.97 ± 0.39	6.81 ± 1.39[a]	6.29 ± 1.07[b]
Insulin (mUI/L)	12.76 ± 16.19	11.76 ± 7.15	7.21 ± 4.93
HOMA2-IR	1.62 ± 1.95	1.59 ± 0.97	1.01 ± 0.67
Triglycerides (mg/dL)	115.02 ± 71.38	110.33 ± 27.84	103.00 ± 40.61
Cholesterol (mg/dl)	192.33 ± 37.81	128.34 ± 23.92[a]	118.81 ± 34.54[b]
HDL-C (mg/dL)	49.13 ± 10.35	23.71 ± 4.64[a]	28.50 ± 6.98[b]
LDL-C (mg/dL)	120.17 ± 39.06	78.56 ± 19.48[a]	69.78 ± 26.21[b]

Subjects were classified according to the samples obtained: serum group of healthy subjects ($n = 16$), non-atherosclerotic mammary artery samples from patients undergoing coronary artery bypass ($n = 13$) and unstable carotid atherosclerotic plaque samples from patients undergoing endarterectomy ($n = 18$). *BMI* body mass index, *HbA1c* glycosylated haemoglobin, *HOMA2-IR* homeostatic model assessment 2- insulin resistance, *HDL-C* high density lipoprotein, *LDL-C* low density lipoprotein. Data are expressed as mean ± SD. p <0.05 are considered statistically significant. [a]refer to the statistically significant differences between coronary patients with non-atherosclerotic mammary artery and serum group of healthy subjects. [b]refer to the statistically significant differences between unstable carotid plaque and serum group of healthy subjects. HOMA-2 is calculated using the HOMA Calculator version 2.2.2 (http://www.dtu.ox.ac.uk)

Adipo/cytokine levels in the secretome

To study the local role of adipo/cytokines in atherosclerosis, we evaluated the presence of adiponectin, visfatin, lipocalin-2, resistin, IL-6 and TNFR2 in secretomes of the unstable carotid atherosclerotic plaque and non-atherosclerotic mammary artery tissue cultures (Table 2). Of all the molecules analysed, visfatin was the only adipo/cytokine that was differently expressed in secretome

Table 2 Adipo/cytokine levels in secretome samples

	Unstable carotid atherosclerotic plaque group	Coronary patients with non-atherosclerotic mammary artery
	($n = 18$)	($n = 13$)
	Mean ± SD	Mean ± SD
Visfatin (ng/µg total protein)	0.100 ± 0.017	0.046 ± 0.012[a]
Adiponectin (µg/µg total protein)	0.311 ± 0.039	0.369 ± 0.096
IL-6 (pg/µg total protein)	0.048 ± 0.012	0.039 ± 0.008
Lipocalin-2 (ng/µg total protein)	0.009 ± 0.002	0.008 ± 0.001
Resistin (ng/µg total protein)	0.001 ± 0.001	0.001 ± 0.001
TNFR2 (ng/µg total protein)	0.007 ± 0.002	0.005 ± 0.001

IL-6 interleukin 6, *TNFR2* tumor necrosis factor receptor 2. Data are expressed as mean ± SD. p <0.05 are considered statistically significant. [a]refer to the statistically significant differences between unstable carotid atherosclerotic plaque and non-atherosclerotic mammary artery group samples. Specifically, visfatin levels were significantly higher in the unstable carotid atherosclerotic plaque than in non-atherosclerotic mammary artery secretomes (Table 2, $p = 0.021$). Conversely, the levels of adiponectin and IL-6 showed no significant differences between the two secretome groups analysed. Finally, the levels of lipocalin-2, resistin and TNFR2 were almost undetectable in the secretome samples. No significant correlations between adipo/cytokines were found.

Circulating Visfatin and adipocytokines levels in serum

As only differences in situ visfatin levels were observed and in order to study whether these differences were only a local effect or if they were also reflected in serum, we measured visfatin circulating levels in the group of patients suffering from atherosclerosis and in a serum group of healthy subjects ($n = 16$). Fig. 1 shows that there were no differences between unstable carotid atherosclerotic plaque and non-atherosclerotic mammary artery group. However, visfatin serum concentration was higher in both unstable carotid atherosclerotic plaque and non-atherosclerotic mammary artery groups than in the serum cohort of healthy subjects ($p = 0.037$ and p = 0.001; respectively). This difference remained significant after adjusting for age, BMI and glucose metabolism.

Then, we analysed the circulating levels of two adipo/cytokines with different profile, pro- and anti-inflammatory (IL-6 and adiponectin, respectively). We found that adiponectin circulating levels were significantly higher in the serum group of healthy subjects (29.20 ± 8.42) than

unstable carotid atherosclerotic plaque group (11.23 ± 1.69, $p = 0.025$) and non-atherosclerotic mammary artery patients (9.26 ± 2.35, $p = 0.031$). However, we observed no differences in the circulating levels of IL-6 between groups. No significant correlations between these adipo/cytokines and visfatin were found.

Discussion

To date, the knowledge of the local action of the adipo/cytokines expressed in secretomes of atherosclerotic plaques is under development. In fact, most secretome studies have been carried out using proteomic techniques [10, 13]. The aim of this study was to analyse the presence of several adipo/cytokines with different profiles, pro- and anti-inflammatory in the secretome of an unstable carotid atherosclerotic plaque with the secretome in a non-atherosclerotic mammary artery. The main finding was that visfatin levels were significantly higher in the unstable carotid atherosclerotic plaque than in non-atherosclerotic mammary artery secretomes, suggesting a possible link between visfatin and unstable carotid atherosclerotic plaque.

Visfatin is a ubiquitous adipokine that is produced in adipose tissue, bone marrow, skeletal muscle, and liver with a physiological role not completely understood [14–16]. In the context of metabolic diseases, most studies have focused on increased circulating levels and adipose tissue expression of visfatin [17, 18]. Also, it was initially proposed as a clinical marker of atherosclerosis, endothelial dysfunction and vascular damage [19]. Also,

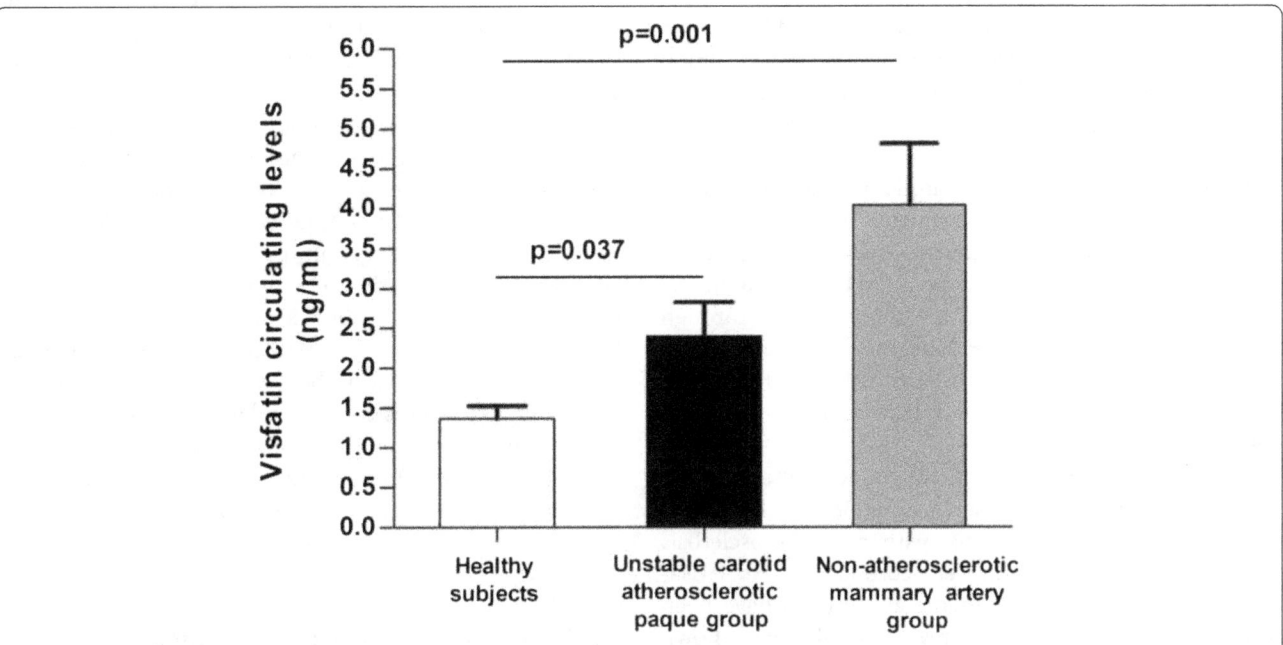

Fig. 1 Visfatin serum levels in different groups: unstable carotid atherosclerotic plaque group ($n = 18$), coronary patients with non-atherosclerotic mammary artery ($n = 13$) and serum cohort of healthy subjects ($n = 16$). $p < 0.05$ were considered statistically significant

visfatin is an active player promoting vascular inflammation, atherosclerosis development and progression, and plaque destabilization [19–21]. As far as the local effect of visfatin on atherosclerotic lesions is concerned, other authors studying the atheroma plaque directly have reported similar results to ours [22–24]. One of the studies that has most similarities with ours has reported that visfatin should be regarded as an inflammatory mediator, localized to foam cell macrophages within unstable atherosclerotic lesions, which potentially plays a role in plaque destabilization [22]. Moreover, Zhou et al. have reported that visfatin induces cholesterol accumulation in macrophages and accelerates the process of atherosclerosis [23]. Apart from the pro-inflammatory effect of visfatin on atherosclerosis, other possible direct mechanisms have been reported: promotion of smooth muscle cell proliferation, alteration of the expression and the activity of matrix metalloproteinases, greater atherosclerotic plaque vulnerability and impairment of endothelial vasodilatory responses [25–28]. The mechanism underlying elevated levels of visfatin in secretomes from unstable atherosclerotic plaques are not known nowadays. However, Dahl et al. have reported enhanced visfatin expression in symptomatic atherosclerotic plaques and also that visfatin had a combined ability of increasing TNF-α as well as to respond with increased expression on TNF-α stimulation. Therefore, this bidirectional interaction between TNF-α and visfatin could represent a pathogenic loop on unstable atherosclerotic lesions [22]. Another study has further demonstrated that the regulation of visfatin in macrophages is related to pro-atherogenic stimuli, including hypoxia, TNF-α and ox-LDL [29].

Although some authors have identified that visfatin is a potential inflammatory mediator in plaque destabilization [22], in our study we only included patients with cerebrovascular ischemia and unstable carotid atherosclerotic plaque. Therefore, we could not compare visfatin levels between stable and unstable carotid plaque secretomes. Although the biological mechanisms involving visfatin in the pathogenesis of atherosclerosis are not well-established, visfatin seems to be an active factor in the development and progression of atherosclerosis through its effects on cytokine and chemokine secretion, macrophage survival, leukocyte recruitment by endothelial cells, vascular smooth muscle inflammation and plaque destabilization [19, 23].

Regarding circulating levels, we found higher visfatin serum concentrations in patients suffering carotid atherosclerosis and coronary patients with non-atherosclerosis mammary artery who underwent coronary revascularisation surgery. In our study, mammary arteries have been used as control arteries, since previous studies have shown its lower incidence of atherosclerosis [30, 31]. However, it is important to remark that although mammary artery patients have non-diseased arterial secretome, they have atherosclerotic coronary disease. Likewise, in recent years, several studies have established positive associations between enhanced circulating visfatin levels and atherogenic inflammatory diseases, which suggest a possible role of visfatin in the atherosclerosis pathogenesis [19, 32]. Specifically, visfatin was associated with infarct-related artery occlusion, and also an association with coronary artery disease was found [33, 34]. On the other hand, some authors claim that high visfatin levels, instead of depicting changes in the atherosclerotic process are more likely to reflect changes in systemic inflammation in patients with cardiovascular disease [19]. Although our local and systemic results reinforce the first hypothesis, additional human studies are needed if these data are to be clarified.

Regarding the other adipo/cytokines, levels of lipocalin-2, resistin and TNFR2 were almost undetectable in the secretome samples. In addition, the levels of adiponectin and IL-6 showed no differences between the two secretome groups analysed. Several studies have described a protective role of adiponectin in cardiovascular diseases [35]. Although we did not find differences between secretome groups, we found higher serum levels of adiponectin in control individuals than in both unstable carotid atherosclerosis and non-atherosclerotic mammary artery patients. Further studies are needed to assess whether adiponectin can have a direct effect in situ by inhibiting the formation of an atherosclerotic plaque. Although IL-6 has been regarded as a pro-inflammatory cytokine that is classically associated with endothelial dysfunction and atherosclerosis [36], we found no differences in secretome or circulating levels between the group of patients suffering from atherosclerosis and the mammary artery. The reason for these discrepancies could be the dissimilarities of the studied populations.

Our results require the following observations. First, we have used mammary arteries as control arteries, since previous studies have shown a lower incidence of atherosclerosis. However, non-atherosclerotic carotid arteries would be the best choice but, unfortunately, are not available. Second, this study was cross-sectional, so it allowed us to detect correlations but not to formulate predictions. Future prospective studies are necessary to elucidate more thoroughly the association between some molecules such as visfatin and atherosclerosis, and also their potential role as new therapeutic approaches and biomarkers of unstable vs. stable plaques. As our study was conducted only including unstable plaques, we could only suggest doing further in order to confirm this hypothesis.

Conclusions

Of all the adipo/cytokines analysed in secretomes, visfatin was the only adipo/cytokine that was higher in unstable carotid artery plaque than in non-atherosclerotic mammary artery secretomes. Regarding visfatin serum levels, there were no differences between unstable carotid atherosclerotic plaque and non-atherosclerotic mammary artery groups. However, these visfatin circulating levels were increased in comparison to serum cohort of healthy subjects. Prospective studies are needed to confirm whether visfatin could play a role as prognostic factor in the stability of atherosclerotic plaque.

Abbreviations
BMI, body mass index; HbA1c, glycosylated hemoglobin; HDL-C, high density lipoprotein; HOMA2-IR, homeostatic model assessment method insulin resistance; IL-6, interleukin 6; LDL-C, low density lipoprotein; PBS, phosphate buffered saline; RPMI, protein-free Roswell Park Memorial Institute medium; TNFR2, tumor necrosis factor receptor 2

Acknowledgments
None.

Funding
This study was supported by the Fondo de Investigación Sanitaria and Fondo Europeo de Desarrollo Regional (FEDER, grant number PI13/00468, to T.A.), the Agència de Gestió d'Ajuts Universitaris i de Recerca (AGAUR 2009 SGR 959 to C.R.), the Grup de Recerca en Medicina Aplicada URV (2010PFR-URV-B2-14 to C.R.) and the Fundación Biociencia.

Authors' contributions
TA and GA were responsible for the study design and finalized the report; EGJ and AB contributed to data interpretation and drafted the manuscript; MC, AA and CA performed the general biochemical determinations; SM participated in technical analysis; VMP, EH, XR, MLC participated in patients selection; CR participated in the overall design. All authors read and approved the final manuscript.

Competing interests
The authors declare that they have no competing interests.

Author details
[1]Grup de Recerca GEMMAIR - Medicina Aplicada. Departament de Medicina i Cirurgia, Universitat Rovira i Virgili (URV), Institut Investigació Sanitària Pere Virgili (IISPV), 43007 Tarragona, Spain. [2]Servei Medicina Interna, Hospital Universitari Joan XXIII, 43007 Tarragona, Spain. [3]Servei Anatomia Patològica, Hospital Universitari Joan XXIII, 43007 Tarragona, Spain. [4]Servei Angiologia i Cirurgia Vascular, Hospital Universitari Joan XXIII, 43007 Tarragona, Spain. [5]Servei de Cirurgia Cardíaca, Hospital Germans Trias i Pujol, 08916 Badalona, Spain.

References
1. Sahin-Efe A, Katsikeris F, Mantzoros CS. Advances in adipokines. Metabolism. 2012;61(12):1659–65.
2. Chang L, Milton H, Eitzman DT, Chen YE. Paradoxical roles of perivascular adipose tissue in atherosclerosis and hypertension. Circ J. 2012;77(1):11–8.
3. Yoo HJ, Choi KM. Adipokines as a novel link between obesity and atherosclerosis. World J Diabetes. 2014;5(3):357–63.
4. Van de Voorde J, Pauwels B, Boydens C, Decaluwé K. Adipocytokines in relation to cardiovascular disease. Metabolism. 2013;62(11):1513–21.
5. Mattu HS, Randeva HS. Role of adipokines in cardiovascular disease. J Endocrinol. 2013;216(1):T17–36.
6. Ntaios G, Gatselis NK, Makaritsis K, Dalekos GN. Adipokines as mediators of endothelial function and atherosclerosis. Atherosclerosis. 2013;227(2):216–21.
7. Anfossi G, Russo I, Doronzo G, Pomero A, Trovati M. Adipocytokines in atherothrombosis: focus on platelets and vascular smooth muscle cells. Mediators Inflamm. 2010;2010:174341.
8. Schneiderman J, Simon AJ, Schroeter MR, Flugelman MY, Konstantinides S, Schaefer K. Leptin receptor is elevated in carotid plaques from neurologically symptomatic patients and positively correlated with augmented macrophage density. J Vasc Surg. 2008;48(5):1146–55.
9. Cho Y, Lee SE, Lee HC, Hur J, Lee S, Youn SW, et al. Adipokine resistin is a key player to modulate monocytes, endothelial cells, and smooth muscle cells, leading to progression of atherosclerosis in rabbit carotid artery. J Am Coll Cardiol. 2011;57(1):99–109.
10. De la Cuesta F, Barderas MG, Calvo E, Zubiri I, Maroto AS, Darde VM, et al. Secretome analysis of atherosclerotic and non-atherosclerotic arteries reveals dynamic extracellular remodeling during pathogenesis. J Proteomics. 2012;75(10):2960–71.
11. Stary HC. Natural history and histological classification of atherosclerotic lesions: an update. Arterioscler Thromb Vasc Biol. 2000;20(5):1177–78.
12. Terra X, Auguet T, Broch M, Sabench F, Hernández M, Pastor RM, et al. Retinol binding protein-4 circulating levels were higher in nonalcoholic fatty liver disease vs. histologically normal liver from morbidly obese women. Obesity (Silver Spring). 2013;21(1):170–7.
13. Durán MC, Martín-Ventura JL, Mas S, Barderas MG, Dardé VM, Jensen ON, et al. Characterization of the human atheroma plaque secretome by proteomic analysis. Methods Mol Biol. 2007;357:141–50.
14. Kato A, Odamaki M, Ishida J, Hishida A. Relationship between serum pre-B cell colony-enhancing factor/Visfatin and atherosclerotic parameters in chronic hemodialysis patients. Am J Nephrol. 2009;29(1):31–5.
15. Chen MP, Chung FM, Chang DM, Tsai JC, Huang HF, Shin SJ, et al. Elevated plasma level of Visfatin/pre-B cell colony-enhancing factor in patients with type 2 diabetes mellitus. J Clin Endocrinol Metab. 2006;91(1):295–9.
16. Goktas Z, Owens S, Boylan M, Syn D, Shen CL, Reed DB, et al. Associations between tissue visfatin/nicotinamide, phosphoribosyltransferase (Nampt), retinol binding protein-4, and vaspin concentrations and insulin resistance in morbidly obese subjects. Mediators Inflamm. 2013;2013:861496.
17. Filippatos TD, Derdemezis CS, Gazi IF, Lagos K, Kiortsis DN, Tselepis AD, et al. Increased plasma visfatin levels in subjects with the metabolic syndrome. Eur J Clin Invest. 2008;38(1):71–2.
18. Ahmed MB, Ismail MI, Meki AR. Relation of osteoprotegerin, visfatin and ghrelin to metabolic syndrome in type 2 diabetic patients. Int J Health Sci (Qassim). 2015;9(2):127–39.
19. Romacho T, Sánchez-Ferrer CF, Peiró C. Visfatin/Nampt: an adipokine with cardiovascular impact. Mediators Inflamm. 2013;2013:946427S.
20. Liu SW, Qiao SB, Yuan JS, Liu DQ. Association of plasma visfatin levels with inflammation, atherosclerosis, and acute coronary syndromes in humans. Clin Endocrinol (Oxf). 2009;71(2):202–7.
21. Kong Q, Xia M, Liang R, Li L, Cu X, Sun Z, et al. Increased serum visfatin as a risk factor for atherosclerosis in patients with ischaemic cerebrovascular disease. Singapore Med J. 2014;55(7):383–87.
22. Dahl TB, Yndestad A, Skjelland M, Øie E, Dahl A, Michelsen A, et al. Increased expression of visfatin in macrophages of human unstable carotid and coronary atherosclerosis: possible role in inflammation and plaque destabilization. Circulation. 2007;115(8):972–80.
23. Zhou F, Pan Y, Huang Z, Jia Y, Zhao X, Chen Y, et al. Visfatin induces cholesterol accumulation in macrophages through up-regulation of scavenger receptor-A and CD36. Cell Stress Chaperones. 2013;18(5):643–52.
24. Chiu CA, Yu TH, Hung WC. Increased expression of visfatin in monocytes and macrophages in male acute myocardial infarction patients. Mediators Inflamm. 2012;2012:469852.
25. Yamawaki H, Hara N, Okada M, Hara Y. Visfatin causes endothelium-dependent relaxation in isolated blood vessels. Biochem Biophys Res Commun. 2009;383(4):503–8.
26. Kim SR, Bae SK, Choi KS, Park SY, Jun HO, Lee JY, et al. Visfatin promotes angiogenesis by activation of extracellular signal-regulated kinase 1/2. Biochem Biophys Res Commun. 2007;357(1):150–6.
27. Vallejo S, Romacho T, Angulo J, Villalobos LA, Cercas E, Leivas A. Visfatin impairs endothelium-dependent relaxation in rat and human mesenteric

microvessels through nicotinamide phosphoribosyltransferase activity. PLoS One. 2011;6(11):e27299.

28. Takebayashi K, Suetsugu M, Wakabayashi S, Aso Y, Inukai T. Association between plasma visfatin and vascular endothelial function in patients with type 2 diabetes mellitus. Metabolism. 2007;56:451–8.

29. Dahl T, Ranheim T, Holm S, Berge R, Aukrust P, Halvorsen P. Nicotinamide phosphoribosyltransferase and lipid accumulation in macrophages. Eur J Clin Invest. 2011;41(10):1098–104.

30. Fonseca DA, Antunes PE, Cotrim MD. Endothelium-dependent vasoactivity of the human internal mammary artery. Coron Artery Dis. 2014;25(3):266–74.

31. Otsuka F, Yahagi K, Sakakura K, Virmani R. Why is the mammary artery so special and what protects it from atherosclerosis? Ann Cardiothorac Surg. 2013;2(4):519–26.

32. Lu YC, Hsu CC, Yu TH, Wang CP, Lu LF, Hung WC, et al. Association between visfatin levels and coronary artery disease in patients with chronic kidnay disease. Iran J Kidney Dis. 2013;7(6):446–52.

33. Tang X, Chen M, Zhang W. Association between elevated visfatin and carotid atherosclerosis in patients with chronic kidney disease. J Cent South Univ (Med Sci). 2013;38(6):553–9.

34. Hung WC, Yu TH, Hsu CC, Lu LF, Chung FM, Tsai IT, et al. Plasma visfatin levels are associated with major adverse cardiovascular events in patients with acute ST-elevation myocardial infarction. Clin Invest Med. 2015;38(3):E100–9.

35. Luo N, Liu J, Chung BH, Yang Q, Klein RL, Garvey WT, et al. Macrophage adiponectin expression improves insulin sensitivity and protects against inflammation and atherosclerosis. Diabetes. 2010;59(4):791–9.

36. Puz P, Lasek-Bal A, Ziaja D, Kazibutowska Z, Ziaja K. Inflammatory markers in patients with internal carotid artery stenosis. Arch Med Sci. 2013;9(2):254–60.

6

Effects of weight management by exercise modes on markers of subclinical atherosclerosis and cardiometabolic profile among women with abdominal obesity

Jina Choo[1]*, Juneyoung Lee[2], Jeong-Hyun Cho[1], Lora E Burke[3], Akira Sekikawa[4] and Sae Young Jae[5]

Abstract

Background: Few studies have examined the differential effects of weight management by exercise mode on subclinical atherosclerosis. We hypothesized that 3 modes of aerobic, resistance, and combination exercises have differential effects on the flow-mediated dilation (FMD), carotid-femoral pulse wave velocity (PWV), and carotid intima-media thickness (IMT) as well as cardiometabolic profile in weight management.

Methods: A randomized, single-blind trial (ISRCTN46069848) was conducted in Seoul, South Korea between November 2011 and December 2012. Randomized participants were 110 women with abdominal obesity (aerobic group n = 50; resistance group n = 30; combination exercise group n = 30). The treatment period was 12 months with 3-month follow up: A diet-alone intervention for the first 3 months and a diet-plus-exercise intervention for the next 9 months according to exercise modes. The exercise training was designed with an intensity of 50-70% heart rate reserve for 3 days a week in 60-minute-long sessions for 9 months, consisting of 30-minute treadmill and 30-minute bike exercises for aerobic group; upper and lower body exercises with an intensity target of 2 sets and 8–12 repetitions for resistance group; 30-minute resistance and consecutive 30-minute aerobic exercises for combination group.

Results: Ninety-two and 49 participants were analyzed for modified intention-to-treat analysis and per-protocol (PP) analysis, respectively. The 3 exercise modes had no significant differential effects on FMD, PWV, and IMT over time; however, the combination group was found to have significantly lower levels of fasting glucose than the aerobic group ($p = .034$) in the PP analysis. Nevertheless, we observed significant time effects such as reductions in PWV ($p = .048$) and IMT ($p = .018$) in cubic and quadratic trends, respectively, and improvements in body weight, waist circumference, low-density and high-density lipoprotein cholesterol levels, fasting glucose levels, and cardiorespiratory fitness in linear, quadratic, or cubic trends.

Conclusions: For women with abdominal obesity, a combination of aerobic and resistance exercises may be preferable to a single exercise mode for effective glucose control. Regardless of exercise mode, exercise interventions combined with dietary interventions in weight management may be beneficial in reducing the risk of subclinical atherosclerosis and cardiometabolic risk.

Background

Abdominal obesity is a risk factor for coronary heart disease (CHD). Prospective cohort studies have reported that an increase in waist circumference is significantly associated with CHD incidence and mortality [1]. In addition, abdominal obesity was found to be associated with subclinical atherosclerotic risk, as assessed by endothelial dysfunction [2], aortic stiffness [3], and carotid atherosclerosis [3,4]. Particularly, the risk for CHD associated with increased waist circumference may be prominent in women [1,5-7], and, in this context, the potential for reducing CHD risk may also be significant in women.

Diet-plus-exercise interventions are commonly recommended for enhancing long-term weight management and reducing CHD risk factors in overweight and obese

* Correspondence: jinachoo@gmail.com
[1]College of Nursing, Korea University, Seoul, South Korea
Full list of author information is available at the end of the article

individuals [8,9]. Empirically, exercise-alone interventions have been found to have weaker effects than diet-plus-exercise interventions on weight loss [10,11]. However, exercise training may have beneficial effects on the regression of subclinical atherosclerosis [12]. A few studies have reported that either aerobic or resistance exercise training improved endothelial dysfunction [13,14], aortic stiffness [15,16], and carotid intima-media thickness (IMT) [17]. However, their effects may differ by exercise modes, i.e., aerobic, resistance, or combination exercise, because each mode leads to different patterns of blood flow and levels of pressure on the endothelium and arterial wall [18,19]. Meanwhile, recent studies have reported that a combination of aerobic and resistance exercises may be more effective on improving anthropometric and cardiometabolic profiles than aerobic or resistance exercise alone [20,21]. In particular, combination exercise was reported to be the most efficacious means of decreasing body weight and waist circumference among overweight and obese adults [20,22] and to have an additional beneficial effect on glucose control compared with either aerobic or resistance exercise for those with type 2 diabetes mellitus [21]. However, there is no information regarding whether the 3 exercise modes, i.e., aerobic, resistance, and combination exercises, have differential effects on markers of subclinical atherosclerosis such as endothelial function, aortic stiffness, or carotid IMT as well as cardiometabolic profile among overweight and obese individuals.

The purpose of the study was to test the hypothesis that aerobic, resistance, and combination exercises in a weight management intervention would have significant differential effects on markers of subclinical atherosclerosis, as measured by brachial flow-mediated dilation (FMD), carotid-femoral pulse wave velocity (PWV) and mean IMT levels at the common carotid artery, and cardiometabolic profile among women with abdominal obesity in the Community-based Heart and Weight Management Trial.

Methods
Study participants and enrollment procedure
We recruited the study subjects from a community (i.e., Seongbuk-Gu) in Seoul, South Korea. The community was characterized as an urban county with a population size of approximately 490,000 residents. Between November 2010 and November 2011, study participants were recruited via poster, leaflet, telephone, and mass mailing advertisements at the municipal health center, churches, universities, and online communities. Eligible participants were invited to an orientation where they were provided a detailed study overview, asked for consent, and screened for additional inclusion criteria. The inclusion criteria were as follows: healthy women aged between 18 and 65 years, elevated waist circumference (≥85 cm) according to the criteria

for abdominal obesity as defined by the Korean Society for the Study of Obesity [23,24], and willingness to be randomly assigned to one of the 3 different exercise modes (i.e., aerobic, resistance, and combination exercise training). The exclusion criteria included current medical conditions such as cardiovascular diseases, diabetes, or cancers; physical limitations restricting exercise ability; current use of hormone therapy; history of participation in a weight loss intervention in the last 1 year; and a weight change in the last 4 weeks prior to participation in our study. Before commencing with the randomization of participants, baseline measurements of body composition (body mass index [BMI] and waist circumference), blood lipids, and fasting glucose were obtained; information regarding sociodemographic and psychosocial variables were obtained through questionnaires. The study was approved by the Institutional Review Board at Korea University (KU-IRB-11-10-A-2). All participants provided written informed consent.

Study design
The Community-based Heart and Weight Management Trial (trial registration no. ISRCTN46069848) includes a randomized 12-month intervention with 3 different exercise groups: aerobic training only, resistance training only, and a combination of aerobic and resistance training. The intervention assignment was carried out using a random allocation computer program (n = 50 for aerobic exercise, n = 30 for resistance exercise, and n = 30 for combination exercise) (Figure 1). Initially, the aerobic exercise group (n = 50) was further divided into 2 groups: one group with (n = 30) and the other group without behavioral therapy (n = 20). However, because there were no significant differences in the outcome variables between both the groups, we pooled the participants of those 2 groups into 1 aerobic exercise group (n = 50) for the present study. This study was a single-blinded trial; assessors of all the outcomes were blinded to participant group assignment, and all outcome data were blinded until the completion of final data entry for the 12-month assessment.

Intervention
We conducted 2 consecutive types of interventions: diet-alone vs. diet-plus-exercise interventions in a sequence over a 12-month weight management program (Figure 2), i.e., a diet-alone intervention for the first 3 months and a diet-plus-exercise intervention for the next 9 months according to exercise modes; for the diet-alone intervention, the 3 groups were asked not to attend any exercise training sessions for the first 3 months.

The exercise intervention over the following 9 months was added to the diet-alone intervention: 60-minute exercise sessions were conducted 3 times a week in a public

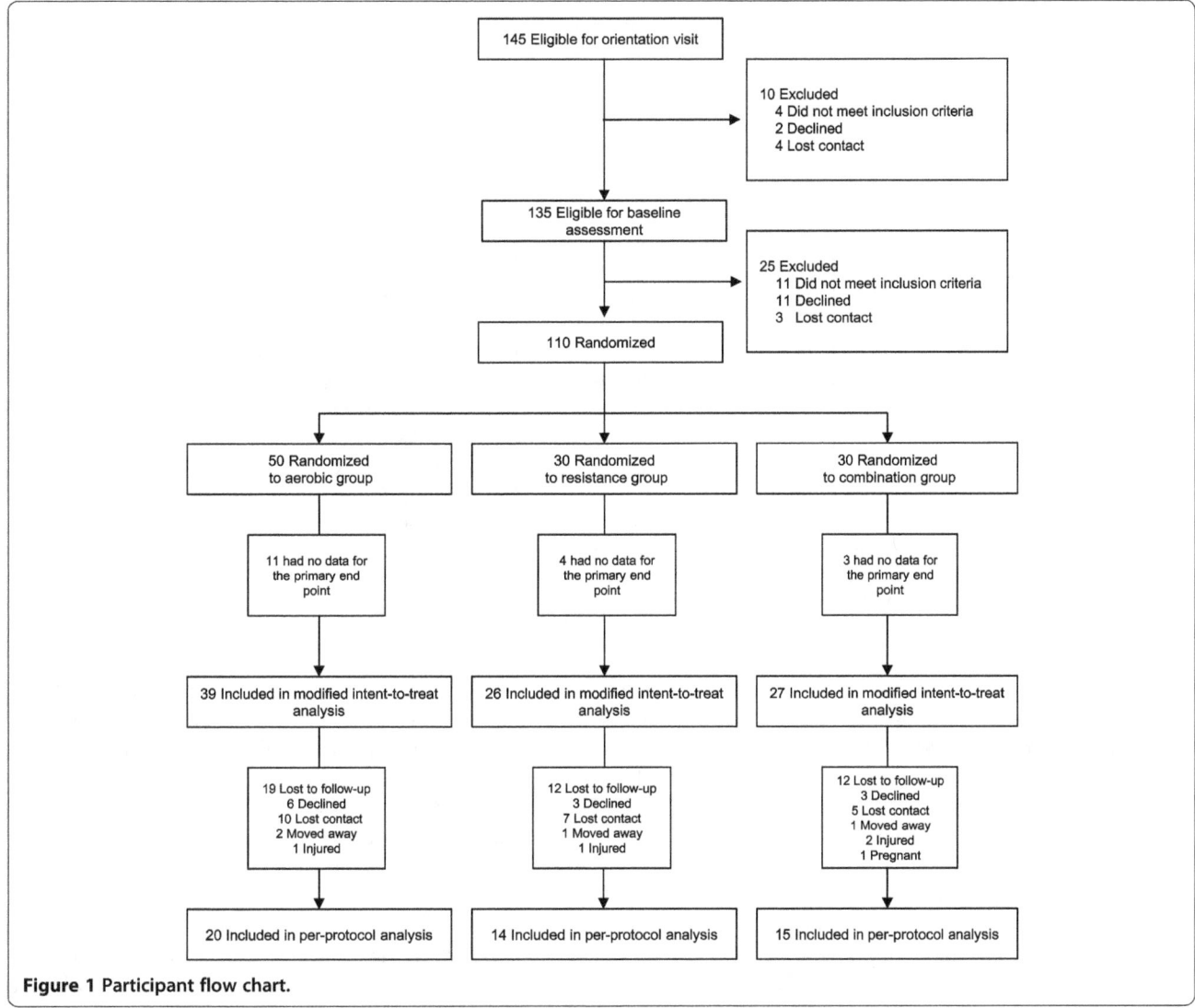

Figure 1 Participant flow chart.

community fitness center under group teaching and supervision of exercise trainers. The aerobic session consisted of 30-minute treadmill exercise and 30-minute bike exercise, with an intensity target of 50–70% of heart rate reserve. The resistance session consisted of both upper and lower body exercises: chest press, lat pull-down, abdominal crunches, back extensions, leg curl, leg extensions, leg press, and calf raise. The load was initially set at 40% and 50% (or 60%) of maximum strength for the upper extremities and lower extremities, respectively. Two sets of 8–12 repetitions were performed during each session. The rest period between each set was less than 90 seconds. The load was progressively increased by 5% every 3 weeks or when subjects could easily perform 15 repetitions. Combination training consisted of 30 minutes of resistance exercise and a consecutive 30-minute session of aerobic exercise (15 minutes on a treadmill and 15 minutes on a bicycle) with 1 set of 8–12 repetitions

for resistance exercise and 50–70% of the heart rate reserve for aerobic exercise.

The diet-alone intervention was administered to all participants, with individualized daily calorie intake (1,200 kcal if the weight was <90.5 kg; 1,500 kcal if the weight was ≥90.5 kg) and fat intake goals (≤25% of total calories), taking into account their baseline body weight measurements. Additionally, all the groups except the aerobic group without behavioral therapy (n = 20) received behavioral counseling (12 sessions of group classes over 6 months) and were also taught the use of established behavior change strategies including goal setting and self-monitoring [25].

Measurements

The primary outcome of the trial was FMD. The secondary outcomes included improvements in other markers of subclinical atherosclerosis (i.e., PWV and carotid IMT),

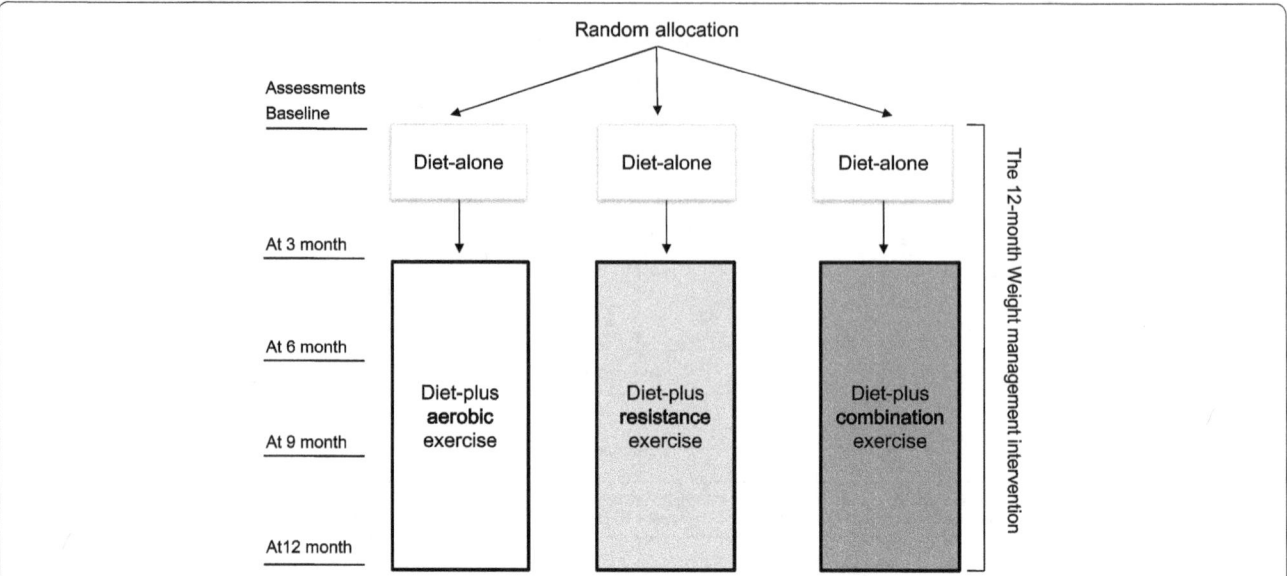

Figure 2 The 12-month weight management intervention in the present study. Following random allocation, a diet-alone intervention for the first 3 months and a diet-plus-exercise intervention according to the exercise modes for the next 9 months were implemented over 12 months. The assessments were conducted at baseline, 3, 6, 9, and 12 months.

anthropometric profile (i.e., body weight and lean body mass), cardiometabolic profile (i.e., waist circumference, systolic blood pressure, total cholesterol, low-density lipoprotein [LDL] cholesterol, high-density lipoprotein [HDL] cholesterol, triglycerides, and fasting glucose), and cardiorespiratory fitness (i.e., maximal oxygen consumption [VO_{2max}]).

All measures were assessed at baseline, 3, 6, and 12 months. Weight was measured after an overnight fast, using the Tanita bioelectrical impedance scale (Tanita Corporation of America, Inc., IL, USA); prior to being weighed, the participants were asked to wear light-weight clothing and take off their shoes. Height was measured using a wall-mounted stadiometer. The BMI was computed as weight (kg)/height (m)^2. Waist circumference (cm) was measured twice using a Gullick II measuring tape at the midpoint between the lowest rib and the iliac crest; the average of 2 measurements was used.

Blood samples were drawn from the antecubital vein in the morning after a 10-hour overnight fast without taking any current medications, including anti-hypertensive or lipid-lowering medications, when participants visited the municipal health center. Participants who took anti-hypertensive (n = 11) or lipid-lowering medications (n = 7) were instructed to take them during the study period. Samples were analyzed using a biochemical auto-analyzer (Hitachi cobas c501; Hitachi, Japan) at the Department of Clinical Laboratory of the municipal health center, in Seoul, South Korea. Total cholesterol and HDL cholesterol levels were measured by a homogeneous enzymatic colorimetric test. The levels of triglycerides and glucose

were measured using the GPO-PAP method and the hexokinase method, respectively. LDL cholesterol level was estimated according to the Friedewald equation [26].

For non-invasive assessment of the FMD, brachial artery dilatation was measured by ultrasonography (ACUSON X 300; Siemens, Mountain View, CA). The brachial artery was imaged in longitudinal sections 5–10 cm proximal to the placement of a blood pressure cuff, just below the antecubital fossa, using a high frequency linear array probe (11.4 MHz). The FMD was measured for 1 minute at baseline and again for 2 minutes after an ischemic stimulus (inflation of a blood pressure cuff around the forearm to 200 mmHg for 5 minutes). The FMD was analyzed using a semi-automated edge detection software system (Brachial Analyzer 5; Medical Imaging Applications, Coralville, IA) to calculate FMD (%) according to the following equation: [(maximum diameter − baseline diameter)/baseline diameter] × 100. A reproducibility (i.e., intraclass correlation coefficient) of 0.95 was achieved within technicians.

Carotid to femoral PWV value was derived to measure central arterial stiffness, using a SphygmoCor®system (AtCor Medical, Sydney, Australia). The distance from the carotid artery sample site to the femoral artery and that from the carotid artery to the suprasternal notch were measured as straight lines with a tape measure. Pulse waves were obtained by applanation tonometry. According to the "foot-to-foot" method, PWV was determined as D/(Δt) (m/s), where Δt is the time difference between carotid-femoral pressure waves, and D is the distance between the 2 arteries. All measurements were taken in duplicate, and the mean values were used for subsequent analysis. Arterial stiffness was measured in accordance with the guidelines of the Clinical Application of Arterial Stiffness, Task Force III. A reproducibility (i.e., intraclass correlation coefficient) of 0.98 was achieved within technicians.

Carotid artery ultrasound imaging was performed using a high-resolution B-mode ultrasound system (ACUSON X 300; Siemens, Mountain View, CA). The IMT was defined as the distance from the leading edge of the lumen-intima interface to the leading edge of the media-adventitia interface of the far wall of the carotid artery. All measurements were made at the end diastole. The carotid IMT of the common carotid artery was determined from a semi-automated measurement obtained 2 cm proximal to the carotid bifurcation. The value for carotid IMT was defined as the mean of the IMT. A reproducibility (i.e., intraclass correlation coefficient) of 0.99 was achieved within technicians.

Cardiorespiratory fitness levels were reported as VO_{2max} values estimated using the Rockport Fitness Walking Test. Participants were administered the 1-mile walk test on an outdoor track in accordance with the protocol of Kline et al. [27].

Statistical analysis

Sample size calculation was based on Olson et al.'s study [13]. The study showed a decreased mean FMD change of 1.4% (standard deviation [SD], 2.32%) at the 12-month follow-up in the control group and an increased mean FMD change of 2.6% (SD, 3.49%) in the resistance group. We considered two-thirds of mean change difference between groups as an effect size for our study because all of our groups received a diet program. To detect a mean difference in FMD of 2.67% by assuming the SD from Olson et al., between any pairs of the 3 groups in our study, at least 21 subjects per group were needed to ensure an 80% power with the Student's t-test and 2-tailed test at the 5% level of significance. Considering the 30% follow-up loss rate during the study period, we initially planned to randomize a total of 90 subjects to 3 study groups (30 participants per group). However, as mentioned in the Study Design section, the actually allocated sample sizes were 50 participants to aerobic, 30 participants to resistance, and 30 participants to the combination exercise group.

To test the homogeneity of exercise groups in terms of baseline measures for sociodemographic, health-related, subclinical atherosclerosis, anthropometric, cardiometabolic, and cardiorespiratory fitness variables, one-way ANOVA, X^2 test, and Fisher's exact test were performed. The modified intention-to-treat (ITT) population, defined as randomized subjects with least 1 FMD measure reported across 4 assessment periods, was used to analyze

the primary outcome variable. This population consisted of 92 (84%) out of 110 randomized participants (Figure 1). The main effects of exercise group and time as well as the interaction effects between exercise group and time were examined using a generalized estimating equation (GEE) model for repeated measures over time. Covariates adjusted for in the GEE model included baseline values and marital status. Per-protocol (PP) analyses were also conducted; the participants involved in this analysis were defined as a subgroup of participants who met the criteria of 100% follow-up by the fifth assessment over 12 months.

All analyses were performed using STATA 10.0 (Stata-Corp LP., USA). A 2-tailed p-value of less than 0.05 was considered statistically significant.

Results

The participants had a mean age of 43.1 years, mean BMI of 28.5 kg/m^2, and mean waist circumference of 94.8 cm (Table 1). Of all participants, 24.5% had an obesity-related condition such as hypertension or dyslipidemia and 29.1% were post-menopausal. Some of the baseline cardiometabolic profile (i.e., waist circumference and total and HDL cholesterol levels) were outside the reference ranges according to the criteria for abdominal obesity in women as defined by the Korean Society for the Study of Obesity [23], criteria of the National Cholesterol Education Program (NCEP) Adult Treatment Panel III (ATP III) [28], and diagnostic criteria for metabolic syndrome according to the NCEP-ATP III [29]. The mean fitness level, as measured by VO_{2max}, was 31.1 mL $\cdot$ kg^{-1} $\cdot$ min^{-1}. The participants in the resistance group were highly likely to be married compared to those in the aerobic or combination exercise groups (F = 6.57, p = .037).

Table 2 summarizes the results for differential effects of exercise mode on outcome variables over time in weight management, i.e., the interaction effects between exercise groups and time on markers of subclinical atherosclerosis and anthropometric and cardiometabolic profiles on the basis of both modified ITT and PP analyses. We did not find significant interaction effects for any of the outcome variables, except for fasting glucose levels. The PP analyses revealed that changes in fasting glucose levels significantly differed by the exercise mode (p = .034); significant reductions in fasting glucose levels were seen in the combination exercise group as compared with that in the aerobic group. Specifically, an additional analysis revealed that such a significant differential effect occurred at 12 months (p = .004), and the changes in fasting glucose levels in the combination exercise group showed a liner trend (p = .014) (data not shown).

Table 3 summarizes the time effects for all the 3 groups on the outcome variables, based on the results of modified ITT and PP analyses. We found significant time effects for PWV (p = .048) and IMT (p = .018). We also

Table 1 Participants' characteristics (N = 110)

	n (%) or mean (SD)				$F/\chi^2/$ Fisher's	P^*
	Total (n = 110)	Aerobic (n = 50)	Resistance (n = 30)	Combination (n = 30)		
Sociodemographic characteristics						
Age, years	43.1 (9.0)	42.2 (9.5)	46.0 (10.0)	41.8 (6.6)	2.16	.120
Married, yes	90 (81.8)	37 (74.0)	29 (97.6)	24 (80.0)	6.57	.037
Education					0.78	.678
Some college or more	66 (60.0)	31 (62.0)	16 (53.3)	19 (63.3)		
High school degree or less	44 (40.0)	19 (38.0)	14 (46.7)	11 (36.7)		
Monthly household income ($)					1.37	.503
<=3,500	61 (55.5)	30 (60.0)	14 (46.7)	17 (56.7)		
> 3,500	49 (44.5)	20 (40.0)	16 (53.3)	13 (43.3)		
Employed, yes	43 (39.1)	19 (38.0)	11 (36.7)	13 (43.3)	0.33	.850
Health-related characteristics						
Obesity-related conditions, yes	27 (24.5)	15 (30.0)	8 (26.7)	4 (13.3)	2.91	.233
Post-menopause, yes	32 (29.1)	15 (30.0)	12 (40.0)	5 (16.7)	4.00	.136
Current smoking, yes	6 (5.5)	2 (4.0)	1 (3.3)	3 (10.0)	1.57	.556
Alcohol drinking (twice or more/week), yes	9 (8.2)	4 (8.0)	2 (6.7)	3 (10.0)	0.36	1.000
Anti-hypertensive medication, yes	11 (10.0)	7 (14.0)	4 (13.3)	0 (0.0)	5.22	.101
Lipid-lowering medication, yes	7 (6.4)	0 (0.0)	5 (16.7)	2 (6.7)	8.74	.007
Markers of subclinical atherosclerosis						
FMD, %	10.76 (3.457)	11.10 (3.263)	9.94 (3.477)	11.08 (3.723)	1.18	.310
PWV, m/sec	7.86 (1.356)	7.77 (1.615)	7.89 (1.210)	7.99 (1.005)	0.24	.784
IMT, mm	0.67 (0.128)	0.68 (0.118)	0.68 (0.131)	0.66 (0.142)	0.32	.724
Anthropometric profile						
Body weight, kg	72.4 (10.55)	72.3 (9.94)	70.8 (10.25)	74.2 (11.86)	0.77	.467
Body mass index, kg/m^2	28.5 (0.36)	28.5 (0.54)	27.9 (0.58)	29.1 (0.79)	0.79	.456
Lean body mass, kg	46.0 (4.76)	46.0 (4.69)	45.5 (5.11)	46.4 (4.63)	0.25	.776
Cardiometabolic profile						
Waist circumference, cm	94.8 (7.80)	94.4 (7.00)	93.8 (7.25)	96.4 (9.46)	0.93	.397
Systolic BP, mmHg	116.5 (13.08)	116.6 (12.97)	117.4 (10.38)	115.6 (15.78)	0.15	.859
Total cholesterol, mg/dL	212.1 (39.74)	214.8 (37.51)	204.5 (45.99)	215.2 (36.81)	0.75	.476
LDL-cholesterol, mg/dL	129.1 (36.39)	130.3 (32.46)	120.2 (42.98)	135.9 (34.75)	1.47	.235
HDL-cholesterol, mg/dL	53.1 (12.61)	53.0 (12.59)	51.6 (15.14)	54.6 (9.78)	0.44	.642
Triglycerides, mg/dL	131.2 (98.40, 73.50)	147.1 (97.10, 205.65)	136.5 (105.05, 177.15)	122.3 (96.13, 146.93)	2.16	.120
Fasting glucose, mg/dL	89.6 (14.45)	90.1 (16.72)	93.6 (14.50)	84.9 (8.05)	2.89	.060
Dietary intake[a]						
Total energy (kcal/day)	1538.2 (446.01)	1498.9 (441.99)	1552.3 (360.01)	1585.8 (525.19)	0.33	.717
Carbohydrates (g/day)	218.5 (64.91)	217.5 (74.77)	216.8 (40.41)	221.6 (68.26)	0.05	.956
Protein (g/day)	65.4 (25.62)	61.9 (18.10)	66.6 (23.40)	69.6 (35.68)	0.82	.445
Lipid (g/day)	45.6 (18.23)	43.3 (17.53)	46.4 (15.78)	48.4 (21.27)	0.68	.508
Cardiorespiratory fitness						
VO$_{2max}$, mL/kg/min	31.1 (6.24)	31.3 (5.80)	30.6 (6.16)	31.3 (7.15)	0.16	.849

BP = blood pressure; FMD = flow mediated dilation; HDL = high-density lipoprotein; LDL = low-density lipoprotein; PWV = pulse wave velocity; IMT = intima media thickness; SD = standard deviation; VO$_{2max}$ = maximal oxygen consumption; Obesity-related conditions include hypertension and dyslipidemia.
*P-values from one-way ANOVA, chi-square or Fisher's exact test as appropriate [a]Analyzed with the sample size (N = 96).

Table 2 Differential effects of exercise mode on markers of subclinical atherosclerosis and anthropometric and cardiometabolic profiles over time

| | Modified intention-to-treat analysis (N = 92) | | | | Per-protocol analysis (N = 49) | | | |
| | Mean (SD) | | | P[a] | Mean (SD) | | | P[a] |
	Aerobic (n = 39)	Resistance (n = 26)	Combination (n = 27)		Aerobic (n = 20)	Resistance (n = 14)	Combination (n = 15)	
FMD (%)				.792				.847
3 M	11.28 (3.50)	10.32 (3.80)	11.02 (3.49)		11.51 (4.02)	10.75 (3.67)	11.32 (3.37)	
6 M	11.55 (3.80)	11.22 (4.43)	11.10 (3.40)		12.38 (4.43)	11.02 (4.39)	11.46 (3.74)	
9 M	11.08 (4.05)	10.89 (4.33)	12.41 (4.27)		11.34 (4.88)	10.05 (4.11)	13.18 (4.34)	
12 M	10.70 (3.75)	11.54 (4.99)	11.30 (4.04)		10.56 (4.15)	11.26 (5.49)	11.20 (4.09)	
PWV (m/sec)				.585				.732
3 M	7.91 (1.18)	7.62 (1.16)	8.11 (1.05)		7.51 (0.77)	7.49 (0.82)	7.81 (1.04)	
6 M	7.83 (1.31)	7.52 (1.15)	7.76 (1.04)		7.36 (0.94)	7.34 (0.75)	7.37 (0.98)	
9 M	7.94 (1.32)	7.70 (1.18)	7.96 (1.01)		7.53 (1.15)	7.60 (0.83)	7.59 (1.02)	
12 M	7.88 (1.30)	7.74 (1.17)	7.96 (0.89)		7.45 (1.00)	7.67 (0.81)	7.61 (0.80)	
IMT (mm)				.574				.379
3 M	0.71 (0.19)	0.72 (0.17)	0.66 (0.10)		0.74 (0.24)	0.72 (0.19)	0.65 (0.09)	
6 M	0.68 (0.15)	0.67 (0.14)	0.64 (0.12)		0.71 (0.18)	0.65 (0.14)	0.65 (0.13)	
9 M	0.69 (0.14)	0.69 (0.14)	0.67 (0.10)		0.73 (0.16)	0.69 (0.13)	0.67 (0.10)	
12 M	0.70 (0.14)	0.70 (0.13)	0.67 (0.11)		0.73 (0.15)	0.71 (0.11)	0.68 (0.12)	
Body weight (kg)				.539				.894
3 M	71.11 (10.69)	67.20 (9.36)	72.62 (12.06)		69.48 (11.63)	64.19 (5.59)	69.06 (8.69)	
6 M	69.48 (11.70)	65.70 (9.45)	71.30 (12.25)		67.14 (12.84)	62.71 (6.27)	66.93 (7.74)	
9 M	69.31 (11.81)	65.60 (9.29)	71.69 (12.25)		65.25 (8.75)	62.64 (6.26)	67.15 (7.87)	
12 M	69.34 (11.84)	65.79 (9.34)	71.75 (12.63)		67.23 (12.70)	62.99 (6.57)	67.25 (8.98)	
Lean body mass (kg)				.717				.637
3 M	45.41 (4.96)	44.44 (5.09)	45.94 (4.95)		44.49 (5.88)	43.50 (4.92)	44.60 (3.81)	
6 M	45.06 (5.28)	44.46 (4.90)	45.90 (4.83)		44.95 (6.34)	43.62 (4.69)	44.38 (3.53)	
9 M	45.03 (5.18)	44.30 (5.02)	45.90 (4.62)		44.25 (4.62)	43.62 (5.05)	44.36 (3.24)	
12 M	44.94 (5.14)	44.29 (4.73)	45.74 (4.76)		44.91 (6.04)	43.61 (4.48)	44.07 (3.45)	
WC (cm)				.790				.825
3 M	93.44 (8.06)	90.14 (8.04)	94.42 (11.36)		91.32 (8.00)	87.26 (4.72)	90.41 (7.11)	
6 M	91.39 (9.41)	87.87 (8.56)	92.83 (12.00)		88.59 (9.67)	84.54 (5.25)	87.46 (7.38)	
9 M	90.77 (9.82)	88.12 (8.11)	93.61 (11.68)		87.61 (8.99)	85.21 (4.68)	88.39 (6.99)	
12 M	91.27 (9.33)	88.78 (7.98)	94.09 (11.58)		89.18 (9.24)	86.44 (4.97)	89.28 (7.33)	
Systolic BP (mmHg)				.935				.838
3 M	115.36 (15.84)	113.10 (11.99)	113.94 (17.98)		114.18 (12.81)	109.07 (9.46)	110.43 (13.70)	
6 M	113.06 (15.46)	112.37 (10.23)	112.74 (17.79)		111.03 (14.66)	111.29 (12.10)	107.53 (11.93)	
9 M	114.62 (14.55)	113.21 (9.53)	112.48 (17.42)		113.33 (13.19)	110.79 (8.74)	106.60 (8.01)	
12 M	113.95 (14.41)	111.94 (10.29)	112.91 (18.64)		112.03 (12.17)	108.43 (9.49)	107.37 (12.45)	
TC (mg/dL)				.517				.689
3 M	197.11 1(44.28)	192.13 (32.70)	201.30 (34.03)		205.07 (51.68)	185.94 (28.42)	191.34 (38.60)	
6 M	195.14 (36.26)	192.95 (35.23)	202.67 (38.54)		198.05 (39.55)	186.59 (28.53)	190.07 (42.89)	
9 M	201.65 (37.10)	202.18 (40.98)	207.30 (38.77)		205.51 (40.42)	203.40 (41.73)	195.81 (43.64)	
12 M	198.86 (42.22)	197.64 (41.46)	201.83 (40.73)		202.53 (50.23)	193.34 (42.04)	185.39 (43.74)	

Table 2 Differential effects of exercise mode on markers of subclinical atherosclerosis and anthropometric and cardiometabolic profiles over time (Continued)

				p				p
LDL-C (mg/dL)				.458				.300
3 M	119.22 (38.47)	114.40 (29.22)	121.88 (36.97)		128.36 (47.15)	111.60 (31.37)	110.59 (40.99)	
6 M	116.65 (30.49)	115.46 (28.85)	124.18 (35.65)		121.73 (35.34)	110.64 (27.77)	112.96 (38.75)	
9 M	121.99 (32.78)	118.19 (39.83)	129.31 (39.32)		127.99 (37.16)	117.66 (46.93)	117.65 (42.97)	
12 M	116.85 (36.74)	116.70 (39.86)	123.48 (39.58)		123.66 (44.04)	113.70 (46.65)	106.80 (39.76)	
HDL-C (mg/dL)				.973				.562
3 M	52.91 (12.29)	49.25 (12.57)	53.58 (10.09)		52.27 (12.55)	46.98 (13.77)	54.99 (11.10)	
6 M	53.74 (13.04)	53.60 q(13.93)	54.79 (10.69)		53.70 (14.45)	51.99 (16.37)	56.19 (12.54)	
9 M	54.52 (12.48)	55.68 (14.20)	56.20 (10.07)		55.78 (13.15)	56.04 (16.64)	59.19 (11.69)	
12 M	57.72 (15.15)	54.69 (13.17)	56.39 (10.35)		59.09 (14.98)	53.51 (14.94)	59.39 (11.96)	
Triglycerides (mg/dL)								.784
3 M	124.90 (59.18)	142.40 (75.42)	129.23 (100.99)		122.18 (43.31)	136.77 (96.43)	128.83 (128.67)	
6 M	123.74 (71.06)	119.47 (57.73)	118.53 (56.25)		113.06 (57.94)	119.85 (69.02)	104.58 (58.74)	
9 M	125.72 (68.76)	141.51 (91.41)	108.93 (50.78)		108.70 (44.08)	148.51 (120.31)	94.87 (52.08)	
12 M	120.88 (70.84)	131.24 (82.54)	109.78 (48.56)		97.81 (38.99)	130.63 (107.88)	96.03 (48.36)	
Fasting glucose (mg/dL)				.413				.034
3 M	88.93 (9.87)	94.54 (19.83)	89.39 (7.69)		86.40 (7.51)	93.54 (12.40)	88.52 (7.78)	
6 M	85.80 (7.90)	91.68 (19.82)	85.67 (7.47)		83.85 (6.56)	89.71 1(12.61)	82.56 (7.86)	
9 M	84.98 (9.76)	93.16 (22.15)	84.97 (8.23)		82.33 (9.23)	94.61 (17.40)	81.33 (8.53)	
12 M	89.78 (8.28)	92.84 (22.41)	86.30 (7.22)		89.26 (7.07)	93.54 (18.33)	81.91 (5.95)*	
VO$_{2max}$ (mL/kg/min)								
3 M	31.77 (5.45)	32.55 (5.04)	32.02 (5.41)	.972	32.72 (3.92)	33.75 (4.57)	33.45 (4.91)	.052
6 M	35.05 (6.72)	34.32 (5.50)	36.36 (6.90)		36.37 (4.77)	35.59 (3.42)	39.27 (4.87)	
9 M	35.62 (6.81)	35.07 (5.89)	34.49 (5.95)		38.24 (5.48)	36.25 (5.14)	36.31 (4.17)	
12 M	34.11 (6.29)	34.61 (6.05)	34.89 (6.45)		35.41 (4.84)	35.82 (5.67)	37.04 (5.28)	

[a]P-values for significance of interaction effects between exercise group and time via the generalized estimating equation.
FMD = flow mediated dilation; PWV = pulse wave velocity; HDL-C = high-density lipoprotein cholesterol; IMT = intima media thickness; LDL-C = low-density lipoprotein cholesterol; SD = standard deviation; TC = total cholesterol; VO$_{2max}$ = maximal oxygen consumption; WC = waist circumference.
*P < .05 is for a significant difference in fasting glucose levels by exercise mode at 12 months.

found significant time effects for body weight (p < .001), lean body mass (p = .040), waist circumference (p < .001), total cholesterol (p = .006), LDL cholesterol (p = .020), and HDL cholesterol levels (p < .001), fasting glucose levels (p < .001), and VO$_{2max}$ (p < .001), based on the modified ITT analysis results. In other words, regardless of the exercise modes, PWV, IMT, body weight, waist circumference, and total and LDL cholesterol levels significantly decreased over time in the diet-plus-exercise intervention; HDL cholesterol level and VO$_{2max}$ significantly increased over time in the diet-plus-exercise intervention. Specifically, changes in body weight, waist circumference, HDL cholesterol level, and VO$_{2max}$ primarily showed linear trends. The IMT and fasting glucose levels showed quadratic curve trends, while PWV and total and LDL cholesterol levels showed cubic curve trends, based on the modified ITT analysis results. The findings from

the PP analyses almost closely matched those from the modified ITT analyses.

Discussion

The exercise mode did not have significant differential effects on FMD, PWV, and IMT in the diet-plus-exercise intervention of a 12-month weight management program. However, the exercise mode had a significant differential effect on fasting glucose levels; combination exercise lowered fasting glucose levels more effectively than aerobic exercise. Meanwhile, there were significant time effects of the diet-plus-exercise intervention, i.e., reductions in PWV and IMT in cubic and quadratic trends, respectively, and improvements in body weight; waist circumference; levels of total, LDL, and HDL cholesterol; and cardiorespiratory fitness in linear, quadratic, or cubic trends.

Effects of weight management by exercise modes on markers of subclinical atherosclerosis...

51

Table 3 Time effects on markers of subclinical atherosclerosis and anthropometric and cardiometabolic profiles

	Modified intention-to-teat analysis (N = 92)		Per-protocol analysis (N = 49)	
	Mean (SD)	P^a	Mean (SD)	P^a
FMD (mm)				
3 M	10.93 (3.57)	.676	11.23 (3.67)	.628
6 M	11.33 (3.84)		1171 (4.17)	
9 M	11.41 (4.20)		11.54 (4.57)	
12 M	11.11 (4.18)		10.93 (4.47)	
PWV (m/sec)				
3 M	7.89 (1.14)	.048‡	7.60 (0.87)	.055
6 M	7.72 (1.19)		7.36 (0.88)	
9 M	7.88 (1.19)		7.57 (1.00)	
12 M	7.87 (1.15)		7.56 (0.88)	
IMT (mm)				
3 M	0.70 (0.16)	.018†‡	0.71 (0.19)	.042
6 M	0.67 (0.14)		0.67 (0.16)	
9 M	0.68 (0.13)		0.70 (0.13)	
12 M	0.69 (0.13)		0.71 (0.13)	
Body weight (kg)				
3 M	70.45 (10.86)	<.001*†‡	67.84 (9.46)	<.001*†‡
6 M	68.95 (11.37)		65.81 (9.87)	
9 M	68.96 (11.41)		65.08 (7.84)	
12 M	69.04 (11.55)		66.03 (10.14)	
Lean body mass (kg)				
3 M	45.29 (4.97)	.040*	44.65 (5.01)	.153
6 M	45.14 (5.02)		44.40 (5.08)	
9 M	45.08 (4.96)		44.10 (4.29)	
12 M	44.99 (4.89)		44.28 (4.86)	
WC (cm)				
3 M	92.80 (9.21)	<.001*†‡	89.88 (7.01)	<.001†
6 M	90.82 (10.10)		87.09 (7.95)	
9 M	90.85 (10.08)		87.14 (7.26)	
12 M	91.39 (9.81)		88.42 (7.60)	
Systolic BP(mmHg)				
3 M	114.30 (15.41)	.245	111.57 (12.21)	.253
6 M	112.77 (14.80)		110.03 (13.00)	
9 M	113.59 (14.18)		110.43 (10.65)	
12 M	113.08 (14.69)		109.57 (11.51)	
TC (mg/dL)				
3 M	196.93 (38.15)	.006‡	195.40 (42.20)	.013‡
6 M	196.73 (36.47)		192.33 (37.43)	
9 M	203.46 (38.37)		201.86 (41.14)	
12 M	199.39 (41.15)		194.66 (45.70)	

Table 3 Time effects on markers of subclinical atherosclerosis and anthropometric and cardiometabolic profiles (Continued)

LDL-C (mg/dL)				
3 M	118.64 (35.38)	.020[‡]	118.13 (41.36)	.034[‡]
6 M	118.52 (31.52)		115.88 (34.15)	
9 M	123.07 (36.68)		121.74 (41.40)	
12 M	118.76 (38.17)		115.65 (43.25)	
HDL-C (mg/dL)				
3 M	52.07 (11.78)	<.001[*]	51.59 (12.63)	<.001[*]
6 M	54.01 (12.54)		53.97 (14.28)	
9 M	55.34 (12.25)		56.92 (13.64)	
12 M	56.47 (13.26)		57.59 (14.06)	
Triglycerides (mg/dL)				
3 M	131.12 (77.41)	.289	128.39 (90.15)	.197
6 M	121.00 (62.72)		112.40 (60.51)	
9 M	125.25 (71.84)		115.99 (77.68)	
12 M	120.55 (68.62)		106.64 (68.35)	
Fasting glucose (mg/dL)				
3 M	90.65 (13.13)	<.001[†]	89.09 (9.52)	.034[*†]
6 M	87.42 (12.54)		85.13 (9.33)	
9 M	87.29 (14.41)		85.60 (13.13)	
12 M	89.62 (13.70)		88.23 (11.93)	
VO$_{2max}$ (mL/kg/min)				
3 M	32.06 (5.27)	<.001[*†‡]	33.23 (4.34)	<.001[*†]
6 M	35.24 (6.44)		37.04 (4.63)	
9 M	35.14 (6.26)		37.05 (4.97)	
12 M	34.48 (6.21)		36.02 (5.15)	

[a]P-values for an equality of mean values across periods; Significance of trend tests: *Linear trend, †Quadratic trend, ‡Cubic trend.
FMD = flow mediated dilation; PWV = pulse wave velocity; IMT = intima media thickness; HDL-C = high-density lipoprotein cholesterol; LDL-C = low-density lipoprotein cholesterol; SD = standard deviation; TC = total cholesterol; VO$_{2max}$ = maximal oxygen consumption; WC = waist circumference.

We found neither differential effects of exercise modes nor time effects of the diet-plus-exercise intervention on FMD in women with abdominal obesity. Several studies have previously reported the beneficial effects of both aerobic and resistance exercise on FMD. Aerobic exercise training is well known to improve FMD [30-32], although only a few studies have reported the effects of aerobic exercise on FMD in obese individuals. Watts et al. [33] reported that FMD was significantly greater among trained obese children compared with untrained obese children after 8 weeks of aerobic exercise training [33]. Similarly, either resistance or combination exercise training may be effective in improving endothelial function, although this was found in small-scale studies, thereby necessitating further confirmation [13,34,35]. In a study of 30 overweight women, Olson et al. [13] reported that FMD improved significantly in a resistance exercise group compared with a control group after a 1-year resistance training intervention [13]. Maiorana et al. [35] reported in a crossover study that a combination of aerobic and

resistance exercise for 8 weeks significantly increased FMD among 16 patients with type 2 diabetes mellitus [35]. Nevertheless, only a few studies have reported the differential effects of exercise mode [36]. Kwon et al. [36] found that aerobic exercise provide greater improvement in FMD than resistance exercise among 40 overweight women with type 2 diabetes mellitus in a comparison study of exercise mode [36].

In the present study, the non-significant differential effects of exercise mode on FMD for women with abdominal obesity may be explained by the complex effects of both exercise and diet in our study design. In previous studies, the effects of exercise training combined with dietary interventions have thus far yielded mixed results among obese individuals. Hamdy et al. [37] reported an improvement in the FMD in 24 obese individuals after a 6-month lifestyle modification consisting of both energy-restricted diet and aerobic exercise training [37]. In contrast, Wycherley et al. [19] did not find any significant improvement in the FMD in 29 obese patients with type II diabetes after a 12-week caloric restriction with aerobic exercise training [19]. Such conflicting findings might be attributable to distinct characteristics of FMD from other measures of subclinical atherosclerosis such as carotid IMT. The Firefighters and their Endothelium study (2005) [38] showed that the FMD had no significant correlation with carotid IMT among middle-aged men who were at low-to-moderate risk of cardiovascular diseases [38]. FMD is a well-standardized measure of endothelial function that is considered an early manifestation of atherosclerosis [39]. Furthermore, FMD is an acute indicator of vascular function, as opposed to carotid IMT, which is a chronic indicator of vascular structural abnormalities. Therefore, changes in FMD may, in part, result from acute influences such as within-individual variations in the exposure to the complex effects of either exercise or diet (i.e., changes in body weight or cardiometabolic risk factors) when they were measured. Meanwhile, non-significant changes in the FMD found in the present study may also be explained by the normal range ($\geq$5.5%) of the FMD values at baseline (10.8%; range, 4.0–18.0% in our data). Swift et al. [31] reported a significant improvement in the FMD in obese women with impaired FMD, but not in those with normal FMD at baseline after a 6-month aerobic exercise training program [31].

We found no differential effect of exercise mode on aortic PWV, but a significant reduction in aortic PWV with the diet-plus-exercise intervention over time. Aerobic exercise training has previously been reported to decrease aortic PWV in a few studies, although the findings were limited to healthy men. Hayashi et al. [40] reported that 16 weeks of aerobic training with moderate-intensity walking and jogging significantly decreased aortic PWV in 17 sedentary middle-aged men [40]. Collier et al. [41] found that aerobic exercise led to a decrease in aortic PWV, whereas resistance exercise led to a significant increase in aortic PWV after 4-week training among 30 middle-aged individuals with prehypertension or stage1 hypertension [41]. However, such increases in aortic PWV with resistance training need to be further clarified. In fact, we did not find any increase in aortic PWV in the resistance exercise group. Similarly, a meta-analysis by Miyachi showed that resistance training may not be associated with increases in aortic PWV in middle-aged subjects [42]. Meanwhile, our data showed that the reduction in aortic PWV peaked at 6 months in the entire intervention and rebounded after the next 6 months in the diet-plus-exercise intervention in a cubic curve trend; this trend appeared to parallel with the weight loss trend in our data. Dengo et al. [43] reported that a reduction in aortic PWV correlated with reductions in total body and abdominal adiposity among overweight and obese adults [43]. In this context, the reduction of aortic PWV may be primarily related to exercise-induced energy expenditure contributing to weight loss rather than exercise mode.

We did not find any differential effect of exercise modes on carotid IMT. Instead, we found a significant regression in carotid IMT with the diet-plus-exercise intervention as a time effect. Similarly, Spence et al. [44] reported that there was no significant differential effect of aerobic versus resistance exercise training on carotid IMT, but there was a significant time effect among 23 young healthy male subjects with 24 weeks of exercise training [44]. Dutheil et al. [17] investigated the effects of combination exercise on carotid IMT according to exercise intensity, and reported that moderate-resistance high-aerobic exercise was more effective for the regression of carotid IMT than moderate-resistance moderate-aerobic exercise [17]. Thus, we speculate that the effects of exercise training on carotid IMT may be influenced by exercise intensity but not by exercise mode.

In our findings, the regression effect of exercise training on carotid IMT (i.e., a time effect) was not linear over time, with a peak at 6 months that was not maintained to 12 months, consistent with the findings of a previous study [45]. There was little evidence for beneficial effects of a lifestyle intervention (i.e., either diet-alone or diet-plus-exercise intervention) on carotid IMT among overweight and obese individuals [45-47]. Fuentes et al. [45] reported a significant regression in carotid IMT over a 24-month follow-up with a diet-induced weight-loss intervention involving 60 obese individuals [45]. Carotid IMT is a vascular measure of structural changes in the carotid arteries, so a reduction in carotid IMT may require long-duration interventions. Thus, the underlying mechanism of these short-term changes in carotid IMT with the diet-plus-exercise intervention need to be further clarified, but we could speculate that the changes are the result of various favorable changes in the cardiometabolic risk factors that occur concomitantly with weight loss induced by the diet-plus-exercise intervention.

Finally, we found a significant differential effect of exercise mode on fasting glucose levels but not on vascular measures (i.e., FMD, PWV, and IMT); specifically, combination of aerobic and resistance exercises was significantly more effective in lowering fasting glucose levels than aerobic exercise alone in the diet-plus-exercise intervention. The beneficial effect of a combination of aerobic and resistance exercises on glucose control has been previously reported only in patients with type 2 diabetes [21,48,49] but not in overweight and obese individuals. Snowling et al. [49] concluded, from their meta-analysis, that aerobic, resistance, and combination exercises had small-to-moderate beneficial effects on glucose control in patients with type 2 diabetes; particularly, compared to aerobic exercise, combination exercise was found to lower fasting glucose levels, albeit to a small extent [49]. Meanwhile, the conflicting effects of exercise mode on fasting glucose levels versus vascular measures may be explained by different exercise-induced physiological responses. The beneficial effect of combination exercise on fasting glucose levels may be attributable to an additional beneficial effect of resistance exercise to aerobic exercise. Physiologically, similar to aerobic exercise, resistance exercise can increase glucose uptake and glycogen repletion in skeletal muscle following exercise by promoting contraction-mediated GLUT4 translocation with increased activation of AMP-activated protein kinase [50]. In this context, both aerobic and resistance exercise may provide a synergistic effect on glucose metabolism. In contrast, non-significant differential effects of exercise mode on vascular measures (i.e., PWV and IMT) may indicate that changes in vascular measures influenced by vascular tone and remodeling with exercise training are not influenced by exercise mode but instead by other components such as exercise intensity or exercise expenditure [17].

This study, to the best of our knowledge, is the first to report on the effects of exercise modes in a weight management intervention on major markers of subclinical atherosclerosis such as endothelial dysfunction, arterial stiffness, and carotid IMT. Nevertheless, this study has several limitations. First, the attrition rate in the study was 55% over 12 months, and this may have led to a bias influencing the validity of results. However, the present study was initiated and implemented as a community-based program and its attrition rate was similar to that in previous studies conducted as community-based programs [51]. Second, of the participants included in the modified ITT analysis (n = 92), 68% had a menstrual cycle. FMD may modulate in response to changing hormonal patterns during the menstrual cycle [52]. Lack of consideration of the effects of the menstrual cycle in vascular measurements might have underestimated or overestimated changes in FMD. Third, since all the participants in present study were Korean women, the results cannot be generalized to men or other ethnic groups.

Conclusions

For women with abdominal obesity, a combination of aerobic and resistance exercise may be preferable to a single mode (i.e., aerobic or resistance exercise) for effective glucose control. Regardless of exercise mode, exercise interventions combined with dietary interventions may be beneficial for reducing the risk of subclinical atherosclerosis and cardiometabolic risk in women with abdominal obesity. Such beneficial effects of exercise training may not be differentiated by exercise mode but by other exercise components such as exercise intensity or expenditure.

Competing interests
The authors declare that they have no competing interests.

Authors' contributions
The authors' contributions were as follows: JC developed the hypothesis of this study and prepared the manuscript draft; JC, JHC, and SYJ were involved in data collection; JC and JL performed the data analyses; SYJ, AS and LEB provided expert consultation on data interpretation and helped to draft the manuscript. All authors were involved in the review and revision of the manuscript and gave approval for the final version to be published.

Acknowledgements
This research was supported by the Basic Science Research Program through the National Research Foundation of Korea (NRF) funded by the Ministry of Education, Science and Technology (No. 2010–0022022).

Author details
[1]College of Nursing, Korea University, Seoul, South Korea. [2]Department of Biostatistics, College of Medicine, Korea University, Seoul, South Korea. [3]School of Nursing and Epidemiology and Clinical and Translational Science Institute, University of Pittsburgh, Pennsylvania, USA. [4]Department of Epidemiology, Graduate School of Public Health, University of Pittsburgh, Pennsylvania, USA. [5]College of Arts and Physical Education, University of Seoul, Seoul, South Korea.

References
1. Flint AJ, Rexrode KM, Hu FB, Glynn RJ, Caspard H, Manson JE, Willett WC, Rimm EB: Body mass index, waist circumference, and risk of coronary heart disease: a prospective study among men and women. *Obes Res Clin Pract* 2010, 4(3):e171–e181.
2. Arcaro G, Zamboni M, Rossi L, Turcato E, Covi G, Armellini F, Bosello O, Lechi A: Body fat distribution predicts the degree of endothelial dysfunction in uncomplicated obesity. *Int J Obes Relat Metab Disord* 1999, 23(9):936–942.
3. Recio-Rodriguez JI, Gomez-Marcos MA, Patino-Alonso MC, Agudo-Conde C, Rodriguez-Sanchez E, Garcia-Ortiz L: Abdominal obesity vs general obesity for identifying arterial stiffness, subclinical atherosclerosis and wave reflection in healthy, diabetics and hypertensive. *BMC Cardiovasc Disord* 2012, 12:3.
4. Asicioglu E, Kahveci A, Arikan H, Koc M, Tuglular S, Ozener CI: Waist circumference is associated with carotid intima media thickness in peritoneal dialysis patients. *Int Urol Nephrol* 2013, 45(5):1437–1443.
5. Rexrode KM, Carey VJ, Hennekens CH, Walters EE, Colditz GA, Stampfer MJ, Willett WC, Manson JE: Abdominal adiposity and coronary heart disease in women. *JAMA* 1998, 280(21):1843–1848.
6. Rexrode KM, Buring JE, Manson JE: Abdominal and total adiposity and risk of coronary heart disease in men. *Int J Obes Relat Metab Disord* 2001, 25(7):1047–1056.
7. Arsenault BJ, Rana JS, Lemieux I, Despres JP, Kastelein JJ, Boekholdt SM, Wareham NJ, Khaw KT: Physical inactivity, abdominal obesity and risk of coronary heart disease in apparently healthy men and women. *Int J Obes (Lond)* 2010, 34(2):340–347.
8. Wu T, Gao X, Chen M, van Dam RM: Long-term effectiveness of diet-plus-exercise interventions vs. diet-only interventions for weight loss: a meta-analysis. *Obes Rev* 2009, 10(3):313–323.
9. Kelley GA, Kelley KS: Effects of diet, aerobic exercise, or both on non-HDL-C in adults: a meta-analysis of randomized controlled trials. *Cholesterol* 2012, 2012:840935.
10. Wing RR, Venditti E, Jakicic JM, Polley BA, Lang W: Lifestyle intervention in overweight individuals with a family history of diabetes. *Diabetes Care* 1998, 21(3):350–359.
11. Hagan RD, Upton SJ, Wong L, Whittam J: The effects of aerobic conditioning and/or caloric restriction in overweight men and women. *Med Sci Sports Exerc* 1986, 18(1):87–94.
12. Beck DT, Martin JS, Casey DP, Braith RW: Exercise training reduces peripheral arterial stiffness and myocardial oxygen demand in young prehypertensive subjects. *Am J Hypertens* 2013, 26(9):1093–1102.
13. Olson TP, Dengel DR, Leon AS, Schmitz KH: Moderate resistance training and vascular health in overweight women. *Med Sci Sports Exerc* 2006, 38(9):1558–1564.
14. Tjonna AE, Stolen TO, Bye A, Volden M, Slordahl SA, Odegard R, Skogvoll E, Wisloff U: Aerobic interval training reduces cardiovascular risk factors

more than a multitreatment approach in overweight adolescents. *Clin Sci (Lond)* 2009, **116**(4):317–326.

15. Guimaraes GV, Ciolac EG, Carvalho VO, D'Avila VM, Bortolotto LA, Bocchi EA: Effects of continuous vs. interval exercise training on blood pressure and arterial stiffness in treated hypertension. *Hypertens Res* 2010, **33**(6):627–632.

16. Goodpaster BH, Delany JP, Otto AD, Kuller L, Vockley J, South-Paul JE, Thomas SB, Brown J, McTigue K, Hames KC, Lang W, Jakicic JM: Effects of diet and physical activity interventions on weight loss and cardiometabolic risk factors in severely obese adults: a randomized trial. *JAMA* 2010, **304**(16):1795–1802.

17. Dutheil F, Lac G, Lesourd B, Chapier R, Walther G, Vinet A, Sapin V, Verney J, Ouchchane L, Duclos M, Obert P, Courteix D, Obert P, Courteix D: Different modalities of exercise to reduce visceral fat mass and cardiovascular risk in metabolic syndrome: the RESOLVE randomized trial. *Int J Cardiol* 2013, **168**(4):3634–3642.

18. McKelvie RS, McCartney N, Tomlinson C, Bauer R, MacDougall JD: Comparison of hemodynamic responses to cycling and resistance exercise in congestive heart failure secondary to ischemic cardiomyopathy. *Am J Cardiol* 1995, **76**(12):977–979.

19. Wycherley TP, Brinkworth GD, Noakes M, Buckley JD, Clifton PM: Effect of caloric restriction with and without exercise training on oxidative stress and endothelial function in obese subjects with type 2 diabetes. *Diabetes Obes Metab* 2008, **10**(11):1062–1073.

20. Schwingshackl L, Dias S, Strasser B, Hoffmann G: Impact of different training modalities on anthropometric and metabolic characteristics in overweight/obese subjects: a systematic review and network meta-analysis. *PLoS One* 2013, **8**(12):e82853.

21. Sigal RJ, Kenny GP, Boule NG, Wells GA, Prud'homme D, Fortier M, Reid RD, Tulloch H, Coyle D, Phillips P, Jennings A, Jaffey J: Effects of aerobic training, resistance training, or both on glycemic control in type 2 diabetes: a randomized trial. *Ann Intern Med* 2007, **147**(6):357–369.

22. Foster-Schubert KE, Alfano CM, Duggan CR, Xiao L, Campbell KL, Kong A, Bain CE, Wang CY, Blackburn GL, McTiernan A: Effect of diet and exercise, alone or combined, on weight and body composition in overweight-to-obese postmenopausal women. *Obesity (Silver Spring)* 2012, **20**(8):1628–1638.

23. Lee SY, Park HS, Kim DJ, Han JH, Kim SM, Cho GJ, Kim DY, Kwon HS, Kim SR, Lee CB, Oh SJ, Park CY, Yoo HJ: Appropriate waist circumference cutoff points for central obesity in Korean adults. *Diabetes Res Clin Pract* 2007, **75**(1):72–80.

24. Cho JH, Jae SY, Choo IL, Choo J: Health-promoting behaviour among women with abdominal obesity: a conceptual link to social support and perceived stress. *J Adv Nurs* 2014, **70**(6):1381–1390.

25. Burke LE, Wang J: Treatment strategies for overweight and obesity. *J Nurs Scholarsh* 2011, **43**(4):368–375.

26. Friedewald WT, Levy RI, Fredrickson DS: Estimation of the concentration of low-density lipoprotein cholesterol in plasma, without use of the preparative ultracentrifuge. *Clin Chem* 1972, **18**(6):499–502.

27. Kline GM, Porcari JP, Hintermeister R, Freedson PS, Ward A, McCarron RF, Ross J, Rippe JM: Estimation of VO2max from a one-mile track walk, gender, age, and body weight. *Med Sci Sports Exerc* 1987, **19**(3):253–259.

28. *Third Report of the Expert Panel on Detection, Evaluation, and Treatment of the High Blood Cholesterol in Adults (Adult Treatment Panel III): Executive Summary*. http://www.nhlbi.nih.gov/guidelines/cholesterol/atp_iii.htm.

29. Grundy SM, Cleeman JI, Daniels SR, Donato KA, Eckel RH, Franklin BA, Gordon DJ, Krauss RM, Savage PJ, Smith SC Jr, Spertus JA, Costa F: Diagnosis and management of the metabolic syndrome: an American Heart Association/National Heart, Lung, and Blood Institute Scientific Statement. *Circulation* 2005, **112**(17):2735–2752.

30. McDermott MM, Ades P, Guralnik JM, Dyer A, Ferrucci L, Liu K, Nelson M, Lloyd-Jones D, Van Horn L, Garside D, Kibbe M, Domanchuk K, Stein JH, Liao Y, Tao H, Green D, Pearce WH, Schneider JR, McPherson D, Laing ST, McCarthy WJ, Shroff A, Criqui MH: Treadmill exercise and resistance training in patients with peripheral arterial disease with and without intermittent claudication: a randomized controlled trial. *JAMA* 2009, **301**(2):165–174.

31. Swift DL, Earnest CP, Blair SN, Church TS: The effect of different doses of aerobic exercise training on endothelial function in postmenopausal women with elevated blood pressure: results from the DREW study. *Br J Sports Med* 2012, **46**(10):753–758.

32. DeSouza CA, Shapiro LF, Clevenger CM, Dinenno FA, Monahan KD, Tanaka H, Seals DR: Regular aerobic exercise prevents and restores age-related declines in endothelium-dependent vasodilation in healthy men. *Circulation* 2000, **102**(12):1351–1357.

33. Watts K, Beye P, Siafarikas A, O'Driscoll G, Jones TW, Davis EA, Green DJ: Effects of exercise training on vascular function in obese children. *J Pediatr* 2004, **144**(5):620–625.

34. Okada S, Hiuge A, Makino H, Nagumo A, Takaki H, Konishi H, Goto Y, Yoshimasa Y, Miyamoto Y: Effect of exercise intervention on endothelial function and incidence of cardiovascular disease in patients with type 2 diabetes. *J Atheroscler Thromb* 2010, **17**(8):828–833.

35. Maiorana A, O'Driscoll G, Cheetham C, Dembo L, Stanton K, Goodman C, Taylor R, Green D: The effect of combined aerobic and resistance exercise training on vascular function in type 2 diabetes. *J Am Coll Cardiol* 2001, **38**(3):860–866.

36. Kwon HR, Min KW, Ahn HJ, Seok HG, Lee JH, Park GS, Han KA: Effects of aerobic exercise vs. resistance training on endothelial function in women with type 2 diabetes mellitus. *Diabetes Metab J* 2011, **35**(4):364–373.

37. Hamdy O, Ledbury S, Mullooly C, Jarema C, Porter S, Ovalle K, Moussa A, Caselli A, Caballero AE, Economides PA, Veves A, Horton ES: Lifestyle modification improves endothelial function in obese subjects with the insulin resistance syndrome. *Diabetes Care* 2003, **26**(7):2119–2125.

38. Yan RT, Anderson TJ, Charbonneau F, Title L, Verma S, Lonn E: Relationship between carotid artery intima-media thickness and brachial artery flow-mediated dilation in middle-aged healthy men. *J Am Coll Cardiol* 2005, **45**(12):1980–1986.

39. Landmesser U, Hornig B, Drexler H: Endothelial function: a critical determinant in atherosclerosis? *Circulation* 2004, **109**(21 Suppl 1):II27–II33.

40. Hayashi K, Sugawara J, Komine H, Maeda S, Yokoi T: Effects of aerobic exercise training on the stiffness of central and peripheral arteries in middle-aged sedentary men. *Jpn J Physiol* 2005, **55**(4):235–239.

41. Collier SR, Kanaley JA, Carhart R Jr, Frechette V, Tobin MM, Hall AK, Luckenbaugh AN, Fernhall B: Effect of 4 weeks of aerobic or resistance exercise training on arterial stiffness, blood flow and blood pressure in pre- and stage-1 hypertensives. *J Hum Hypertens* 2008, **22**(10):678–686.

42. Miyachi M: Effects of resistance training on arterial stiffness: a meta-analysis. *Br J Sports Med* 2013, **47**(6):393–396.

43. Dengo AL, Dennis EA, Orr JS, Marinik EL, Ehrlich E, Davy BM, Davy KP: Arterial destiffening with weight loss in overweight and obese middle-aged and older adults. *Hypertension* 2010, **55**(4):855–861.

44. Spence AL, Carter HH, Naylor LH, Green DJ: A prospective randomized longitudinal study involving 6 months of endurance or resistance exercise: conduit artery adaptation in humans. *J Physiol* 2013, **591**(Pt 5):1265–1275.

45. de las Fuentes L, Waggoner AD, Mohammed BS, Stein RI, Miller BV 3rd, Foster GD, Wyatt HR, Klein S, Davila-Roman VG: Effect of moderate diet-induced weight loss and weight regain on cardiovascular structure and function. *J Am Coll Cardiol* 2009, **54**(25)):2376–2381.

46. Mavri A, Stegnar M, Sentocnik JT, Videcnik V: Impact of weight reduction on early carotid atherosclerosis in obese premenopausal women. *Obes Res* 2001, **9**(9):511–516.

47. Thijssen DH, Cable NT, Green DJ: Impact of exercise training on arterial wall thickness in humans. *Clin Sci (Lond)* 2012, **122**(7):311–322.

48. Church TS, Blair SN, Cocreham S, Johannsen N, Johnson W, Kramer K, Mikus CR, Myers V, Nauta M, Rodarte RQ, Sparks L, Thompson A, Earnest CP: Effects of aerobic and resistance training on hemoglobin A1c levels in patients with type 2 diabetes: a randomized controlled trial. *JAMA* 2010, **304**(20):2253–2262.

49. Snowling NJ, Hopkins WG: Effects of different modes of exercise training on glucose control and risk factors for complications in type 2 diabetic patients: a meta-analysis. *Diabetes Care* 2006, **29**(11):2518–2527.

50. Dreyer HC, Drummond MJ, Glynn EL, Fujita S, Chinkes DL, Volpi E, Rasmussen BB: Resistance exercise increases human skeletal muscle AS160/TBC1D4 phosphorylation in association with enhanced leg glucose uptake during postexercise recovery. *J Appl Physiol* 2008, **105**(6):1967–1974.

51. Graffagnino CL, Falko JM, La Londe M, Schaumburg J, Hyek MF, Shaffer LE, Snow R, Caulin-Glaser T: Effect of a community-based weight management program on weight loss and cardiovascular disease risk factors. *Obesity (Silver Spring)* 2006, **14**(2):280–288.

52. Williams MR, Westerman RA, Kingwell BA, Paige J, Blombery PA, Sudhir K, Komesaroff PA: Variations in endothelial function and arterial compliance during the menstrual cycle. *J Clin Endocrinol Metab* 2001, **86**(11):5389–5395.

7

Impact of carotid atherosclerosis detection on physician and patient behavior in the management of type 2 diabetes mellitus

In-Kyung Jeong[1], Sin-Gon Kim[2], Dong Hyeok Cho[3], Chong Hwa Kim[4], Chul Sik Kim[5], Won-Young Lee[6], Kyu-Chang Won[7] and Doo-Man Kim[8*]

Abstract

Background: This study compared carotid ultrasound (CUS) and traditional risk calculations in determining cardiovascular disease (CVD) risk in patients with type 2 diabetes mellitus (DM) and investigated whether awareness of CVD affects patient and/or physician behavior.

Methods: In this prospective, observational, multicenter study, 797 participants with type 2 diabetes were assessed using CUS, the United Kingdom Prospective Diabetes Study Risk Engine (UKPDSRE) calculator, and the Framingham Risk Score (FRS) algorithm. Health-related behaviors and physician treatments were compared at baseline and at 6 months after assessment.

Results: According to CUS, 43.5 % of the participants were at high risk (compared to 10.6 % and 4.3 % using the UKPDSRE and FRS approaches, respectively). Interestingly, 31.5 % of the patients with low risk scores according to the UKPDSRE calculator and 35.8 % of the patients with low risk scores according to the FRS algorithm were found to be at high risk according to CUS. The proportion of patients who achieved target LDL-C levels significantly increased after CUS. Moreover, increased awareness of atherosclerosis through CUS findings significantly altered physician treatment patterns and patient health-related behaviors.

Conclusions: Carotid atherosclerosis was detected in more than 30 % of all participants with low or intermediate risk stratification scores. Improved awareness of atherosclerosis through CUS findings had a positive impact on both patient and physician behavior, resulting in improved CV risk management.

Keywords: Behavior, Cardiovascular disease, Carotid atherosclerosis, Diabetes mellitus, Type 2

Background

Cardiovascular disease (CVD) is a major cause of mortality and morbidity in patients with type 2 diabetes mellitus (DM), making early diagnosis and treatment of atherosclerosis extremely important [1]. However, most patients with diabetes with subclinical atherosclerosis are asymptomatic [2]. In addition, the prevalence of silent myocardial ischemia (MI) is much higher in patients with diabetes compared to the general population [3]. Thus, in order to provide optimal medical therapy to prevent future cardiac events, identification of patients who are at high risk for CVD is of prime importance. The current guidelines on CVD prevention recommend targeted management of CV risk factors after assessment using one of the many available methods, even in asymptomatic patients.

Cardiovascular disease risk analysis can be performed using well-known risk-stratification approaches, including

* Correspondence: dm@hallym.or.kr; dmjmsy@hanmail.net
[8]Department of Internal Medicine, Kangdong Sacred Heart Hospital, Hallym University Medical Center, Gil-Dong, Gangdong-Gu, Seoul, South Korea
Full list of author information is available at the end of the article

the Framingham Risk Score (FRS) algorithm [4] and the United Kingdom Prospective Diabetes Study Risk Engine (UKPDSRE) calculator [5]. The results of the FRS and UKPDSRE approaches, which include traditional CV risk factors, generally correlate with coronary heart disease risk [4]. However, a substantial number of people with low (<10 %) to intermediate (10–20 %) FRS scores go on to develop atherosclerosis [6]. Previous reports have also demonstrated that the UKPDSRE lacks adequate sensitivity and specificity for detection of subclinical atherosclerosis [7]. Therefore, additional tools are needed to improve CV risk assessment.

Recent investigations have shown that noninvasive techniques, such as carotid intima media thickness (CIMT), presence of plaque, coronary artery calcium score (CACS), ankle-brachial index (ABI), and aortic pulse wave velocity may accurately detect subclinical atherosclerosis that is associated with the development of cardiovascular or cerebrovascular diseases [8]. These studies have shown that imaging modalities are the best method for detecting the presence and extent of atherosclerosis. As such, it is important to conduct imaging studies in all patients regardless of the presence of traditional CV risk factors, such as hypertension, dyslipidemia, and diabetes mellitus, in order to comprehensively identify patients who are at risk for developing CVD. We chose to focus our study on CIMT because CUS is feasible in all individuals, dose not involve exposure to radiation, and is relatively inexpensive. When using imaging studies, a CACS >0, stenosis >50th percentile, or the presence of plaque are considered to be positive findings. These findings suggest a high risk of developing CVD according to the guidelines from the Screening for Heart Attack Prevention and Education (SHAPE), published by the Association for Eradication of Heart Attack (AEHA) [9].

However, the outcomes of this guideline have not yet been compared to those of the traditional guideline. Therefore, we analyzed the prevalences of abnormal carotid ultrasound (CUS) findings and compared them to traditional risk stratification results obtained using the FRS and UKPDSRE approaches.

Although physicians provide comprehensive treatment for diabetes, hypertension, and dyslipidemia, patient drug compliance is critical for optimal outcomes. If a physician assesses CVD risk and uses these results to educate the patient about ways to prevent CVD, the patient may implement lifestyle modifications or improve his/her drug compliance. However, no studies have yet investigated the effect of assessing subclinical atherosclerosis on patient behavior, or whether awareness of subclinical atherosclerosis alters physician treatment patterns.

Here we explored how two distinct assessment methods varied in their estimation of CV risk, a non-invasive imaging test (CUS) and traditional risk calculators (UKPDSRE, FRS). We also examined how awareness of being at high risk for CVD affected physician treatment patterns as well as patient behavior with respect to risk management. Our hypothesis was that receiving an explanation of CUS results, along with proper education about mitigating risk factors, would have a favorable effect on patient behavior and physician treatment plans.

Methods

This prospective, observational, multicenter study included 797 patients with type 2 DM aged >40 years who had never undergone a carotid ultrasound examination. Participants were recruited from 24 hospitals in Korea. We excluded patients who had previously undergone carotid artery ultrasound, or who had a history of coronary artery disease, symptomatic congestive heart failure, coronary revascularization, cerebrovascular disease, stroke, transient ischemic attack, or documented peripheral vascular disease (e.g. peripheral artery disease, abdominal aneurysm, or carotid artery stenosis). The investigation protocol was approved by the institutional review boards of each institution involved in the study. After obtaining informed written consent, the height, weight, and body mass index (BMI) (weight/height^2, kg/m^2) of each patient were measured. Blood pressure was measured using a standard mercury sphygmomanometer. All patients were interviewed prior to CUS examination. Questionnaires were administered using one-on-one interviews and self-reporting techniques to collect data on smoking; alcohol use; stress; dietary habits; physical activity; past history of hypertension, dyslipidemia, and atrial fibrillation; medication compliance; and family history of CVD. The validated Korean version [10] of Morsky's self-reported questionnaire [11] was used to assess medication compliance. Levels of fasting plasma glucose, HbA$_{1C}$, total cholesterol (TC), triglyceride (TG), high-density lipoprotein cholesterol (HDL-C), and low-density lipoprotein cholesterol (LDL-C); current medications; and the microalbumin-to-creatinine ratio within the past 1 month were collected by reviewing patient medical records.

All subjects were assessed by CUS. Carotid intimal-media thickness (IMT) was measured with the patient in the supine position. A high-resolution B-mode ultrasound machine with a 7.5-MHz transducer was used on the bilateral segments of the carotid arteries. The carotid IMT was measured on the posterior far wall of the left carotid artery. At least 4 measurements were taken, each about 1 cm proximal to the bifurcation. Positive criteria for carotid atherosclerosis were defined as ≥1 mm of intima medial thickness or the presence of plaque.

Although CUS was performed separately in the 24 different hospitals, each used a standardized protocol recommended by the Mannheim carotid IMT consensus report [12]. In addition, to adjust for potential intercenter variations due to different sonographers, every hospital used Intimascope software (Media Cross Co, Ltd, Tokyo, Japan) for measurement. This software performs automated IMT measurements based on an algorithm that delineates the lumen-intima and media adventitial interfaces [13].

Patients were stratified by risk using the UKPDSRE and FRS assessments. A total of 622 patients provided all required information to be assessed by the UKPDSRE calculator and 648 patients provided sufficient information to be assessed by the FRS algorithm. A total of 622 patients were assessed by CUS, UKPDSRE, and FRS. The UKPDS calculator classified subjects into low (<15 %), intermediate (15–30 %), or high (>30 %) 10-year risk levels for CVD based on age, sex, duration of diabetes, smoking, systolic blood pressure, total cholesterol, HDL, ethnicity, and HbA_{1C} [4]. The FRS algorithm categorized subjects into low (<10 %), intermediate (10–19 %), or high (≤20 %) 10-year risk levels for symptomatic CVD according to age, sex, lipid levels, blood pressure, smoking, and presence of diabetes [5].

Blood samples were collected six months after carotid IMT assessment to measure levels of TC, HDL-C, TG, and LDL-C. Patients were also re-examined for changes in responses to interview questions, physician prescriptions, and patient behaviors.

All statistical analyses were completed using SAS (version 9.2, USA). All data are presented as means ± standard deviations (SDs) or as numbers (percentages). To compare clinical characteristics between the two groups, an independent t-test was used for continuous variables and a chi-squared test was used for categorical variables. Multiple logistic regression analysis was used to analyze the association between carotid IMT and CVD risk factors. A paired t-test was used to measure changes in patient behavior before and after they were informed about their subclinical carotid atherosclerosis risk. Differences with a p-level <0.05 were considered statistically significant.

Results

Baseline characteristics of the subjects with type 2 DM

Table 1 summarizes the clinical and laboratory measurements of the subjects with type 2 DM included in this study. The mean patient age was 60 years and the mean BMI was 25.1 ± 3.1 kg/m^2. Half of the subjects had a >10-year duration since diagnosis with type 2 DM.

According to patient questionnaires, the most frequent co-morbidities were hypertension (50.69 %) and dyslipidemia (37.5 %) (not shown in Table 1). Examination of medical records revealed that antihypertensive drugs, statins, and antiplatelet agents were prescribed to 43.3 %, 42.3 %, and 41.2 % of all patients, respectively. Approximately 20 % of the patients were current smokers. The mean HbA_{1C} level was 60 ± 18.6 mmol/mol. The mean LDL-C level was 2.57 ± 0.86 mmol/L.

Estimated cardiovascular risk of the subjects

In total, 42.9 % of the subjects with diabetes had a positive finding for atherosclerosis according to carotid US (Table 1). Of the 622 patients assessed using the UKPDS calculator, 43.6 % were positive for atherosclerosis according to carotid US. The UKPDS risk calculator determined that 343 (55.2 %) patients were at low risk for CVD, 213 (34.2 %) patients were at intermediate risk for CVD, and 66 (10.6 %) patients were at high risk for CVD. The FRS algorithm determined that 425 (65.6 %) patients were at low risk for CVD, 195 (30.1 %) patients were at intermediate risk for CVD, and 28 (4.3 %) patients were at high risk for CVD (Table 1). The 10-year risk of CVD was higher in the UKPDS high-risk group compared to the FRS high-risk group (10.6 % vs. 4.3 %, $p < 0.0001$).

We also calculated the UKPDS and FRS cutoff points for the prediction of positive CUS (IMT > 1 mm). The UKPDS cutoff was 14.52 (sensitivity 66.38 %, specificity 61.99 %) and the FRS cutoff was 14 (sensitivity 72.75 %, specificity 46.62 %).

There was a significant correlation between CV risk score and carotid IMT. The correlation coefficient between UKPDS score and mean IMT was 0.295 ($p < 0.001$). The correlation coefficient between FRS score and mean IMT was 0.227 ($p < 0.001$).

We next investigated whether the UKPDSRE or FRS calculator is a superior predictor of positive CUS. The area under the UKPDSRE ROC curve was 0.677 (95 % CI, 0.635, 0.719), while the area under the FRS ROC curve was 0.629 (95 % CI, 0.584, 0.672); this difference was significant ($P = 0.001$). Therefore, the UKPDSRE calculator was better at predicting positive CUS than the FRS algorithm.

Patient clinical characteristics according to positive carotid ultrasound findings

Patients with positive carotid ultrasound findings were significantly older (63.5 ± 9.0 vs. 57.9 ± 9.2 years), had a longer duration of diabetes (9.0 ± 7.6 vs. 7.4 ± 6.7 years), used more antihypertensive medication (50.0 vs. 38.2 %) and antiplatelet agents (46.2 vs. 37.4 %), and had higher log hs-CRP levels (-1.4 ± 1.7 vs. -1.0 ± 1.8 mg/L) compared to subjects with negative carotid US findings

Table 1 Baseline clinical characteristics of patients with versus without subclinical atherosclerosis

		Atherosclerosis Findings via Carotid IMT		
	Total (N = 797)	Negative (N = 455)	Positive (N = 342)	*P-value
Age (years)	60.0 ± 9.5	57.9 ± 9.2	63.5 ± 9.0	<0.001
Sex (percent male)	395 (49.6)	227 (49.9)	175 (51.2)	0.721
BMI (kg/m^2)	25.1 ± 3.1	25.3 ± 3.4	24.9 ± 3.0	0.067
Waist circumference (cm)	87.2 ± 8.2	87.6 ± 8.6	86.7 ± 7.6	0.164
Blood pressure (mmHg)				
Systolic	125.3 ± 14.5	124.5 ± 14.7	126.5 ± 14.2	0.060
Diastolic	75.3 ± 10.1	75.7 ± 9.6	74.7 ± 10.6	0.170
DM duration (years)	8.1 ± 7.1	7.4 ± 6.7	9.0 ± 7.6	0.002
Medication use [N (%)]				
Antihypertensive drug	345 (43.3)	174 (38.2)	171 (50.0)	0.001
Statin	337 (42.3)	195 (42.9)	142 (41.5)	0.705
Antiplatelet agent	328 (41.2)	170 (37.4)	158 (46.2)	0.012
Current smoker (%)	153 (19.2)	81 (17.9)	72 (21.1)	0.253
Glucose (mmol/L)	8.1 ± 2.8	8.0 ± 2.7	8.2 ± 3.0	0.591
HbA1C (mmol/mol)	60 ± 18.6	60 ± 17.5	61 ± 19.7	0.417
Log hs-CRP (mg/L)	−1.2 ± 1.8	−1.4 ± 1.7	−1.0 ± 1.8	0.017
Total cholesterol (mmol/L)	4.4 ± 1.0	4.4 ± 1.0	4.5 ± 1.0	0.710
Triglycerides (mmol/L)	1.7 ± 1.1	1.7 ± 1.2	1.7 ± 1.0	0.884
LDL-C (mmol/L)	2.6 ± 0.9	2.5 ± 0.9	2.6 ± 0.8	0.284
HDL-C (mmol/L)	1.2 ± 0.4	1.3 ± 0.3	1.2 ± 0.4	0.594
UKPDS risk engine score	16.8 ± 12.1	13.3 ± 8.7	20.4 ± 13.6	<0.001
UKPDS risk engine (%) (N = 622)				
High	66 (10.6)	15 (4.3)	51 (18.8)	
Intermediate	213 (34.2)	101 (28.8)	112 (41.3)	<0.001
Low	343 (55.2)	235 (67.0)	108 (39.9)	
Framingham risk score	7.7 ± 6.4	6.2 ± 5.7	9.20 ± 7.1	<0.001
Framingham risk engine (%) (N = 648)				
High	28 (4.3)	6 (1.6)	22 (7.8)	
Intermediate	195 (30.1)	88 (24.0)	107 (38.1)	<0.001
Low	425 (65.6)	273 (74.4)	152 (54.1)	

IMT intima medial thickness, *BMI* body mass index, *DM* diabetes mellitus, *CRP* C-reactive protein, *LDL-C* low-density lipoprotein cholesterol, *HDL* high-density lipoprotein cholesterol, *UKPDS* United Kingdom Prospective Diabetes Study
*P-value: comparison of clinical data between patients who were negative versus positive for carotid atherosclerosis according to carotid IMT

(Table 1). Furthermore, the UKPDSRE and FRS scores were higher in subjects with positive carotid IMT findings. In addition, the percentages of high risk patients as classified by the UKPDSRE and FRS systems were higher for subjects with positive carotid IMT findings compared to subjects with negative findings (18.8 vs. 4.3 % and 7.8 vs. 1.7 %, respectively) (Table 1).

Multiple logistic regression analysis was next performed to investigate the associations between CV risk factors and abnormal carotid US findings after adjusting for age and sex. Carotid IMT was positively correlated with LDL-C level. There was a trend towards a positive association between ex- and current smokers and positive carotid IMT findings. No significant associations were noted between positive CUS findings and BP, BMI, DM duration, HbA$_{1C}$, UKPDSRE score, or FRS score (Table 2).

Prevalence of carotid atherosclerosis according to risk stratification scores

According to the UKPDS risk engine, the prevalences of positive carotid US findings were 31.5 % in the low-risk group, 52.6 % in the intermediate-risk group, and 77.3 % in the high-risk group. According to the

Table 2 Associations between carotid intima medial thickness and cardiovascular disease risk factors[a]

	OR	95 % CI	P-value
BMI	1.051	0.945, 1.169	0.835
Systolic blood pressure	1.010	0.994, 1.027	0.219
DM duration	0.997	0.963, 1.033	0.887
Ex & current smokers	1.771	0.907, 3.459	0.094
HbA$_{1C}$	1.006	0.843, 1.201	0.946
Triglycerides	1.002	0.999, 1.005	0.142
LDL-C	1.018	1.003, 1.032	0.017
HDL-C	1.013	0.985, 1.042	0.360
UKPDS risk engine score	27.003	0.057, 999.999	0.294
Framingham risk score	0.971	0.900, 1.047	0.441

OR odds ratio, *CI* confidence interval, *BMI* body mass index, *DM* diabetes mellitus, *LDL-C* low-density lipoprotein cholesterol, *HDL* high-density lipoprotein cholesterol, *UKPDS* United Kingdom Prospective Diabetes Study
[a]Values adjusted for age and sex

FRS algorithm, the prevalences of abnormal carotid US findings were 35.8 % in the low-risk group, 54.9 % in the intermediate-risk group, and 78.6 % in the high-risk group (Fig. 1). Overall, about one-third of the patients in both low-risk groups had a positive finding according to carotid US. On the other hand, only about 20 % of the patients in both high-risk groups had a negative finding according to carotid US (Fig. 1).

Factors contributing to the discrepancy between UKPDS risk engine stratification and carotid US findings

In total, 39.9 % of subjects with a positive CUS finding were classified as low-risk according to the UKPDSRE calculator (Table 1). To identify the factors that were associated with abnormal CUS findings in patients

assessed by the UKPDSRE calculator, we compared the clinical parameters of patients with negative versus positive CUS findings in each risk-stratified group. In the low-risk group, patients with positive CUS findings were significantly older and had a significantly lower waist circumference, lower diastolic BP, a higher prevalence of hypertension and dyslipidemia, and a higher prevalence of antihypertensive medication use compared to subjects with negative CUS findings. In the intermediate-risk group, positive CUS findings were associated with increased age, female sex, and higher hs-CRP levels compared to subjects with negative CUS findings. In the high-risk group, no significant associations were observed between any parameter and positive CUS findings between the two groups (Additional file 1: Table S1). This finding may be due to the relatively small number of subjects in the high-risk group.

Changes in treatment patterns after CUS measurements

Changes in physician prescriptions were investigated at 6 months after the initial CUS measurements. Awareness of high-risk CUS findings significantly altered physician treatment patterns ($p = 0.011$) for managing major CV risk factors. In addition, significant increases in the addition and dosages of anti-hypertensive drugs ($p = 0.013$) and antiplatelet agents ($p = 0.003$) were observed in patients with positive CUS findings (Table 3).

The percentage of subjects who achieved the target LDL-C goal (<2.59 mmol/L) was significantly higher 6 months after CUS examination in patients with negative CUS findings and also in patients with positive CUS findings (Table 3). Abnormal CUS findings affected physician behavior regardless of patient risk level according to the UKPDSRE calculator. A significant change in treatment patterns for antihypertensive drug use (7.0 vs. 14.6 %) was observed in patients with positive CUS findings who were identified as low-risk according to the UKPDS calculator.

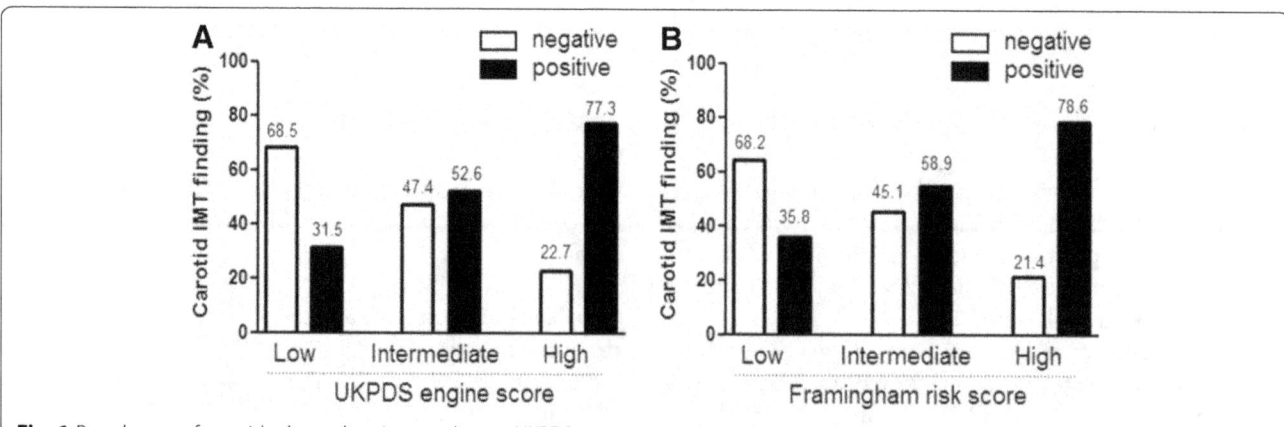

Fig. 1 Prevalences of carotid atherosclerosis according to UKPDS engine score (**a**) and Framingham risk score (**b**). Open bar: negative findings from carotid ultrasound. Black bar: positive findings from carotid ultrasound

Table 3 Changes in treatment patterns after knowledge of subclinical carotid atherosclerosis results

	Carotid Artery Ultrasound Findings		P-value
	Negative, N (%) $N = 455$	Positive, N (%) $N = 342$	
Treatment pattern			
Changed	96 (24.7)	107 (33.4)	0.011
Additional medications			
Anti-hypertensive drugs	32 (8.3)	45 (18.1)	0.013
Lipid-lowering drugs	52 (13.4)	44 (13.8)	0.893
Antiplatelet agents	26 (6.7)	43 (13.4)	0.003
Achievement of treatment target goals			
BP (<130/80 mmHg)			
At baseline	210 (49.1) (N = 428)	142 (46.3) (N = 307)	0.452
After 6 months	199 (46.5) (N = 428)	139 (45.3) (N = 307)	0.744
Baseline vs. 6 months	$P = 0.389$	$P = 0.785$	
LDL-C (<2.59 mmol/L)			
At baseline	112 (57.7) (N = 194)	80 (55.6) (N = 144)	0.690
After 6 months	130 (67.0) (N = 194)	105 (72.9) (N = 144)	0.243
Baseline vs. 6 months	$P = 0.022$	$P < 0.001$	
Calculated LDL[a] (<2.59 mmol/L)			
At baseline	125 (56.8) (N = 220)	96 (56.8) (N = 169)	0.998
After 6 months	157 (71.4) (N = 220)	126 (74.6) (N = 169)	0.483
Baseline vs. 6 months	$P = 0.022$	$P < 0.001$	

BP blood pressure, LDL-C low-density lipoprotein cholesterol
[a]Calculated LDL = total cholesterol – (triglyceride/5) – HDL

A significant change in treatment patterns for antiplatelet agent use (0 vs. 22.0 %) was also observed in patients with positive CUS findings who were identified as high-risk according to the UKPDSRE calculator (Additional file 1: Table S2).

Changes in patient behavior after education based on carotid US results

Interviews were performed 6 months after patients were informed of their carotid US results. Overall, patients who were informed of their CUS results exhibited significant changes in their health-related behaviors. For example, the rates of smoking cessation and dietary changes ($p < 0.005$ each) were both increased at the 6-month follow-up visit. Moreover, the percentage of patients who had quit smoking had significantly increased and the amount of soup intake had reduced significantly at six months after the CUS examination (Fig. 2). This finding suggests that the patients tried to reduce their salt intake by decreasing their soup consumption.

Discussion
Our results suggest that CUS can identify CVD-vulnerable patients out of the population of patients with type 2 DM with low-risk or intermediate-risk stratification

scores. In addition, improved awareness of CVD risk based on carotid IMT results can improve CV risk management by increasing the prevention efforts of both physicians and patients.

According to CUS, 271 (43.5 %) patients were at high risk for CVD. In contrast, only 66 (10.6 %) and 28 (4.3 %) patients were at high risk for CVD according to the UKPDSRE calculator and the FRS algorithm, respectively. We also found that more high-risk patients were identified using the UKPDSRE calculator compared to the FRS algorithm (10.6 vs. 4.5 %, $p < 0.0001$). This finding was not surprising, since the UKPDS risk engine was developed especially for use with patients with diabetes [5]. As such, this method has a higher prognostic value for coronary heart disease in patients newly diagnosed with type 2 diabetes [14]. Also, the UKPDSRE calculator provided the highest odds ratios for predicting carotid atherosclerosis in Korean patients with type 2 diabetes compared to the FRS and the SCORE methods [15]. However, the prevalences of positive CUS findings were very similar in the low-risk (31.5 % vs. 35.8 %), intermediate-risk (52.6 % vs. 54.9 %), and high-risk (77.3 % vs. 78.6 %) groups for both the UKPDS risk engine and the FRS algorithm, respectively (Fig. 1).

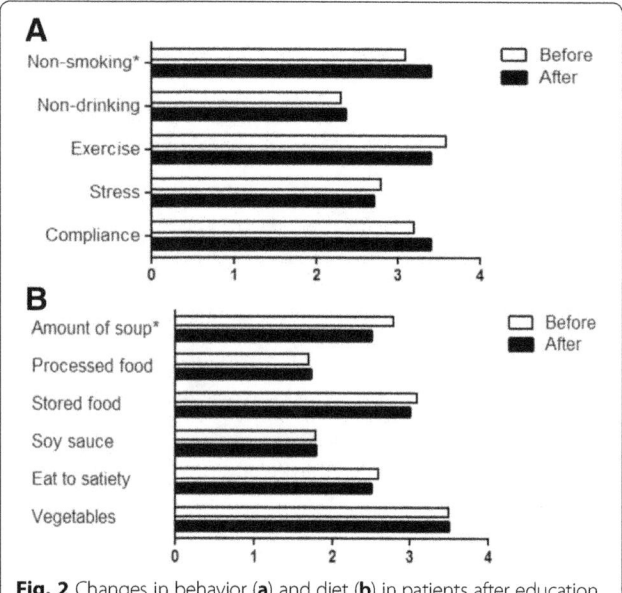

Fig. 2 Changes in behavior (**a**) and diet (**b**) in patients after education based on carotid US results. [※: *p* < 0.05 between behavior before (open bar) and after (black bar) awareness of positive findings from carotid ultrasound]

The FRS and UKPDSRE approaches, both of which include traditional CV risk factors, have been validated for predicting CV risk in Asian populations [15–17]. Although the results of these approaches are generally correlated with subclinical atherosclerosis, the majority of CVD events occur in patients with low or intermediate risk of CVD [4]. To our surprise, one-third of the low-risk patients according to both the UKPDSRE and FRS classifications had a positive CUS finding. Of the patients classified as low-risk based on their UKPDSRE score, 39.9 % had a positive CUS finding. One previous study found that 32.8 % of all women and 40.5 % of all men with low (<10 %) to intermediate (10–20 %) risk of CVD according to the FRS algorithm had subclinical atherosclerosis [6]. Analysis of factors related to atherosclerosis in the low-risk group indicated that positive CUS findings were significantly associated with older age, higher prevalences of hypertension and dyslipidemia, and a higher prevalence of antihypertensive medication history.

Carotid IMT and the presence of carotid plaque are important markers of subclinical atherosclerosis that can be used to predict cardiovascular morbidity. Many epidemiology studies, such as the Atherosclerosis Risk in Communities (ARIC) study [18] and the Insulin Resistance Atherosclerosis Study (IRAS) [19], have demonstrated that age, male sex, smoking, hypertension, dyslipidemia, and postmenopausal status are independent correlates of carotid atherosclerosis. In particular, Chin et al. [20] showed that LDL-C levels in males and HDL-C levels in females were risk factors for IMT progression among patients

newly diagnosed with type 2 diabetes. We found that old age, diabetes duration, percentage of antihypertensive medication use, antiplatelet agent use, and log hs-CRP level were significantly higher in patients with positive CUS findings. After adjustment for age and sex, LDL-C was an independent correlate of subclinical carotid atherosclerosis. These data suggest that LDL-C should be managed to protect or delay the progression of atherosclerosis. Therefore, comprehensive management of CV risk factors and patient adherence to the treatment plan may prevent or delay the progression of atherosclerosis.

We also assessed how patient lifestyle and physician prescriptions changed after receiving the CUS results, as well as how knowing these results affected the achievement of target lipid and BP levels after 6 months. Among the patients with positive CUS findings, significant increases in the use or dosage of anti-hypertensive drugs and antiplatelet agents were observed compared to those in patients with negative CUS findings. We speculate that learning that a patient had subclinical atherosclerosis of the carotid artery may have encouraged physicians to more intensively manage patient risk factors for atherosclerosis. In addition, this intervention was associated with a significant improvement in the achievement of target LDL-C levels, even though a change in medication prescriptions related to hypercholesterolemia was not observed. This finding implies that medication compliance for lipid-lowering drugs might increase after patients receive their CUS findings, regardless of whether these findings are negative or positive. Hong et al. [21] reported that among asymptomatic patients with hypertension, atherosclerosis detection by CUS significantly increased the proportion of patients who achieved their target LDL-C levels compared to patients who received a negative CUS finding. However, we found that patient knowledge of CUS findings improved outcomes, regardless of whether the results were positive or negative. As such, we propose that CUS is a beneficial tool for increasing adherence to lipid-lowering drug regimens as part of CV risk management in patients with type 2 diabetes.

Patient behaviors also changed significantly after the patients received their CUS results. Specifically, patients who underwent CUS examination subsequently reduced smoking and salt intake (for the latter, by reducing soup consumption). We infer that since consumption of Korean soup or stew has been shown to be associated with high salt intake [22], patients made an effort to reduce their salt intake by decreasing their soup consumption. Thus, our data indicate that knowledge of carotid US results and subsequent explanation of the relevant CVD risks is a useful approach for enabling patients to achieve the recommended lifestyle modifications. Furthermore, CUS is a very helpful tool that enables patients to better understand their atherosclerosis status, particularly when CUS imaging results are employed. Our results thus indicate that explanation of CUS results assists patients with diabetes and their physicians to achieve patient therapeutic targets through behavior changes and medication plan alterations.

This study did have some limitations. First, the study period was only 6 months, which is a relatively short period of time for full evaluation of CVD event outcomes. Second, although our results indicated that awareness of CUS results may positively influence physician management of CV risk factors and patient behavior, correlation does not imply causality. Third, we did not evaluate the quality or area of the carotid plaques found by CUS. Several studies have shown that the quality of plaque and the plaque area are more strongly predictive of CV events than IMT [23, 24]. Fourth, we defined a positive CUS finding as an IMT $\geq$ 1 mm or the presence of plaque. We chose these criteria based on several large clinical studies (e.g. the ARIC study and studies performed in Finland) that compared the hazard ratios between CIMT $\geq$ 1 mm and < 1 mm [25–27]. Specifically, the ARIC study showed that the hazard ratio comparing extreme mean CIMT ($\geq$1 mm) to not extreme CIMT (<1 mm) was 5.07 for women and 1.85 for men. Above 1 mm, the CV event rates were elevated [26]. However, this cutoff point was derived from a non-Asian population. To more accurately predict CV risk in future studies, a more comprehensive investigation of the optimal CIMT cutoff point to predict CV risk in an Asian population would be beneficial. Finally, all subjects in the present study were Asian, and thus our findings may not be applicable to other populations.

Conclusions

Our data indicate that CUS screening is an effective method for identifying patients with subclinical atherosclerosis, even among patients considered to be low-risk according to the UKPDRES or FRS approach. In addition, educating patients with type 2 DM about their atherosclerosis risk as determined by their CUS results may result in improved management of CV risk factors.

Abbreviations
AEHA: Association for Eradication of Heart Attack; BMI: Body mass index; CUS: Carotid ultrasound; CVD: Cardiovascular disease; DM: Diabetes mellitus; FRS: Framingham risk score; HDL-C: High-density lipoprotein cholesterol; IMT: Intima media thickness; LDL-C: Low-density lipoprotein cholesterol; MI: Myocardial ischemia; SD: Standard deviation; SHAPE: Screening for heart attack prevention and education; TC: Total cholesterol; TG: Triglyceride; UKPDS: United Kingdom Prospective Diabetes Study Risk Engine

Acknowledgments
The authors wish to thank the following medical groups and diabetes education centers for their collaboration: Kangbuk Samsung Hospital, Cheil General Hospital, Chung-Ang University Yong-San Hospital, Chung-Ang University Hospital, Myongji Hospital, Korea University Anam Hospital, Hallym University Chuncheon Sacred Heart Hospital, Sejong General Hospital, Hallym University Kangnam Sacred Heart Hospital, Samsung Medical Center, Gang Nam Severance Hospital, Hallym University Kangdong Sacred Heart Hospital, Bundang Cha Hospital, Hallym University Sacred Heart Hospital, Kyung Hee University Hospital at Gangdong, Chonnam National University Hospital, Chonbuk National University Hospital, Keimyung University Dongsan Hospital, Gyeongsang National University Hospital, Yeungnam University Hospital, Daegu Catholic University Medical Center, Pusan National University Hospital, Kosin University Gospel Hospital, and Inje University Pusan Paik Hospital.

Funding
This study was funded by Pfizer Pharmaceuticals Korea Ltd. The funding source was involved in the study design, collection of data, or interpretation of results.

Authors' contributions
IKJ reviewed the data and wrote the manuscript. SGK, DHC, CHK, CSK, WYL, and KCW performed research and contributed to discussions. DMK reviewed and edited the manuscript. All authors read and approved the final manuscript.

Competing interests
The authors declare that they have no competing interests.

Ethical approval and consent to participate
All procedures involving human participants performed in this study were in accordance with the ethical standards of the relevant institutional and/or national research committees and with the 1964 Helsinki Declaration and its later amendments or comparable ethical standards.
This study has received ethical approval by institutional review board of each hospital : Kangbuk Samsung Hospital, Cheil General Hospital, Chung-Ang University Yong-San Hospital, Chung-Ang University Hospital, Myongji Hospital, Korea University Anam Hospital, Hallym University Chuncheon Sacred Heart Hospital, Sejong General Hospital, Hallym University Kangnam Sacred Heart Hospital, Samsung Medical Center, Gang Nam Severance Hospital, Hallym University Kangdong Sacred Heart Hospital, Bundang Cha Hospital, Hallym University Sacred Heart Hospital, Kyung Hee University Hospital at Gangdong, Chonnam National University Hospital, Chonbuk National University Hospital, Keimyung University Dongsan Hospital, Gyeongsang National University Hospital, Yeungnam University Hospital, Daegu Catholic University Medical Center, Pusan National University Hospital, Kosin University Gospel Hospital, and Inje University Pusan Paik Hospital. Informed consent was obtained from all participants included in the study.

Author details
[1]Department of Endocrinology and Metabolism, Kyung Hee University School of Medicine, Kyung Hee University Hospital at Gangdong, Seoul, South Korea. [2]Korea University Anam Hospital, Seoul, South Korea. [3]Chonnam National University Hospital, Gwangju, South Korea. [4]Sejong General Hospital, Gyeonggi-do, South Korea. [5]Hallym University Sacred Heart Hospital, Gyeonggi-do, South Korea. [6]Kangbuk Samsung Hospital, Seoul, South Korea. [7]Yeungnam University Medical Center, Daegu, South Korea. [8]Department of Internal Medicine, Kangdong Sacred Heart Hospital, Hallym University Medical Center, Gil-Dong, Gangdong-Gu, Seoul, South Korea.

References
1. Wild S, Roglic G, Green A, Sicree R, King H. Global prevalence of diabetes: estimate for the year 2000 and projections for 2030. Diabetes Care. 2004;27: 1047–53.
2. Nesto RW, Phillips RT, Kett KG, Hill T, Perper E, Young E, et al. Angina and exertional myocardial ischemia in diabetic and nondiabetic patients. Ann Intern Med. 1998;108:170–5.
3. Valensi P, Lorgis L, Cottin Y. Prevalence, incidence, predictive factors and

prognosis of silent myocardial infarction: a review of the literature. Arch Cardiovasc Dis. 2011;104:178–88.

4. Wilson PWF, D'Agostino RB, Levy D, Belanger AM, Silbershatz H, Kannel WB. Prediction of coronary heart disease using risk factor categories. Circulation. 1998;97:1837–47.

5. Stevens RJ, Kothari V, Adler AI, Stratton IM, United Kingdom Prospective Diabetes Study (UKPDS) Group. The UKPDS risk engine: a model for the risk of coronary heart disease in Type II diabetes (UKPDS 56). Clin Sci (Lond). 2001;101:671–9.

6. Postley JE, Perez A, Wong ND, Gardin JM. Prevalence and distribution of sub-clinical atherosclerosis by screening vascular ultrasound in low and intermediate risk adults: the New York physicians study. J Am Soc Echocardiogr. 2009;22:1145–51.

7. Yeboah J, Erbel R, Delaney JC, Nance R, Guo M, Bertoni AG, Budoff M, Moebus S, Jöckel KH, Burke GL, Wong ND, Lehmann N, Herrington DM, Möhlenkamp S, Greenland P. Development of a new diabetes risk prediction tool for incident coronary heart disease events: the Multi-Ethnic Study of Atherosclerosis and the Heinz Nixdorf Recall Study. Atherosclerosis. 2014;236(2):411–7.

8. Simon A, Chironi G, Levenson J. Performance of Subclinical Arterial Disease Detection as a Screening Test for Coronary Heart Disease. Hypertension. 2006;48:392–6.

9. Naghavi M, Falk E, Hecht HS, Jamieson MJ, Kaul S, Berman D, SHAPE Task Force, et al. From Vulnerable Plaque to Vulnerable Patient-Part III: Executive Summary of the Screening for Heart Attack Prevention and Education (SHAPE) Task Force Report. Am J Cardiol. 2006;98 suppl:2H–15H.

10. Kim SW, Kim MY, Yoo TW, Huh BR. Concurrent validity of the Korean version of self reported questionnaire. J Korean Acad Fam Med. 1995;16:172–80.

11. Morisky DE, Levine DM, Green LW, Shapiro S, Russell RP, Smith CR. Five-year blood pressure control and mortality following health education for hypertensive patients. Am J Public Health. 1983;73:153–62.

12. Touboul PJ, Hennerici MG, Meairs S, Adams H, Amarenco P, Desvarieux M, et al. Mannheim intimamedia thickness consensus. Cerebrovasc Dis. 2004;18:346–9.

13. O'Leary DH, Polak JF, Wolfson Jr SK, Bond MG, Bommer W, Shelth S, Psaty BM, Sharrett AR, Manolio TA. Use of sonography to evaluate carotid atherosclerosis in the elderly: the Cardiovascular Health Study: CHS Collaborative Research Group. Stroke. 1991;22:1155–63.

14. Guzder RN, Gatling W, Mullee MA, Mehta RL, Byrne CD. Prognostic value of the Framingham cardiovascular risk equation and the UKPDS risk engine for coronary heart disease in newly diagnosed Type 2 diabetes: results from a United Kingdom study. Diabet Med. 2005;22:554–62.

15. Ahn HR, Shin MH, Yun WJ, Kim HY, Lee YH, Kweon SS, et al. Comparison of the Framingham Risk Score, UKPDS Risk Engine, and SCORE for Predicting Carotid Atherosclerosis and Peripheral Arterial Disease in Korean Type 2 Diabetic Patients. Korean J Fam Med. 2011;32:189–96.

16. Chia YC, Gray SY, Ching SM, Lim HM, Chinna K. Validation of the Framingham general cardiovascular risk score in a multiethnic Asian population : a retrospective cohort study. BMJ Open. 2015;19:e007324.

17. Tanaka S, Tanaka S, Iimuro S, Yamashita H, Katayama S, Akanuma Y, Yamada N, Araki A, Ito H, Sone H, Ohashi Y, Japan Diabetes Complication Study Group, Japanese Elderly Diabetes Intervention Trial Group. Predicting macro-and microvascular complications in type 2 diabetes: the Japan Diabetes Complications Study/the Japanese Elderly Diabetes Intervention Trial risk engine. Diabetes Care. 2013;36:1193–9.

18. Heiss G, Sharrett AR, Barnes R, Chambless LE, Szklo M, Zizola C. Carotid atherosclerosis measured by B-mode ultrasound in populations: associations with cardiovascular risk factors in the ARIC Study. Am J Epidemiol. 1991;134:250–6.

19. Wagenknecht LE, D'Agostino Jr R, Savage PJ, O'Leary DH, Saad MF, Haffner SM. Duration of diabetes and carotid wall thickness: the Insulin Resistance Atherosclerosis Study (IRAS). Stroke. 1997;28:999–1005.

20. Chin SW, Hwang JK, Rhee SY, Chon S, Hwang YC, Oh SJ, et al. Risk Factors for Progression of Intima-Media Thickness of Carotid Arteries: A 2-Year Follow-up Study in Patients with Newly Diagnosed Type 2 Diabetes. Diabetes Metab J. 2013;37(5):48–54.

21. Hong SJ, Chang HJ, Song K, Hong GR, Park SW, Kang HJ, et al. Impact of atherosclerosis detection by carotid ultrasound on physician behavior and risk-factor management in asymptomatic hypertensive subjects. Clin Cardiol. 2014;37(2):91–6.

22. Kim YC, Koo HS, Kim S, Chin HJ. Estimation of daily salt intake through a 24-hour urine collection in Pohang, Korea. J Korean Med Sci. 2014;20(S2):S87–90.

23. Spence JD, Eliasziw M, Di Cicco M, Hackam DG, Galil R, Lohmann T. Carotid plaque area: a tool for targeting and evaluating vascular preventive therapy. Stroke. 2002;33:2916–22.

24. Johnsen SH, Mathiesen EB, Joakimsen O, Stensland E, Wilsgaard T, Løchen ML, et al. Carotid atherosclerosis is a stronger predictor of myocardial infarction in women than in men: a 6-year follow-up study of 6226 persons: the Tromsø Study. Stroke. 2007;38:2873–80.

25. Naqvi TZ, Lee MS. Carotid intima-media thickness and plaque in cardiovascular risk assessment. JACC Cardiovasc Imaging. 2014;7(10):1025–38.

26. Chambless LE, Heiss G, Folsom AR, Rosamond W, Szklo M, Sharrett AR, Clegg LX. Association of coronary heart disease incidence with carotid arterial wall thickness and major risk factors: the Atherosclerosis Risk in Communities (ARIC) Study, 1987–1993. Am J Epidemiol. 1997;46(6):483–94.

27. Salonen R, Salonen JT. Determinants of carotid intima-media thickness: a population-based ultrasonography study in eastern Finnish men. J Intern Med. 1991;229(3):225–31.

8

Macrophage migration inhibitory factor promoter polymorphisms (−794 CATT5−8): Relationship with soluble MIF levels in coronary atherosclerotic disease subjects

Lu Qian[1†], Xiao-Yan Wang[2†], Saroj Thapa[1], Lu-yuan Tao[1], Shao-Ze Wu[1], Gao-Jiang Luo[2], Lu-Ping Wang[1], Jiao-Ni Wang[1], Jie Wang[1], Ji Li[1], Ji-Fei Tang[1*] and Kang-Ting Ji[1*] (iD)

Abstract

Background: We analyzed the relationship of −794 CATT5−8 MIF polymorphisms with soluble MIF in Coronary Atherosclerotic Disease (CAD) patients.

Methods: A total of 256 patients selected, on which 186 normal-coronary and 70 Coronary artery disease subjects, were recruited in the study (Retrospectively registered). Genotyping of −794 CATT5−8 polymorphisms were performed by PCR and DNA sequencing. Serum MIF levels were measured using an ELISA kit. Patients were classified by coronary angiogram, and CAD based on Gensini's integral degree (angiographic scoring system).

Results: The allele frequency and genotype frequency of −794 CATT5−8 did not show any differences in normal-coronary subjects and CAD subjects. In CAD patients, serum MIF levels was lower in CATT (5) subjects than in CATT (7) subjects, while the genotype of −794 CATT5−8 did not show differences in serum MIF levels. In addition, we found a decrease in serum MIF levels in carriers of the (5/5) genotypes the −794 CATT5−8 MIF polymorphisms, although it was not significant. There was no relationship of CAD class and the allele frequency of −794 CATT5−8.

Conclusions: This study found no association between CAD class and −794 CATT5−8 MIF polymorphisms with soluble MIF levels in CAD Subjects.

Keywords: Macrophage Migration Inhibitory Factor, Gene polymorphisms, Coronary Atherosclerotic Disease, Gensini's degree integral

Background

Coronary Atherosclerotic Disease (CAD) is characterized by atherosclerotic plaques in the vascular wall that results in vascular stenosis or plaque disruption with acute thrombotic occlusion. It occurs due to gradual cholesterol and fibrous tissue plaque in the wall of coronary artery over long period [1]. Various risk factors have been identified for CAD, such as smoking, hypercholesterolemia, hypertension, and diabetes [2].

Evidence suggests that CAD is an inflammatory process with chronic inflammation of vessel wall infiltrated by circulating immune cells, such as monocytes and macrophages [3]. Macrophage migration inhibitory factor (MIF) is a homotrimer protein with a molecular weight of 37.5 kDa, which can promote the inflammation [4]. The first experimental studies that utilized pure recombinant MIF and neutralizing antibodies established that MIF played a critical role in the inflammatory cascade leading to endotoxic shock and death [5] . Soon thereafter, it was found that the macrophage, which had been considered historically to be the "target" of MIF action, was in fact a significant source of MIF production. In the case of the

* Correspondence: jefftang@medmail.com; ziguanger@163.com
†Equal contributors
[1]Department of Cardiology, the Second Affiliated Hospital, Wenzhou Medical University, Wenzhou, Zhejiang 325000, China
Full list of author information is available at the end of the article

macrophage, MIF promotes TNFα production, which leads to further MIF release and a re-entrant activation pathway that is required for the optimal expression of TNFα and other pro-inflammatory mediators [6]. MIF is expressed in several cell types, including monocytes, macrophages, vascular smooth muscle cells (SMCs), and cardiomyocytes [6–8].

As described by Jie Wu et al. [9], the MIF gene maps to chromosome 21q22.33 in human (2119 bp). There are four polymorphisms that have been mainly reported in the human MIF gene, including three Single Nucleotide Polymorphisms (SNPs) at positions –173 (rs755622), +254 (rs2096525), and +656 (rs2070766) and a 794CATT5–8 microsatellite polymorphism. Loci rs2096525 and rs2070766 are located in introns, whereas rs755622 and –794CATT5–8 are located in the promoter region of MIF [9] . Earlier studies have found that circulating MIF levels are elevated in ulcerative colitis (UC) [10], psoriasis [9] and tuberculosis (TB) [11]. Since these diseases are accompanied by persistent inflammation of varying degrees, it is possible that MIF may play a role in the development of these diseases.

Previous studies have reported that the plasma MIF level of CAD group was higher than non-CAD patients and the plasma MIF level was related to the stability of the plaque [12]. Also, we demonstrated a close association between the polymorphism of MIF on the –173 position and CAD [12]. The aim of this study was to investigate the relationship between –794 CATT5–8 MIF polymorphisms and soluble MIF levels in CAD patients.

Methods

Subjects

A total of 256 subjects were enrolled, including 186 without CAD and 70 with CAD subjects, in the period from 06/2012 to 12/2012 in our inpatient department. All patients underwent coronary angiography (CAG) interpreted by one independent radiologist. Stenosis of the left main artery [13], Left Anterior Descending (LAD) branch, Right Coronary Artery (RCA), and other major branches were evaluated. CAD patients had the evidence of atherosclerosis (i.e., ≥ 50% luminal stenosis) in at least one coronary artery or major branch segment in their epicardial coronary tree. Patients in the control group had no luminal stenosis at CAG. Patients were excluded if they had acute inflammatory diseases, tumors, autoimmune disease and severe hepatic and renal dysfunction. All participants were of Han ethnicity living in Wenzhou, a southeastern coastal city of China. This protocol was approved by the Research Ethics Committee of Wenzhou Medical University

(registration number L-2013-03). All authors have identified individual participants after data collection.

Gensini score

The severity of CAD was determined by Gensini scoring system which has been previously described [14]. Briefly, if any branches of main coronary artery Left Main Artery (LM), LAD, Left Circumflex Coronary Artery (LCX) and RCA has stenosis reaching 1–24% of the internal lumen diameter, 1 point is given. Similarly, 2 is given for 25–49% stenosis, 4 for 50–74%, 8 for 75–90%, 16 for 91–99% and 32 for 100% or total occlusion. Depending on the lesion location, the single lesion score and the coefficient, the final Gensini total score was calculated.

Human genomic DNA extraction

A blood sample of 5 mL was collected into a tube containing ethylene diamine tetra acetic acid (EDTA) from the radial artery. After centrifugation, plasma was collected and stored at –80 °C until use. Genomic DNA was extracted from cells by a DNA extraction kit (Tiangen Company, Beijing, China). The isolated DNA was also stored at –80 °C.

MIF – 794 CATT5–8 genotyping

Polymorphism was genotyped by sequencing of polymerase chain reaction (PCR) product as reported previously [4, 15]. The forward primer was 5-TTGCACCTATCAGAGACC-3 and the reverse primer was 5-TCCACTAATGGTAAACTCG-3. These primers were designed to amplify a 207 bp segment of the MIF promoter region. PCR was carried out in a volume of 25 µl. The reaction conditions of PCR were as follows: initial denaturation at 95 °C for 5 min, followed by 35 cycles at 95 °C for 30 s, 60 °C for 30 s, and 72 °C for 1 min, with final extension at

Table 1 Clinical and biochemical characteristics by study group

	Control group (n = 186)	CHD group (n = 70)	F/x²	P value
Mean age(year)[a]	60.78 ± 9.26	66.71 + 10.25	1.24	0.081
Gander[b] (male/female)	84/102	44/26	6.37	0.012
cigarette smoking(%)[b]	31.6%	33.3%	0.236	0.627
Drinking(%)[b]	18.3%	24.3%	0.677	0.41
Hypertension(%)[b,c]	66.7%	68.6%	0.054	0.817
Hyperlipidemia(%)[b,d]	16.7%	37.1%	6.76	0.009
Diabetes(%)[b,e]	3.3%	7.1%	0.92	0.337

[a]Data presented as mean ± SD. Student's t-test
[b]Chi-square
[c]blood pressure ≥ 140/90 mmHg
[d]LDL-C ≥ 120mg/dl
[e]FPG ≥ 7.0 mmol/l and/or OGTT 2 h FPG ≥ 11.1 mmol/l

Table 2 Genotype and allele frequencies of −794 CATT5–8 MIF polymorphisms

Polymorphisms	Genotypes/ alleles	CHD group $n = 70$	Control group $n = 186$	x^2	P value[a]
−794CATT	5/5	11(15.7)	31(17.6)		
	6/6	16(22.9)	30(17.0)		
	7/7	3(4.3)	7(4.0)		
	5/6	22(31.4)	56(31.8)		
	5/7	10(14.3)	24(13.6)		
	6/7	8(11.4)	26(14.8)		
	6/8	0(0)	1(0.54)	0.464	0.834
	5	54(38.6)	132(35.5)		
	6	62(44.3)	190(51.1)		
	7	24(17.1)	49(13.2)		
	8	0(0)	1(0.27)	0.003	0.959

[a]Chi-square test x^2

72 °C for 10 min. PCR products were revealed by agarose gel electrophoresis.

Genomic DNA was extracted from blood collected into tubes containing EDTA. The DNA of individuals previously sequenced was used as a template to generate control DNA fragments, using BigDye Terminator v1.1, in order to correlate the fragment size observed on the ABI 310 analyzer with the number of CATT repeats in the test samples [16]. (Sequenced by Shanghai Hybio BioTechnology Co., Ltd.).

Analysis of serum MIF levels

The plasma concentrations of MIF were measured using an enzyme linked immunosorbent assay (ELISA) kit according to the manufacturer's instructions (R&D, USA).

Statistic analyses

MIF genotype and allele frequencies were analyzed using SPSS17.0 statistical software. The allele and genotype distributions were estimated by gene counting, and distribution of the polymorphic variants was tested against Hardy–Weinberg (H–W) equilibrium by χ2 analysis. Plasma MIF concentrations were expressed as means ± SD. For comparisons between two groups, we determined the significance of differences between means by t-tests. Comparisons between multiple groups were performed by ANOVA. $P \leq 0.05$ was considered statistically significant.

Results

Frequencies of MIF − 794 alleles and genotypes of CAD patients and controls

There were no significant differences in age, cigarette smoking, drinking hypertension, and diabetes except gender, ($P > 0.05$) (Table 1) between the CAD patients and the control. Both CAD patients and controls were in Hardy-Weinberg equilibrium with MIF −794CATT5–8 genotypes' distribution ($P > 0.05$). There were seven kinds of genotypes and four kinds of alleles in these two groups (Table 2). The comparative analysis of genotype and allele frequencies of −794 CATT5–8 polymorphisms between groups did not show significant differences ($P > 0.05$).

The plasma concentration of MIF

The plasma MIF concentration of CAD group was 65.75 ± 6.32 µg/L, significantly higher than that of non-CAD group (51.13 ± 7.33µg/L, $P < 0.05$), as we known before [12]. MIF serum levels were similar among CATT (5), CATT (6), and CATT (7) allele carriers. (Table 3).

In CAD patients the plasma MIF concentration of the carriers of CATT(5) allele was significantly lower than that of the CATT(7) allele carriers ($P < 0.05$) (Fig. 1a). When MIF serum levels were compared among CAD patients with different genotypes, we did not observe significant difference. In the CAD patients, the plasma MIF concentration was lower in the CATT(5/5) group than CATT(6/6) and CATT(7/7) groups but the difference was not statically significant ($P > 0.05$) (Fig. 1b). While in normal-coronary subjects, we did not observe a correlation between MIF serum levels with allele and genotypes ($P > 0.05$) (data not shown).

Table 3 The plasma MIF concentration

	CHD group (n = 70)	Control group (n = 186)	P* value	
mean concentration of MIF + SD	65.75 ± 6.32	51.13 ± 7.33		
median of MIF	65.66	50.01	0.00	
	alleles 5 (2n = 186)	alleles 6 (2n = 252)	alleles 7 (2n = 73)	P[#] value
mean concentration of MIF + SD	58.68 + 7.80	60.22 + 9.77	62.09 + 5.32	
median of MIF	58.275 + 1.42	59.75 + 0.98	61.79 + 0.51	0.373

*Student's t-test
[#]Chi-square test x^2

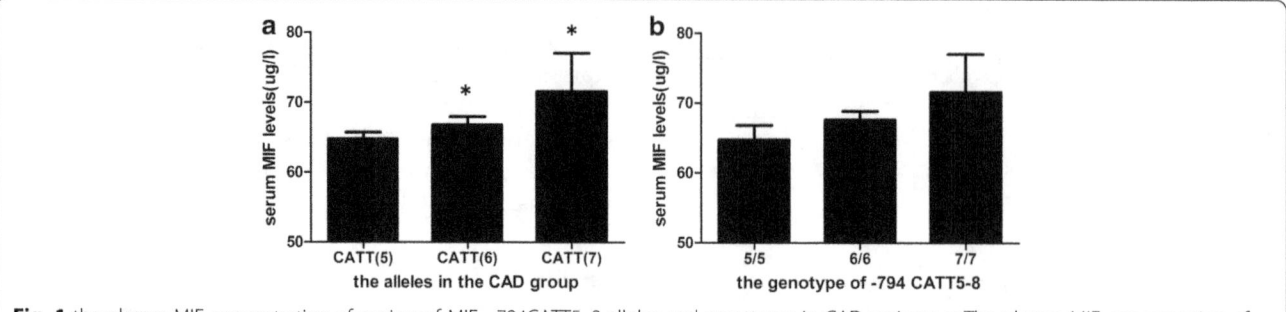

Fig. 1 the plasma MIF concentration of carriers of MIF −794CATT5–8 alleles and genotypes in CAD patients. **a** The plasma MIF concentration of the carriers of CATT(5) allele was significantly lower than that of the CATT(7) allele carriers ($P < 0.05$). **b** The plasma MIF concentration was lower in the CATT(5/5) group than CATT(6/6) and CATT(7/7) groups but the difference was not statically significant ($P > 0.05$)

Frequencies of MIF− CATT$_{5-8}$ alleles among CAD patients
Patients were classified into three subgroups according to the Gensini system. There was no difference in MIF–CATT5–8 allele frequency in CAD patients with different scores (Table 4).

Discussion

Despite the improvements in medical treatments and subsequent survival rates, CAD is still the leading cause of death worldwide [1]. In addition, it is well documented that there is strong relationship between many genetic variants and environmental factor in CAD. Therefore, the knowledge of genetic mechanisms of CAD is helpful to develop new disease prevention and treatment strategies.

Polymorphism of MIF on the −173 position has been reported in several inflammatory diseases, including ulcerative colitis (UC) [10], psoriasis [9] and tuberculosis (TB) [11]. Several studies have reported the association between MIF794CATT gene polymorphism, MIF protein level and CAD. For example in Western Mexico, MIF794CATT (6/7) genotype was found to correlate with the onset of acute coronary syndrome [17]. Lan et al. reported that discovered polymorphism of the MIF gene was associated with the severity of carotid atherosclerotic plaque [18]. In the present study, MIF794CATT gene polymorphism and CAD incidence were not significantly correlated, but in

the CAD patients, CATT (5) allele carriers had lower serum MIF concentration than the other two groups. Indeed, in vitro studies found that, CATT (5) allele has the lowest level of basic and stimulated MIF promoter activity when compared to the CATT (6) and CATT (7) alleles [16, 19]. However, it is still unknown which transcription factors regulate the expression of MIF by binding to CATT gene promoter region [20].

We found that serum MIF concentrations were significantly higher in CAD patients than the non-CAD patients, which is inconsistence with the previous finding that increased incidence MIF protein concentration is related to increased incidence of CAD [12]. However, MIF794CATT5−8 allele were not associated with the severity of CAD.

Our study is based at single center and the cases are limited because of time and geographical restrictions. Further studies with bigger sample size and patients from more cities are needed to confirm this primary conclusion.

Conclusion

To sum up, there is no significant correlation between the polymorphism of 794CATT gene and the severity of CAD.

Table 4 the relationship between CHD class and the allele frequency of MIF-794 CATT$_{5-8}$

CHD class (Gensini's intergral degree)	the allele frequency of MIF-794 CATT$_{5-8}$	
	5	6
≦20	16	10
20–40	14	10
≧40	13	4
x^2	1.55	
P^a value	0.46	

[a]Chi-square test

Abbreviations
CAD: Coronary Atherosclerotic Disease; CAG: Coronary Angiography; EDTA: Ethylene Diamine Tetra Acetic Acid; ELISA: Enzyme Linked Immunosorbent Assay; LAD: Left Anterior Descending; LCX: Left Circumflex Coronary Artery; LM: Left Main Artery; MIF: Migration Inhibitory Factor; PCR: Polymerase Chain Reaction; RCA: Right Coronary Artery; SMCs: Vascular smooth muscle cells; SNPs: Single Nucleotide Polymorphism; TB: Tuberculosis; UC: Ulcerative Colitis

Acknowledgements
Not applicable.

Funding
The authors disclosed receipt of the following financial support for the research and authorship of this article: National Natural Science Foundation of China [Nos. 81,573,185], Natural Science Foundation of Zhejiang Province

[Nos. 2014C33163], Wenzhou Municipal Science and Technology Bureau [Nos. H20140001, Nos.Y20130167].

Authors' contributions

LQ: research design, perform experiments, collect data and analysis of data, draft manuscript. XW: perform experiments, collect data and analysis of data. ST: perform experiments, draft manuscript. LT: perform experiments, collect data and analysis of data. SW: perform experiments, collect data and analysis of data. GL: collect data, draft manuscript. LW: perform experiments, collect data and analysis of data. JW1(Jiao-Ni Wang): perform experiments, collect data and analysis of data. JW2(Jie Wang): collect data and analysis of data. JL: research design, revising manuscript. JT: research design, draft manuscript. KJ: research design, draft manuscript. All authors read and approved the final manuscript.

Competing interests

The authors declare that there is no conflict of interests regarding the publication of this paper.

Author details

[1]Department of Cardiology, the Second Affiliated Hospital, Wenzhou Medical University, Wenzhou, Zhejiang 325000, China. [2]Department of Cardiology, Yiwu Central Hospital, Yiwu 322000, China.

References

1. Zaiying Lu NZ, Xie Y, Hu P. Internal medicine: People's medical publishing house; 2008. p. 274.
2. Rifai N, Ridker PM. Inflammatory markers and coronary heart disease. Curr Opin Lipidol. 2002;13(4):383–9.
3. Pamukcu B, Lip GY, Devitt A, et al. The role of monocytes in atherosclerotic coronary artery disease. Ann Med. 2010;42(6):394–403.
4. Leng L, Bucala R. Insight into the biology of macrophage migration inhibitory factor (MIF) revealed by the cloning of its cell surface receptor. Cell Res. 2006;16(2):162–8.
5. Bernhagen J, Calandra T, Mitchell RA, et al. MIF is a pituitary-derived cytokine that potentiates lethal endotoxaemia. Nature. 1993;365(6448):756–9.
6. Calandra T, Bernhagen J, Mitchell RA, et al. The macrophage is an important and previously unrecognized source of macrophage migration inhibitory factor. J Exp Med. 1994;179(6):1895–902.
7. Burger-Kentischer A, Goebel H, Seiler R, et al. Expression of macrophage migration inhibitory factor in different stages of human atherosclerosis. Circulation. 2002;105(13):1561–6.
8. Willis MS, Carlson DL, Dimaio JM, et al. Macrophage migration inhibitory factor mediates late cardiac dysfunction after burn injury. Am J Phys Heart Circ Phys. 2005;288(2):H795–804.
9. Wu J, Chen F, Zhang X, et al. Association of MIF promoter polymorphisms with psoriasis in a Han population in northeastern China. J Dermatol Sci. 2009;53(3):212–5.
10. Shiroeda H, Tahara T, Nakamura M, et al. Association between functional promoter polymorphisms of macrophage migration inhibitory factor (MIF) gene and ulcerative colitis in Japan. Cytokine. 2010;51(2):173–7.
11. Li Y, Zeng Z, Deng S. Study of the relationship between human MIF level, MIF-794CATT5-8 microsatellite polymorphism, and susceptibility to tuberculosis in Southwest China. Braz J Infect Dis. 2012;16(4):383–6.
12. Ji K, Wang X, Li J, et al. Macrophage migration inhibitory factor polymorphism is associated with susceptibility to inflammatory coronary heart disease. Biomed Res Int. 2015;2015:315174.
13. Barton A, Lamb R, Symmons D, et al. Macrophage migration inhibitory factor (MIF) gene polymorphism is associated with susceptibility to but not severity of inflammatory polyarthritis. Genes Immun. 2003;4(7):487–91.
14. Gensini GG. A more meaningful scoring system for determining the severity of coronary heart disease. Am J Cardiol. 1983;51(3):606.
15. Eriksson EE. Mechanisms of leukocyte recruitment to atherosclerotic lesions: future prospects. Curr Opin Lipidol. 2004;15(5):553–8.
16. Baugh JA, Chitnis S, Donnelly SC, et al. A functional promoter polymorphism in the macrophage migration inhibitory factor (MIF) gene associated with disease severity in rheumatoid arthritis. Genes Immun. 2002;3(3):170–6.
17. Valdes-Alvarado E, Munoz-Valle JF, Valle Y, et al. Association between the −794 (CATT)5–8 MIF gene polymorphism and susceptibility to acute coronary syndrome in a western Mexican population; 2014. p. 704854.
18. Lan MY, Chang YY, Chen WH, et al. Association between MIF gene polymorphisms and carotid artery atherosclerosis. Biochem Biophys Res Commun. 2013;435(2):319–22.
19. Renner P, Roger T, Bochud PY, et al. A functional microsatellite of the macrophage migration inhibitory factor gene associated with meningococcal disease. FASEB J. 2012;26(2):907–16.
20. Radstake TR, Sweep FC, Welsing P, et al. Correlation of rheumatoid arthritis severity with the genetic functional variants and circulating levels of macrophage migration inhibitory factor. Arthritis Rheum. 2005;52(10):3020–9.

9

The difference between Asian and Western in the effect of LDL-C lowering therapy on coronary atherosclerotic plaque

Yu-Feng Li[1†], Quan-Zhou Feng[1*†], Wen-Qian Gao[2†], Xiu-Jing Zhang[3†], Ya Huang[1] and Yun-Dai Chen[1*]

Abstract

Background: The different effects of LDL-C levels and statins therapy on coronary atherosclerotic plaque between Western and Asian remain to be settled.

Methods: PubMed, EMBASE, and Cochrane databases were searched from Jan. 2000 to Sep. 2014 for randomized controlled or blinded end-points trials assessing the effects of LDL-C lowering therapy on regression of coronary atherosclerotic plaque (CAP) in patients with coronary heart disease by intravascular ultrasound. The significance of plaques regression was assessed by computing standardized mean difference (SMD) of the volume of CAP between the baseline and follow-up.

Results: Twenty trials (ten in the West and ten in Asia) were identified. For Westerns, Mean lowering LDL-C by 49.4% and/or to level 61.9 mg/dL in the group of patients with baseline mean LDL-C 123.2 mg/dL could significantly reduce the volume of CAP at follow up (SMD −0.156 mm^3, 95% CI −0.248 ∼ −0.064, $p = 0.001$). LDL-C lowering by rosuvastatin (mean 40 mg daily) could significantly decrease the volumes of CAP at follow up. For Asians, Mean lowering LDL-C by 36.1% and/or to level 84.0 mg/dL with baseline mean LDL-C 134.2 mg/dL could significantly reduce the volume of CAP at follow up (SMD −0.211 mm^3, 95% CI −0.331 ∼ −0.092, $p = 0.001$). LDL-C lowering by rosuvastatin (mean 14.1 mg daily) and atorvastatin (mean 18.9 mg daily) could significantly decrease the volumes of CAP at follow up.

Conclusions: There was a different effect of LDL-C lowering on CAP between Westerns and Asians. For regressing CAP, Asians need lower dosage of statins or lower intensity LDL-C lowering therapy than Westerns.

Keywords: Low-density lipoprotein-cholesterol, Coronary atherosclerotic plaque, Intravascular ultrasound, Coronary artery disease, Western, Asian

Background

Atherosclerotic plaque is the hallmark and cornerstone of atherosclerotic disease. Disruption of coronary atherosclerotic plaque (CAP) may lead to sudden cardiac death, acute myocardial infarction, or unstable angina [1]. Intravascular ultrasound (IVUS) is considered to be gold standard for measurement of atherosclerotic plaque [2].

The meta-analysis of twenty trials evaluated the effects of LDL-C lowering on CAP indicated that intensive LDL-C lowering with statins could slow atherosclerotic plaque progression and lead to plaque regression [3]. But the meta-analysis did not investigate the effects of LDL-C lowering on CAP in different race.

In this meta-analysis, we investigated the difference between Western and Asian in the effect of LDL-C lowering therapy on the progression of the CAP from the current trials on LDL-C lowering therapy retarding the progression of the CAP and identified the different targets of LDL-C that result in the regression of the CAP for Western and Asian.

Methods

Materials and methods of this meta-analysis were detailed in the paper by Gao et al. [3].

* Correspondence: fqz301@yahoo.com; cyundai@medmail.com.cn
†Equal contributors
[1]The Department of Cardiology, Chinese PLA General Hospital, Fuxing Road 28, Beijing 100853, China
Full list of author information is available at the end of the article

Search strategy and selection criteria

An electronic literature search was performed to identify all relevant studies published in PubMed, EMBASE, and Cochrane databases in the English language from Jan. 1, 2000 to Sep. 13, 2014, using the terms "atherosclerosis" and "cholesterol blood level". Trials were included using the criteria as: 1) randomized controlled or prospective, blinded end-points trials, and its primary end point was CAP change detected by IVUS; 2) report of LDL-C levels at baseline and follow-up; 3) data on the volume of CAP at baseline and follow-up, and volume of CAP was calculated as vessel volume minus lumen volume; Exclusion criteria were: 1) only CAP area or volume index or percent atheroma volume were detected; 2) the levels of LDL-C at baseline or follow-up were not provided; and 3) target plaques were unstable.

Data extraction and quality assessment

Two investigators independently reviewed all potentially eligible studies and collected data on patient and study characteristics, and any disagreement was resolved by consensus. The primary end point of this study was the volume change of CAP detected by IVUS. Quality assessments of trials were evaluated with Jadad quality scale.

Data synthesis and analysis

Volume changes of CAP from baseline to follow-up were analyzed using standardized mean differences (SMD).

Volume changes of plaque in every arm were used for pooled analysis. The trials were firstly grouped into group Western and Asian according to the location of the trials. Then, according to the levels and the reducing percentage of LDL-C at follow-up, the arms were grouped to following groups: ≤ 70, $>70 \leq 100$ HP, $>70 \leq 100$ MP, $>70 \leq 100$ LP, >100 mg/dL; and <0, $\geq 0 < 30$, $\geq 30 < 40$, $\geq 40 < 50$, $\geq 50\%$ respectively [3], to investigate the effect of different levels of LDL-C at follow up on CAPs. According to statins, the arms were grouped to: rosuvastatin, atorvastatin, pitavastatin, simvastatin, fluvastatin and pravastatin groups, to investigate the effect of different statins on CAPs. The volume of CAP at follow up was compared with that at baseline to evaluate effect of LDL-C levels on regression of CAP.

Heterogeneity across trials (arms) was assessed via a standard χ^2 test with significance being set at $p < 0.10$ and also assessed by means of I^2 statistic with significance being set at $I^2 > 50\%$. Pooled analyses were calculated using fixed-effect models, whereas random-effect models were applied in case of significant heterogeneity across trials (arms). Sensitivity analyses (exclusion of one study at one time) were performed to determine the stability of the results. Publication bias was assessed using the Egger regression asymmetry test. Statistical analyses were performed using STATA software 12.0 (StataCorp, College Station, Texas).

All continuous variables were expressed as mean ± SD, and continuous variables were compared between the Western and Asian groups using Student's t test (SigmaStat 3.5). A P value <0.05 was considered to be statistically significant.

Results

Eligible studies

The flow of selecting studies for the meta-analysis was shown in Figure 1. Briefly, of the initial 673 articles, one hundred and twenty-two of abstracts were reviewed, resulting in exclusion of 102 articles, and 20 articles were reviewed in full text, resulting in exclusion of 10 trials and inclusion of 18 additional trials cited in the 20 articles. Twenty two RCTs [4-25] and six blinded end-points trial [26-31] were carefully evaluated, and eight trials [4,8,9,18,19,21,27,31] were excluded because of specific the index of plaque or lack of some data. Sixteen RCT (ESTABLISH [11], REVERSAL [10], A-PLUS [5], ACTIVATE [6], ILLUSTRATE [7], JAPAN-ACS [20], REACH [14], SATURN [16], ARTMAP [17], ERASE [23], STRADIVARIUS [24], PERISCOPE [25], and trials by Yokoyama M [12], by Kawasaki M [13], by Hong MK [15], and Tani S [22]) and four blinded end-points trial (ASTEROID [26], COSMOS [29], trial by Jensen LO [28] and trial by Nasu K [30]) were finally analyzed.

The characteristics of the included trials were as same as in the study [3] and shown in Table 1. Briefly, among the 20 trials, 10 trials are completed in European, America and Australia [10,5-7,16,23-26,28], 10 in Asia [20,11-15,17,22,29,30], and there were 15 trials assessing statins (statin vs. usual care in 6 trials [11-14,22,30]; intensive statin vs. moderate statin treatment in 5 trials [10,15-17,20]; follow up vs baseline in 3 trial [26,28,29], before acute coronary syndrome (ACS) vs after ACS in one trial [23]), 2 trials assessing enzyme acyl–coenzyme A: cholesterol acyltransferase (ACAT) inhibition [5,6], one trial assessing cholesteryl ester transfer protein (CETP) inhibitor torcetrapib [7], one trial assessing a decreasing obesity drug: rimonabant [24], and one trial assessing glucose-lowering agents [25]. Overall, 5910 patients with coronary heart disease (CHD) underwent serial IVUS examination for evaluating regression of CAP. Follow-up periods ranged from 2 to 24 months. The levels of LDL-C of each arm at baseline and follow-up were shown in Table 2.

Risk of bias of included studies, evaluated through Cochrane's methods, showed an overall acceptable quality of selected trials (Figures 2 and 3).

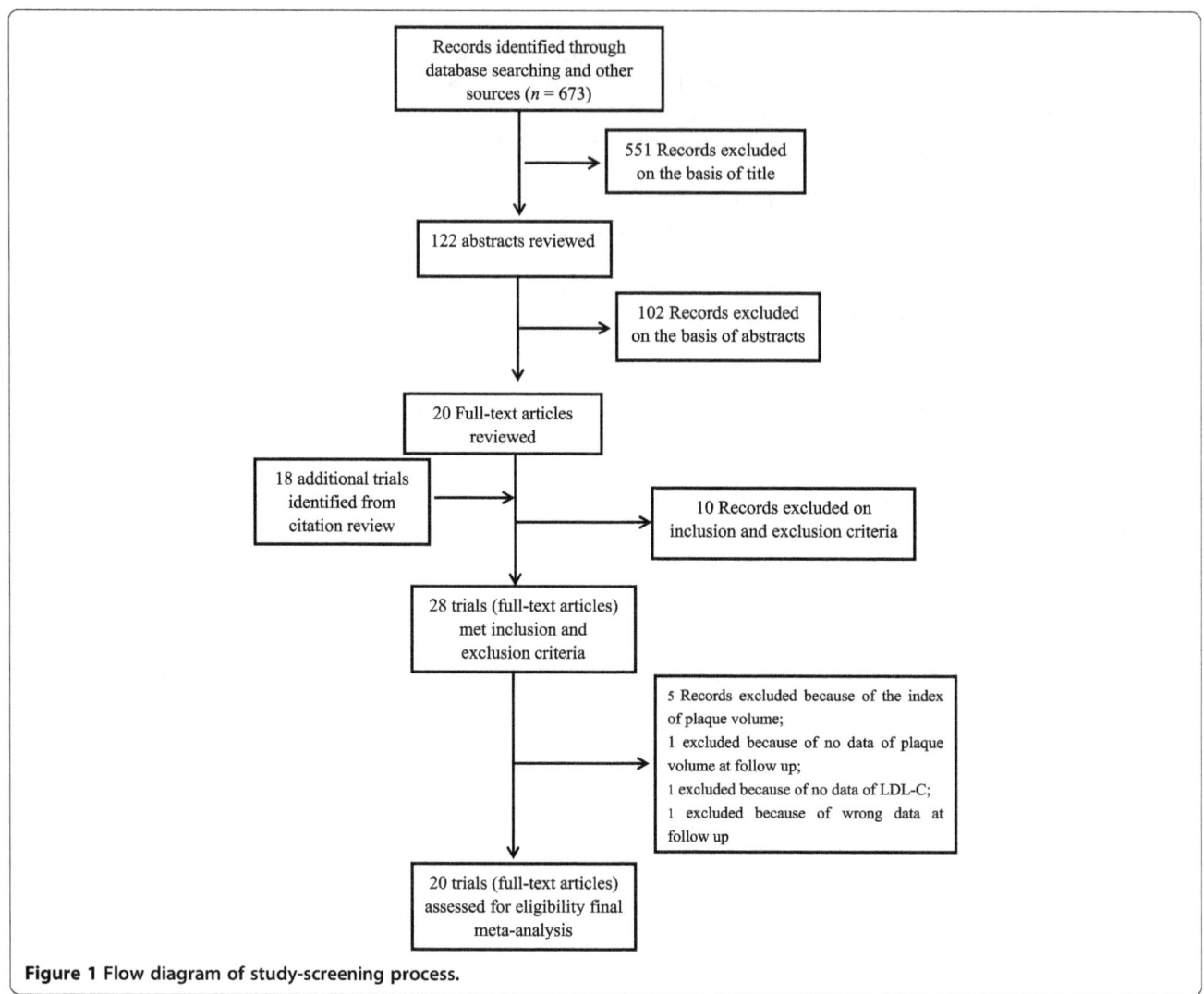

Figure 1 Flow diagram of study-screening process.

The effect of the levels of LDL-C at follow-up on regression of coronary atherosclerotic plaque in Western and Asian

For Western, meta-analysis indicated that LDL-C lowering in group ≤70 mg/dL could lead to regression of CAP, but LDL-C lowering in group >70 ≤ 100 HP, >70 ≤ 100 MP, >70 ≤ 100 LP and >100 mg/dL could not (Figure 4, Table 3).

In group ≤70 mg/dL (including three arms) with mean 23.1 months of follow up, the volumes of CAP (160.6 mm^3) at follow up were significantly decreased, compared with the volumes (171.4 mm^3) at baseline [SMD –0.156 mm^3, 95% CI (confidence interval) -0.248 ~ –0.064, p = 0.001]. There was no significant heterogeneity among arms (χ^2 for heterogeneity = 0.33, p =0.886, I^2 = 0%).

Sensitivity analyses suggested that LDL-C lowering in group ≤70 mg/dL could lead to regression of CAP with reduction of the CAP volume ranged from –0.139 mm^3 (SMD, 95% CI: –0.257 ~ –0.021) when the arm of 2006 ASTEROID Ros was omitted to –0.175 mm^3 (SMD,

95% CI: –0.317 ~ –0.034) when the arm of 2011 SATURN Ros was omitted. No publication bias was found, the values of p by Egger's test was 0.789.

For Asian, according to the levels of LDL-C at follow-up, the arms were grouped to three groups: ≤70, >70 ≤ 100 HP and >100 mg/dL.

LDL-C lowering in group ≤70 mg/dL and >70 ≤ 100 HP could lead to regression of CAP, but LDL-C lowering in group >100 mg/dL could not (Figure 5, Table 3).

In group ≤70 mg/dL (including four arms) with mean 6.9 months of follow up and group >70 ≤ 100HP mg/dL (including eight arms) with mean 11.0 months of follow up, the volumes of CAP (179.9, 87.5 mm^3 respectively) at follow up were significantly decreased, compared with the volumes (192.2, 96.4 mm^3 respectively) at baseline [SMD –0.157 mm^3, 95% CI –0.307 ~ –0.008, p = 0.039; SMD –0.211 mm^3, 95% CI –0.331 ~ –0.092, p = 0.001; respectively]. There was no significant heterogeneity among arms (χ^2 for heterogeneity = 0.24, p =0.955,

Table 1 Features of participating trials

Authors and trial name	Trial type and location	Objective	Year	N T/C	Study population	LDL-C at follow up	LDL-C reducing percentage	Treatments	Follow up	Main Results or Conclusion
Okazaki S[11]; ESTABLISH	RCT: prospective, open-label, randomized, single center study, Japan	Effects of statins on changes in plaque by IVUS	2004	24/24	ACS	70/119	-44/-0.004	Ato 20 vs Diet	6	Plaque volume was sigificantly reduced in the Ato group compared with the control group.
Nissen SE[10], REVERSAL	RCT: Double-blind, randomized active control multicenter trial: USA	Effects of statins (intensive or moderate) on changes in plaque by IVUS	2004	253/249	CAD	79/110	-46/-25	Ato 80 vs Pra40	18	Ato reduced progression of coronary plaque compared with Pra. Compared with baseline values, Ato had no change in atheroma burden, whereas patients treated with Pra showed progression of coronary plaque.
Tardif JC[5]; A-PLUS	RCT: international, multicenter, double-blind, placebo-controlled, randomized trial. Canada, USA	Effects of different dosage of avasimibe on changes in plaque by IVUS	2004	108/98/117/109	CAD	100/102/101/91	7.8/9.1/10.9/1.7	Ava50, 250, and 750 vs Placebo on the basis of LDL-C < 125	18	Avasimibe did not favorably alter coronary atherosclerosis as assessed by IVUS.
Jensen LO[28]	Open non placebo controlled serial investigation; blinded end-points. Denmark	To investigate the effect of lipid lowering by simvastatin on coronary atherosclerotic plaque volumes and lumen.	2004	40	CAD	85	-46.3	Sim 40	15	Lipid-lowering therapy with Sim is associated with a significant plaque regression in coronary arteries.
Yokoyama M[12]	RCT: randomized, single center. Japan	Effects of statins on changes in plaque by IVUS	2005	29/30	stabl angina	87/124	-35/-0.075	Ato 10 vs Diet	6	Treatment with Ato may reduce volumes of coronary plaques.
Kawasaki M[13]	RCT: randomization, open-label, single-center study. Japan	Effects of statins on changes in plaque by IVUS	2005	17/18/17	stable angina	95/102/149	-39/-32/-0.02	Ato 20, Pra 20 vs Diet	6	Treatment with Ato and Pra may not significantly reduce volumes of coronary plaques.
Tani S[22]	RCT: a prospective, single-center, randomized, open trial. Japan	Investigated the effects of pravastatin on the serum levels of MDA-LDL and coronary atherosclerosis.	2005	52/23	stable angina	104/120	-20/-2.4	Pra 10-20 vs con	6	Plaque volume was significantly reduced in the Pra group compared with the control group.
Nissen SE[6], ACTIVATE	RCT: randomized, multicenter. USA	Effects of pactimibe on changes in plaque by IVUS	2006	206/202	CAD	91/86	-9.6/-14.9	Pac100 vs Placebo	18	Pac is not an effective strategy for limiting atherosclerosis and may promote atherogenesis.
Nissen SE[26], ASTEROID	Prospective, open-label blinded end-points. USA, Germany, France, Canada	Effects of Statins with different levels of LDL-C on changes in plaque by IVUS	2006	349	CAD	61	-53.2	Ros 40	24	Therapy using Ros can result in significant regression of atherosclerosis.

Table 1 Features of participating trials *(Continued)*

		Year							
Yamada T[14]; REACH	RCT: open-labeled, randomized, multicenter study, Japan	2007	26/32	stable angina	83/115	−43/0	Ato 5 vs Con	12	Ato treatment prevented the further progression of atherosclerosis by maintaining LDL-C below 100 mg/dll in patients with CHD.
Nissen SE[7]; ILLUSTRATE	RCT: prospective, randomized, multicenter, double-blind clinical trial. North America or Europe	2007	446/464	CAD	87/70	6.6/-13.3	Ato10-80 vs Ato + Tor 60 on the basis of LDL-C ≤ 100 by Ato	24	The Tor was associated with a substantial increase in HDL-C and decrease in LDL –C, and there was no significant decrease in the progression of coronary atherosclerosis.
Nissen SE[25]; PERISCOPE	RCT: prospective, randomized, multicenter, double-blind clinical trial. USA	2008	181/179	CAD,DM	96.1/95.6	1.8/2.2	Gli1-4 mg vs Pio 15-45 mg on bases of statins therapy	18	In patients with type 2 diabetes and CAD, treatment with Pio resulted in a significantly lower rate of progression of coronary atherosclerosis compared with Gli.
Nissen SE[24], STRADIVARIUS	RCT: Randomized, double-blinded, placebo -controlled, 2-group, parallel-group trial. North America, Europe, and Australia	2008	335/341	CAD, Obesity	87.6/86.3	−4.7/-3.6	Rim 20 mg vs Placebo on bases of statins therapy	18	Rim can reduce progression of coronary plaque, and increase HDL-C levels, decrease triglyceride levels.
Hiro T[20]; JAPAN-ACS	RCT: prospective, randomized, open-label, parallel group, multicenter. Japan	2009	127/125	ACS	84/81	−36/-36	Ato 20 vs Pit 4	10	The administration of Pit or Ato in patients with ACS equivalently resulted in significant regression of coronary plaque volume.
Takayama T; COSMOS[29]	Prospective, open-label blinded end-points multicenter trial. Japan	2009	126	stable angina	83	−38.6	Ros <20	14	Ros exerted significant regression of coronary plaque volume in Japanese patients with stable CAD.
Rodés-Cabau; ERASE[23]	RCT: multicenter randomized placebo-controlled. Canada	2009	38/36	ACS	77/63	8.5/-37	Before ACS vs After ACS	<2	Newly initiated statin therapy is associated with rapid regression of coronary atherosclerosis.
Nasu K[30]	Prospective and multicenter study with nonrandomized and non-blinded design, but blinded end. Japan	2009	40/39	stable angina	98.1/121	−32.3/-1.1	Flu 60 vs Con	12	One-year lipid-lowering therapy by Flu showed significant regression of plaque volume.

Table 1 Features of participating trials (Continued)

Study	Design	Objective	Year	T/C	Disease		LDL-C (%)	Treatment	Months	Conclusion
Hong MK[15]	RCT: randomized control trial. Korea.	Evaluated the effects of statin treatments for each component of coronary plaques.	2009	50/50	stable angina	78/64	−34.5/−44.8	Sim 20 vs Ros 10	12	Statin treatments might be associated with significant changes in necrotic core and fibrofatty plaque volume.
Nicholls SJ; SATURN[16]	RCT: a prospective, randomized, multicenter, double-blind clinical trial. USA	Compare the effect of these two intensive statin regimens on the progression of coronary atherosclerosis.	2011	519/520	CHD	70.2/62.6	−41.5/−47.8	Ato 80 vs Ros 40	24	Maximal doses of Ros and Ato resulted in significant regression of coronary atherosclerosis.
Lee CW[17]; ARTMAP	RCT: a prospective, single-center, open-label, randomized comparison trial. Korea.	Compared the effects of atorvastatin 20 mg/day versus rosuvastatin 10 mg/day on mild coronary atherosclerotic plaques.	2012	143/128	stable angina	56/53	−47/−49	Ato 20 vs Ros 10	6	Usual doses of Ato and Ros induced significant regression of coronary atherosclerosis in statin-naive patients.

Abbreviations: T Treatment, C Control, RCT randomized controlled trials, IVUS Intravascular ultrasound, CAD Coronary artery disease, ACS Acute coronary syndrome, CHD Coronary heart disease, Ato Atorvastatin, Ros Rosuvastatin, Pra Pravastatin, Pit Pitavastatin, Sim Simvastatin, Flu Fluvastatin, Con Control, Pac Pactimibe, Tor Torcetrapib, Ava 50, 250, 750, Avasimibe 50, 250, 750 mg, T/C Treat/Control, Gli Glimepiride, Pio Pioglitazone, Rim Rimonabant.

Table 2 The levels of LDL-C at baseline and follow up in each arm of included trials

Authors	Trial name	Management in each arm	N	LDL-C level	
				At baseline	At follow-up
Tardif JC	A-PLUS	Avasimibe50	108	92.8 ± 1.7	100*
Tardif JC	A-PLUS	Avasimibe250	98	93.4 ± 1.6	101.9*
Tardif JC	A-PLUS	Avasimibe750	117	91.4 ± 1.6	101.4*
Tardif JC	A-PLUS	Placebo	109	89.6 ± 1.6	91.1*
Okazaki S	ESTABLISH	Control	24	123.9 ± 35.3	119.4 ± 24.6
Okazaki S	ESTABLISH	Atorvastatin	24	124.6 ± 34.5	70.0 ± 25.0
Yokoyama M		Control	30	131.5 ± 23#	124.5 ± 24.1#
Yokoyama M		Atorvastatin	29	133 ± 13	87 ± 29
Nissen SE	REVERSAL	Atorvastatin	253	150.2 ± 27.9	78.9 ± 30.2
Nissen SE	REVERSAL	Pravastatin	249	150.2 ± 25.9	110.4 ± 25.8
Nissen SE	ACTIVATE	Pactimibe	206	101.4 ± 27.7	91.3
Nissen SE	ACTIVATE	Placebo	202	101.5 ± 31.1	86.4
Nissen SE	ILLUSTRATE	Atorvastatin	446	84.3 ± 18.9	87.2 ± 22.6
Nissen SE	ILLUSTRATE	Atorva + torcetrapib	464	83.1 ± 19.7	70.1 ± 25.4
Kawasaki M		Control	17	152 ± 20	149 ± 24
Kawasaki M		Pravastatin	18	149 ± 19	102 ± 13
Kawasaki M		Atorvastatin	17	155 ± 22	95 ± 15
Hiro T	JAPAN-ACS	Pitavastatin	125	130.9 ± 33.3	81.1 ± 23.4
Hiro T	JAPAN-ACS	Atorvastatin	127	133.8 ± 31.4	84.1 ± 27.4
Nissen SE	ASTEROID	Rosuvastatin	349	130.4 ± 34.3	60.8 ± 20.0
Takayama T	COSMOS	Rosuvastatin	126	140.2 ± 31.5	82.9 ± 18.7
Lee CW	ARTMAP	Atorvastatin	143	110 ± 31	56 ± 18
Lee CW	ARTMAP	Rosuvastatin	128	109 ± 31	53 ± 18
Yamada T	REACH	Atorvastatin	26	123 ± 17	83 ± 22
Yamada T	REACH	Control	32	115 ± 14	115 ± 30
Nasu K		Fluvastatin	40	144.9 ± 31.5	98.1 ± 12.7
Nasu K		Control	39	122.3 ± 18.9	121.0 ± 21.2
Nicholls SJ	SATURN	Atorvastatin	519	119.9 ± 28.9	70.2 ± 1.0
Nicholls SJ	SATURN	Rosuvastatin	520	120.0 ± 27.3	62.6 ± 1.0
Hong MK		Simvastatin	50	119 ± 30	78 ± 20
Hong MK		Rosuvastatin	50	116 ± 28	64 ± 21
Tani S		Pravastatin	52	130 ± 38	104 ± 20
Tani S		Control	23	123 ± 28	120 ± 30
Rodés-C Bef	ERASE	Statins before ACS	38	71 ± 23	77 ± 25
Rodés-C Aft	ERASE	Statins after ACS	36	100 ± 30	63 ± 17
Jensen LO		Simvastatin	40	158.7 ± 30.6	85.1 ± 22.1
Nissen SE	PERISCOPE	Statins + Gli	181	94.4 ± 32.9	96.1 ± 30.4
Nissen SE	PERISCOPE	Statins + Pio	179	93.5 ± 30.7	95.6 ± 28.9
Nissen SE	STRADIVARIUS	Statins + Rim	335	91.9 ± 27.9	87.6 ± 30.5
Nissen SE	STRADIVARIUS	Statins + Con	341	89.5 ± 32.2	86.3 ± 30.3

Note: *calculated on the bases of baseline levels and change percentage at follow up[5].
#calculated according to Figure 2 in the paper[12].

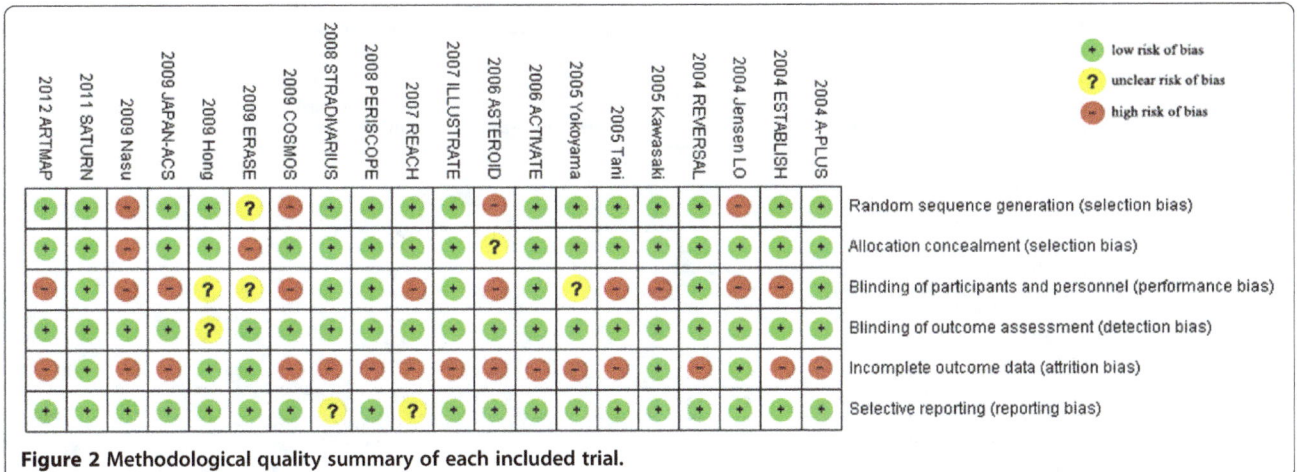

Figure 2 Methodological quality summary of each included trial.

$I^2 = 0\%$ for group ≤70 mg/dL; χ^2 for heterogeneity = 2.68, p =0.913, $I^2 = 0\%$ for group >70 ≤ 100HP mg/dL).

Sensitivity analyses suggested that LDL-C lowering in group >70 ≤ 100 HP mg/dL could lead to regression of CAP with reduction of the CAP volume ranged from −0.177 mm³ (SMD, 95% CI: −0.314 ~ −0.040) when the arm of 2009 JAPAN-ACS Ato was omitted to −0.231 mm³ (SMD, 95% CI: −0.368 ~ −0.094) when the arm of 2009 COSMOS Ros was omitted; but that LDL-C lowering in group ≤ 70 mg/dL could not significantly lead to regression of CAP with reduction of the CAP volume when the arm of 2012 ARTMAP Ros or 2012 ARTMAP Ato was omitted (Table 3).

No publication bias was found, the values of p by Egger's test for group ≤70 and >70 ≤ 100HP mg/dL were 0.970, 0.083 respectively.

The effect of the LDL-C reducing percentage at follow-up on regression of CAP in Western and Asian

For Western, meta-analysis showed that LDL-C lowering in group ≥40 < 50, ≥50% could lead to regression of CAP, but LDL-C lowering in group <0, ≥0 < 30% and ≥30 < 40 could not (Figure 6, Table 3).

In group ≥40 < 50% (including four arms) with mean 22.6 months of follow up, the volumes of CAP (143.1 mm³) at follow up were significantly decreased, compared with the volumes (148.8 mm³) at baseline (SMD −0.095 mm³, 95% CI −0.171 ~ −0.019, p = 0.014). There was no significant heterogeneity among arms (χ^2 for heterogeneity = 1.64, P = 0.651, I^2 = 0%).

Sensitivity analyses showed that LDL-C lowering in group ≥40 < 50 could still lead to regression of CAP with reduction of the plaque volume ranged from −0.065 mm³ (95% CI −0.163 ~ 0.032) when the arm of 2011 SATURN Ros was omitted to −0.116 mm³ (SMD, 95% CI −0.201 ~ −0.032) when 2004 REVERSAL Ato was omitted. Publication bias analysis suggested the values of p by Egger's test were 0.804.

In group group <0, ≥0 < 30% and ≥30 < 40, meta-analysis were showed in Table 3.

For Asian, according to the reducing percentage of LDL-C at follow-up, the arms were grouped to following groups: ≥0 < 30, ≥30 < 40, ≥40 < 50.

LDL-C lowering in group ≥30 < 40, ≥40 < 50% could lead to regression of CAP, but LDL-C lowering in group ≥0 < 30% could not (Figure 7, Table 3).

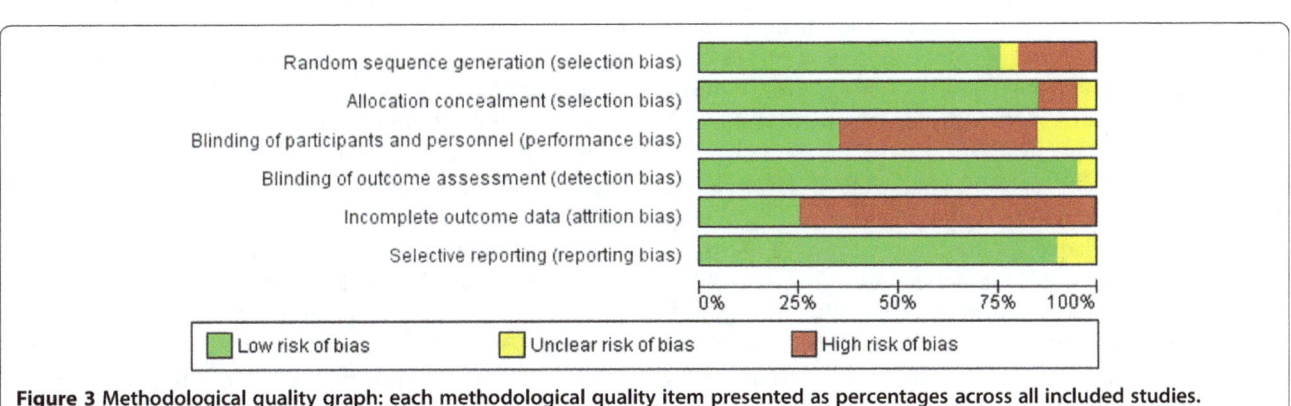

Figure 3 Methodological quality graph: each methodological quality item presented as percentages across all included studies.

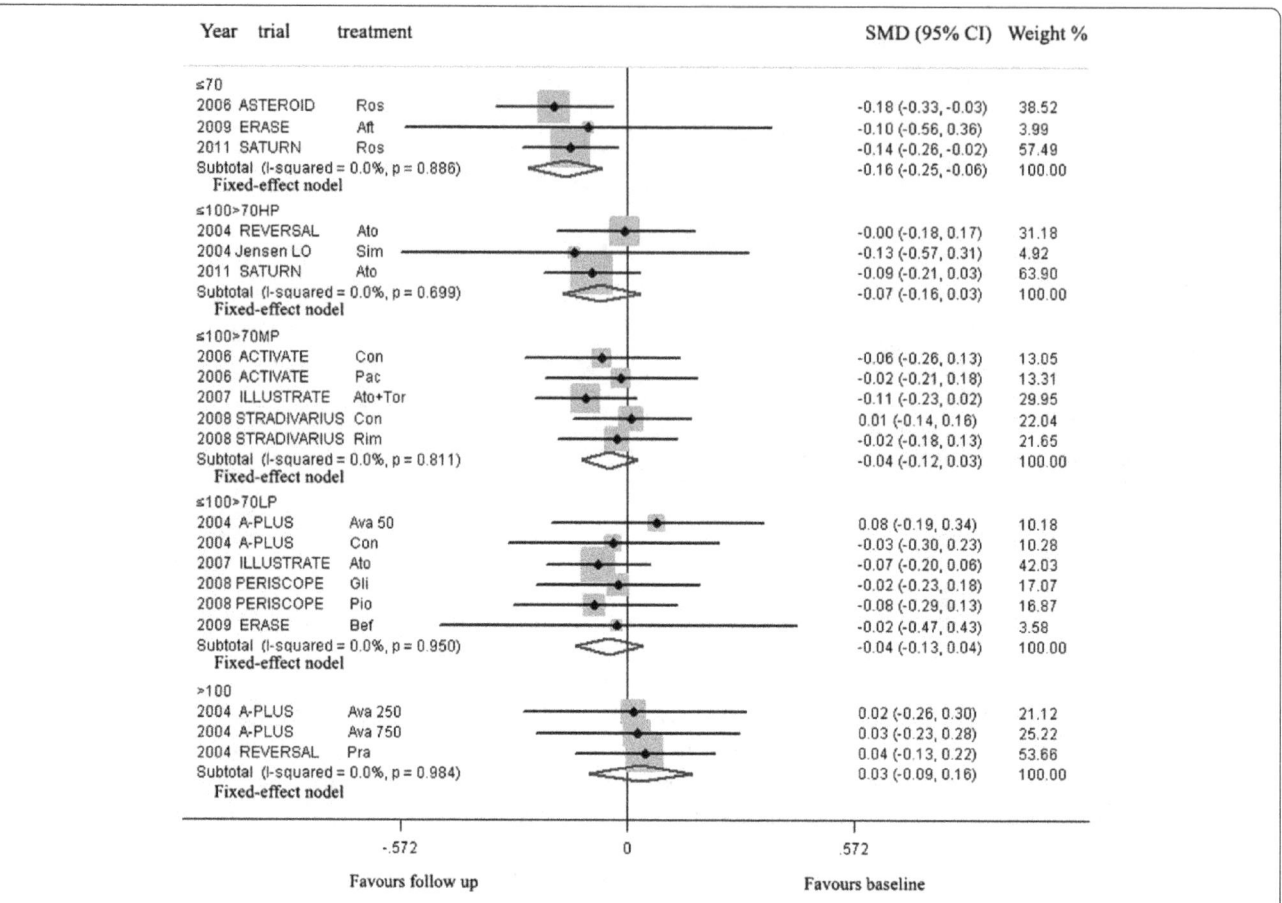

Figure 4 Meta- analysis of the effects of reduction levels of LDL-C at follow up on the regression of coronary atherosclerotic plaque in **Western.** Abbreviations: Ato, Atorvastatin; Ros, Rosuvastatin; Pra, Pravastatin; Pit, Pitavastatin; Sim, Simvastatin; Flu, Fluvastatin; Con, Control; Pac, Pactimibe; Tor, Torcetrapib, Ava 50, 250, 750, Avasimibe 50, 250, 750 mg; Bef, before ACS; Aft, after ACS; Gli, Glimepiride; Pio, Pioglitazone; Rim, Rimonabant.

In group $\geq 30 < 40\%$ (including nine arms) with mean 10.9 months of follow up, and group $\geq 40 < 50\%$ (including four arms) with mean 6.9 months of follow up, the volumes of CAP (90.0, 179.9 mm^3 respectively) at follow up were significantly decreased, compared with the volumes (98.6, 192.2 mm^3 respectively) at baseline (SMD -0.206 mm^3, 95% CI $-0.324 \sim -0.088$, $p = 0.001$; SMD -0.157 mm^3, 95% CI $-0.307 \sim -0.008$, $p = 0.039$; respectively). There was no significant heterogeneity among arms (χ^2 for heterogeneity = 2.91, $P = 0.840$, $I^2 = 0\%$; χ^2 for heterogeneity = 0.33, $p = 0.955$, $I^2 = 0\%$; for group $\geq 30 < 40$, and group $\geq 40 < 50$ respectively).

Sensitivity analyses showed that LDL-C lowering in group $\geq 30 < 40\%$ could still lead to regression of CAP with reduction of the plaque volume ranged from -0.172 mm^3 (95% CI $-0.306 \sim -0.038$) when the arm of 2009 JAPAN-ACS Ato was omitted to -0.223 mm^3 (SMD, 95% CI $-0.357 \sim -0.089$) when 2009 COSMOS Ros was omitted. Publication bias analysis suggested that bias was significant with 0.004 of p value by Egger's test.

Mean levels of LDL-C at baseline and follow up, mean reducing percentage of LDL-C in each group were showed in Table 4.

The effect of lowering LDL-C by statins on regression of coronary atherosclerotic plaque in Western and Asian

For Western, atorvastatin, rosuvastatin, pravastatin and simvastatin were used in trials to investigate the effects of LDL-C lowering on CAP. Meta-analysis indicated that LDL-C lowering by rosuvastatin could lead to regression of CAP, but LDL-C lowering by atorvastatin, pravastatin, and simvastatin could not (Figure 8, Table 5).

LDL-C lowering by rosuvastatin (mean 40.0 mg daily for mean 24 months) could significantly decrease the volumes of CAP at follow up, compared with the volumes at baseline (SMD -0.158 mm^3, 95% CI: $-0.253 \sim -0.064$, $p = 0.001$). There was no significant heterogeneity among arms (χ^2 for heterogeneity = 0.18, $p = 0.672$, $I^2 = 0\%$).

Table 3 Results of meta-analysis in each group and mean CAP volume in each group at baseline and follow up in Western and Asian

Group		Included arms (case)	CAP volume at baseline (mm³)	CAP volume at follow up (mm³)	Pooled SMD (95% CI, p)	Heterogeneity test χ² test (p)	I²	Sensitivity analyses Lower SMD (95% CI)	Upper SMD (95% CI)	Egger's test
	<70 mg	3(905)	171.4±32.7	160.6±29.7	−0.156(−0.248~−0.064, 0.001)	0.33(0.886)	0	−0.139(−0.257~−0.021) Without 2006 ASTEROID Ros	−0.175(−0.317~−0.034) Without 2011 SATURN Ros	0.789
	>70≤100 HPmg	3(812)	151.9±30.4	147.9±31.9	−0.065(−0.136~0.032, 0.189)	0.71(0.699)	0			0.987
	>70≤100 MPmg	5(1548)	195.8±2.3	191.8±4.7	−0.045(−0.115~−0.026, 0.215)	1.59(0.811)	0			0.500
	>70≤100 LPmg	6(1061)	201.2±15.1	197.3±15.0	−0.045(−0.130~0.040, 0.301)	1.14(0.950)	0			0.241
Western	>100 mg	3(464)	197.6±3.5	201.1±1.9	0.034(−0.094~0.163, 0.601)	0.03(0.984)	0			
	>50%	1(349)	212.2±81.3	197.5±79.1	−0.183(−0.332~−0.035, 0.016)					
	>40≤50%	4(1332)	148.8±24.0	143.1±25.6	−0.095(−0.171~−0.019, 0.014)	1.64(0.651)	0	−0.065(−0.163~0.032) Without 2011 SATURN Ros	−0.116(−0.201~−0.032) Without 2004 REVERSAL Ato	0.804
	>30≤40%	1(36)	169.1±77.3	161.5±75.2	−0.099(−0.561~0.363, 0.675)	0.00(0.000)	0			
	>0≤30%	6(1797)	195.6±2.1	192.9±5.1	−0.032(−0.098~0.033, 0.335)	2.45(0.784)	0			
	<0%	8(1276)	201.2±13.8	198.3±13.8	−0.034(−0.111~0.044, 0.396)	1.55(0.981)	0			0.087
	<70 mg	4(345)	192.2±59.9	179.9±53.0	−0.157(−0.307~−0.008, 0.039)	0.24(0.955)	0	−0.126(−0.314~0.063) Without 2012 ARTMAP Ros	−0.187(−0.383~0.008) Without 2012 ARTMAP Ato	0.970
	>70≤100 HPmg	8(540)	96.4±99.3	87.5±92.0	−0.211(−0.331~−0.092, 0.001)	2.68(0.913)	0	−0.177(−0.314~−0.040) Without 2009 JAPAN-ACS Ato	−0.231(−0.368~−0.094) Without 2009 COSMOS Ros	0.083
Asian	>100 mg	8(235)	133.0±139.6	134.3±143.8	−0.029(−0.210~0.152, 0.750)	2.14(0.952)	0			
	>40≤50%	4(345)	192.2±56.9	179.9±53.0	−0.157(−0.307~−0.008, 0.039)	0.33(0.955)	0	−0.126(−0.314~0.063) Without 2012 ARTMAP Ros	−0.187(−0.383~0.008) Without 2012 ARTMAP Ato	0.970
	>30≤40%	9(558)	98.6±98.5	90.0±91.6	−0.206(−0.324~−0.088, 0.001)	2.91(0.840)	0	−0.172(−0.306~−0.038) Without 2009 JAPAN-ACS Ato	−0.223(−0.357~−0.089) Without 2009 COSMOS Ros	0.004
	>0≤30%	7(217)	130.2±144.9	131.8±149.4	−0.028(−0.216~0.161, 0.773)	2.14(0.907)	0			

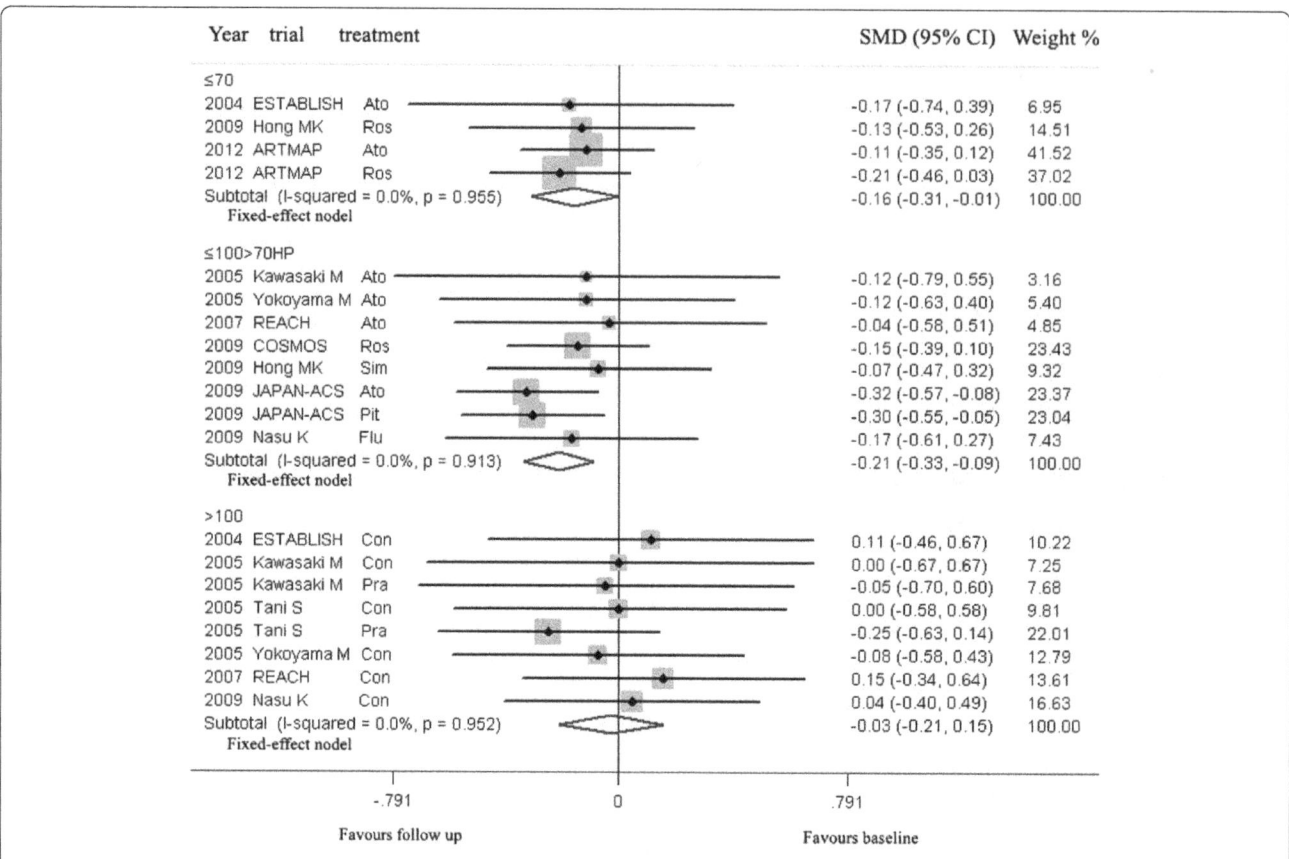

Figure 5 Meta- analysis of the effects of reduction levels of LDL-C at follow up on the regression of coronary atherosclerotic plaque in Asian. Abbreviation as in Figure 4.

Sensitivity analyses suggested that lowering LDL-C by rosuvastatin could lead to regression of CAP with reduction of the plaque volume ranged from -0.142 mm^3 (SMD, 95% CI: $-0.263 \sim -0.020$) when the arm of 2006 ASTEROID Ros was omitted to -0.183 mm^3 (SMD, 95% CI: $-0.332 \sim -0.035$) when the arm of 2011 SATURN Ros was omitted. But publication bias was found, the values of p by Egger's test was 0.000 (Table 5).

For Asian, atorvastatin, rosuvastatin, pitavastatin, pravastatin, fluvastatin and simvastatin were used in trials to investigate the effects of LDL-C lowering on CAP. Meta-analysis indicated that LDL-C lowering by rosuvastatin, atorvastatin could lead to regression of CAP, but LDL-C lowering by pitavastatin, pravastatin, fluvastatin and simvastatin could not (Figure 9, Table 5).

LDL-C lowering by rosuvastatin (mean 14.1 mg daily for mean 10.3 months), atorvastatin (mean 18.9 mg daily for mean 7.8 months) could significantly decrease the volumes of CAP at follow up, compared with the volumes at baseline (SMD -0.172 mm^3, 95% CI: $-0.331 \sim -0.012$, $p = 0.035$; SMD -0.185, 95% CI: $-0.330 \sim -0.040$, $p = 0.013$; respectively). There was no significant heterogeneity among arms (χ^2 for heterogeneity = 0.17, $p = 0.917$, $I^2 = 0\%$

for rosuvastatin; χ^2 for heterogeneity = 1.94, $p = 0.858$, $I^2 = 0\%$ for atorvastatin).

Sensitivity analyses suggested that lowering LDL-C by rosuvastatin could not significantly lead to regression of CAP when the arm of 2012 ARTMAP Ros or 2009 COSMOS Ros was omitted. Also, Lowering LDL-C by atorvastatin could not significantly lead to regression of CAP when the arm of 2009 JAPAN-ACS Ato was omitted. No publication bias was found, the values of p by Egger's test for rosuvastatin and atorvastatin group were 0.660, 0.456 respectively (Table 5).

Intensity of lowering LDL-C by different statins was shown in Table 6. Rosuvastatin and atorvastatin could reduce LDL-C by more than 40%.

The difference between Western and Asian in usage of statins

The meta analysis showed that rosuvastatin and atorvastatin can regress CAP (Table 5). LDL-C levels, intensity of lowering LDL-C by rosuvastatin and atorvastatin, its dosage and duration were compared between Western and Asian (Table 7). Intensity of lowering LDL-C by rosuvastatin and atorvastatin in Western group were

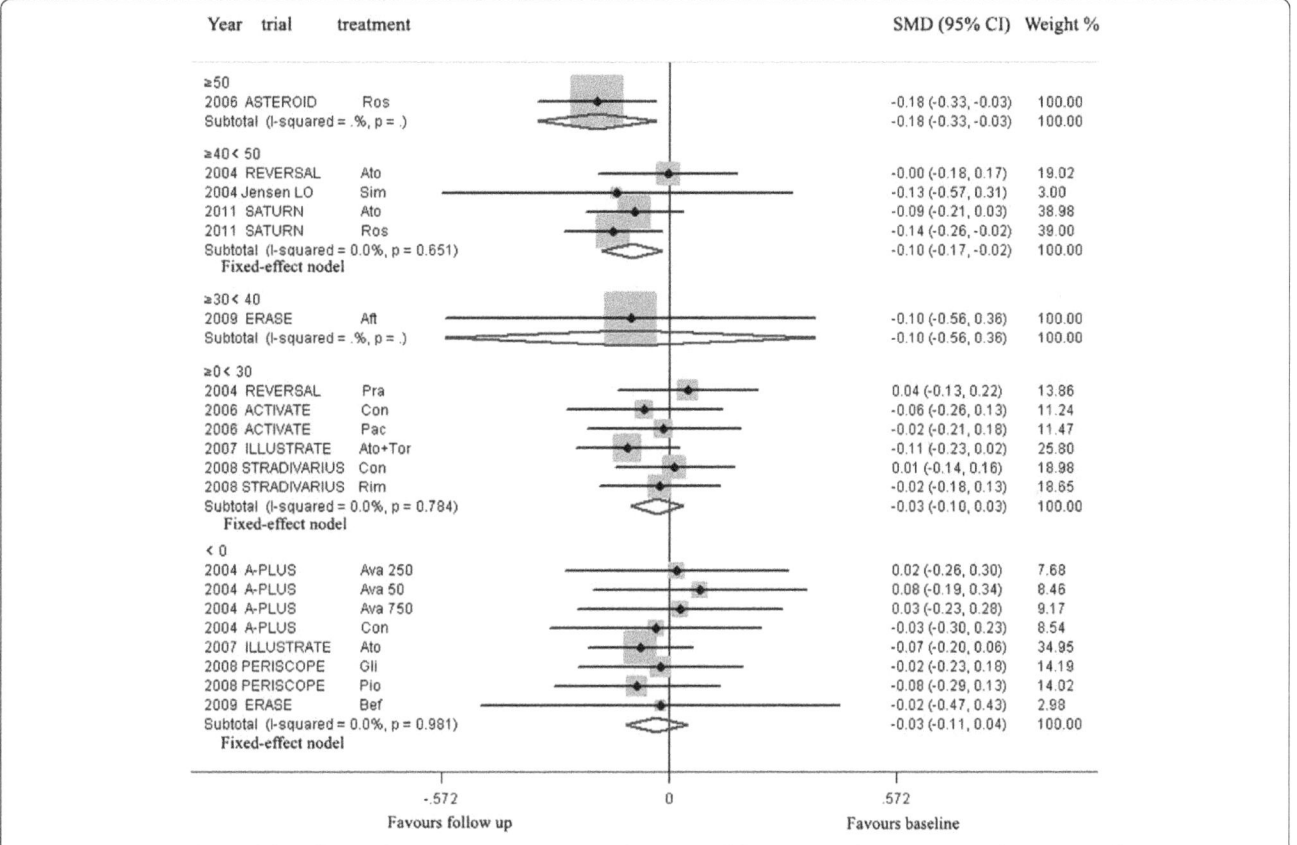

Figure 6 Meta- analysis of the effects of reduction percentages of LDL-C at follow up on the regression of coronary atherosclerotic plaque in Western. Abbreviation as in Figure 4.

similar to that in Asian group, but the dosages of rosuvastatin and atorvastatin in Asian group were significantly lower than those in Western group, and the duration of statins administration in Asian group were significantly shorter than those in Western, as showed in Table 7.

Discussion

This meta-analysis revealed that intensive LDL-C lowering can regress CAP both in Western and Asian. For regressing CAP, the dosage of statins administrated in Westerns was different from that in Asians. Asians need lower dosage of atorvastatin or rosuvastatin than Westerns though there was no difference between Westerns and Asians in pharmacokinetic and pharmacodynamic study [32,33].

The effect difference of LDL-C lowering on CAP between Western and Asian

For Western including American, Canadian, German, French, English, Australian and Dane [10,5-7,16,23-26,28], the meta-analysis (Table 3) in subgroup ≤70 mg and ≥40 < 50% of Western indicated that LDL-C level

lowering to <69.3 mg or reducing by > 45% for 22.6 months of follow up (Table 4) could lead to regression of CAP, but the meta-analysis (Table 3) in subgroup >70 ≤ 100 HP mg of Western showed that LDL-C level lowering to 73.2 mg or reducing by 43.6% for 21.7 months of follow up (Table 4) was not enough for regressing CAP.

For Asian including Japanese and Korean [20,11-15, 17,22,29,30], the meta-analysis in subgroup ≤70 mg and ≥40 < 50% of Asian indicated that LDL-C level lowering to 57.0 mg or reducing by 47.2% for 6.9 months of follow up could lead to regression of CAP, but sensitivity analyses showed that LDL-C lowering in this two subgroup could not significantly lead to regression of CAP when the arm of 2012 ARTMAP Ros or 2012 ARTMAP Ato was omitted (Table 3). The meta-analysis in subgroup ≥ 30 < 40% of Asian indicated that LDL-C level lowering to 84.6 mg or reducing by 36.0% for 10.9 months of follow up could also lead to regression of CAP, but publication bias was significant. The meta-analysis in subgroup >70 ≤ 100HP mg of Asian with good sensitivity and no publication bias indicated that LDL-C level lowering to 84.0 mg or reducing

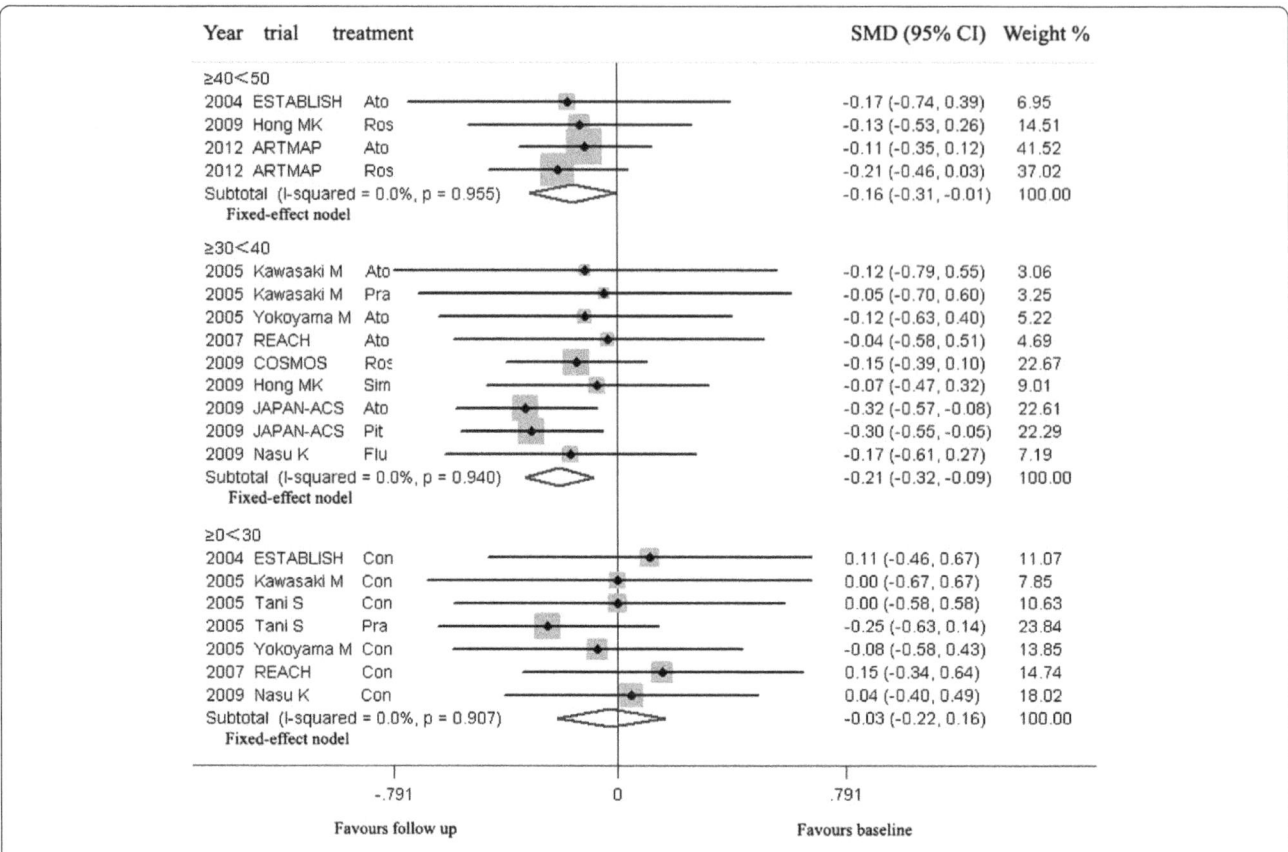

Figure 7 Meta- analysis of the effects of reduction percentages of LDL-C at follow up on the regression of coronary atherosclerotic plaque in Asian. Abbreviation as in Figure 4.

by 36.1% for 11 months of follow up with could lead to regression of CAP (Table 3).

Taken all the results of meta-analysis together, for Western, it was recommended that LDL-C level might be reduced by >45% or to a target level < 69 mg/dL for regressing CAP; for Asian, LDL-C level might be reduced by >36% or to a target level < 84 mg/dL.

Different effects of statins on Westerns and Asians

Whether statins has different effect on Westerns and Asians remains to be settled.

The study by Lee E et al. [34] and MEGA Study [35] suggested statins have different effects on Westerns and Asians. In 2005, Lee E et al. [34] prospectively examined the pharmacokinetics of rosuvastatin in White and Asian individuals living in Singapore, and reported that plasma exposure to rosuvastatin and its metabolites was significantly higher in Chinese, Malay, and Asian-Indian subjects compared with Western subjects living in the same environment. But the mechanisms underlying ethnic differences in rosuvastatin disposition remain to be unearthed [36]. MEGA Study [35]

indicated that a small dose of pravastatin that was half the dose administered to western patients, reduced LDL-C by 19-22% (which is lower than that reductions of 23–35% in western patients), but could substantially reduce the risk of coronary heart disease in Japanese.

But two meta-analysis did not demonstrate the difference of rosuvastatin and atorvastatin on Westerns and Asians. The meta-analysis including the 36 trials of pharmacodynamics of rosuvastatin in Western and Asian hypercholesterolemia patients did not confirm that there was significant difference in the exposure-response relationship for LDL-C reduction between Westerners and Asians [33].The meta-analysis including 22 pharmacokinetic studies also demonstrated no differences in the systemic exposure to atorvastatin between Asian and Caucasian subjects [32].

Our meta-analysis revealed that there were difference of rosuvastatin and atorvastatin in lowering LDL-C and regressing CAP between Westerns and Asians. The meta-analysis of rosuvastatin including 2 trials with 869 Western patients indicated that 40 mg of rosuvastatin daily for 24 months with reducing LDL-C by 49.9% could regress CAP. But the meta-analysis of

Table 4 Levels and reducing percentage of LDL-C and duration in each group in Western and Asian (Mean ± SD)

Group		N	Mean LDL-C at baseline (mg)	Mean LDL-C at follow up (mg)	Mean reducing percentage	Actual range of reducing percentage	Duration (month)
Western	≤70 mg	905	123.2 ± 6.9	61.9 ± 0.9	49.4 ± 3.5	37 ~ 53	23.1 ± 4.3
	>70 ≤ 100 HPmg	812	131.3 ± 15.2	73.6 ± 4.8	43.2 ± 2.2	41.5 ~ 46.7	21.7 ± 3.1
	>70 ≤ 100 MPmg	1548	91.3 ± 6.9	82.4 ± 8.2	9.0 ± 4.5	3.6 ~ 14.9	19.8 ± 2.7
	>70 ≤ 100 LPmg	1061	88.5 ± 5.5	91.5 ± 5.4	−4.7 ± 2.5	−1.7 ~ −8.5	19.9 ± 4.5
	>100 mg	464	123.4 ± 28.9	106.3 ± 4.4	8.7 ± 17.5	−10.9 ~ 25.0	18.0 ± 0.0
	>50%	349	130.4 ± 0.0	60.8 ± 0.0	53.4 ± 0.0	53.4 ~ 53.4	24.0 ± 0.0
	>40 ≤ 50%	1332	126.9 ± 13.1	69.3 ± 6.5	45.0 ± 2.8	41.5 ~ 47.8	22.6 ± 2.7
	>30 ≤ 40%	36	100.2 ± 30.2	63.1 ± 17.4	37.0	37 ~ 37	2.0 ± 0.0
	>0 ≤ 30%	1797	99.4 ± 21.4	86.2 ± 12.2	11.2 ± 6.9	3.6 ~ 25.0	19.5 ± 2.6
	<0%	1276	89.1 ± 5.3	93.2 ± 6.2	−5.6 ± 3.1	−1.7 ~ −10.9	19.6 ± 4.2
Asian	≤70 mg	345	111.5 ± 4.3	57.0 ± 5.0	47.2 ± 1.7	44 ~ 49	6.9 ± 2.1
	>70 ≤ 100 HPmg	540	134.2 ± 7.8	84.0 ± 5.0	36.1 ± 1.8	32.3 ~ 39.0	11.0 ± 2.2
	>100 mg	235	128.6 ± 10.5	117.2 ± 11.9	7.3 ± 10.7	0 ~ 32	7.8 ± 2.8
	>40 ≤ 50%	345	111.5 ± 4.3	57.0 ± 5.0	47.2 ± 1.7	44 ~ 49	6.9 ± 2.1
	>30 ≤ 40%	558	134.7 ± 8.1	84.6 ± 5.8	36.0 ± 1.9	32 ~ 39	10.9 ± 2.4
	>0 ≤ 30%	217	126.9 ± 9.1	118.3 ± 11.5	5.3 ± 8.3	0 ~ 20.0	8.0 ± 2.8

rosuvastatin including 3 trials with 304 Asian patients showed that 14.1 mg of rosuvastatin daily for 10.3 months with reducing LDL-C by 44.0% could also regress CAP though the result of sensitivity analyses is not as good as that in Western (Table 5). The meta-analysis of atorvastatin including 2 trials with 772 Western patients showed that 80 mg of atorvastatin daily for 22 months with reducing LDL-C by 43.0% could not significantly regress CAP. But the meta-analysis of atorvastatin including 6 trials with 366

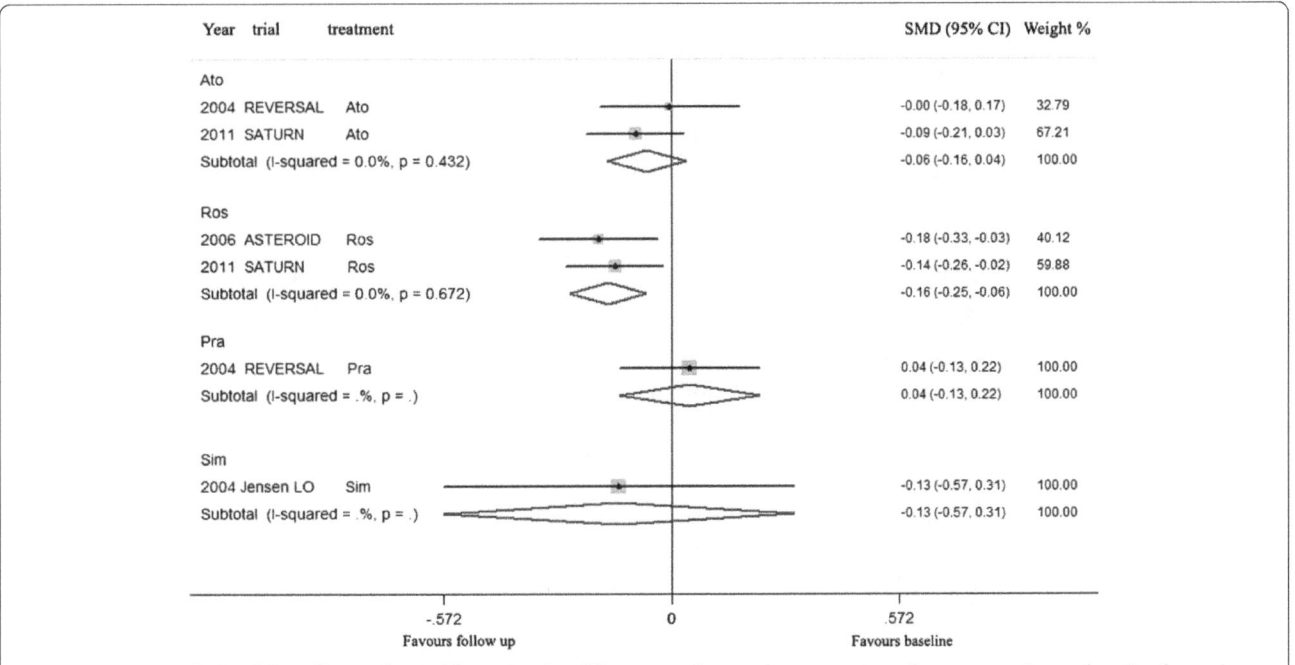

Figure 8 Meta- analysis of the effects of LDL-C lowering by different statins on the regression of coronary atherosclerotic plaque in **Western.** Abbreviation as in Figure 4.

Table 5 Results of meta-analysis in different statins groups in Western and Asian

Group		Included arms (and case)	Pooled SMD (95% CI, p)	Heterogeneity test		Sensitivity analyses		Egger's test
				χ^2 test (p)	I^2	Lower SMD (95% CI)	Upper SMD (95% CI)	
Western	Rosuvastatin	2(869)	−0.158(−0.253 ~ −0.064, 0.001)	0.18(0.672)	0	−0.142 (−0.263 ~ −0.020) Without 2006 ASTEROID Ros	−0.183 (−0.332 ~ −0.035) Without 2011 SATURN Ros	0.000
	Atorvastatin	2(772)	−0.062(−0.162 ~ 0.038, 0.225)	0.62(0.432)	0			0.000
	Pravastatin	1(249)	0.045(−0.131 ~ 0.221, 0.616)					
	Simvastatin	1(40)	−0.133(−0.572 ~ 0.306, 0.552)					
Asian	Rosuvastatin	3(304)	−0.172(−0.331 ~ −0.012, 0.035)	0.17(0.917)	0	−0.143 (−0.352 ~ 0.066) Without 2012 ARTMAP Ros	−0.189 (−0.397 ~ 0.019) Without 2009 COSMOS Ros	0.660
	Atorvastatin	6(366)	−0.185(−0.330 ~ −0.040, 0.013)	1.94(0.858)	0	−0.113 (−0.292 ~ 0.068) Without 2009 JAPAN-ACS Ato	−0.230 (−0.417 ~ −0.044) Without 2012 ARTMAP Ato	0.456
	Pravastatin	2(70)	−0.197(−0.529 ~ 0.135, 0.245)	0.26(0.608)	0			
	Pitavastatin	1(125)	−0.304(−0.553 ~ −0.055, 0.017)					
	Fluvastatin	1(40)	−0.169(−0.608 ~ 0.270, 0.450)					
	Simvastatin	1(50)	−0.074(−0.467 ~ 0.318, 0.710)					

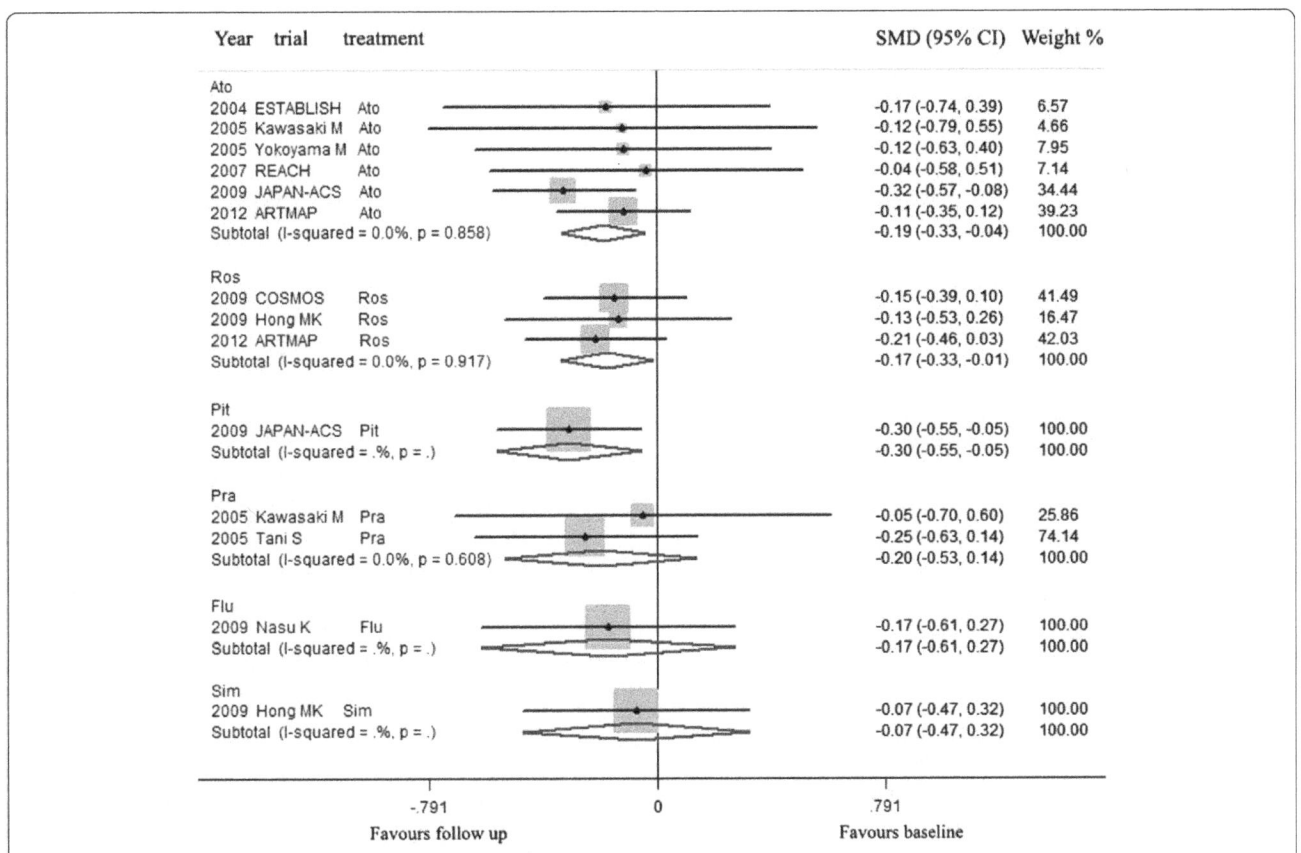

Figure 9 Meta- analysis of the effects of LDL-C lowering by different statins on the regression of coronary atherosclerotic plaque in **Asian.** Abbreviation as in Figure 4.

Asian patients demonstrated that 18.9 mg of atorvastatin daily for 7.8 months with reducing LDL-C by 40.7% could significantly regress CAP though the result of sensitivity analyses is not as good as that expected (Table 5).

Comparison between Western and Asian in using rosuvastatin and atorvastatin indicated that the dosages of rosuvastatin and atorvastatin in Asian group were significantly lower than those in Western (Table 7).

Table 6 Levels and reducing percentage of LDL-C, dosage and duration in different statin group in Western and Asian (Mean ± SD)

Group		N	Age	MeanLDL-C at baseline (mg)	MeanLDL-C at follow up (mg)	Mean reducing percentage	Statin dosage (mg)	Duration (month)
Western	Rosuvastatin	869	57.8 ± 0.6	124.2 ± 5.1	61.9 ± 0.9	49.9 ± 2.6	40.0 ± 0.0	24.0 ± 0.0
	Atorvastatin	772	57.2 ± 1.0	129.8 ± 14.2	73.1 ± 4.1	43.0 ± 2.1	80.0 ± 0.0	22.0 ± 2.8
	Pravastatin	249	56.6 ± 0.0	150.2 ± 0.0	110.4 ± 0.0	25.0 ± 0.0	40.0 ± 0.0	18.0 ± 0.0
	Simvastatin	40	57.7 ± 0.0	158.7 ± 0.0	85.1 ± 0.0	46.7 ± 0.0	40.0 ± 0.0	25.0 ± 0.0
Asian	Rosuvastatin	304	58.9 ± 3.3	123.1 ± 14.6	67.2 ± 13.8	44.0 ± 4.8	14.1 ± 4.9	10.3 ± 3.7
	Atorvastatin	366	60.9 ± 3.0	124.1 ± 12.7	72.9 ± 14.2	40.7 ± 5.5	18.9 ± 2.9	7.8 ± 2.2
	Pitavastatin	125	62.5 ± 11.5	130.9 ± 33.3	81.1 ± 23.4	36.2 ± 19.5	4	8 ~ 12
	Pravastatin	70	64.0 ± 1.8	134.9 ± 8.4	130.5 ± 0.9	23.1 ± 5.3	16.3 ± 2.2	6.0 ± 0.0
	Fluvastatin	40	63.0 ± 10.0	144.9 ± 31.5	98.1 ± 12.7	32.3	60	12
	Simvastatin	50	58.0 ± 0.0	119.0 ± 0.0	78.0 ± 0.0	34.5 ± 0.0	20.0 ± 0.0	12.0 ± 0.0

Table 7 Comparison between Western and Asian in rosuvastatin and atorvastatin

	Rosuvastatin			Atorvastatin		
	Western	Asian	p	Western	Asian	p
N/arm	869/2	304/3		772/2	366/6	
Mean LDL-C at baseline (mg)	124.2 ± 5.1	123.1 ± 14.6	0.928	129.8 ± 14.2	124.1 ± 12.7	0.610
Mean LDL-C at follow up (mg)	61.9 ± 0.9	67.2 ± 13.8	0.642	73.1 ± 4.1	72.9 ± 14.2	0.986
LDL-C Mean reducing percentage	49.9 ± 2.6	44.0 ± 4.8	0.221	43.0 ± 2.1	40.7 ± 5.5	0.600
Statin dosage (mg)	40.0 ± 0.0	14.1 ± 4.9	0.006	80.0 ± 0.0	18.9 ± 2.9	<0.001
Duration (month)	24.0 ± 0.0	10.3 ± 3.7	0.016	22.0 ± 2.8	7.8 ± 2.2	<0.001

Based on this meta-analysis, reducing LDL-C by >40% in Westerns need atorvastatin 80 mg or rosuvastatin 40 mg, but in Asians need only atorvastatin 18.9 mg or rosuvastatin 14.1 mg. For regressing CAP, 40 mg of rosuvastatin might be daily administrated in Western for 24 months; 14.1 mg of rosuvastatin or 18.9 mg of atorvastatin might be daily administrated in Asian for 10.7 or 7.8 months respectively.

Study limitation

As with the meta-analysis [3], this study has some limitations. There might be publication bias, difference of the method detected and follow up duration. But those differences in measurements and plaque selection did not affect the change of the target plaque with LDL-C levels. So, it has little effect on homogeneous of studies, and on the relationship between CAP change and LDL-C level. But the trials of single statin on LDL-C and CAP of specific population (for example, 2 trials about atorvastatin on Western with 727 participants or 6 on Asian with 366 in Table 5) were limited, the effect of statin on specific population remains to be investigated. The duration of follow up between Western and Asian was different (Table 4, 6 and 7), and treatment duration might have some effect on CAP regression. But the trials from Asian and Western were respectively meta-analysed in this study. Therefore, the difference in follow-up duration between Asian and Western did not influence the results of the meta-analysis. The CAP regression in short period of statins therapy in Asian suggested that the CAPs in Asian were easily regressed by statins.

This meta-analysis did not investigate the effect of reduction of LDL-C on adverse cardiovascular events because all participants of the included trial must be alive at follow up. But in the Extended-ESTABLISH study, the incidence of adverse cardiovascular events in statin group with CAP regression were reduced to half that seen in the control group [37]. In the Extended JAPAN-ACS study [38], there was no significantly different association of incidence of adverse cardiovascular events with the CAP regression extent, but that greater external elastic membrane volume regression (<–6.56%) had a significantly lower incidence of cumulative events than the lesser suggested the importance of CAP regression in reducing adverse cardiovascular events. A meta-analysis [39] included 7864 CAD patients showed that rates of plaque volume regression were significantly associated with the incidence of MI or revascularization.

Conclusions

LDL-C lowering therapy has a different effect on atherosclerotic plaque between Westerns and Asians. This systemic review demonstrated that there is a different effect of LDL-C lowering on CAP between Westerns and Asians. For regressing CAP, Asians need lower dosage of statins or lower intensity LDL-C lowering therapy (by >36%) than Westerns (by 45%).

Abbreviations
ACAT: Acyl–coenzyme A: cholesterol acyltransferase; ACS: Acute coronary syndrome; ATP III: Adult Treatment Panel III; CAD: Coronary artery disease; CAG: Coronary angiography; CAP: Coronary atherosclerotic plaque; CETP: Cholesteryl ester transfer protein; CHD: Coronary heart disease; IVUS: Intravascular ultrasound; CI: Confidence interval; LDL-C: Low-density lipoprotein cholesterol; RCT: Randomized controlled trial; SMD: Standardized mean differences.

Competing interests
The authors declare that they have no competing interests. This study was not funded.

Authors' contributions
LYF, FQZ, GWQ and ZXJ carried out data extraction, participated in the analysis and drafted the manuscript. CYD and HY participated in the design of the study, helped to draft the manuscript, and participated in its statistical analysis. All authors read and approved the final manuscript.

Author details
[1]The Department of Cardiology, Chinese PLA General Hospital, Fuxing Road 28, Beijing 100853, China. [2]The First Department of Geriatric Cardiology, Chinese PLA General Hospital, Beijing 100853, China. [3]The First Clinics, Administrative and Supportive Bureau, Chinese PLA General Logistics Department, Jia 14, Fuxing Road 22, Beijing 100842, China.

References

1. Falk E, Shah PK, Fuster V. Coronary plaque disruption. Circulation. 1995;92:657–71.
2. Nissen SE, Yock P. Intravascular ultrasound: novel pathophysiological insights and current clinical applications. Circulation. 2001;103:604–16.
3. Gao WQ, Feng QZ, Li YF, Li YX, Huang Y, Chen YM, et al. Systematic study of the effects of lowering low-density lipoprotein-cholesterol on regression of coronary atherosclerotic plaques using intravascular ultrasound. BMC Cardiovasc Disord. 2014;14:60.
4. Schartl M, Bocksch W, Koschyk DH, Voelker W, Karsch KR, Kreuzer J, et al. Use of intravascular ultrasound to compare effects of different strategies of lipid-lowering therapy on plaque volume and composition in patients with coronary artery disease. Circulation. 2001;104:387–92.
5. Tardif JC, Gregoire J, L'Allier PL, Anderson TJ, Bertrand O, Reeves F, et al. Effects of the acyl coenzyme A:cholesterol acyltransferase inhibitor avasimibe on human atherosclerotic lesions. Circulation. 2004;110:3372–7.
6. Nissen SE, Tuzcu EM, Brewer HB, Sipahi I, Nicholls SJ, Ganz P, et al. Effect of ACAT inhibition on the progression of coronary atherosclerosis. N Engl J Med. 2006;354:1253–63.
7. Nissen SE, Tardif JC, Nicholls SJ, Revkin JH, Shear CL, Duggan WT, et al. Effect of torcetrapib on the progression of coronary atherosclerosis. N Engl J Med. 2007;356:1304–16.
8. Nozue T, Yamamoto S, Tohyama S, Umezawa S, Kunishima T, Sato A, et al. Statin treatment for coronary artery plaque composition based on intravascular ultrasound radiofrequency data analysis. Am Heart J. 2012;163:191–9.e1.
9. Zhang X, Wang H, Liu S, Gong P, Lin J, Lu J, et al. Intensive-dose atorvastatin regimen halts progression of atherosclerotic plaques in new-onset unstable angina with borderline vulnerable plaque lesions. J Cardiovasc Pharmacol Ther. 2013;18:119–25.
10. Nissen SE, Tuzcu EM, Schoenhagen P, Brown BG, Ganz P, Vogel RA, et al. Effect of intensive compared with moderate lipid-lowering therapy on progression of coronary atherosclerosis: a randomized controlled trial. JAMA. 2004;291:1071–80.
11. Okazaki S, Yokoyama T, Miyauchi K, Shimada K, Kurata T, Sato H, et al. Early statin treatment in patients with acute coronary syndrome: demonstration of the beneficial effect on atherosclerotic lesions by serial volumetric intravascular ultrasound analysis during half a year after coronary event: the ESTABLISH Study. Circulation. 2004;110:1061–8.
12. Yokoyama M, Komiyama N, Courtney BK, Nakayama T, Namikawa S, Kuriyama N, et al. Plasma low-density lipoprotein reduction and structural effects on coronary atherosclerotic plaques by atorvastatin as clinically assessed with intravascular ultrasound radio-frequency signal analysis: a randomized prospective study. Am Heart J. 2005;150:287.
13. Kawasaki M, Sano K, Okubo M, Yokoyama H, Ito Y, Murata I, et al. Volumetric quantitative analysis of tissue characteristics of coronary plaques after statin therapy using three-dimensional integrated backscatter intravascular ultrasound. J Am Coll Cardiol. 2005;45:1946–53.
14. Yamada T, Azuma A, Sasaki S, Sawada T, Matsubara H. Randomized evaluation of atorvastatin in patients with coronary heart disease: a serial intravascular ultrasound study. Circ J. 2007;71:1845–50.
15. Hong MK, Park DW, Lee CW, Lee SW, Kim YH, Kang DH, et al. Effects of statin treatments on coronary plaques assessed by volumetric virtual histology intravascular ultrasound analysis. JACC Cardiovasc Interv. 2009;2:679–88.
16. Nicholls SJ, Ballantyne CM, Barter PJ, Chapman MJ, Erbel RM, Libby P, et al. Effect of two intensive statin regimens on progression of coronary disease. N Engl J Med. 2011;365:2078–87.
17. Lee CW, Kang SJ, Ahn JM, Song HG, Lee JY, Kim WJ, et al. Comparison of effects of atorvastatin (20 mg) versus rosuvastatin (10 mg) therapy on mild coronary atherosclerotic plaques (from the ARTMAP trial). Am J Cardiol. 2012;109:1700–4.
18. Hong YJ, Jeong MH, Hachinohe D, Ahmed K, Choi YH, Cho SH, et al. Comparison of effects of rosuvastatin and atorvastatin on plaque regression in Korean patients with untreated intermediate coronary stenosis. Circ J. 2011;75:398–406.
19. Kovarnik T, Mintz GS, Skalicka H, Kral A, Horak J, Skulec R, et al. Virtual histology evaluation of atherosclerosis regression during atorvastatin and ezetimibe administration: HEAVEN study. Circ J. 2012;76:176–83.
20. Hiro T, Kimura T, Morimoto T, Miyauchi K, Nakagawa Y, Yamagishi M, et al. Effect of intensive statin therapy on regression of coronary atherosclerosis in patients with acute coronary syndrome: a multicenter randomized trial evaluated by volumetric intravascular ultrasound using pitavastatin versus atorvastatin (JAPAN-ACS [Japan assessment of pitavastatin and atorvastatin in acute coronary syndrome] study). J Am Coll Cardiol. 2009;54:293–302.
21. Petronio AS, Amoroso G, Limbruno U, Papini B, De Carlo M, Micheli A, et al. Simvastatin does not inhibit intimal hyperplasia and restenosis but promotes plaque regression in normocholesterolemic patients undergoing coronary stenting: a randomized study with intravascular ultrasound. Am Heart J. 2005;149:520–6.
22. Tani S, Watanabe I, Anazawa T, Kawamata H, Tachibana E, Furukawa K, et al. Effect of pravastatin on malondialdehyde-modified low-density lipoprotein levels and coronary plaque regression as determined by three-dimensional intravascular ultrasound. Am J Cardiol. 2005;96:1089–94.
23. Rodes-Cabau J, Tardif JC, Cossette M, Bertrand OF, Ibrahim R, Larose E, et al. Acute effects of statin therapy on coronary atherosclerosis following an acute coronary syndrome. Am J Cardiol. 2009;104:750–7.
24. Nissen SE, Nicholls SJ, Wolski K, Rodes-Cabau J, Cannon CP, Deanfield JE, et al. Effect of rimonabant on progression of atherosclerosis in patients with abdominal obesity and coronary artery disease: the STRADIVARIUS randomized controlled trial. JAMA. 2008;299:1547–60.
25. Nissen SE, Nicholls SJ, Wolski K, Nesto R, Kupfer S, Perez A, et al. Comparison of pioglitazone vs glimepiride on progression of coronary atherosclerosis in patients with type 2 diabetes: the PERISCOPE randomized controlled trial. JAMA. 2008;299:1561–73.
26. Nissen SE, Nicholls SJ, Sipahi I, Libby P, Raichlen JS, Ballantyne CM, et al. Effect of very high-intensity statin therapy on regression of coronary atherosclerosis: the ASTEROID trial. JAMA. 2006;295:1556–65.
27. Matsuzaki M, Hiramori K, Imaizumi T, Kitabatake A, Hishida H, Nomura M, et al. Intravascular ultrasound evaluation of coronary plaque regression by low density lipoprotein-apheresis in familial hypercholesterolemia: the Low Density Lipoprotein-Apheresis Coronary Morphology and Reserve Trial (LACMART). J Am Coll Cardiol. 2002;40:220–7.
28. Jensen LO, Thayssen P, Pedersen KE, Stender S, Haghfelt T. Regression of coronary atherosclerosis by simvastatin: a serial intravascular ultrasound study. Circulation. 2004;110:265–70.
29. Takayama T, Hiro T, Yamagishi M, Daida H, Hirayama A, Saito S, et al. Effect of rosuvastatin on coronary atheroma in stable coronary artery disease: multicenter coronary atherosclerosis study measuring effects of rosuvastatin using intravascular ultrasound in Japanese subjects (COSMOS). Circ J. 2009;73:2110–7.
30. Nasu K, Tsuchikane E, Katoh O, Tanaka N, Kimura M, Ehara M, et al. Effect of fluvastatin on progression of coronary atherosclerotic plaque evaluated by virtual histology intravascular ultrasound. JACC Cardiovasc Interv. 2009;2:689–96.
31. Hattori K, Ozaki Y, Ismail TF, Okumura M, Naruse H, Kan S, et al. Impact of statin therapy on plaque characteristics as assessed by serial OCT, grayscale and integrated backscatter-IVUS. JACC Cardiovasc Imaging. 2012;5:169–77.
32. Gandelman K, Fung GL, Messig M, Laskey R. Systemic exposure to atorvastatin between Asian and Caucasian subjects: a combined analysis of 22 studies. Am J Ther. 2012;19:164–73.
33. Yang J, Li LJ, Wang K, He YC, Sheng YC, Xu L, et al. Race differences: modeling the pharmacodynamics of rosuvastatin in Western and Asian hypercholesterolemia patients. Acta Pharmacol Sin. 2011;32:116–25.
34. Lee E, Ryan S, Birmingham B, Zalikowski J, March R, Ambrose H, et al. Rosuvastatin pharmacokinetics and pharmacogenetics in white and Asian subjects residing in the same environment. Clin Pharmacol Ther. 2005;78:330–41.
35. Nakamura H, Arakawa K, Itakura H, Kitabatake A, Goto Y, Toyota T, et al. Primary prevention of cardiovascular disease with pravastatin in Japan (MEGA Study): a prospective randomised controlled trial. Lancet. 2006;368:1155–63.
36. Tirona RG. Ethnic differences in statin disposition. Clin Pharmacol Ther. 2005;78:311–6.
37. Dohi T, Miyauchi K, Okazaki S, Yokoyama T, Yanagisawa N, Tamura H, et al. Early intensive statin treatment for six months improves long-term clinical outcomes in patients with acute coronary syndrome (Extended-ESTABLISH trial): a follow-up study. Atherosclerosis. 2010;210:497–502.

Systematic study of the effects of lowering low-density lipoprotein-cholesterol on regression of coronary atherosclerotic plaques using intravascular ultrasound

Wen-Qian Gao[1,2†], Quan-Zhou Feng[1*†], Yu-Feng Li[1†], Yuan-Xin Li[3], Ya Huang[1], Yan-Ming Chen[1], Bo Yang[1] and Cai-Yi Lu[1*]

Abstract

Background: Conflicting results currently exist on the effects of LDL-C levels and statins therapy on coronary atherosclerotic plaque, and the target level of LDL-C resulting in the regression of the coronary atherosclerotic plaques has not been settled.

Methods: PubMed, EMBASE, and Cochrane databases were searched from Jan. 2000 to Jan. 2014 for randomized controlled or blinded end-points trials assessing the effects of LDL-C lowering therapy on regression of coronary atherosclerotic plaque (CAP) in patients with coronary heart disease by intravascular ultrasound. Data concerning the study design, patient characteristics, and outcomes were extracted. The significance of plaques regression was assessed by computing standardized mean difference (SMD) of the volume of CAP between the baseline and follow-up. SMD were calculated using fixed or random effects models.

Results: Twenty trials including 5910 patients with coronary heart disease were identified. Mean lowering LDL-C by 45.4% and to level 66.8 mg/dL in the group of patients with baseline mean LDL-C 123.7 mg/dL, mean lowering LDL-C by 48.8% and to level 60.6 mg/dL in the group of patients with baseline mean LDL-C 120 mg/dL, and mean lowering LDL-C by 40.4% and to level 77.8 mg/dL in the group of patients with baseline mean LDL-C 132.4 mg/dL could significantly reduce the volume of CAP at follow up (SMD -0.108 mm^3, 95% CI $-0.176 \sim -0.040$, $p = 0.002$; SMD -0.156 mm^3, 95% CI $-0.235 \sim -0.078$, $p = 0.000$; SMD -0.123 mm^3, 95% CI $-0.199 \sim -0.048$, $p = 0.001$; respectively). LDL-C lowering by rosuvastatin (mean 33 mg daily) and atorvastatin (mean 60 mg daily) could significantly decrease the volumes of CAP at follow up (SMD -0.162 mm^3, 95% CI: $-0.234 \sim -0.081$, $p = 0.000$; SMD -0.101, 95% CI: $-0.184 \sim -0.019$, $p = 0.016$; respectively). The mean duration of follow up was from $17 \sim 21$ months.

Conclusions: Intensive lowering LDL-C (rosuvastatin mean 33 mg daily and atorvastatin mean 60 mg daily) with >17 months of duration could lead to the regression of CAP, LDL-C level should be reduced by >40% or to a target level <78 mg/dL for regressing CAP.

Keywords: Low-density lipoprotein-cholesterol, Coronary atherosclerotic plaque, Intravascular ultrasound, Coronary artery disease

* Correspondence: fqz301@yahoo.com; cylu2000@126.com
†Equal contributors
[1]The Department of Cardiology, Chinese PLA General Hospital, Beijing 100853, China
Full list of author information is available at the end of the article

Background

It is universally accepted that high serum concentrations of low-density lipoprotein cholesterol (LDL-C) can lead to atherosclerosis and accelerate the progression of atherosclerosis which is main causes of coronary artery disease [1]. Disruption of coronary atherosclerotic plaque (CAP) with subsequent thrombus formation may lead to sudden cardiac death, acute myocardial infarction, or unstable angina [2]. The evidence showed that reducing LDL-C can prevent coronary heart disease (CHD) and improve survival of CHD based on results from multiple randomized controlled trials (RCTs) [3,4].

For many years coronary angiography (CAG) has been the gold standard method for the investigation of the anatomy of coronary arteries and measure the efficacy of anti-atherosclerotic drug therapies [5,6]. But changes in CAG are measured only in the vascular lumen and not in the vessel wall [7], where the atherosclerotic process is located. Intravascular ultrasound (IVUS) is superior to angiography in the detection of early plaque formation and changes in plaque volume [8-10]. Through IVUS, Takagi et al. found that pravastatin lowered serum cholesterol levels and reduced the progression of CAP in patients with elevated serum cholesterol levels in 1997 [11]. Since then, multiple RCTs and no RCT about the effect of lowering LDL-C therapy on the regression of coronary atherosclerosis have been performed [12-16]. But the results varied with the RCTs: intensive LDL-C lowering therapy could reduce the progression of the plaques [12]; the mild LDL-C lowering did not [14-16]. The meta-analysis by Bedi et al. [17] evaluated the effects of LDL-C lowering on CAP by comparing statins with control therapy, and demonstrated that treatment with statins could slow atherosclerotic plaque progression and lead to plaque regression. The meta-analysis by Tian et al. [18] showed that CAP could be regressed in group of patients with <100 mg of LDL-C level at follow up. But so far, there are no systematic reviews of the effects of LDL-C levels on CAP, and the targets of LDL-C level that could result in the regression of the plaques have not been settled.

In this study, we conducted meta-analyses to summarize findings from the current trials on LDL-C lowering therapy retarding the progression of the CAP and to identify the targets of LDL-C resulting in the regression of the CAP for guiding the LDL-C lowering therapy. Effect of different statins on the progression of the CAP was also investigated.

Methods

Search strategy and selection criteria

An electronic literature search was performed to identify all relevant studies published in PubMed, EMBASE, and Cochrane databases in the English language from Jan. 1, 2000 to Jan. 1, 2014, using the terms "atherosclerosis" and "cholesterol blood level". The references of the studies were also searched for relevant studies. Studies were included using the following criteria: 1) randomized controlled or prospective, blinded end-points trials in which patients with CHD were assigned to LDL-C lowering therapy or placebo, and its primary end point was CAP change detected by IVUS; 2) report of LDL-C levels at baseline and follow-up (in each arm) or the level of LDL-C which can be calculated from the data in the paper (as in the trial by Yokoyama M [15], in which the LDL-C concentrations in control arm were directly extracted from the figure); 3) data on the volume of CAP, detected in IVUS at baseline and follow-up (in each arm), and volume of CAP was calculated as vessel volume minus lumen volume; Exclusion criteria were: 1) only CAP area or volume index or percent atheroma volume were detected by IVUS; 2) the levels of LDL-C at baseline or follow-up were not provided; and 3) target plaques were unstable.

Data extraction and quality assessment

Two investigators independently reviewed all potentially eligible studies and collected data on patient and study characteristics (author, year, design, sample size, the measures of LDL-C lowering, LDL-C levels, follow-up duration, and plaque volume), and any disagreement was resolved by consensus. The primary end point of this study was progression or regression of CAP detected by IVUS. Quality assessments were evaluated with Jadad quality scale [19].

Data synthesis and analysis

Continuous variables (change of CAP volume from baseline to follow-up) were analyzed using standardized mean differences (SMD).

The trials may have control arm and multiple active treatment arms, changes of plaque volume in every arms were used for pooled analysis. According to the levels and the reducing percentage of LDL-C at follow-up, the arms were grouped to following groups: ≤70, >70 ≤ 100HP (>70 ≤ 100 mg and reducing percentage ≥30%), >70 ≤ 100MP (>70 ≤ 100 mg and reducing percentage ≥0 < 30%), >70 ≤ 100LP (>70 ≤ 100 mg and reducing percentage <0%), >100 mg/dL; and <0, ≥0 < 30, ≥30 < 40, ≥40 < 50, ≥50% respectively, to investigate the effect of different levels of LDL-C at follow up on CAPs. According to different statins, the arms were grouped to following groups: rosuvastatin, atorvastatin , pitavastatin, simvastatin, fluvastatin and pravastatin group, to investigate the effect of different statins on CAPs. The volume of CAP at follow up was compared with that at baseline to evaluate effect of LDL-C levels on regression of CAP.

Heterogeneity across trials (arms) was assessed via a standard χ^2 test with significance being set at $p < 0.10$ and also assessed by means of I^2 statistic with significance being set at $I^2 > 50\%$. Pooled analyses were calculated using fixed-effect models, whereas random-effect models were applied in case of significant heterogeneity across studies (arms). Sensitivity analyses (exclusion of one study at one time) were performed to determine the stability of the overall effects of LDL-C levels. Additionally, publication bias was assessed using the Egger regression asymmetry test. Mean LDL-C level and follow up duration of groups were calculated by descriptive statistics. A two-sided p values < 0.05 was considered statistically significant. Statistical analyses were performed using STATA software 12.0 (StataCorp, College Station, Texas) and Review Manager V5.2 (Copenhagen: The Nordic Cochrane Centre, The Cochrane Collaboration, 2012).

Results
Eligible studies

The flow of selecting studies for the meta-analysis is shown in Figure 1. Briefly, of the initial 647 articles, one hundred and twenty of abstracts were reviewed, resulting in exclusion of 100 articles, and 20 articles were reviewed in full text, resulting in exclusion of 10 trials and inclusion of 18 additional trials. Twenty two RCTs [12-16,20-31], [32-36] and six blinded end-points trial [37-42] were carefully evaluated. Five trials were excluded because of specific the index of plaque (volume index in TRUTH [24], trial by Kovarnik T [31], by Hattori K [42], and by Petronio AS [32]; area in LACMART [38]); GAIN [20] excluded because of no data of plaque volume at follow up; trial by Zhang X [25] excluded because of no data of LDL-C; trial by Hong YJ [30] excluded because of wrong data at follow up. Sixteen RCT (ESTABLISH [14], REVERSAL [13], A-PLUS [21], ACTIVATE

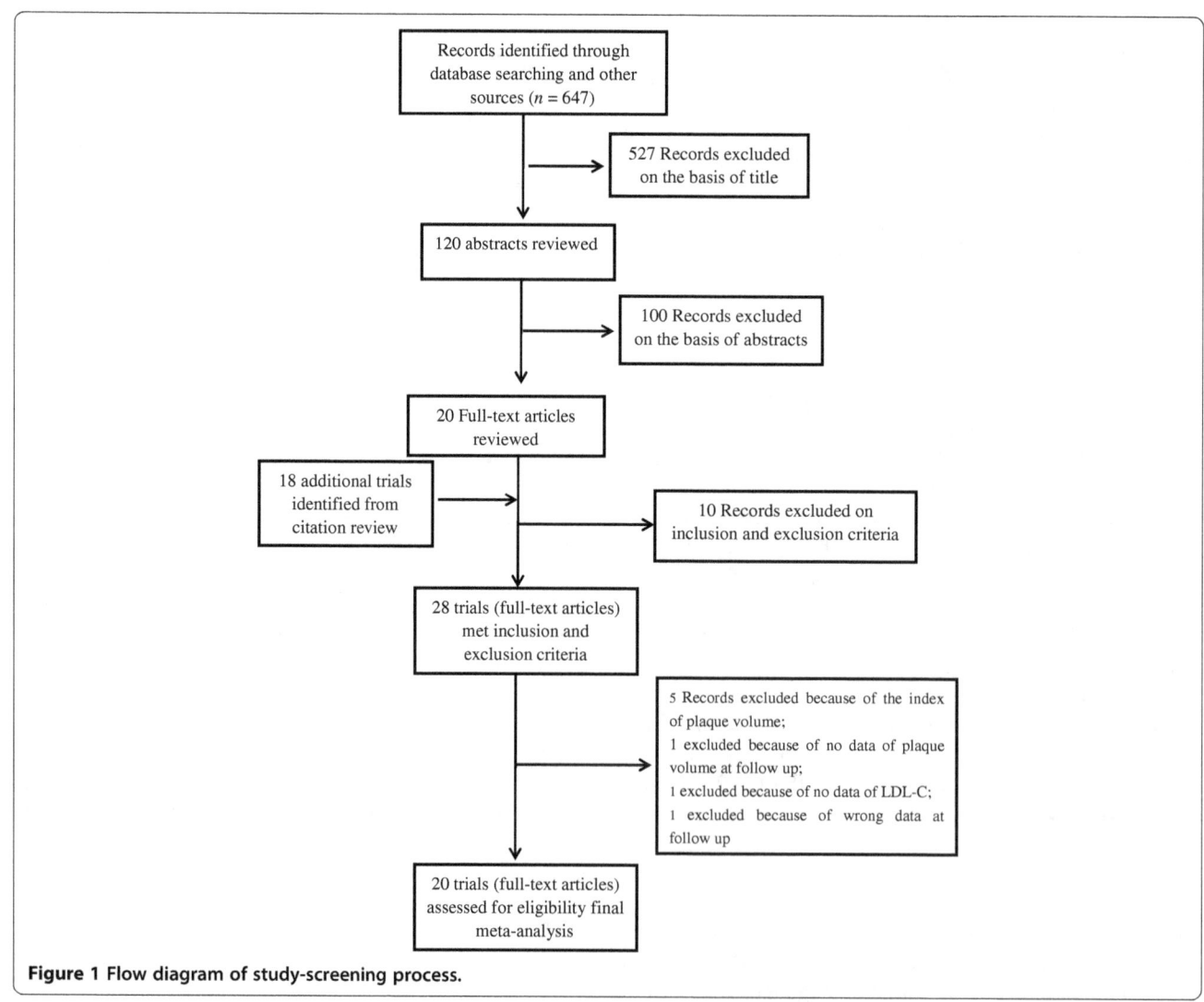

Figure 1 Flow diagram of study-screening process.

[22], ILLUSTRATE [23], JAPAN-ACS [12], REACH [26], SATURN [28], ARTMAP [29], ERASE [34], STRADIVARIUS [35], PERISCOPE [36], and trials by Yokoyama M [15], by Kawasaki M [16], by Hong MK [27], and Tani S [33]) and four blinded end-points trial (ASTEROID [37], COSMOS [40], trial by Jensen LO [39] and trial by Nasu K [41]) were finally analyzed.

The characteristics of the included trials were shown in Table 1. Among the 20 trials, there were 15 trials assessing statins (statin vs. usual care in 6 trials [14-16,26,33,41]; intensive statin vs. moderate statin treatment in 5 trials [12,13,27-29]; follow up vs baseline in 3 trial [37,39,40], before acute coronary syndrome (ACS) vs after ACS in one trial [34]), 2 trials assessing enzyme acyl–coenzyme A: cholesterol acyltransferase (ACAT) inhibition (vs. placebo, both on the basis of mean LDL-C < 102 after background lipid-lowering therapy with statins in 62-79% of patients) [21,22], one trial assessing cholesteryl ester transfer protein (CETP) inhibitor torcetrapib (vs. statins on the basis of LDL-C ≤ 100 by statins) [23], one trial assessing a decreasing obesity drug: rimonabant (vs. placebo, on the basis of statins therapy) [35], and one trial assessing glucose-lowering agents (pioglitazone vs glimepiride on the basis of statins therapy) [36]. In three trials [12,14,34] with acute coronary syndrome, all target plaques were selected in non-culprit vessels. Overall, 5910 patients with CHD underwent serial IVUS examination for evaluating regression of CAP. Follow-up periods ranged from 2 to 24 months. The levels of LDL-C of each arm at baseline and follow-up were shown in Table 2.

Risk of bias of included studies, evaluated through Cochrane's methods, showed an overall acceptable quality of selected trials (Figures 2 and 3).

The effect of the levels of LDL-C at follow-up on regression of coronary atherosclerotic plaque

LDL-C lowering in group ≤70 and >70 ≤ 100HP mg/dL could lead to regression of CAP, but LDL-C lowering in group >70 ≤ 100MP, >70 ≤ 100LP and >100 mg/dL could not (Figure 4, Table 3).

In group ≤70 mg/dL (including seven arms) with mean 18.6 months of follow up and group >70 ≤ 100HP mg/dL (including eleven arms) with mean 17.4 months of follow up, the volumes of CAP (125.9, 123.8 mm^3 respectively) at follow up were significantly decreased, compared with the volumes (177.1, 129.7 mm^3 respectively) at baseline [SMD –0.156 mm^3, 95% CI (confidence interval) -0.235 ~ –0.078, $p = 0.000$; SMD –0.123 mm^3, 95% CI –0.199 ~ –0.048, $p = 0.001$; respectively]. There was no significant heterogeneity among arms (χ^2 for heterogeneity = 0.57, p =0.997, I^2 = 0% for group ≤70 mg/dL; χ^2 for heterogeneity = 6.83, p =0.741, I^2 = 0% for group >70 ≤ 100HP mg/dL).

Sensitivity analyses suggested that LDL-C lowering in group ≤70 and >70 ≤ 100HP mg/dL could lead to regression of CAP with reduction of the CAP volume ranged from –0.146 mm^3 (SMD, 95% CI: –0.238 ~ –0.054) when the arm of 2006 ASTEROID Ros was omitted to –0.167 mm^3 (SMD, 95% CI: –0.270 ~ –0.064) when the arm of 2011 SATURN Ros was omitted; and from –0.103 mm^3 (SMD, 95% CI: –0.182 ~ –0.024) when the arm of 2009 JAPAN-ACS Ato was omitted to –0.151 mm^3 (SMD, 95% CI: –0.235 ~ –0.067) when the arm of 2004 REVERSAL Ato was omitted. No publication bias was found, the values of p by Egger's test for group ≤70 and >70 ≤ 100HP mg/dL were 0.835, 0.501 respectively.

In group >100 mg/dL (including eleven arms) with mean 14.6 months of follow up, the volume of CAP at follow up was not significantly increased, compared with the volumes at baseline (SMD 0.013 mm^3, 95% CI –0.092 ~ 0.118, $p = 0.809$). There was no significant heterogeneity among arms (χ^2 for heterogeneity = 2.49, p =0.991, I^2 = 0%).

Sensitivity analyses suggested that LDL-C lowering to >100 mg/dL at follow-up could still not lead to regression of CAP with reduction of the plaque volume ranged from –0.005 mm^3 (95% CI –0.136 ~ 0.126) when the arm of 2004 REVERSAL Pro was omitted to 0.034 mm^3 (SMD, 95% CI –0.075 ~ 0.143) when 2005 Tani S Pra was omitted. No publication bias was observed from the values of p (0.566) by Egger's test.

Mean levels of LDL-C at baseline and follow up and mean reducing percentage of LDL-C in group ≤70, >70 ≤ 100HP, >70 ≤ 100MP, >70 ≤ 100LP and >100 mg/dL were showed in Table 4.

The effect of the LDL-C reducing percentage at follow-up on regression of CAP

LDL-C lowering in group ≥30 < 40, ≥40 < 50, ≥50% could lead to regression of CAP, but LDL-C lowering in group <0 and ≥0 < 30% could not (Figure 5, Table 3).

In group ≥30 < 40% (including ten arms) with mean 10.3 months of follow up, and group ≥40 < 50% (including eight arms) with mean 19.4 months of follow up, the volumes of CAP (94.3, 150.7 mm^3 respectively) at follow up were significantly decreased, compared with the volumes (102.9, 157.8 mm^3 respectively) at baseline (SMD –0.199 mm^3, 95% CI –0.314 ~ –0.085, $p = 0.001$; SMD –0.108 mm^3, 95% CI –0.176 ~ –0.040, $p = 0.002$; respectively). There was no significant heterogeneity among arms (χ^2 for heterogeneity = 3.10, $P = 0.960$, I^2 = 0%; χ^2 for heterogeneity = 2.50, p =0.927, I^2 = 0%; for group ≥30 < 40, and group ≥40 < 50 respectively).

Sensitivity analyses showed that LDL-C lowering in group ≥30 < 40% and group ≥40 < 50 could still lead to regression of CAP with reduction of the plaque volume ranged from –0.166 mm^3 (95% CI –0.295 ~ –0.038) when the arm of 2009 JAPAN-ACS Ato was omitted

Table 1 Features of participating trials

Authors and trial name	Trial type and location	Objective	Year	N T/C	Study population	LDL-C at follow up	LDL-C reducing percentage	Treatments	Follow up	Main Results or Conclusion
Okazaki S [14]; ESTABLISH	RCT: prospective, open-label, randomized, single center study. Japan	Effects of statins on changes in plaque by IVUS	2004	24/24	ACS	70/119	-44/-0.004	Ato 20 vs Diet	6	Plaque volume was sigificantly reduced in the Ato group compared with the control group.
Nissen SE [13]; REVERSAL	RCT: Double-blind, randomized active control multicenter trial; USA	Effects of statins (intensive or moderate) on changes in plaque by IVUS	2004	253/249	CAD	79/110	-46/-25	Ato 80 vs Pra40	18	Ato reduced progression of coronary plaque compared with Pra. Compared with baseline values, Ato had no change in atheroma burden, whereas patients treated with Pra showed progression of coronary plaque.
Tardif JC [21]; A-PLUS	RCT: international, multicenter, double-blind, placebo-controlled, randomized trial. Canada, USA	Effects of different dosage of avasimibe on changes in plaque by IVUS	2004	108/98/ 117/109	CAD	100/102/ 101/91	7.8/9.1/ 10.9/1.7	Ava50, 250, and 750 vs Placebo on the basis of LDL-C<125	18	Avasimibe did not favorably alter coronary atherosclerosis as assessed by IVUS.
Jensen LO [39]	Open non placebo controlled serial investigation; blinded end-points. Denmark	To investigate the effect of lipid lowering by simvastatin on coronary atherosclerotic plaque volumes and lumen.	2004	40	CAD	85	-46.3	Sim 40	15	Lipid-lowering therapy with Sim is associated with a significant plaque regression in coronary arteries.
Yokoyama M [15]	RCT: randomized, single center. Japan	Effects of statins on changes in plaque by IVU	2005	29/30	Stable angina	87/124	-35/-0.075	Ato 10 vs Diet	6	Treatment with Ato may reduce volumes of coronary plaques.
Kawasaki M [16]	RCT: randomization, open-label, single-center study. Japan	Effects of statins on changes in plaque by IVUS	2005	17/18/17	Stable angina	95/102/149	-39/-32/-0.02	Ato 20, Pra 20 vs Diet	6	Treatment with Ato and Pra may not significantly reduce volumes of coronary plaques.
Tani S [33]	RCT: a prospective, single-center, randomized, open trial. Japan	Investigated the effects of pravastatin on the serum levels of MDA-LDL and coronary atherosclerosis.	2005	52/23	Stable angina	104/120	-20/-2.4	Pra 10-20 vs con	6	Plaque volume was sigificantly reduced in the Pra group compared with the control group.
Nissen SE [22]; ACTIVATE	RCT: randomized, multicenter. USA	Effects of pactimibe on changes in plaque by IVUS	2006	206/202	CAD	91/86	-9.6/-14.9	Pac100 vs Placebo	18	Pac is not an effective strategy for limiting atherosclerosis and may promote atherogenesis.

Table 1 Features of participating trials *(Continued)*

Study	Design	Year	N	Condition	Baseline	LDL change	Treatment	Months	Conclusion
Nissen SE [37]; ASTEROID	Prospective, open-label blinded end-points. USA, Germany, France, Canada	2006	349	CAD	61	-53.2	Ros 40	24	Therapy using Ros can result in significant regression of atherosclerosis.
Yamada T [26]; REACH	RCT: open-labeled, randomized, multicenter study. Japan	2007	26/32	Stable angina	83/115	-43/0	Ato 5 vs Con	12	Ato treatment prevented the further progression of atherosclerosis by maintaining LDL-C below 100 mg/dl in patients with CHD.
Nissen SE [23]; ILLUSTRATE	RCT: prospective, randomized, multicenter, double-blind clinical trial. North America or Europe	2007	446/464	CAD	87/70	6.6/-13.3	Ato10-80 vs Ato+Tor 60 on the basis of LDL-C≤100 by Ato	24	The Tor was associated with a substantial increase in HDL-C and decrease in LDL–C, and there was no significant decrease in the progression of coronary atherosclerosis.
Nissen SE [36]; PERISCOPE	RCT: prospective, randomized, multicenter, double-blind clinical trial. USA	2008	181/179	CAD, DM	96.1/95.6	1.8/2.2	Gli1-4 mg vs Pio 15-45 mg on bases of statins therapy	18	In patients with type 2 diabetes and CAD, treatment with Pio resulted in a significantly lower rate of progression of coronary atherosclerosis compared with Gli.
Nissen SE [35]; STRADIVARIUS	RCT: Randomized, double-blinded, placebo-controlled, 2-group, parallel-group trial. North America, Europe, and Australia	2008	335/341	CAD, Obesity	87.6/86.3	-4.7/-3.6	Rim 20 mg vs Placebo on bases of statins therapy	18	Rim can reduce progression of coronary plaque, and increase HDL-C levels, decrease triglyceride levels.
Hiro T [12]; JAPAN-ACS	RCT: prospective, randomized, open-label, parallel group, multicenter. Japan	2009	127/125	ACS	84/81	-36/-36	Ato 20 vs Pit 4	10	The administration of Pit or Ato in patients with ACS equivalently resulted in significant regression of coronary plaque volume.
Takayama T; COSMOS [40]	Prospective, open-label blinded end-points multicenter trial. Japan	2009	126	Stable angina	83	-38.6	Ros <20	14	Ros exerted significant regression of coronary plaque volume in Japanese patients with stable CAD.

Table 1 Features of participating trials *(Continued)*

Rodés-Cabau; ERASE [34]	RCT: multicenter randomized placebo-controlled. Canada	Evaluate the early effects of newly initiated statin therapy on coronary atherosclerosis as evaluated by IVUS.	2009	38/36	ACS	77/63	8.5/-37	Before ACS vs After ACS	<2	Newly initiated statin therapy is associated with rapid regression of coronary atherosclerosis.
Nasu K [41]	Prospective and multicenter study with nonrandomized and non-blinded design, but blinded end. Japan	Evaluate the effect of treatment with statins on the progression of coronary atherosclerotic plaques of a nonculprit vessel by serial IVUS.	2009	40/39	Stable angina	98.1/121	-32.3/-1.1	Flu 60 vs Con	12	One-year lipid-lowering therapy by Flu showed significant regression of plaque volume.
Hong MK [27]	RCT: randomized control trial. Korea.	Evaluated the effects of statin treatments for each component of coronary plaques.	2009	50/50	Stable angina	78/64	-34.5/-44.8	Sim 20 vs Ros 10	12	Statin treatments might be associated with significant changes in necrotic core and fibrofatty plaque volume.
Nicholls SJ; SATURN [28]	RCT: a prospective, randomized, multicenter, double-blind clinical trial. USA	Compare the effect of these two intensive statin regimens on the progression of coronary atherosclerosis.	2011	519/520	CHD	70.2/62.6	-41.5/-47.8	Ato 80 vs Ros 40	24	Maximal doses of Ros and Ato resulted in significant regression of coronary atherosclerosis.
Lee CW [29]; ARTMAP	RCT: a prospective, single-center, open-label, randomized comparison trial. Korea.	Compared the effects of atorvastatin 20 mg/day versus rosuvastatin 10 mg/day on mild coronary atherosclerotic plaques.	2012	143/128	Stable angina	56/53	-47/-49	Ato 20 vs Ros 10	6	Usual doses of Ato and Ros induced significant regression of coronary atherosclerosis in statin-naive patients.

Abbreviations: RCT, randomized controlled trials; T, treatment group; C, control group IVUS, Intravascular ultrasound; CAD, Coronary artery disease; ACS, Acute coronary syndrome; CHD, Coronary heart disease; Ato, Atorvastatin; Ros, Rosuvastatin; Pra, Pravastatin; Pit, Pitavastatin; Flu, Fluvastatin; Sim, Simvastatin; Con, Control; Pac, Pactimibe; Tor, Torcetrapib, Ava 50, 250, 750, Avasimibe 50, 250, 750 mg; T/C, Treat/Control; Gli, Glimepiride; Pio, Pioglitazone; Rim, Rimonabant.

Table 2 The levels of LDL-C at baseline and follow up in each arm of included trials

Authors	Trial name	Management in each arm	N	LDL-C level	
				At Baseline	At Follow-up
Tardif JC	A-PLUS	Avasimibe50	108	92.8 ± 1.7	100*
Tardif JC	A-PLUS	Avasimibe250	98	93.4 ± 1.6	101.9*
Tardif JC	A-PLUS	Avasimibe750	117	91.4 ± 1.6	101.4*
Tardif JC	A-PLUS	Placebo	109	89.6 ± 1.6	91.1*
Okazaki S	ESTABLISH	Control	24	123.9 ± 35.3	119.4 ± 24.6
Okazaki S	ESTABLISH	Atorvastatin	24	124.6 ± 34.5	70.0 ± 25.0
Yokoyama M		Control	30	131.5 ± 23#	124.5 ± 24.1#
Yokoyama M		Atorvastatin	29	133 ± 13	87 ± 29
Nissen SE	REVERSAL	Atorvastatin	253	150.2 ± 27.9	78.9 ± 30.2
Nissen SE	REVERSAL	Pravastatin	249	150.2 ± 25.9	110.4 ± 25.8
Nissen SE	ACTIVATE	Pactimibe	206	101.4 ± 27.7	91.3
Nissen SE	ACTIVATE	Placebo	202	101.5 ± 31.1	86.4
Nissen SE	ILLUSTRATE	Atorvastatin	446	84.3 ± 18.9	87.2 ± 22.6
Nissen SE	ILLUSTRATE	Atorva+torcetrapib	464	83.1 ± 19.7	70.1 ± 25.4
Kawasaki M		Control	17	152 ± 20	149 ± 24
Kawasaki M		Pravastatin	18	149 ± 19	102 ± 13
Kawasaki M		Atorvastatin	17	155 ± 22	95 ± 15
Hiro T	JAPAN-ACS	Pitavastatin	125	130.9 ± 33.3	81.1 ± 23.4
Hiro T	JAPAN-ACS	Atorvastatin	127	133.8 ± 31.4	84.1 ± 27.4
Nissen SE	ASTEROID	Rosuvastatin	349	130.4 ± 34.3	60.8 ± 20.0
Takayama T	COSMOS	Rosuvastatin	126	140.2±31.5	82.9±18.7
Lee CW	ARTMAP	Atorvastatin	143	110 ± 31	56 ± 18
Lee CW	ARTMAP	Rosuvastatin	128	109 ± 31	53±18
Yamada T	REACH	Atorvastatin	26	123 ± 17	83 ± 22
Yamada T	REACH	Control	32	115 ± 14	115 ± 30
Nasu K		Fluvastatin	40	144.9 ± 31.5	98.1 ± 12.7
Nasu K		Control	39	122.3 ± 18.9	121.0 ± 21.2
Nicholls SJ	SATURN	Atorvastatin	519	119.9 ± 28.9	70.2 ± 1.0
Nicholls SJ	SATURN	Rosuvastatin	520	120.0 ± 27.3	62.6 ± 1.0
Hong MK		Simvastatin	50	119 ± 30	78 ± 20
Hong MK		Rosuvastatin	50	116 ± 28	64 ± 21
Tani S		Pravastatin	52	130 ± 38	104 ± 20
Tani S		Control	23	123 ± 28	120 ± 30
Rodés-C Bef	ERASE	Statins before ACS	38	71 ± 23	77 ± 25
Rodés-C Aft	ERASE	Statins after ACS	36	100 ± 30	63 ± 17
Jensen LO		Simvastatin	40	158.7 ± 30.6	85.1 ± 22.1
Nissen SE	PERISCOPE	Statins+Gli	181	94.4 ± 32.9	96.1 ± 30.4
Nissen SE	PERISCOPE	Statins+Pio	179	93.5 ± 30.7	95.6 ± 28.9
Nissen SE	STRADIVARIUS	Statins+Rim	335	91.9 ± 27.9	87.6 ± 30.5
Nissen SE	STRADIVARIUS	Statins+Con	341	89.5 ± 32.2	86.3 ± 30.3

Note: *calculated on the bases of baseline levels and change percentage at follow up [21].
calculated according to Figure 2 in the paper [15].

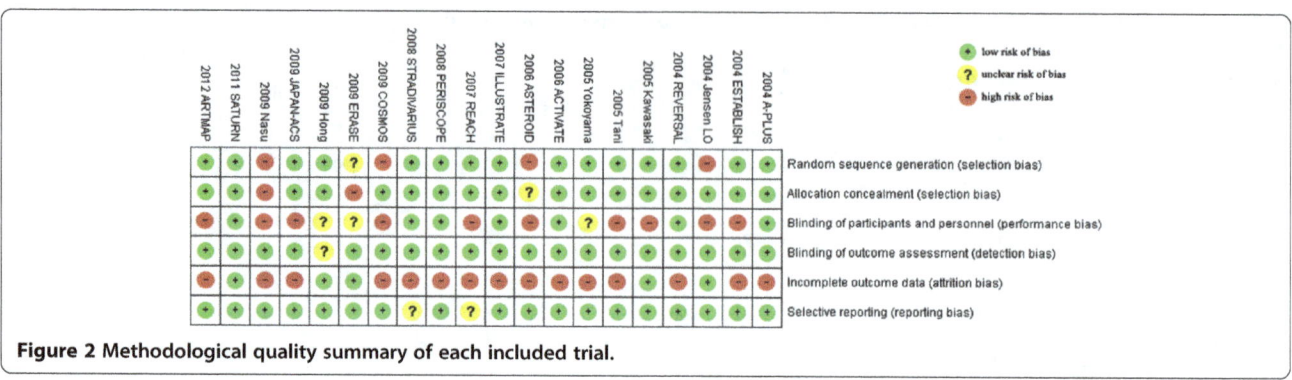

Figure 2 Methodological quality summary of each included trial.

to -0.214 mm^3 (SMD, 95% CI $-0.342 \sim -0.085$) when 2009 COSMOS Ros was omitted; from -0.093 mm^3 (95% CI $-0.174 \sim -0.011$) when the arm of 2011 SATURN Ros was omitted to -0.126 mm^3 (SMD, 95% CI $-0.200 \sim -0.053$) when 2004 REVERSAL Ato was omitted respectively. Publication bias analysis suggested the values of p by Egger's test were 0.024, 0.605 for group $\geq 30 < 40$, and group $\geq 40 < 50$ respectively.

In group <0 with mean 19.6 months of follow up and group $\geq 0 < 30\%$ with mean 18.3 months of follow up, the volume of CAP at follow up was not significantly decreased, compared with the volumes at baseline (SMD -0.034 mm^3, 95% CI $-0.111 \sim 0.044$, $p = 0.396$; SMD -0.032 mm^3, 95% CI $-0.093 \sim 0.030$, $p = 0.315$ respectively). There was no significant heterogeneity among arms (χ^2 for heterogeneity = 1.55, $p = 0.981$, $I^2 = 0\%$ for group $<0\%$; χ^2 for heterogeneity = 4.59, $p = 0.970$, $I^2 = 0\%$ for group $\geq 0 < 30\%$).

Sensitivity analyses showed that LDL-C lowering in group $\geq 0 < 30\%$ could not still significantly decrease the volume of CAP with reduction of the CAP volume ranged from -0.010 mm^3 (SMD, 95% CI: $-0.080 \sim 0.061$) when the arm of 2007 ILLUSTRATE Ato + Tor was omitted to -0.042 mm^3 (SMD, 95% CI: $-0.108 \sim 0.024$) when the arm of 2004 REVERSAL Pro was omitted. No publication bias was found, the values of p by Egger's test for group $\geq 0 < 30\%$ were 0.537.

Mean levels of LDL-C at baseline and follow up, mean reducing percentage of LDL-C in group <0, $\geq 0 < 30$, $\geq 30 < 40$, $\geq 40 < 50$ and $\geq 50\%$, were showed in Table 4.

The effect of lowering LDL-C by statins on regression of coronary atherosclerotic plaque

LDL-C lowering by rosuvastatin, atorvastatin and pitavastatin in group ≤ 70 and $>70 \leq 100$HP mg/dL could lead to regression of CAP, but LDL-C lowering by simvastatin, fluvastatin and pravastatin could not (Figure 6, Table 5).

LDL-C lowering by rosuvastatin (mean 33.3 mg daily for mean 20 months), atorvastatin (mean 60.3 mg daily for mean 17 months) and pitavastatin (4 mg daily for $8 \sim 12$ months) in group ≤ 70 and $>70 \leq 100$HP mg/dL could significantly decrease the volumes of CAP at follow up, compared with the volumes at baseline (SMD -0.162 mm^3, 95% CI: $-0.234 \sim -0.081$, $p = 0.000$; SMD -0.101, 95% CI: $-0.184 \sim -0.019$, $p = 0.016$; SMD -0.304 mm^3, 95% CI: $-0.553 \sim -0.055$, $p = 0.017$; respectively). There was no significant heterogeneity among arms (χ^2 for heterogeneity = 0.37, $p = 0.985$, $I^2 = 0\%$ for rosuvastatin; χ^2 for heterogeneity = 4.44, $p = 0.728$, $I^2 = 0\%$ for atorvastatin.

Sensitivity analyses suggested that lowering LDL-C by rosuvastatin could lead to regression of CAP with reduction of the plaque volume ranged from -0.153 mm^3 (SMD, 95% CI: $-0.249 \sim -0.056$) when the arm of 2006 ASTEROID Ros was omitted to -0.178 mm^3 (SMD, 95%

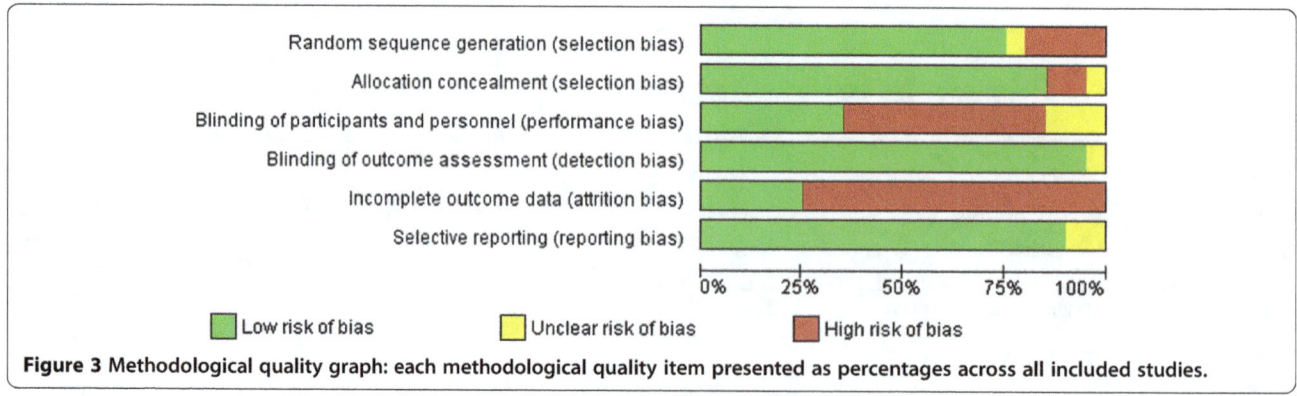

Figure 3 Methodological quality graph: each methodological quality item presented as percentages across all included studies.

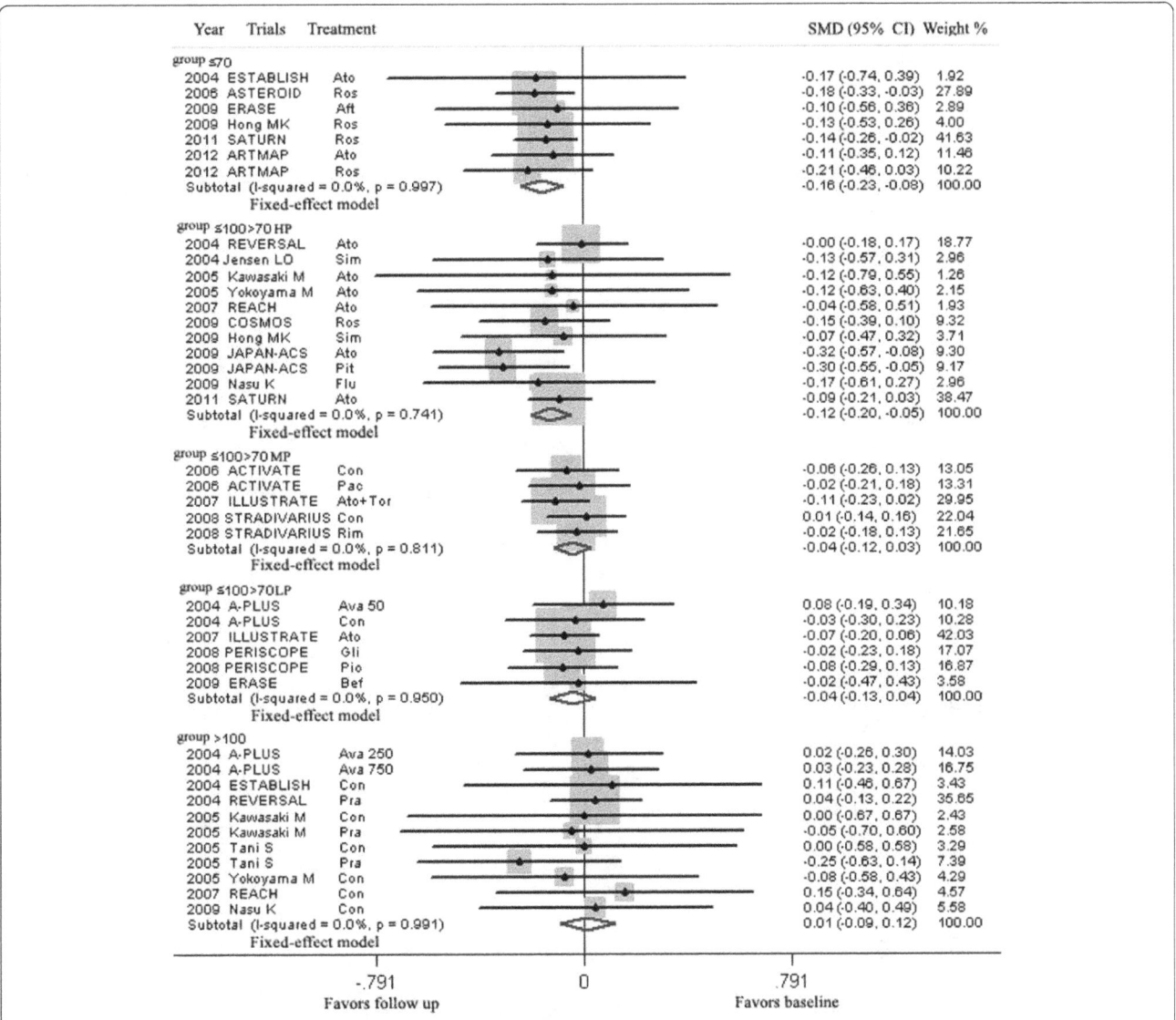

Figure 4 Meta-analysis of the effects of reduction levels of LDL-C at follow up on the regression of coronary atherosclerotic plaque.

Abbreviations: Ato, Atorvastatin; Ros, Rosuvastatin; Pra, Pravastatin; Pit, Pitavastatin; Sim, Simvastatin; Flu, Fluvastatin; Con, Control; Pac, Pactimibe; Tor, Torcetrapib, Ava 50, 250, 750, Avasimibe 50, 250, 750 mg; Bef, before ACS; Aft, after ACS; Gli, Glimepiride; Pio, Pioglitazone; Rim, Rimonabant.

CI: −0.287 ~ −0.069) when the arm of 2011 SATURN Ros was omitted. Lowering LDL-C by atorvastatin could, but not significantly, lead to regression of CAP when the arm of 2009 JAPAN-ACS Ato was omitted (SMD: −0.075 mm³, 95% CI: −0.162 ~ 0.012). No publication bias was found, the values of p by Egger's test for rosuvastatin and atorvastatin group were 0.770, 0.582 respectively (Table 5).

Intensity of lowering LDL-C by different statins was shown in Table 6. Rosuvastatin and atorvastatin could reduce LDL-C by more than 40%.

Discussion
Feature of this meta-analysis
This meta-analysis broke though the limit of single trial, and pooled arms together according to the levels of LDL-C at follow up in the arms, regardless of the measures of lowering LDL-C: treating arm (statins, ACAT inhibitor, CETP inhibitor, decreasing obesity drug, and glucose-lowering agents) and control arms (dietary restriction, moderate LDL-C lowering by statin); intensive and moderate LDL-C lowering. The volumes of CAP at follow up were compared with those at baseline in the same arms to evaluate the regression of the CAPs, this meta-analysis really reflected the change of the plaques volume with the change of LDL-C levels.

Our meta-analysis results indicated that intensive lowering LDL-C in group ≤70, >70 ≤ 100HP mg/dL (mean follow up LDL-C, mean duration of follow up: 60.6 mg/dL, 18.6 months; 77.8 mg/ dL, 17.4 months respectively), ≥30 < 40, ≥40 < 50 and ≥50% (mean LDL-C reducing, mean

Table 3 Results of meta-analysis in each group and mean CAP volume in each group at baseline and follow up

Group	Included arms (case)	CAP Volume at Baseline (mm³)	CAP Volume at Follow up (mm³)	Pooled SMD (95% CI, p)	Heterogeneity test χ² test (p)	I^2	Sensitivity analyses Lower SMD (95% CI)	Upper SMD (95% CI)	Egger's test
≤70 mg	7 (1250)	177.1±41.9	125.9±38.6	-0.156 (-0.235~ -0.078, 0.000)	0.57 (0.997)	0	-0.146 (-0.238~ -0.054) Without 2006 ASTEROID Ros	-0.167 (-0.270~ -0.064) Without 2011 SATURN Ros	0.835
>70≤100HP mg	11 (1352)	129.7±72.3	123.8±69.8	-0.123 (-0.199~ -0.048, 0.001)	6.83 (0.741)	0	-0.103 (-0.182~ -0.024) Without 2009 JAPAN-ACS Ato	-0.151 (-0.235~ -0.067) Without 2004 REVERSAL Ato	0.501
>70≤100MP mg	5 (1548)	195.8±2.3	191.8±4.7	-0.045 (-0.115~ -0.026, 0.215)	1.59 (0.811)	0	-0.016 (-0.103~ -0.066) Without 2007 ILLUSTRATE Ato+Tor	-0.061 (-0.140~ -0.019) Without 2008 STRADIVARIUS Con	0.500
>70≤100LP mg	6 (1061)	201.2±15.1	197.3±15.0	-0.045 (-0.130~0.040, 0.301)	1.14 (0.950)	0	-0.024 (-0.136~ 0.087) Without 2007 ILLUSTRATE Ato	-0.059 (-0.148~ 0.031) Without 2004 A-PLUS Ava 50	0.241
>100 mg	10 (669)	175.9±86.4	178.7±89.1	0.017 (-0.090~0.124, 0.757)	2.37 (0.984)	0	-0.000 (-0.135~ 0.136) Without 2004 REVERSAL Pro	0.039 (-0.073~ 0.151) Without 2005 Tani S Pra	0.692
<0%	8 (1276)	201.2±13.8	198.3±13.8	-0.034 (-0.111~ 0.044, 0.396)	1.55 (0.981)	0	-0.012 (-0.109~ 0.084) Without 2007 ILLUSTRATE Ato	-0.044 (-0.125~ 0.037) Without 2004 A-PLUS Ava 50	0.087
>0≤30%	13 (2014)	188.6±51.7	186.3±52.7	-0.032 (-0.093~ 0.030, 0.315)	4.59 (0.970)	0	-0.010 (-0.080~ 0.061) Without 2007 ILLUSTRATE Ato+Tor	-0.042 (-0.108~ 0.024) Without 2004 REVERSAL Pra	0.537
>30≤40%	10 (594)	102.9±96.9	94.3±90.4	-0.199 (-0.314~ -0.085, 0.001)	3.10 (0.960)	0	-0.166 (-0.295~ -0.038) Without 2009 JAPAN-ACS Ato	-0.214 (-0.342~ -0.085) Without 2009 COSMOS Ros	0.024
>40≤50%	8 (1677)	157.8±37.8	150.7±36.3	-0.108 (-0.176~ -0.040, 0.002)	2.50 (0.927)	0	-0.093 (-0.174~ -0.011) Without 2011 SATURN Ros	-0.126 (-0.200~ -0.053) Without 2004 REVERSAL Ato	0.605
>50%	1 (349)	212.2±81.3	197.5±79.1	-0.183 (-0.332~ -0.035, 0.016)					

Table 4 Levels and reducing percentage of LDL-C and duration in each group

Group	N	Mean LDL-C at Baseline (mg)	Mean LDL-C at Follow up (mg)	Mean Reducing percentage	Actual range of reducing percentage	Duration (month)
≤70 mg	1250	120.0±8.2	60.6±3.5	48.8±3.3	37~53.2	18.6±8.2
>70≤100HP mg	1352	132.4±12.9	77.8±7.0	40.4±4.0	32.3~46.7	17.4±5.9
>70≤100MP mg	1548	91.3±6.9	82.4±8.2	9.1±4.5	3.6~14.9	19.8±2.7
>70≤100LP mg	1061	88.5±5.5	91.5±5.4	-4.7±2.5	-1.7~-8.5	19.9±4.5
>100 mg	699	125.1±24.4	110.0±9.3	8.3±15.6	-10.9~32	14.6±5.1
<0%	1276	89.1±5.3	93.2±6.2	-5.6±3.1	-1.7~-10.9	19.6±4.2
>0≤30%	2014	102.4±22.1	89.7±15.7	10.6±7.3	0~25	18.3±4.5
>30≤40%	594	132.6±11.4	83.3±7.7	36.1±1.9	32~39	10.3±3.1
>40≤50%	1677	123.7±13.4	66.8±8.0	45.4±2.8	41.5~49	19.4±6.9
>50%	349	130.4±34.3	60.8±20.0	53.2	53.2	24

duration of follow up: 36.1%, 10.3 months; 45.4%, 19.4 months; 53.2%, 24 months respectively) could lead to the regression of CAP; that moderate lowering LDL-C in group >70 ≤ 100MP mg/dL (mean LDL-C reducing by 9.1%, mean 19.8 months of follow up), >100 (mean follow up LDL-C 110.0 and mean 14.6 months of follow up) mg/dL and ≥0 < 30% (mean LDL-C reducing by 10.6%, mean 18.3 months of follow up) could not lead to the regression; and that intensive lowering LDL-C, by mean 48% with rosuvastatin, and by mean 42% with atorvastatin, could regress CAP. The sensitivity analysis confirmed the effect of the LDL-C change on the volume of the plaque.

The importance of intensive lowing LDL-C on regression of CAP and LDL-C target of this meta-analysis

In the trials that evaluated the effects of LDL-C lowering on atheroma progression by IVUS, the effects varied with level of LDL-C at follow up. In group ≤70 mg, ≥30 < 40% and ≥40 < 50%, the LDL-C at baseline in most trials (including ESTABLISH [14], REVERSAL [13], JAPAN-ACS [12], ASTEROID [37], COSMOS [40], trial by Kawasaki M [16] and by Nasu K [41]) were >120 mg. In ASTEROID [37], COSMOS [40], JAPAN-ACS [12] trial and fluvastatin arm of the trial by Nasu K [41] with respective the mean LDL-C level 60.8 mg, 82.9 mg, 81-84 mg and 98 mg (53.2%, 38.6%, 36% and 32.3% reduction of level of LDL-C) at follow up, it was showed that CAP could be regressed with intensive statin therapy. In ESTABLISH [14] and REVERSAL [13], the mean reducing percent of LDL-C at follow up in the statin treatment arms were 44% and 46% respectively, the volumes of CAPs at follow up were not significantly decreased, compared with those in baseline. In the trails by Yokoyama M [15] and Kawasaki M [16], mean reducing percentage of LDL-C at follow up was 35% for atorvastatin arm of the trial by Yokoyama M [15], 32% for pravastatin arm of the trial by Kawasaki M [16] and 39% for atorvastatin arm of the trial by Kawasaki M [16], the volume of CAPs at

follow up were also not significantly decreased, compared with that at baseline. Pooled these arms with follow up LDL-C ≤70 mg or reducing >30% together, these meta-analysis showed that the CAPs could be regressed in group ≤70 mg, ≥30 < 40% and ≥40 < 50%. Because of publication bias in group ≥30 < 40% (Table 3), the level of LDL-C in this group could not be recommended for regressing CAP. Based on the mean level and reducing percentage of LDL-C in group ≤70 mg and ≥40 < 50% (60.6 ± 3.5 mg, 48.8 ± 3.3%; 66.8 ± 8.0 mg, 45.4 ± 2.8%, in Table 4), the meta-analysis in group ≤70 mg and ≥40 < 50% suggested that for regressing CAP, LDL-C should be reduced by >45% or to a target level ≤ 66 mg/dL.

In trials with 18–24 months of non-statin (ACAT inhibitor, decreasing obesity drugs and glucose-lowering agents) treatment, although the levels of LDL-C at follow up in some arms (ACTIVATE [22], STRADIVARIUS [35], PERISCOPE [36], and A-PLUS [21] with daily 50 mg of avasimibe) were >70 ≤ 100 mg/dL, the LDL-C lowering percentage at follow up in the arms were below 30% because the levels of LDL-C at baseline were <95 mg/dL. In ILLUSTRATE trial [23], after treatment with atorvastatin to reduce levels of LDL-C to less than 100 mg/dL, patients were randomly assigned to receive either atorvastatin monotherapy or atorvastatin plus 60 mg of torcetrapib daily. After 24 months, the reduction of LDL-C in both arms was <24% and the progression of CAP was not halted. In trial [34,35] with statins treatment and baseline LDL-C < 110 mg, if the LDL-C lowering percentage at follow up were <24%, the CAP was also not regressed. The meta analysis with six arms in group >70 ≤ 100LP mg/dL and five arms in group >70 ≤ 100MP mg/dL did not show that only >70 ≤ 100 mg/dL of LDL-C level but <30% reduction at follow up could lead to regression of CAP, which further confirmed the importance of intensively lowering LDL-C in regression of CAP. Though LDL-C at follow up in some trials [13,15,16,26,27,39] of LDL-C lowering by statins was >70 ≤ 100 mg/dL and

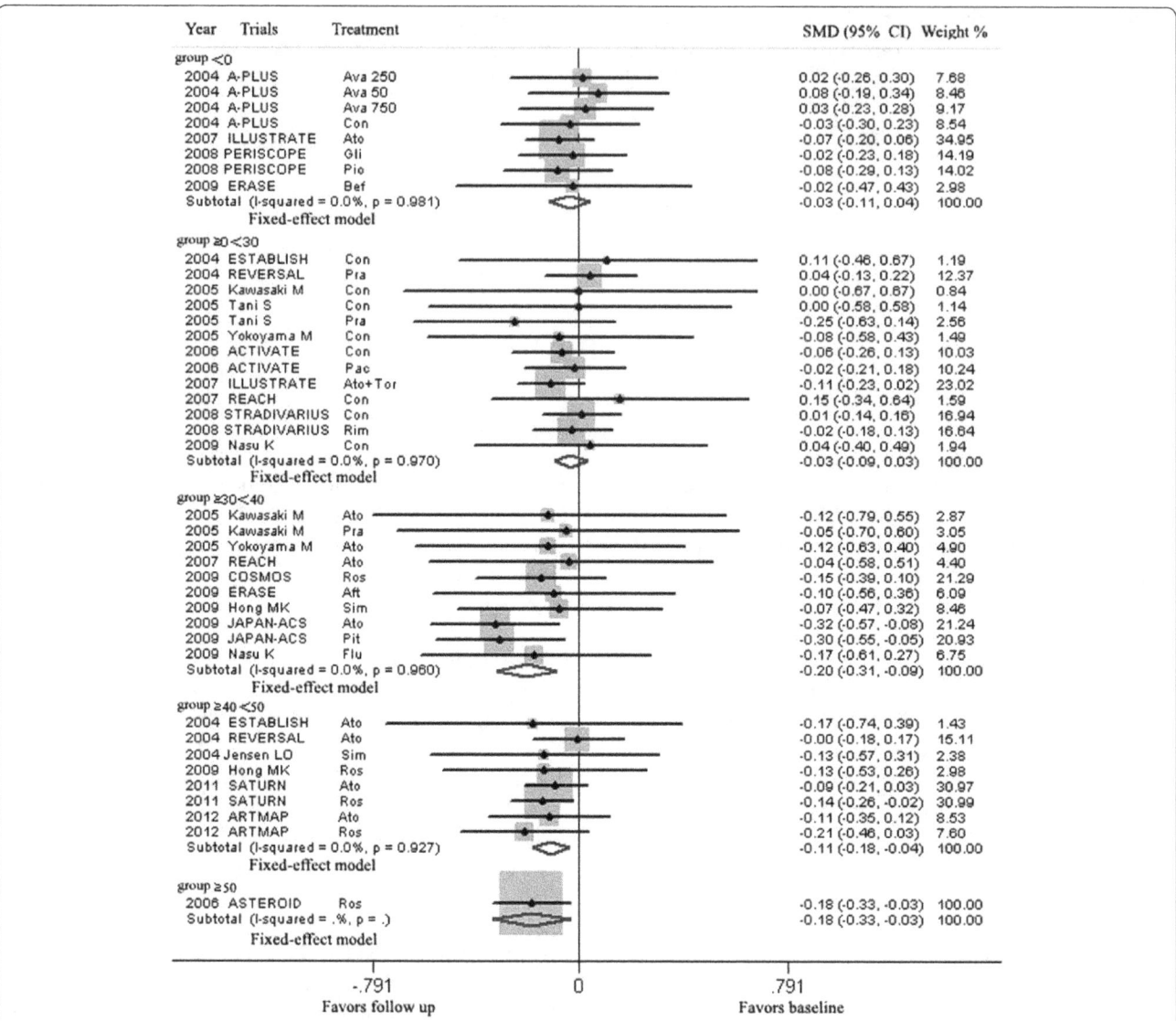

Figure 5 Meta-analysis of the effects of reduction percentages of LDL-C at follow up on the regression of coronary atherosclerotic plaque.
Abbreviations: Ato, Atorvastatin; Ros, Rosuvastatin; Pra, Pravastatin; Pit, Pitavastatin; Sim, Simvastatin; Flu, Fluvastatin; Con, Control; Pac, Pactimibe; Tor, Torcetrapib, Ava 50, 250, 750, Avasimibe 50, 250, 750 mg; Bef, before ACS; Aft, after ACS; Gli, Glimepiride; Pio, Pioglitazone; Rim, Rimonabant.

reducing >30%, the CAP in the trials was also not regressed. Included eleven arms with baseline LDL-C > 130.0 mg/dL, follow up LDL-C >70 ≤ 100 mg/dL and LDL-C reducing >30% (in group >70 ≤ 100HP mg), this meta-analysis suggested that LDL-C reducing >40% or to target 77.8 mg could regress CAP (Table 4). The meta-analysis in group >70 ≤ 100HP, >70 ≤ 100MP and >70 ≤ 100LP mg/dL indicated that LDL-C reducing percentage, not lowering absolute value of LDL-C at follow up, was important for regressing CAP.

Although rosuvastatin, atorvastatin, pitavastatin, simvastatin, and fluvastatin in some trials could reduce LDL-C level to ≤100 mg or by 30%, the meta-analysis indicated that rosuvastatin, atorvastatin and pitavastatin (mean lowering LDL-C by 48.4%, 42.3% and 36.2% respectively) could

regress the CAPs, and simvastatin with mean lowering LDL-C by 39.9% could not. The role of pitavastatin in regressing CAPs remains to be verified because the role was from only one RCT with 125 cases [12]. Pravastatin with mean lowering LDL-C by 24.6% could not regress the CAPs either. Fluvastatin with mean lowering LDL-C by 32.3% in the blinded endpoint trial with 40 patients can regress the CAP [41], but meta-analysis indicated that fluvastatin could not regress the CAP. The reason that pravastatin and fluvastatin in this meta–analysis can not regress the CAPs might be attributed to their low-intensity of lowering LDL-C and low dosage which can not reduce LDL-C by >40%.

Taken all the results of meta-analysis together, it was recommended that LDL-C level should be reduced by >40% or to a target level < 78 mg/dL for regressing CAP.

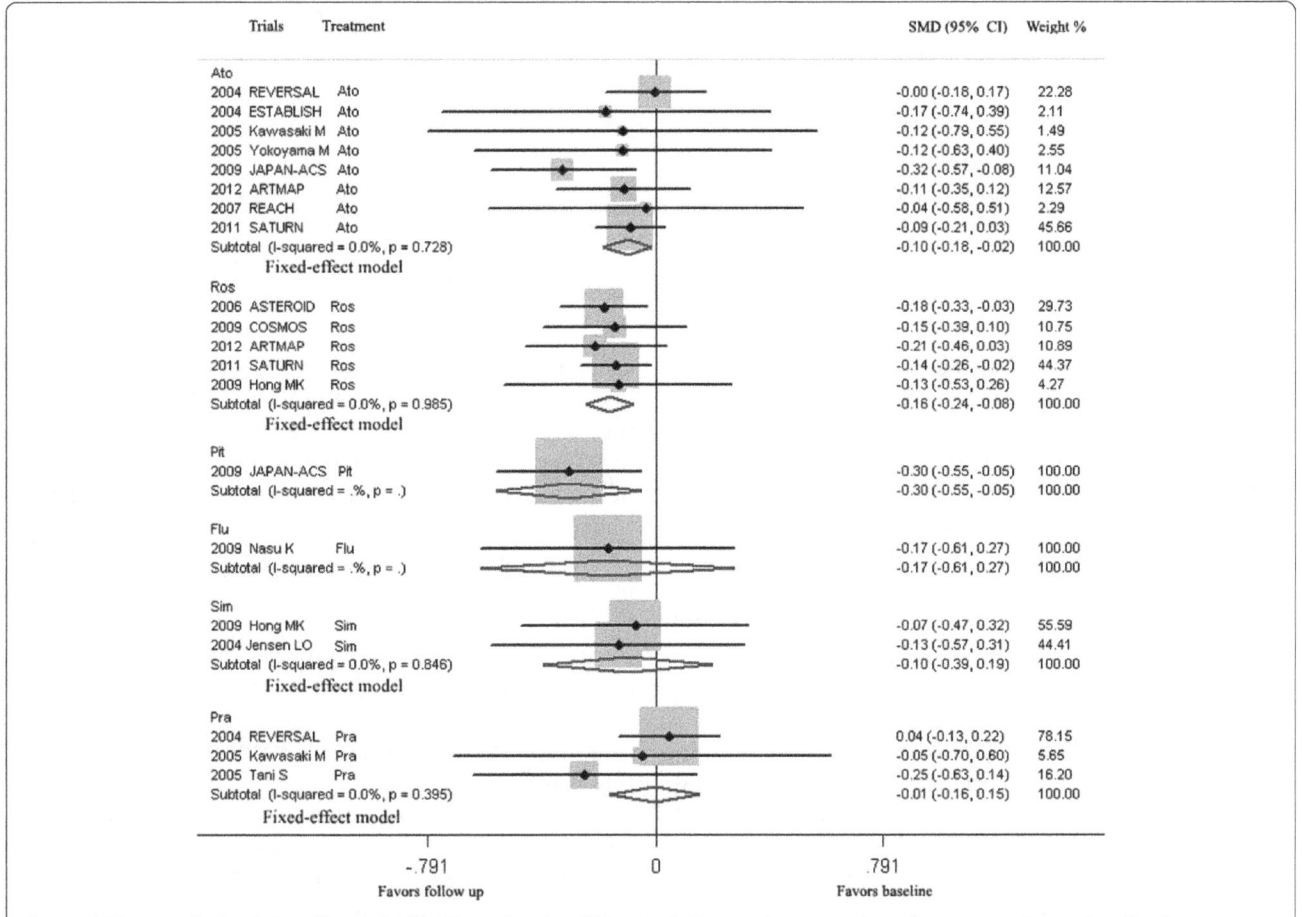

Figure 6 Meta-analysis of the effects of LDL-C lowering by different statins on the regression of coronary atherosclerotic plaque.

Abbreviations: Ato, Atorvastatin; Ros, Rosuvastatin; Pra, Pravastatin; Pit, Pitavastatin; Sim, Simvastatin; Flu, Fluvastatin; Con, Control; Pac, Pactimibe; Tor, Torcetrapib, Ava 50, 250, 750, Avasimibe 50, 250, 750 mg; Bef, before ACS; Aft, after ACS; Gli, Glimepiride; Pio, Pioglitazone; Rim, Rimonabant.

The difference of LDL-C target level between this meta-analysis and current guidelines

The patients included in this meta-analysis were coronary heart disease. According to 2004 the guideline of the Adult Treatment Panel III (ATP III) of the National Cholesterol Education Program [43] and 2011 ESC/EAS Guidelines for the management of dyslipidaemias [1], this group of patients belongs to very high risk category, and the recommended targets of LDL-C should be less than 70 mg/dL or 30-40% reduction from baseline in

Table 5 Results of meta-analysis in different statins groups

Group	Included arms (and case)	Pooled SMD (95% CI, p)	Heterogeneity test		Sensitivity analyses		Egger's test
			χ^2 test (p)	I^2	Lower SMD (95% CI)	Upper SMD (95% CI)	
Rosuvastatin	5 (1173)	-0.162 (-0.234~ -0.081, 0.000)	0.37 (0.985)	0	-0.153 (-0.249~-0.056) Without 2006 ASTEROID Ros	-0.178 (-0.287~-0.069) Without 2011 SATURN Ros	0.770
Atorvastatin	8 (1138)	-0.101 (-0.184~ -0.019, 0.016)	4.44 (0.728)	0	-0.075 (-0.162~0.012) Without 2009 JAPAN-ACS Ato	-0.132 (-0.225~-0.038) Without 2004 REVERSAL Ato	0.582
Pitavastatin	1 (125)	-0.304 (-0.553~-0.055, 0.017)					
Fluvastatin	1 (40)	-0.169 (-0.608~0.270, 0.450)					
Simvastatin	2 (90)	-0.10 (-0.393~ 0.192, 0.501)	0.04 (0.846)	0	-0.074 (-0.467~0.318) Without 2004 Jensen LO Sim	-0.133 (-0.572~0.360) Without 2009 Hong MK Sim	0.000
Pravastatin	3 (319)	-0.008 (-0.163~0.147, 0.920)	1.86 (0.395)	0	-0.005 (-0.165~0.154) Without 2005 Kawasaki M Pra	0.039 (-0.131~0.208) Without 2005 Tani S Pra	0.528

Table 6 Levels and reducing percentage of LDL-C, dosage and duration in different statin group

Group	N	Age	MeanLDL-C at Baseline (mg)	MeanLDL-C at Follow up (mg)	Mean Reducing percentage	Statin dosage (mg)	Duration (month)
Rosuvastatin	1173	58.1±1.8	123.9±8.6	63.3±7.4	48.4±4.2	33.3±11.6	20.5±6.3
Atorvastatin	1138	58.4±2.5	128.0±14.0	73.0±8.7	42.3±3.7	60.3±28.6	17.5±7.1
Pitavastatin	125	62.5±11.5	130.9±33.3	81.1±23.4	36.2±19.5	4	8~12
Fluvastatin	40	63.0±10.0	144.9±31.5	98.1±12.7	32.3	60	12
Simvastatin	90	57.9±0.1	136.61±5.3	81.2±3.5	39.9±6.1	28.9±10.0	17.8±6.5
Pravastatin	319	58.2±3.2	146.8±7.4	108.9±2.9	24.6±2.6	34.8±9.9	15.4±5.0

ATP III, and less than 70 mg/dL or a ≥50% reduction in 2011 ESC/EAS Guidelines. The target levels for subjects at very high risk in the both guidelines are extrapolated from several clinical trials [43], mainly from the meta-analysis by Cholesterol Treatment Trialists' Collaborators [44], which indicated that absolute benefit of LDL-C lowering related chiefly to the absolute reduction of LDL-C, and the risk reductions are proportional to the absolute LDL-C reductions, but the meta-analysis did not provide target level of LDL-C for the benefit in terms of cardiovascular disease reduction [44]. According to 2013 ACC/AHA blood cholesterol guideline [45], this group of patients should be treated with high-intensity statin (atorvastatin 40–80 mg daily or rosuvastatin 20–40 mg daily), which was the intensity of statin suggested in this meta-analysis (Table 6).

The results of our meta-analysis imply that the patients with CHD should be intensively treated with statins (rosuvastatin 33 mg or atorvastatin 60 mg daily) to reduce the level of LDL-C by >40% or to a target level <78 mg/dL for regressing CAP, which have a little different to the guidelines. These different targets level of LDL-C might be due to different observational index: cardiovascular events for both guidelines, CAP volume for this meta-analysis. Moreover, our target is directly from meta-analysis, the target of 2011 ESC/EAS Guidelines is from extrapolation of meta-analysis, not a direct data. Our meta-analysis revealed the relation between the regression of coronary artery disease and LDL-C level from the view of pathological anatomy. Published meta-analysis [17,18] about CAP by IVUS did not review the relationship between LDL-C level and CAP.

Study limitation
The results of this analysis were obtained by pooling data from twenty clinical trials. As with any meta-analysis, this study has some limitations. Firstly, though no publication bias was observed by Egger's test there may be a potential of publication bias because only published data were included. Secondly, the methodology used for measurement of coronary atheroma might not be the same in the studies. The plaques volume may be

calculated from slices with 1 mm apart for a length of 10 mm vessel in some trials [13,15,22,23,27-29,37], or 0.1-0.3 mm-apart for a length of 10–50 mm vessel in other trials [12,21,33,39,40], which might affect accuracy of plaque measurement. There were some differences in selecting plaque: some trials assessed the plaque in non-culprit vessel, while others assessed non-culprit plaque in a culprit vessel [12,14,34], which assured the plaque was stable. Our study focus on target plaque change, i.e. plaque regression or progression, those differences in measurements and plaque selection did not affect the change of the target plaque with LDL-C levels. So, it has little effect on homogeneous of studies, and this detection bias was very much limited from values of P in χ^2 test and I^2 in each group. Thirdly, follow up duration might have some effects of the changes of CAP. Fourthly, other cardiovascular risk factors but LDL-C levels, for example, demographic characteristics such as age, gender and ethnicity, might also affect the effect of LDL-C on CAP, and the effects of these factors on CAP remain to be investigated in future.

Implication for practice
This meta-analysis investigated the effect of reduction of LDL-C only on the regression of the plaque, not on reduction of cardiovascular events. In fact, all the included trial have no the data about death because only the alive have IVUS data at follow up. But in four-year of the OLIVUS-Ex [46], it was found that patients with annual atheroma progression had more adverse cardio- and cerebrovascular events than the rest of the population. A meta-analysis [47] included 7864 CAD patients showed that rates of plaque volume regression were significantly associated with the incidence of MI or revascularization, and it was concluded that regression of atherosclerotic coronary plaque volume in stable CAD patients may represent a surrogate for myocardial infarction and repeat revascularization. Plaque in CAD, as blood pressure level in hypertension, is not major adverse cardiac events, but does be an important surrogate. Therefore, the conclusion of this meta-analysis not only applies to guide LDL-C lowering therapy for regressing CAP, may also apply to guide LDL-C lowering therapy for reducing

major adverse cardio- and cerebrovascular events. Furthermore, high level of LDL-C plays a crucial role in the formation of atherosclerotic plaque, but LDL-C level is not unique risk factor for atherosclerotic plaque. Hypertension is another important risk factor for the formation of plaque [48,49]. Smoking cessation, administrating β-blockers, anti-hypertension therapy might play some role in slowing progression of CAP [48,50-52]. The trend of CAP regression in group <0% might attribute to these non-LDL-C reducing factors.

Conclusions

Atherosclerotic plaque extension and disruption are basic mechanism of atherosclerotic cardio- and cerebrovascular disease. Stabling and regressing atherosclerotic plaque play an important role in preventing cardio- and cerebrovascular disease. Pooled the twenty trials with CAP detected by gold standard: IVUS, this systemic review demonstrated that intensive lowering LDL-C (rosuvastatin mean 33 mg daily and atorvastatin mean 60 mg daily) with >17 months of duration could lead to the regression of coronary atherosclerotic plaque, LDL-C level should be reduced by >40% or to a target level < 78 mg/dL for regressing CAP.

Abbreviations
LDL-C: Low-density lipoprotein cholesterol; CAP: Coronary atherosclerotic plaque; CHD: Coronary heart disease; RCT: Randomized controlled trial; CAG: Coronary angiography; IVUS: Intravascular ultrasound; SMD: Standardized mean differences; ACS: Acute coronary syndrome; ACAT: Acyl–coenzyme A:cholesterol acyltransferase; CETP: Cholesteryl ester transfer protein; CI: Confidence interval; ATP III: Adult Treatment Panel III; CAD: Coronary artery disease.

Competing interests
The authors declare that they have no competing interests. This study was not funded.

Authors' contributions
GWQ, FQZ and LYF carried out data extraction, participated in the analysis and drafted the manuscript. LYX and LCY participated in the design of the study and helped to draft the manuscript. HY, CYM and YB conceived the study, and participated in its statistical analysis. All authors read and approved the final manuscript.

Author details
[1]The Department of Cardiology, Chinese PLA General Hospital, Beijing 100853, China. [2]The First Department of Geriatric Cardiology, Chinese PLA General Hospital, Beijing 100853, China. [3]Navy Wangshoulu Clinics, Xicui Road, Beijing 100036, China.

References
1. Reiner Z, Catapano AL, De Backer G, Graham I, Taskinen MR, Wiklund O, Agewall S, Alegria E, Chapman MJ, Durrington P, Erdine S, Halcox J, Hobbs R, Kjekshus J, Filardi PP, Riccardi G, Storey RF, Wood D: ESC/EAS Guidelines for the management of dyslipidaemias: the Task Force for the management of dyslipidaemias of the European Society of Cardiology (ESC) and the European Atherosclerosis Society (EAS). Eur Heart J 2011, 32:1769–1818.
2. Falk E, Shah PK, Fuster V: Coronary plaque disruption. Circulation 1995, 92:657–671.
3. The Long-Term Intervention with Pravastatin in Ischaemic Disease (LIPID) Study Group: Prevention of cardiovascular events and death with pravastatin in patients with coronary heart disease and a broad range of initial cholesterol levels. N Engl J Med 1998, 339:1349–1357.
4. Scandinavian Simvastatin Survival Study Group: Randomised trial of cholesterol lowering in 4444 patients with coronary heart disease: the Scandinavian Simvastatin Survival Study (4S). Lancet 1994, 344:1383–1389.
5. Brown G, Albers JJ, Fisher LD, Schaefer SM, Lin JT, Kaplan C, Zhao XQ, Bisson BD, Fitzpatrick VF, Dodge HT: Regression of coronary artery disease as a result of intensive lipid-lowering therapy in men with high levels of apolipoprotein B. N Engl J Med 1990, 323:1289–1298.
6. Blankenhorn DH, Azen SP, Kramsch DM, Mack WJ, Cashin-Hemphill L, Hodis HN, DeBoer LW, Mahrer PR, Masteller MJ, Vailas LI, Alaupovic P, Hirsch LJ: Coronary angiographic changes with lovastatin therapy. The Monitored Atherosclerosis Regression Study (MARS). Ann Intern Med 1993, 119:969–976.
7. Thomas AC, Davies MJ, Dilly S, Dilly N, Franc F: Potential errors in the estimation of coronary arterial stenosis from clinical arteriography with reference to the shape of the coronary arterial lumen. Br Heart J 1986, 55:129–139.
8. Hausmann D, Johnson JA, Sudhir K, Mullen WL, Friedrich G, Fitzgerald PJ, Chou TM, Ports TA, Kane JP, Malloy MJ, Yock PG: Angiographically silent atherosclerosis detected by intravascular ultrasound in patients with familial hypercholesterolemia and familial combined hyperlipidemia: correlation with high density lipoproteins. J Am Coll Cardiol 1996, 27:1562–1570.
9. Mintz GS, Painter JA, Pichard AD, Kent KM, Satler LF, Popma JJ, Chuang YC, Bucher TA, Sokolowicz LE, Leon MB: Atherosclerosis in angiographically "normal" coronary artery reference segments: an intravascular ultrasound study with clinical correlations. J Am Coll Cardiol 1995, 25:1479–1485.
10. Nissen SE, Yock P: Intravascular ultrasound: novel pathophysiological insights and current clinical applications. Circulation 2001, 103:604–616.
11. Takagi T, Yoshida K, Akasaka T, Hozumi T, Morioka S, Yoshikawa J: Intravascular ultrasound analysis of reduction in progression of coronary narrowing by treatment with pravastatin. Am J Cardiol 1997, 79:1673–1676.
12. Hiro T, Kimura T, Morimoto T, Miyauchi K, Nakagawa Y, Yamagishi M, Ozaki Y, Kimura K, Saito S, Yamaguchi T, Daida H, Matsuzaki M: Effect of intensive statin therapy on regression of coronary atherosclerosis in patients with acute coronary syndrome: a multicenter randomized trial evaluated by volumetric intravascular ultrasound using pitavastatin versus atorvastatin (JAPAN-ACS [Japan assessment of pitavastatin and atorvastatin in acute coronary syndrome] study). J Am Coll Cardiol 2009, 54:293–302.
13. Nissen SE, Tuzcu EM, Schoenhagen P, Brown BG, Ganz P, Vogel RA, Crowe T, Howard G, Cooper CJ, Brodie B, Grines CL, DeMaria AN: Effect of intensive compared with moderate lipid-lowering therapy on progression of coronary atherosclerosis: a randomized controlled trial. JAMA 2004, 291:1071–1080.
14. Okazaki S, Yokoyama T, Miyauchi K, Shimada K, Kurata T, Sato H, Daida H: Early statin treatment in patients with acute coronary syndrome: demonstration of the beneficial effect on atherosclerotic lesions by serial volumetric intravascular ultrasound analysis during half a year after coronary event: the ESTABLISH Study. Circulation 2004, 110:1061–1068.
15. Yokoyama M, Komiyama N, Courtney BK, Nakayama T, Namikawa S, Kuriyama N, Koizumi T, Nameki M, Fitzgerald PJ, Komuro I: Plasma low-density lipoprotein reduction and structural effects on coronary atherosclerotic plaques by atorvastatin as clinically assessed with intravascular ultrasound radio-frequency signal analysis: a randomized prospective study. Am Heart J 2005, 150:287.
16. Kawasaki M, Sano K, Okubo M, Yokoyama H, Ito Y, Murata I, Tsuchiya K, Minatoguchi S, Zhou X, Fujita H, Fujiwara H: Volumetric quantitative analysis of tissue characteristics of coronary plaques after statin therapy using three-dimensional integrated backscatter intravascular ultrasound. J Am Coll Cardiol 2005, 45:1946–1953.
17. Bedi U, Singh M, Singh P, Molnar J, Khosla S, Arora R: Effects of statins on progression of coronary artery disease as measured by intravascular ultrasound. J Clin Hypertens (Greenwich) 2011, 13:492–496.
18. Tian J, Gu X, Sun Y, Ban X, Xiao Y, Hu S, Yu B: Effect of statin therapy on the progression of coronary atherosclerosis. BMC Cardiovasc Disord 2012, 12:70.
19. Jadad AR, Moore RA, Carroll D, Jenkinson C, Reynolds DJ, Gavaghan DJ, McQuay HJ: Assessing the quality of reports of randomized clinical trials: is blinding necessary? Control Clin Trials 1996, 17:1–12.

20. Schartl M, Bocksch W, Koschyk DH, Voelker W, Karsch KR, Kreuzer J, Hausmann D, Beckmann S, Gross M: Use of intravascular ultrasound to compare effects of different strategies of lipid-lowering therapy on plaque volume and composition in patients with coronary artery disease. *Circulation* 2001, 104:387–392.

21. Tardif JC, Gregoire J, L'Allier PL, Anderson TJ, Bertrand O, Reeves F, Title LM, Alfonso F, Schampaert E, Hassan A, McLain R, Pressler ML, Ibrahim R, Lesperance J, Blue J, Heinonen T, Rodes-Cabau J: Effects of the acyl coenzyme A: cholesterol acyltransferase inhibitor avasimibe on human atherosclerotic lesions. *Circulation* 2004, 110:3372–3377.

22. Nissen SE, Tuzcu EM, Brewer HB, Sipahi I, Nicholls SJ, Ganz P, Schoenhagen P, Waters DD, Pepine CJ, Crowe TD, Davidson MH, Deanfield JE, Wisniewski LM, Hanyok JJ, Kassalow LM: Effect of ACAT inhibition on the progression of coronary atherosclerosis. *N Engl J Med* 2006, 354:1253–1263.

23. Nissen SE, Tardif JC, Nicholls SJ, Revkin JH, Shear CL, Duggan WT, Ruzyllo W, Bachinsky WB, Lasala GP, Tuzcu EM: Effect of torcetrapib on the progression of coronary atherosclerosis. *N Engl J Med* 2007, 356:1304–1316.

24. Nozue T, Yamamoto S, Tohyama S, Umezawa S, Kunishima T, Sato A, Miyake S, Takeyama Y, Morino Y, Yamauchi T, Muramatsu T, Hibi K, Sozu T, Terashima M, Michishita I: Statin treatment for coronary artery plaque composition based on intravascular ultrasound radiofrequency data analysis. *Am Heart J* 2012, 163:191–199. e1.

25. Zhang X, Wang H, Liu S, Gong P, Lin J, Lu J, Qiu J, Lu X: Intensive-dose atorvastatin regimen halts progression of atherosclerotic plaques in new-onset unstable angina with borderline vulnerable plaque lesions. *J Cardiovasc Pharmacol Ther* 2013, 18:119–125.

26. Yamada T, Azuma A, Sasaki S, Sawada T, Matsubara H: Randomized evaluation of atorvastatin in patients with coronary heart disease: a serial intravascular ultrasound study. *Circ J* 2007, 71:1845–1850.

27. Hong MK, Park DW, Lee CW, Lee SW, Kim YH, Kang DH, Song JK, Kim JJ, Park SW, Park SJ: Effects of statin treatments on coronary plaques assessed by volumetric virtual histology intravascular ultrasound analysis. *JACC Cardiovasc Interv* 2009, 2:679–688.

28. Nicholls SJ, Ballantyne CM, Barter PJ, Chapman MJ, Erbel RM, Libby P, Raichlen JS, Uno K, Borgman M, Wolski K, Nissen SE: Effect of two intensive statin regimens on progression of coronary disease. *N Engl J Med* 2011, 365:2078–2087.

29. Lee CW, Kang SJ, Ahn JM, Song HG, Lee JY, Kim WJ, Park DW, Lee SW, Kim YH, Park SW, Park SJ: Comparison of effects of atorvastatin (20 mg) versus rosuvastatin (10 mg) therapy on mild coronary atherosclerotic plaques (from the ARTMAP trial). *Am J Cardiol* 2012, 109:1700–1704.

30. Hong YJ, Jeong MH, Hachinohe D, Ahmed K, Choi YH, Cho SH, Hwang SH, Ko JS, Lee MG, Park KH, Sim DS, Yoon NS, Yoon HJ, Kim KH, Park HW, Kim JH, Ahn Y, Cho JG, Park JC, Kang JC: Comparison of effects of rosuvastatin and atorvastatin on plaque regression in Korean patients with untreated intermediate coronary stenosis. *Circ J* 2011, 75:398–406.

31. Kovarnik T, Mintz GS, Skalicka H, Kral A, Horak J, Skulec R, Uhrova J, Martasek P, Downe RW, Wahle A, Sonka M, Mrazek V, Aschermann M, Linhart A: Virtual histology evaluation of atherosclerosis regression during atorvastatin and ezetimibe administration: HEAVEN study. *Circ J* 2012, 76:176–183.

32. Petronio AS, Amoroso G, Limbruno U, Papini B, De Carlo M, Micheli A, Ciabatti N, Mariani M: Simvastatin does not inhibit intimal hyperplasia and restenosis but promotes plaque regression in normocholesterolemic patients undergoing coronary stenting: a randomized study with intravascular ultrasound. *Am Heart J* 2005, 149:520–526.

33. Tani S, Watanabe I, Anazawa T, Kawamata H, Tachibana E, Furukawa K, Sato Y, Nagao K, Kanmatsuse K, Kushiro T: Effect of pravastatin on malondialdehyde-modified low-density lipoprotein levels and coronary plaque regression as determined by three-dimensional intravascular ultrasound. *Am J Cardiol* 2005, 96:1089–1094.

34. Rodes-Cabau J, Tardif JC, Cossette M, Bertrand OF, Ibrahim R, Larose E, Gregoire J, L'allier PL, Guertin MC: Acute effects of statin therapy on coronary atherosclerosis following an acute coronary syndrome. *Am J Cardiol* 2009, 104:750–757.

35. Nissen SE, Nicholls SJ, Wolski K, Rodes-Cabau J, Cannon CP, Deanfield JE, Despres JP, Kastelein JJ, Steinhubl SR, Kapadia S, Yasin M, Ruzyllo W, Gaudin C, Job B, Hu B, Bhatt DL, Lincoff AM, Tuzcu EM: Effect of rimonabant on progression of atherosclerosis in patients with abdominal obesity and coronary artery disease: the STRADIVARIUS randomized controlled trial. *JAMA* 2008, 299:1547–1560.

36. Nissen SE, Nicholls SJ, Wolski K, Nesto R, Kupfer S, Perez A, Jure H, De Larochelliere R, Staniloae CS, Mavromatis K, Saw J, Hu B, Lincoff AM, Tuzcu EM: Comparison of pioglitazone vs glimepiride on progression of coronary atherosclerosis in patients with type 2 diabetes: the PERISCOPE randomized controlled trial. *JAMA* 2008, 299:1561–1573.

37. Nissen SE, Nicholls SJ, Sipahi I, Libby P, Raichlen JS, Ballantyne CM, Davignon J, Erbel R, Fruchart JC, Tardif JC, Schoenhagen P, Crowe T, Cain V, Wolski K, Goormastic M, Tuzcu EM: Effect of very high-intensity statin therapy on regression of coronary atherosclerosis: the ASTEROID trial. *JAMA* 2006, 295:1556–1565.

38. Matsuzaki M, Hiramori K, Imaizumi T, Kitabatake A, Hishida H, Nomura M, Fujii T, Sakuma I, Fukami K, Honda T, Ogawa H, Yamagishi M: Intravascular ultrasound evaluation of coronary plaque regression by low density lipoprotein-apheresis in familial hypercholesterolemia: the Low Density Lipoprotein-Apheresis Coronary Morphology and Reserve Trial (LACMART). *J Am Coll Cardiol* 2002, 40:220–227.

39. Jensen LO, Thayssen P, Pedersen KE, Stender S, Haghfelt T: Regression of coronary atherosclerosis by simvastatin: a serial intravascular ultrasound study. *Circulation* 2004, 110:265–270.

40. Takayama T, Hiro T, Yamagishi M, Daida H, Hirayama A, Saito S, Yamaguchi T, Matsuzaki M: Effect of rosuvastatin on coronary atheroma in stable coronary artery disease: multicenter coronary atherosclerosis study measuring effects of rosuvastatin using intravascular ultrasound in Japanese subjects (COSMOS). *Circ J* 2009, 73:2110–2117.

41. Nasu K, Tsuchikane E, Katoh O, Tanaka N, Kimura M, Ehara M, Kinoshita Y, Matsubara T, Matsuo H, Asakura K, Asakura Y, Terashima M, Takayama T, Honye J, Hirayama A, Saito S, Suzuki T: Effect of fluvastatin on progression of coronary atherosclerotic plaque evaluated by virtual histology intravascular ultrasound. *JACC Cardiovasc Interv* 2009, 2:689–696.

42. Hattori K, Ozaki Y, Ismail TF, Okumura M, Naruse H, Kan S, Ishikawa M, Kawai T, Ohta M, Kawai H, Hashimoto T, Takagi Y, Ishii J, Serruys PW, Narula J: Impact of statin therapy on plaque characteristics as assessed by serial OCT, grayscale and integrated backscatter-IVUS. *JACC Cardiovasc Imaging* 2012, 5:169–177.

43. Grundy SM, Cleeman JI, Merz CN, Brewer HB Jr, Clark LT, Hunninghake DB, Pasternak RC, Smith SC Jr, Stone NJ: Implications of recent clinical trials for the National Cholesterol Education Program Adult Treatment Panel III guidelines. *Circulation* 2004, 110:227–239.

44. Baigent C, Keech A, Kearney PM, Blackwell L, Buck G, Pollicino C, Kirby A, Sourjina T, Peto R, Collins R, Simes R: Efficacy and safety of cholesterol-lowering treatment: prospective meta-analysis of data from 90,056 participants in 14 randomised trials of statins. *Lancet* 2005, 366:1267–1278.

45. Stone NJ, Robinson J, Lichtenstein AH, Merz CN, Blum CB, Eckel RH, Goldberg AC, Gordon D, Levy D, Lloyd-Jones DM, McBride P, Schwartz JS, Shero ST, Smith SC Jr, Watson K, Wilson PW: 2013 ACC/AHA Guideline on the Treatment of Blood Cholesterol to Reduce Atherosclerotic Cardiovascular Risk in Adults: A Report of the American College of Cardiology/American Heart Association Task Force on Practice Guidelines. *Circulation* 2013, 00:000.

46. Hirohata A, Yamamoto K, Miyoshi T, Hatanaka K, Hirohata S, Yamawaki H, Komatsubara I, Hirose E, Kobayashi Y, Ohkawa K, Ohara M, Takafuji H, Sano F, Toyama Y, Kusachi S, Ohe T, Ito H: Four-year clinical outcomes of the OLIVUS-Ex (impact of Olmesartan on progression of coronary atherosclerosis: evaluation by intravascular ultrasound) extension trial. *Atherosclerosis* 2012, 220:134–138.

47. D'Ascenzo F, Agostoni P, Abbate A, Castagno D, Lipinski MJ, Vetrovec GW, Frati G, Presutti DG, Quadri G, Moretti C, Gaita F, Zoccai GB: Atherosclerotic coronary plaque regression and the risk of adverse cardiovascular events: a meta-regression of randomized clinical trials. *Atherosclerosis* 2013, 226:178–185.

48. Nissen SE, Tuzcu EM, Libby P, Thompson PD, Ghali M, Garza D, Berman L, Shi H, Buebendorf E, Topol EJ: Effect of antihypertensive agents on cardiovascular events in patients with coronary disease and normal blood pressure: the CAMELOT study: a randomized controlled trial. *JAMA* 2004, 292:2217–2225.

49. Hirohata A, Yamamoto K, Miyoshi T, Hatanaka K, Hirohata S, Yamawaki H, Komatsubara I, Murakami M, Hirose E, Sato S, Ohkawa K, Ishizawa M, Yamaji H, Kawamura H, Kusachi S, Murakami T, Hina K, Ohe T: Impact of olmesartan on progression of coronary atherosclerosis a serial volumetric intravascular ultrasound analysis from the OLIVUS (impact of OLmesarten on progression of coronary atherosclerosis: evaluation by intravascular ultrasound) trial. *J Am Coll Cardiol* 2010, 55:976–982.

50. Redgrave JN, Lovett JK, Rothwell PM: **Histological features of symptomatic carotid plaques in relation to age and smoking: the oxford plaque study.** *Stroke* 2010, **41**:2288–2294.

51. Heidland UE, Strauer BE: **Left ventricular muscle mass and elevated heart rate are associated with coronary plaque disruption.** *Circulation* 2001, **104**:1477–1482.

52. Sipahi I, Tuzcu EM, Wolski KE, Nicholls SJ, Schoenhagen P, Hu B, Balog C, Shishehbor M, Magyar WA, Crowe TD, Kapadia S, Nissen SE: **Beta-blockers and progression of coronary atherosclerosis: pooled analysis of 4 intravascular ultrasonography trials.** *Ann Intern Med* 2007, **147**:10–18.

11

Prevalence and treatment of atherogenic dyslipidemia in the primary prevention of cardiovascular disease in Europe

Julian P. Halcox[1*], José R. Banegas[2], Carine Roy[3], Jean Dallongeville[4], Guy De Backer[5], Eliseo Guallar[6], Joep Perk[7], David Hajage[3], Karin M. Henriksson[8] and Claudio Borghi[9]

Abstract

Background: Atherogenic dyslipidemia is associated with poor cardiovascular outcomes, yet markers of this condition are often ignored in clinical practice. Here, we address a clear evidence gap by assessing the prevalence and treatment of two markers of atherogenic dyslipidemia: elevated triglyceride levels and low levels of high-density lipoprotein cholesterol.

Methods: This cross-sectional observational study assessed the prevalence of two atherogenic dyslipidemia markers, high triglyceride levels and low high-density lipoprotein cholesterol levels, in the study population from the European Study on Cardiovascular Risk Prevention and Management in Usual Daily Practice (EURIKA; N = 7641; of whom 51.6% were female and 95.6% were White/Caucasian). The EURIKA population included European patients, aged at least 50 years with at least one cardiovascular risk factor but no history of cardiovascular disease.

Results: Over 20% of patients from the EURIKA population have either triglyceride or high-density lipoprotein cholesterol levels characteristic of atherogenic dyslipidemia. Furthermore, the proportions of patients with one of these markers were higher in subpopulations with type 2 diabetes mellitus or those already calculated to be at high risk of cardiovascular disease. Approximately 55% of the EURIKA population who have markers of atherogenic dyslipidemia are not receiving lipid-lowering therapy.

Conclusions: A considerable proportion of patients with at least one major cardiovascular risk factor in the primary cardiovascular disease prevention setting have markers of atherogenic dyslipidemia. The majority of these patients are not receiving optimal treatment, as specified in international guidelines, and thus their risk of developing cardiovascular disease is possibly underestimated.

Keywords: Atherogenic dyslipidemia, Cardiovascular disease, Epidemiology, Risk factors/global assessment

* Correspondence: j.p.j.halcox@swansea.ac.uk
[1]Institute of Life Sciences 2, Swansea University College of Medicine, Singleton Park, Swansea SA2 8PP, UK
Full list of author information is available at the end of the article

Background

Although considerable progress has been made in understanding and treating associated risk factors, cardiovascular disease (CVD) remains the leading cause of death among adults under the age of 75 years in Europe [1]. Traditionally recognized risk factors for CVD include age, male sex, smoking, lack of exercise, obesity, hypertension, high levels of low-density lipoprotein cholesterol (LDL-C), type 2 diabetes mellitus (T2DM), and familial predisposition [2]. In addition, other factors, including atherogenic dyslipidemia, and elevated lipoprotein(a) or C-reactive protein (CRP) levels, may also be important considerations when estimating patients' overall CVD risk [2–9]. Atherogenic dyslipidemia has been characterized as a combination of elevated LDL-C and triglyceride (TG) levels, decreased high-density lipoprotein cholesterol (HDL-C) levels, and a preponderance of small-dense LDL-C particles [10]. Here, we use data from the European Study on Cardiovascular Risk Prevention and Management in Usual Daily Practice (EURIKA, ClinicalTrials.gov identifier: NCT00882336), a cross-sectional observational study including data on patients from 12 European countries with at least one traditional CVD risk factor but no history of cardiovascular events [11, 12], to assess the prevalence and treatment of two markers of atherogenic dyslipidemia: elevated TG levels and low HDL-C levels. We have previously assessed the prevalence of elevated levels of CRP in the EURIKA population [9]. Among patients without T2DM not receiving a statin, approximately half had CRP levels of at least 2 mg/l. The impact of CRP and markers of atherogenic dyslipidemia on CVD risk is often underestimated in clinical practice, with a lack of evidence for the prevalence and treatment of the latter. TG and CRP levels are not taken into account in global cardiovascular risk calculators, such as the Systematic Coronary Risk Evaluation (SCORE) algorithm [13] and the risk calculator developed alongside the American College of Cardiology/American Heart Association (ACC/AHA) 2013 guidelines [14].

Methods

Study design and participants

EURIKA was a cross-sectional study carried out in 12 European countries (Austria, Belgium, France, Germany, Greece, Norway, Russia, Spain, Sweden, Switzerland, Turkey, and the UK) [11]. Included patients were aged 50 years or older and had at least one risk factor for CVD but no history of cardiovascular events. Data collection started in May 2009 and ended in January 2010, with a 3-month data-collection period for each country. The study protocol was approved by the appropriate clinical research ethics committees in each participating country, and all patients provided signed informed consent. The methods for the study have been reported

in detail elsewhere [12]. Briefly, the study sample was selected in a two-stage process that involved the random selection of both physicians and patients [12, 15]. In the first stage, primary care physicians (PCPs) and specialists involved in CVD prevention (including cardiologists, endocrinologists, and internal medicine specialists) were randomly selected for invitation to participate using the OneKey database (Cegedim Dendrite, Boulogne-Billancourt, France) [16]. In total, 809 physicians (approximately 60 per country) agreed to participate in EURIKA, 64% of whom were PCPs [15]. In the second stage, participating physicians sequentially invited patients who met the selection criteria (aged ≥50 years, who were free from CVD but with at least one major cardiovascular risk factor [dyslipidemia, hypertension, current smoker, T2DM, or obesity]). Hypertension was defined as having a systolic blood pressure (SBP) of at least 140 mmHg, a diastolic blood pressure (DBP) of at least 90 mmHg, or receiving treatment with antihypertensive medications. Approximately 600 patients were included per country, with a final sample size of 7641.

Assessment of CVD risk factors

Demographic information and other details of participating patients were gathered from medical records and patient interviews. For each patient, a physical examination was conducted, blood pressure measured, and a 12-h fasting blood sample collected within 1 day of the initial outpatient consultation [12]. Blood pressure was measured under standardized conditions, and blood sample analysis was performed at a central laboratory (BioAnalytical Research Corporation, Ghent, Belgium), with the exception of patients in Russia (approximately 5% of the total patient population), for whom a laboratory analysis was performed locally. HDL-C concentration was measured using a modified enzymatic method, total cholesterol concentration using the cholesterol oxidase/p-aminophenazone (CHOD-PAP) method, TG concentration using the glycerol-3-phosphate-oxidase/p-aminophenazone (GPO-PAP) method, and CRP levels using a high-sensitivity immunoturbidimetric method (all using the Roche Modular P chemistry analyzer [Roche Diagnostics, Indianapolis, IN, USA]). LDL-C concentration was calculated by the Friedewald formula [17]. The ACC/AHA risk calculator was used to calculate 10-year CVD risk scores, and the version of the SCORE algorithm updated to consider patients' total cholesterol and HDL-C levels as independent variables (SCORE-HDL) [6, 13, 14, 18]. Patients were considered to be at high CVD risk if they had a score of at least 7.5% when using the ACC/AHA risk calculator, or at least 5% when using the SCORE-HDL algorithm.

High TG levels were defined as those of at least 2.3 mmol/l (200 mg/dl), and low HDL-C levels as those lower than 1.0 mmol/l (40 mg/dl) in men and lower than 1.3 mmol/l (50 mg/dl) in women. For statin treatment, therapy was categorized as low or moderate intensity (pravastatin 5–40 mg/day, simvastatin 2.5–80 mg/day, lovastatin 10–80 mg/day, fluvastatin 10–80 mg/day, atorvastatin 5–40 mg/day, or rosuvastatin 5–20 mg/day), or high intensity (atorvastatin ≥40 mg/day or rosuvastatin ≥20 mg/day).

Statistical analyses

Data are presented as mean and standard deviation for continuous variables, and as frequency and percentage for categorical variables. Comparisons between groups were performed using Student's *t*-tests for normally distributed continuous variables, Mann–Whitney U tests for continuous variables that were not normally distributed, and χ^2 or Fisher's exact tests for categorical variables, as appropriate. A *p* value below 0.05 was considered significant. Multivariate logistic regression was performed to assess factors associated with high TG and/ or low HDL-C levels. Variables considered in the multivariate analysis included country of origin, age, sex, hypertension, obesity, T2DM status, smoking status, total cholesterol levels, CRP levels, use of β-blockers, use of α-adrenergic antagonists, and use of diuretics. A stepwise (bidirectional) selection method was used to keep only those variables statistically significantly associated at the *p* < 0.05 level in the final model. Statistical analyses were performed using SAS version 9.2 (SAS Institute Inc., Cary, NC, USA).

Results

Overall patient characteristics

The EURIKA study population consisted of 7641 patients with a mean age of 63.2 years, of whom 48.4% were men and of whom 95.6% were White/Caucasian (Table 1). Mean body mass index (BMI) was 28.9 kg/m^2, 21.0% of patients were current smokers, and 26.8% of participants had T2DM. Mean alcohol consumption of the EURIKA study population was 5.7 units/week, and 19.8% of patients reported undertaking no physical exercise. Almost three-quarters (72.8%) of patients had hypertension.

Prevalence of high TG and/or low HDL-C levels

Among the overall population that included treated and untreated patients, a total of 1591 patients (20.8%) were classified as having high TG levels (≥ 2.3 mmol/l), 1691 (22.1%) had low HDL-C levels (men: < 1.0 mmol/l; women: < 1.3 mmol/l), and 759 (9.9%) had both high TG and low HDL-C levels (Table 1; Fig. 1). A very small proportion of patients in the overall population had very high TG levels (> 5 mmol/L [1.9%]; > 10 mmol/L [0.3%]). Similarly, only 0.1% of the EURIKA population

had very low HDL-C levels (< 0.5 mmol/L). The mean ages of patients in the subpopulations with high TG levels, low HDL-C levels, or both were similar to that of the overall population, as were mean SBP, DBP, and the proportions of patients with hypertension. There were higher proportions of patients classified as obese (BMI ≥ 30 kg/m^2) in the subpopulations with high TG levels, low HDL-C levels, or both than in the overall population. There was a higher proportion of men with high TG levels than women in the patient population; conversely, the proportion of women was higher among patients with low HDL-C levels when compared with men. The proportion of patients who had T2DM was higher among patients with markers of atherogenic dyslipidemia than in the overall population. There were patients within the EURIKA population, both male and female, exceeding the recommended weekly limit of alcohol consumption. There were similar proportions of patients undertaking no physical exercise in the subpopulations with high TG levels, low HDL-C levels, or both to those in the overall population. We observed cross-country variation in the proportions of patients with markers of atherogenic dyslipidemia (Additional file 1: Table S1).

Treatment of high TG and/or low HDL-C levels

With regard to treatment, over half of patients in the overall population and in the subpopulations with markers of atherogenic dyslipidemia were not receiving any form of lipid-lowering therapy (LLT, Table 1). Of patients receiving LLT, most were receiving a statin alone. Only small proportions of patients were receiving ezetimibe, a fibrate, or nicotinic acid. Of those patients receiving a statin, most were receiving a low- or moderate-intensity statin; only a small proportion of patients (≤ 5%) were receiving a high-intensity statin (Fig. 2).

Differences in the prevalence of high TG and/or low HDL-C levels according to statin treatment, T2DM, and CVD risk status

Patients in the overall population were described according to whether or not they were receiving statin therapy, and then further stratified according to the presence or absence of T2DM, and then, among patients without T2DM, overall CVD risk assessed using either the ACC/AHA or SCORE-HDL risk calculators [6, 14]. Higher proportions of patients with T2DM were found to have high TG and/or low HDL-C levels than patients without T2DM (Fig. 3). Among patients without T2DM, greater proportions of patients in the higher overall CVD risk categories had high TG and/or low HDL-C levels than patients in lower overall CVD risk categories. These trends were observed in both statin-treated and non-statin-treated patients. Given that the SCORE-HDL and

Table 1 Patient characteristics and treatment

	Overall (N = 7641)	High TG (n = 1591)	Low HDL-C (n = 1691)	High TG and low HDL-C (n = 759)
Age (year)	63.2 (9.0)	61.5 (8.4)	62.0 (8.8)	60.8 (8.5)
Sex				
Male (n, %)	3696 (48.4)	903 (56.8)	623 (36.8)	330 (43.5)
Female (n, %)	3945 (51.6)	688 (43.2)	1068 (63.2)	429 (56.5)
Race				
White/Caucasian (n, %)	6675 (95.6)	1408 (94.9)	1515 (94.3)	681 (94.7)
Middle East/North African (n, %)	74 (1.1)	15 (1.01)	23 (1.4)	9 (1.3)
South Asian (n, %)	63 (0.9)	16 (1.01)	21 (1.3)	6 (0.8)
Other Asian countries (n, %)	34 (0.5)	10 (0.7)	8 (0.5)	2 (0.3)
South American origin (n, %)	22 (0.3)	6 (0.4)	8 (0.5)	4 (0.6)
Sub-Saharan (n, %)	15 (0.2)	1 (0.1)	2 (0.1)	1 (0.1)
Caribbean (n, %)	14 (0.2)	2 (0.1)	2 (0.1)	1 (0.1)
Other (n, %)	82 (1.2)	26 (1.8)	28 (1.7)	15 (2.1)
Current smoker (n, %)	1608 (21.0)	393 (24.7)	397 (23.5)	201 (26.5)
BMI (kg/m^2)	28.9 (5.5)	30.6 (5.4)	30.9 (5.8)	31.3 (5.4)
≥ 30 kg/m^2 (n, %)	2788 (37.0)	783 (49.6)	858 (50.7)	410 (54.0)
T2DM[a] (n, %)	2046 (26.8)	562 (35.3)	617 (36.5)	305 (40.2)
Blood pressure				
Hypertension[b] (n, %)	5559 (72.8)	1193 (75.2)	1278 (75.6)	564 (74.3)
SBP (mmHg)	135.1 (16.6)	136.9 (16.7)	135.5 (17.1)	136.0 (17.0)
DBP (mmHg)	80.9 (9.9)	82.3 (10.1)	81.7 (10.0)	82.5 (9.9)
Serum lipid levels				
TC (mmol/l)	5.5 (1.1)	5.9 (1.2)	5.2 (1.2)	5.7 (1.2)
LDL-C (mmol/l)	3.2 (1.0)	3.3 (1.1)	3.1 (1.0)	3.2 (1.0)
Non-HDL-C (mmol/l)	4.0 (1.1)	4.7 (1.2)	4.2 (1.2)	4.7 (1.2)
TG (mmol/l)	1.8 (1.3)	3.4 (1.9)	2.6 (2.0)	3.8 (2.5)
HDL-C (mmol/l)	1.4 (0.4)	1.2 (0.3)	1.0 (0.2)	1.0 (0.2)
CRP (mg/l)	4.2 (8.7)	4.4 (6.3)	6.0 (12.2)	5.0 (7.5)
LLT				
At least one LLT (n, %)	3278 (42.9)	757 (47.6)	749 (44.3)	349 (46.0)
Statin alone (n, %)	2862 (37.5)	598 (37.6)	617 (36.5)	258 (34.0)
Statin + other LLT (n, %)	178 (2.3)	74 (4.7)	57 (3.4)	43 (5.7)
Other LLT alone (n, %)	238 (3.1)	85 (5.3)	75 (4.4)	48 (6.3)
Ezetimibe (n, %)	151 (2.0)	57 (3.6)	45 (2.7)	35 (4.6)
Fibrate (n, %)	220 (2.9)	84 (5.3)	68 (4.0)	45 (5.9)
Nicotinic acid (n, %)	6 (0.1)	3 (0.2)	4 (0.2)	3 (0.4)
Alcohol consumption[c]				
(units/week)	5.7 (11.3)	6.4 (12.2)	3.2 (6.4)	3.6 (6.8)
> 14 units/week (male; n, %)	529 (17.8)	129 (18.0)	47 (9.6)	27 (10.3)
> 7 units/week (female; n, %)	272 (8.9)	49 (9.4)	43 (5.5)	22 (6.9)

Table 1 Patient characteristics and treatment *(Continued)*

Physical exercise				
No exercise (*n*, %)	1489 (19.8)	368 (23.5)	406 (24.3)	191 (25.5)
Only light physical activity per week (*n*, %)	3782 (50.2)	807 (51.5)	910 (54.6)	403 (53.8)
Heavy physical activity 1–2 times per week (*n*, %)	1232 (16.4)	220 (14.1)	203 (12.2)	90 (12.0)
Heavy physical activity ≥3 times per week (*n*, %)	1026 (13.6)	171 (10.9)	149 (8.9)	65 (8.7)

Data are mean (standard deviation) unless otherwise indicated
High TG: ≥ 2.3 mmol/l. Low HDL-C: < 1.0 mmol/l in men and <1.3 mmol/l in women
[a]Considered present if the diagnosis was documented in the medical records
[b]SBP ≥ 140 mmHg, DBP ≥ 90 mmHg, or receiving antihypertensive medication
[c]Moderate alcohol consumption of 14 units/week (male) and 7 units/week (female) is outlined in the 2016 ESC/EAS guidelines for management of dyslipidemias [3]
Abbreviations: BMI body mass index, *CRP* C-reactive protein, *DBP* diastolic blood pressure, *HDL-C* high-density lipoprotein cholesterol, *LDL-C* low-density lipoprotein cholesterol, *LLT* lipid-lowering therapy, *SBP* systolic blood pressure, *T2DM* type 2 diabetes mellitus, *TC* total cholesterol, *TG* triglyceride

ACC/AHA risk calculators are valid only for assessing risk in routine clinical practice in patients up to 65 and 79 years of age, respectively, we went further in our analysis and stratified according to these age limits (Additional file 2: Figure S1 and Additional file 3: Figure S2). For the subgroups of patients up to the age of 65 years (SCORE-HDL) and 79 years (ACC/AHA), the proportions of patients with high TG and/or low HDL-C levels were similar to or slightly larger than the corresponding CVD risk groups for the whole population.

Factors associated with high TG and/or low HDL-C levels

Factors significantly associated with high TG levels, low HDL-C levels, or both were assessed using multivariate analysis ($p < 0.0001$; Fig. 4). Female sex was positively associated with low HDL-C status but negatively associated with high TG levels. Other cardiovascular risk factors, including T2DM, obesity, smoking, and hypertension (indicated by the use of β-blockers) were positively associated

with markers of atherogenic dyslipidemia. The association of markers of atherogenic dyslipidemia with CRP levels was found to be significant only after adjusting for confounding factors among patients with low HDL-C levels. Some variation in patients' likelihood of having markers of atherogenic dyslipidemia was seen between countries of origin, when assessed relative to the UK.

Association between high TG and/or low HDL-C levels and CRP

In the overall population, mean CRP was 4.2 mg/l, and this was increased in patients with high TG levels (4.4 mg/l), low HDL-C levels (6.0 mg/l), and both (5.0 mg/l) (Table 1). Patients in the overall population with high TG levels and/or low HDL-C levels were categorized by plasma CRP concentrations into two subpopulations: CRP lower than 1 mg/l, 1–< 3 mg/l, or at least 3 mg/l; and CRP lower than 2 mg/l or at least 2 mg/l. Greater proportions of patients had CRP levels of either

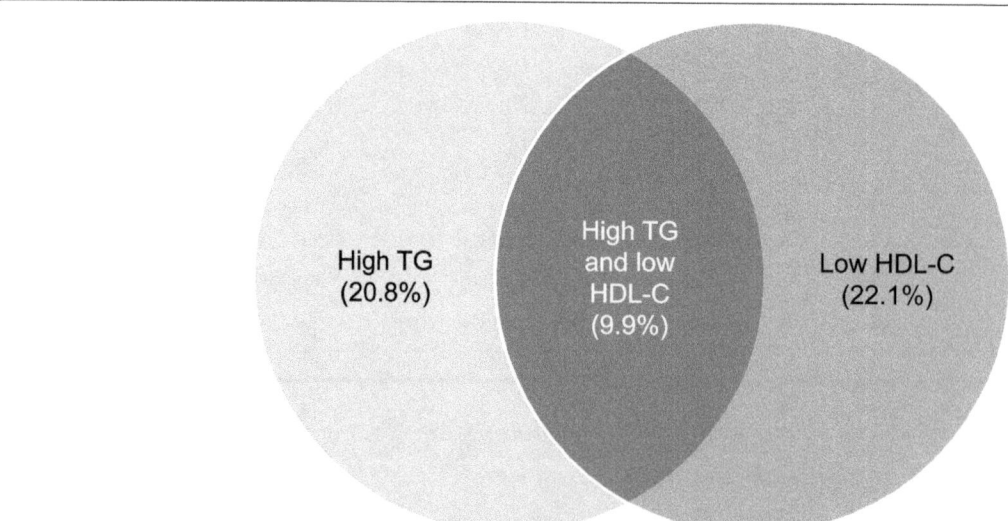

Fig. 1 Prevalence of high TG and/or low HDL-C levels in the EURIKA population. Percentages indicated are of the total EURIKA population (*N* = 7641). High TG: ≥ 2.3 mmol/l. Low HDL-C: < 1.0 mmol/l in men and < 1.3 mmol/l in women *Abbreviations: EURIKA* European Study on Cardiovascular Risk Prevention and Management in Usual Daily Practice, *HDL-C* high-density lipoprotein cholesterol, *TG* triglyceride

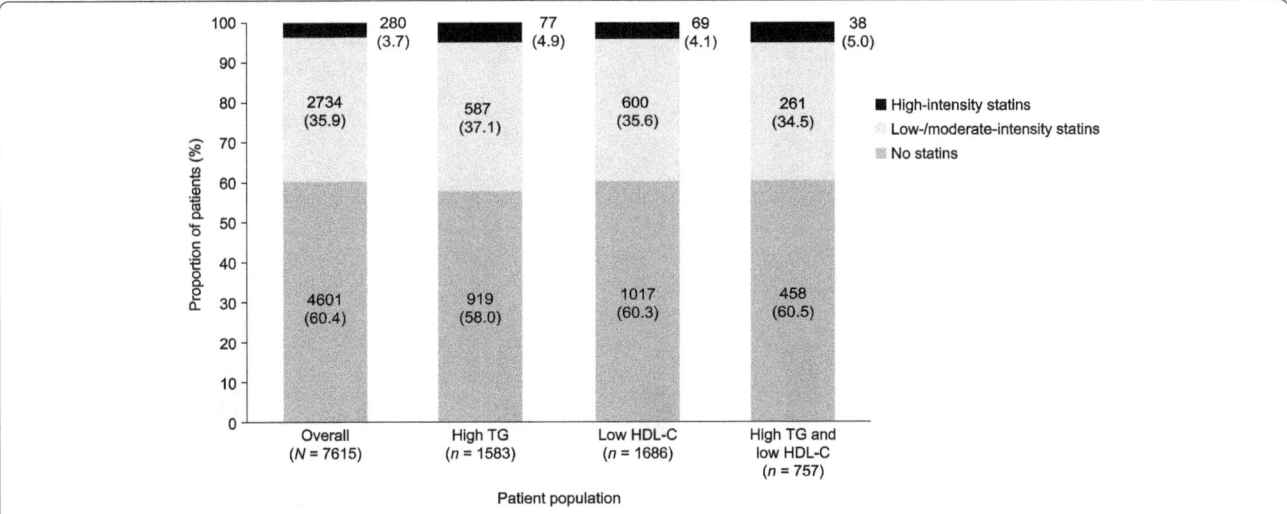

Fig. 2 Proportion of patients treated with or without statins according to markers of atherogenic dyslipidemia. Data were missing for 26 patients in the overall population, 8 patients in the high TG group, 5 patients in the low HDL-C group, and 2 patients in the high TG and low HDL-C group. Data within bars are *n* (%). High TG: ≥ 2.3 mmol/l. Low HDL-C: < 1.0 mmol/l in men and < 1.3 mmol/l in women. *Abbreviations: HDL-C* high-density lipoprotein cholesterol, *TG* triglyceride

at least 2 mg/l or at least 3 mg/l among those with high TG levels and/or low HDL-C levels than in the overall population, with between approximately 60 and 70% of patients with markers of atherogenic dyslipidemia having CRP levels of at least 2 mg/l, and between 45 and 50% having CRP levels of at least 3 mg/l (Fig. 5).

Discussion

We have analyzed the number of patients with high levels of TG and/or low levels of HDL-C, two markers of atherogenic dyslipidemia, in the large clinical EUR-IKA population. We have shown that 20.8% of patients had high TG levels, 22.1% had low HDL-C levels, and 9.9% had both high TG and low HDL-C levels. Very few patients in our cohort had very high TG levels or very low HDL-C levels; it is likely that other comorbidities or underlying genetic factors may affect these individuals. Our analysis also reveals that the proportion of patients with T2DM (who are already considered to be at high risk of CVD) with high TG and/or low HDL-C levels is higher than that of patients without T2DM. In addition, when categorizing patients without T2DM according to the ACC/AHA or SCORE-HDL risk calculators, larger proportions of patients with high TG and/or low HDL-C levels are in the higher risk categories than in the lower risk categories. Cross-country variation in the proportions of patients with high TG and/or low HDL-C levels was observed and could be a consequence of genetic, cultural or socio-economic factors that have been discussed elsewhere [11]. We are unable to provide definitive explanations in the analysis presented here. Our multivariate analysis revealed that female sex was positively associated with low HDL-C status, which may

reflect the specific selection criteria for the EURIKA population as females have higher HDL-C levels than males in the general population. Thus, our data suggest that European women with at least one cardiovascular risk factor but no history of cardiovascular disease are actually more likely than men to have a low HDL-C status.

The EURIKA study has provided important insights into the effectiveness of current practices related to primary CVD prevention in Europe [9, 11, 19]. The primary analysis of the EURIKA data demonstrated that a substantial proportion of patients had CVD risk factors that remained uncontrolled, despite receiving treatment [11]. A follow-up analysis of CRP levels in the EURIKA population revealed that among patients without T2DM who were not receiving statin treatment, more than one-third had CRP levels of at least 3 mg/l, while almost half had CRP levels of at least 2 mg/l [9]. Here, our analysis of CRP levels demonstrates that a greater proportion of patients with high TG and/or low HDL-C levels also have low-grade inflammation, evident by elevated CRP levels, than in the overall at-risk population. These patients are likely to be at an even higher risk of CVD than those with either atherogenic dyslipidemia or elevated CRP levels alone.

We have previously reported on the proportions of patients in EURIKA who were not receiving any form of LLT and who had uncontrolled LDL-C levels [19]. Elevated LDL-C levels are among the primary causal risk factors for cardiovascular disease, and are a component of the atherogenic dyslipidemia profile [2]. Over one-third of patients defined as being at high risk of CVD in our previous analysis were not receiving any form of

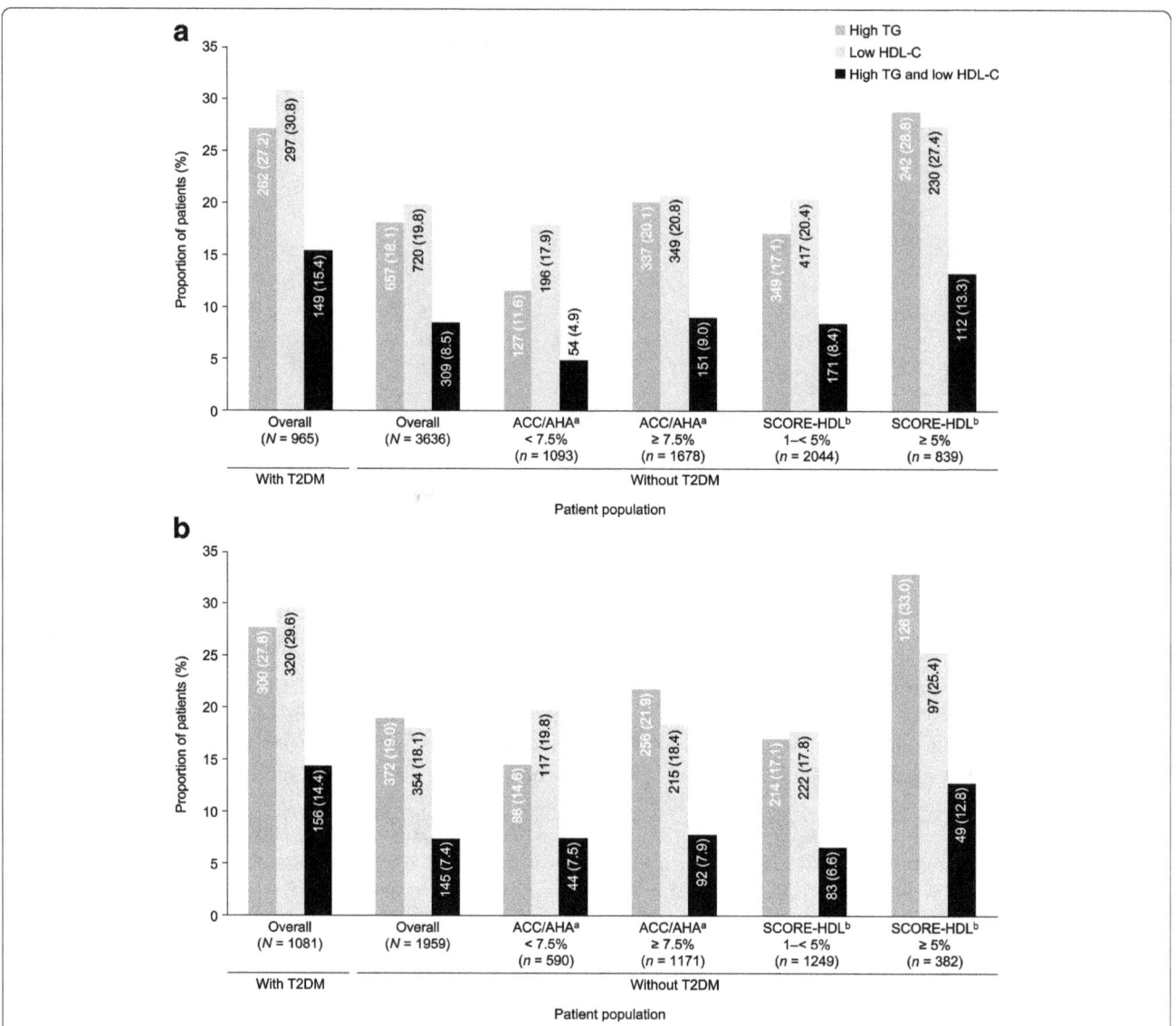

Fig. 3 Proportion of patients with markers of atherogenic dyslipidemia, according to T2DM status and CVD risk. (**a**) Non-statin - treated patients; (**b**) statin-treated patients. Data within bars are n (%). High TG: ≥ 2.3 mmol/l. Low HDL-C: < 1.0 mmol/l in men and < 1.3 mmol/l in women. [a]ACC/AHA risk calculator [14]. [b]SCORE-HDL risk calculator [6, 18]. *Abbreviations: ACC* American College of Cardiology, *AHA* American Heart Association, *CVD* cardiovascular disease, *HDL-C* high-density lipoprotein cholesterol, *SCORE-HDL* Systematic Coronary Risk Evaluation-high-density lipoprotein, *T2DM* type 2 diabetes mellitus, *TG* triglyceride

LLT [19]. Moreover, LDL-C levels were controlled in only 40% of these patients at high risk of CVD who were receiving LLT [19]. Findings from the Centralized Pan-Regional Surveys on the Undertreatment of Hypercholesterolemia (CEPHEUS) were similar; only 49.4% of patients achieved their recommended LDL-C levels [20]. A literature review from 2004 also reported a widespread failure in the attainment of recommended lipid levels in patients treated with LLT [21]. Similarly, in the current analysis, we observed that approximately 55% of patients with high TG levels, low HDL-C levels, or both were not taking any form of LLT. Furthermore, of those patients treated with statins, the majority were using low-

intensity statins. These observations build on our previous arguments that there is a clear opportunity to improve rates of treatment for primary CVD prevention, and for patients with dyslipidemia in particular.

Whether or not TG levels are a causal risk factor for CVD is debated [22, 23]; patients with high TG levels often have additional CVD risk factors; TG levels in human plasma are highly variable and are strongly associated with low HDL-C levels, which makes it difficult to separate the contributions of these two components [22–25]. Nevertheless, several population studies and meta-analyses have shown a significant link between TG levels and CVD risk, independent of other CVD risk

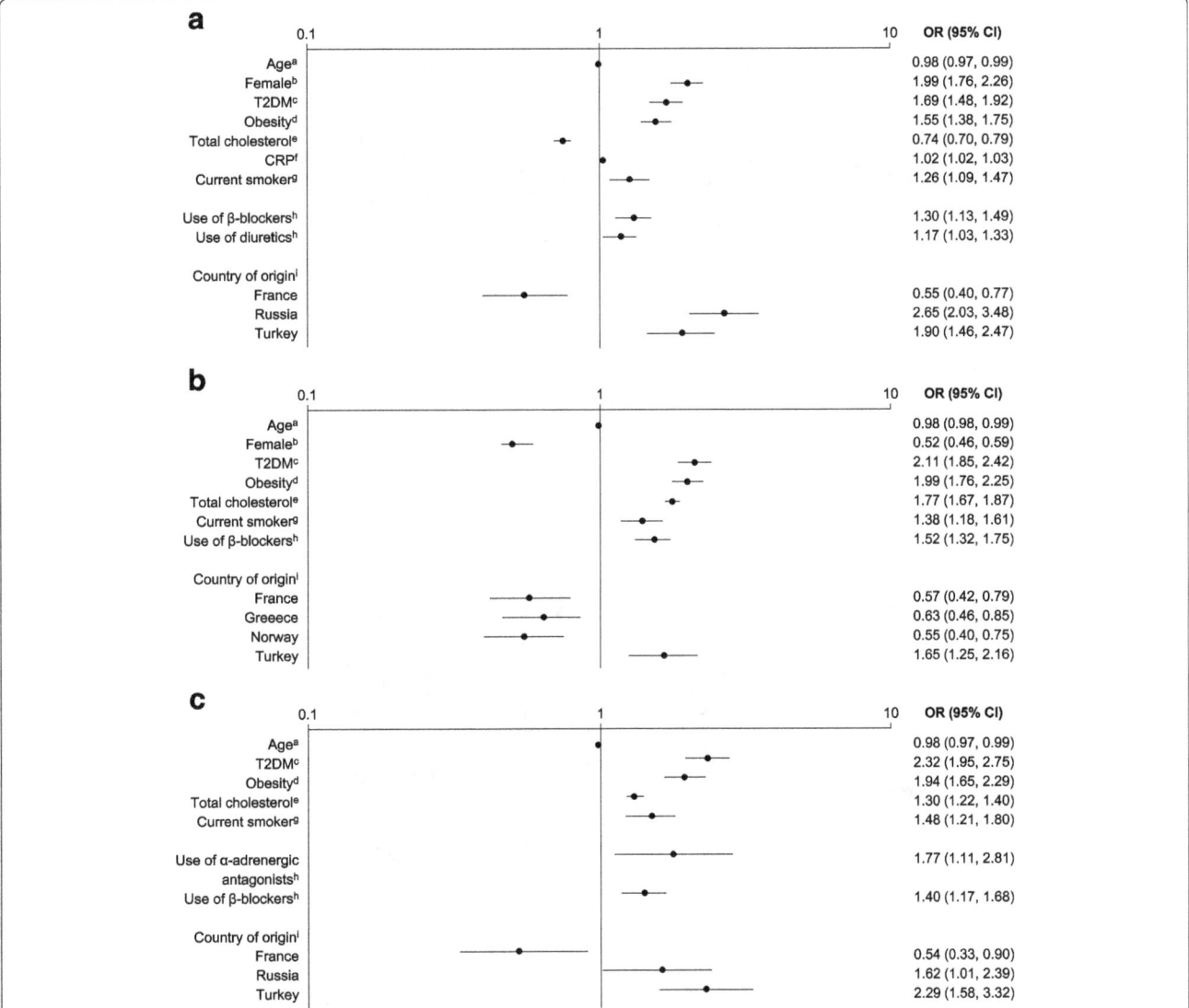

Fig. 4 Multivariate analysis of factors associated with markers of atherogenic dyslipidemia. (**a**) Low HDL-C levels; (**b**) high TG levels; (**c**) low HDL-C and high TG levels. $p < 0.0001$ for all factors. Countries of origin with an OR that was not significant have been omitted. [a]Per year. [b]Relative to male participants. [c]Relative to not having T2DM. [d]BMI $\geq$ 30 kg/m^2, relative to not being obese. [e]Per mmol/l. [f]Per mg/l. [g]Relative to never smoking. [h]Relative to non-use. [i]Relative to the UK. *Abbreviations: BMI* body mass index, *CI* confidence interval, *CRP* C-reactive protein, *HDL-C* high-density lipoprotein cholesterol, *OR* odds ratio, *T2DM* type 2 diabetes mellitus, *TG* triglyceride

factors, including HDL-C levels [26–28]. A topic of debate has been whether measuring non-fasting TG levels is a better predictor of CVD than measuring fasting TG levels, with some studies showing a stronger association between non-fasting TG levels and CVD risk than fasting TG levels [24, 29]. European guidelines have previously recommended the measurement of fasting TG levels, as was done in EURIKA, owing to a lack of standardization of non-fasting TG measurements [30]. Guidelines recommend lifestyle interventions in patients with moderately elevated TG levels (e.g. reduction in alcohol consumption, dietary modifications, or increased aerobic exercise) [23]. A reduction in alcohol consumption is of particular importance, as patients with elevated TG levels are likely to experience further increases from consuming even small quantities of alcohol [3]. Our analysis reveals that within the EURIKA population, small proportions of patients with elevated TG levels are consuming more units of alcohol than the recommended weekly limit. Furthermore, almost 20% of the overall population reported undertaking no physical exercise. In patients with TG levels above 500 mg/dl, pharmacological intervention in the form of fibrates, niacins, or omega-3 fish oils should be considered [23].

The EURIKA study has the strength of allowing analysis of data from a large sample of patients from

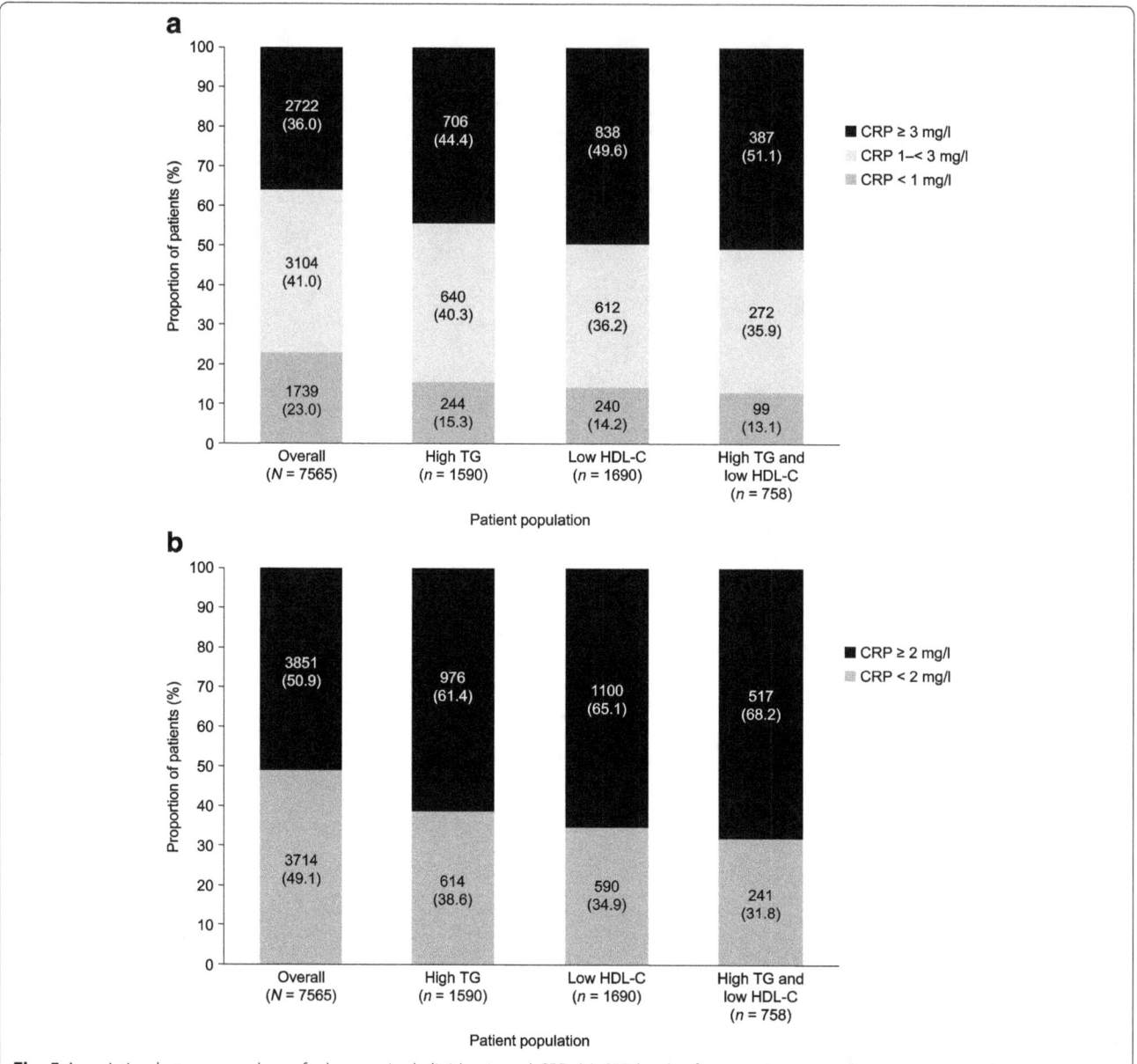

Fig. 5 Association between markers of atherogenic dyslipidemia and CRP. (**a**) CRP levels of < 1 mg/L, 1–< 3 mg/L or ≥ 3 mg/L; (**b**) CRP levels < 2 mg/L or ≥ 2 mg/L. Data were missing for 76 patients in the overall population, and for 1 patient in each of the dyslipidemia groups. Data within bars are *n* (%). High TG: ≥ 2.3 mmol/l. Low HDL-C: < 1.0 mmol/l in men and < 1.3 mmol/l in women. *Abbreviations: CRP* C-reactive protein, *HDL-C* high-density lipoprotein cholesterol, *TG* triglyceride

multiple European countries according to standardized procedures. Almost all blood samples were analyzed at the same location, with the exception of patients from Russia. A limitation of the study, however, is that it is cross-sectional, and therefore does not allow conclusions to be drawn regarding the longitudinal association of individual factors with CVD risk. The EURIKA study recruited individuals over 50 years of age with at least one major CVD risk factor, including dyslipidemia. Therefore, the proportion of patients identified with low HDL-C and high TG levels is likely to be greater than in

people of the same age in the general population. Previous cohort studies investigating the predictive power of HDL-C levels in CVD risk have measured HDL-C using precipitation methods. In EURIKA, HDL-C levels were measured using an enzymatic method; it has been demonstrated that enzymatic methods result in higher recorded HDL-C levels than precipitation methods [31]. Therefore, it is possible that we have underestimated the proportion of the cohort with low HDL-C levels. The participation rate among invited physicians was also low; however, potential patient selection bias is likely to have been reduced by the high participation rate among invited patients, and the randomized method of patient selection. Finally, we did not calculate the ratio of TG to HDL-C concentrations in the EURIKA study; however, this marker has been proposed to correlate with insulin resistance and thus could be used to identify patients at risk of CVD [32].

Conclusions

A considerable proportion of primary prevention patients at risk of CVD in routine clinical practice have high levels of TG and low levels of HDL-C. Many of these patients also have evidence of elevated CRP levels, reflecting low-grade inflammation. Therefore, these patients' absolute CVD risk may be underestimated by current European and US global risk calculators. These patients may benefit from more intensive or better-tailored treatment options to address their overall CVD risk, in accordance with evidence-based guidelines.

Additional files

Additional file 1: Table S1. Prevalence of high TG and/or low HDL-C levels in the EURIKA population by country. Data are (n, %). High TG: ≥ 2.3 mmol/l. Low HDL-C: < 1.0 mmol/l in men and <1.3 mmol/l in women. Abbreviations: HDL-C high-density lipoprotein cholesterol, TG triglyceride (DOCX 15 kb)

Additional file 2: Figure S1. Proportion of non-statin-treated patients with markers of atherogenic dyslipidemia, according to T2DM status, CVD risk, and age: (a) according to SCORE-HDL categories; (b) according to ACC/AHA categories. Data within bars are n (%). High TG: ≥ 2.3 mmol/l. Low HDL-C: < 1.0 mmol/l in men and <1.3 mmol/l in women. Abbreviations: ACC American College of Cardiology, AHA American Heart Association, CVD cardiovascular disease, HDL-C high-density lipoprotein cholesterol, SCORE-HDL Systematic Coronary Risk Evaluation-high-density lipoprotein, T2DM type 2 diabetes mellitus, TG triglycerides (PDF 1099 kb)

Additional file 3: Figure S2. Proportion of statin-treated patients with markers of atherogenic dyslipidemia, according to T2DM status, CVD risk and age: (a) according to SCORE-HDL categories; (b) according to ACC/AHA categories. Data within bars are n (%). High TG: ≥ 2.3 mmol/l. Low HDL-C: < 1.0 mmol/l in men and <1.3 mmol/l in women. Abbreviations: ACC American College of Cardiology, AHA American Heart Association, CVD cardiovascular disease, HDL-C high-density lipoprotein cholesterol, SCORE-HDL Systematic Coronary Risk Evaluation-high-density lipoprotein, T2DM type 2 diabetes mellitus, TG triglycerides (PDF 1090 kb)

Abbreviations
ACC: American College of Cardiology; AHA: American Heart Association; BMI: Body mass index; CEPHEUS: Centralized Pan-Regional Surveys on the Undertreatment of Hypercholesterolemia; CI: Confidence interval; CRP: C-reactive protein; CVD: Cardiovascular disease; DBP: Diastolic blood pressure; EURIKA: European Study on Cardiovascular Risk Prevention and Management in Usual Daily Practice; HDL-C: High-density lipoprotein cholesterol; LDL-C: Low-density lipoprotein cholesterol; LLT: Lipid-lowering therapy; OR: Odds ratio; PCP: Primary care physician; SBP: Systolic blood pressure; SCORE: Systematic Coronary Risk Evaluation; SCORE-HDL: Systematic Coronary Risk Evaluation-high-density lipoprotein; T2DM: Type 2 diabetes mellitus; TC: Total cholesterol; TG: Triglyceride

Acknowledgments
Writing support was provided by Gary Male, PhD from Oxford PharmaGenesis, Oxford, UK and was funded by AstraZeneca.

Funding
The EURIKA study was funded by AstraZeneca. The study was run by an independent academic steering committee, which worked under rules agreed a priori that allowed intellectual input of the funder (i.e. the funder contributed ideas to the study design, data analysis, and preparation of the manuscript) while granting the executive and decision making role to the committee. The authors had full access to all data and had final responsibility for the contents of the manuscript and the decision to submit it for publication.

Authors' contributions
Conceived and designed the experiments: JPH, JB, CR, JD, GDB, EG, JP, DH, KMH, CB. Performed the experiments: JPH, JB, CR, JD, GDB, EG, JP, DH, KMH, CB. Analyzed the data: JPH, CR, DH. Wrote the paper: JPH, JB, CR, JD, GDB, EG, JP, DH, KMH, CB. All authors read and approved the final manuscript.

Competing interests
Julian P. Halcox has received speaker and consulting fees from Abbot Products and AstraZeneca; Claudio Borghi has received speaker and consulting fees from Amgen, Menarini, Novartis, Roche, Sanofi, Servier, and Takeda; Carine Roy has received research funding from AstraZeneca; Jean Dallongeville has received fees from AstraZeneca, Bayer, and Merck Sharp & Dohme. Karin M. Henriksson was an employee of AstraZeneca when this manuscript was initiated but has since retired from this position. The other authors declare that they have no competing interests.

Ethics approval and consent to participate
The study protocol was approved by the appropriate clinical research ethics committees in each participating country, and all patients provided signed informed consent. The study protocol has been approved by the appropriate clinical research ethics committees in each participating country, and complies with the local regulations for clinical research. Specifically, the protocol was approved by the following ethics committees: Ethics Committee of Hospital Barmherzige Brüder, Vienna, Austria; Ethics Committee University Hospital, Ghent, Belgium; National Commission on Informatics and Liberties, Paris, France; Ethics Committee of the Friedrich-Alexander-University Erlangen-Nuremberg, Germany; Scientific Council of University General Hospital of Ioannina, and the National Organization for Medicines (EOF), Greece; Regional Committee for Ethics in Medicine and Research Sor-øst B (REK Sor-øst B), Oslo, Norway; Independent Interdisciplinary Ethics Committee, Moscow, Russia; Clinical Research Ethics Committee of La Paz University Hospital, Madrid, Spain; Ethics Committee of the University Hospital of Linköping, Sweden; Ethics Committee for Ambulatory Clinical Research, Medical Association of Geneva, Switzerland; Research Ethics Committee of Medical Faculty, Gazi University, Ankara, Turkey; Brent Primary Care Trust Applied Research Unit, National Health Service, London, UK.

Author details
[1]Institute of Life Sciences 2, Swansea University College of Medicine, Singleton Park, Swansea SA2 8PP, UK. [2]Department of Preventive Medicine and Public Health, School of Medicine, Universidad Autónoma de Madrid/IdiPaz and CIBER of Epidemiology and Public Health (CIBERESP), Madrid, Spain. [3]INSERM CIC-EC 1425 and Département d'Épidémiologie et Recherche Clinique, Assistance Publique–Hôpitaux de Paris, Hôpital Bichat, Paris, France. [4]INSERM U 744, Institut Pasteur de Lille, Université Lille-Nord de France, Lille, France. [5]Department of Public Health, University of Ghent, Ghent, Belgium. [6]Departments of Epidemiology and Medicine and Welch Center of Prevention, Epidemiology and Clinical Research, Johns Hopkins Bloomberg School of Public Health, Baltimore, MD, USA. [7]School of Health and Caring Sciences, Linnaeus University, Kalmar, Sweden. [8]Department of Medical Sciences, Uppsala University, Uppsala, Sweden. [9]Department of Internal Medicine, Ageing and Clinical Nephrology, University of Bologna, Bologna, Italy.

References

1. European cardiovascular disease statistics http://www.ehnheart.org/cvd-statistics.html Accessed 18 Oct 2016.

2. Piepoli MF, Hoes AW, Agewall S, Albus C, Brotons C, Catapano AL, et al. European guidelines on cardiovascular disease prevention in clinical practice: the sixth joint Task Force of the European Society of Cardiology and Other Societies on cardiovascular disease prevention in clinical practice (constituted by representatives of 10 societies and by invited experts): developed with the special contribution of the European Association for Cardiovascular Prevention & rehabilitation (EACPR). Eur Heart J. 2016;37(29): 2315–81.

3. Catapano AL, Graham I, De Backer G, Wiklund O, Chapman MJ, Drexel H, et al. ESC/EAS guidelines for the Management of Dyslipidaemias: the Task Force for the Management of Dyslipidaemias of the European Society of Cardiology (ESC) and European Atherosclerosis Society (EAS) developed with the special contribution of the European Association for Cardiovascular Prevention & Rehabilitation (EACPR). Atherosclerosis. 2016;253:281–344.

4. Nordestgaard BG, Varbo A. Triglycerides and cardiovascular disease. Lancet. 2014;384(9943):626–35.

5. Chapman MJ, Ginsberg HN, Amarenco P, Andreotti F, Boren J, Catapano AL, et al. Triglyceride-rich lipoproteins and high-density lipoprotein cholesterol in patients at high risk of cardiovascular disease: evidence and guidance for management. Eur Heart J. 2011;32(11):1345–61.

6. Cooney MT, Dudina A, De Bacquer D, Fitzgerald A, Conroy R, Sans S, et al. How much does HDL cholesterol add to risk estimation? A report from the SCORE investigators. Eur J Cardiovasc Prev Rehabil. 2009;16(3):304–14.

7. Cooney MT, Dudina A, De Bacquer D, Wilhelmsen L, Sans S, Menotti A, et al. HDL cholesterol protects against cardiovascular disease in both genders, at all ages and at all levels of risk. Atherosclerosis. 2009;206(2):611–6.

8. Danesh J, Wheeler JG, Hirschfield GM, Eda S, Eiriksdottir G, Rumley A, et al. C-reactive protein and other circulating markers of inflammation in the prediction of coronary heart disease. N Engl J Med. 2004;350(14):1387–97.

9. Halcox JP, Roy C, Tubach F, Banegas JR, Dallongeville J, De Backer G, et al. C-reactive protein levels in patients at cardiovascular risk: EURIKA study. BMC Cardiovasc Disord. 2014;14:25.

10. Grundy SM. Small LDL, atherogenic dyslipidemia, and the metabolic syndrome. Circulation. 1997;95(1):1–4.

11. Banegas JR, Lopez-Garcia E, Dallongeville J, Guallar E, Halcox JP, Borghi C, et al. Achievement of treatment goals for primary prevention of cardiovascular disease in clinical practice across Europe: the EURIKA study. Eur Heart J. 2011;32(17):2143–52.

12. Rodriguez-Artalejo F, Guallar E, Borghi C, Dallongeville J, De Backer G, Halcox JP, et al. Rationale and methods of the European study on cardiovascular risk prevention and Management in Daily Practice (EURIKA). BMC Public Health. 2010;10:382.

13. Conroy RM, Pyorala K, Fitzgerald AP, Sans S, Menotti A, De Backer G, et al. Estimation of ten-year risk of fatal cardiovascular disease in Europe: the SCORE project. Eur Heart J. 2003;24(11):987–1003.

14. Goff DC, Jr., Lloyd-Jones DM, Bennett G, Coady S, D'Agostino RB, Sr., Gibbons R, et al. 2013 ACC/AHA guideline on the assessment of cardiovascular risk: a report of the American College of Cardiology/ American Heart Association Task Force on practice guidelines. Circulation. 2014;129(25 Suppl. 2):S49–73.

15. Dallongeville J, Banegas JR, Tubach F, Guallar E, Borghi C, De Backer G, et al. Survey of physicians' practices in the control of cardiovascular risk factors: the EURIKA study. Eur J Cardiovasc Prev Rehabil. 2011;19(3):541–50.

16. OneKey [http://www.i-marches.com/index.php?id=onekey].

17. Friedewald WT, Levy RI, Fredrickson DS. Estimation of the concentration of low-density lipoprotein cholesterol in plasma, without use of the preparative ultracentrifuge. Clin Chem. 1972;18(6):499–502.

18. HeartScore – a unique and interactive risk prediction and management system http://www.escardio.org/Education/Practice-Tools/CVD-prevention-toolbox/HeartScore. Accessed 18 Oct 2016.

19. Halcox JP, Tubach F, Lopez-Garcia E, De Backer G, Borghi C, Dallongeville J, et al. Low rates of both lipid-lowering therapy use and achievement of low-density lipoprotein cholesterol targets in individuals at high-risk for cardiovascular disease across Europe. PLoS One. 2015;10(2):e0115270.

20. Chiang CE, Ferrieres J, Gotcheva NN, Raal FJ, Shehab A, Sung J, et al. Suboptimal control of lipid levels: results from 29 countries participating in the Centralized pan-Regional Surveys on the Undertreatment of Hypercholesterolemia (CEPHEUS). J Atheroscler Thromb. 2016;23(5):567–87.

21. Schwandt P, Brady AJ. Achieving lipid goals in Europe: how large is the treatment gap? Expert Rev Cardiovasc Ther. 2004;2(3):431–49.

22. Harchaoui KE, Visser ME, Kastelein JJ, Stroes ES, Dallinga-Thie GM. Triglycerides and cardiovascular risk. Curr Cardiol Rev. 2009;5(3):216–22.

23. Miller M, Stone NJ, Ballantyne C, Bittner V, Criqui MH, Ginsberg HN, et al. Triglycerides and cardiovascular disease: a scientific statement from the American Heart Association. Circulation. 2011;123(20):2292–333.

24. Mora S, Rifai N, Buring JE, Ridker PM. Fasting compared with nonfasting lipids and apolipoproteins for predicting incident cardiovascular events. Circulation. 2008;118(10):993–1001.

25. Ginsberg HN, Bonds DE, Lovato LC, Crouse JR, Elam MB, Linz PE, et al. Evolution of the lipid trial protocol of the action to control cardiovascular risk in diabetes (ACCORD) trial. Am J Cardiol. 2007;99(12A):56i–67i.

26. Assmann G, Schulte H, Funke H, von Eckardstein A. The emergence of triglycerides as a significant independent risk factor in coronary artery disease. Eur Heart J. 1998;(19 Supp. Mat):M8–14.

27. Jeppesen J, Hein HO, Suadicani P, Gyntelberg F. Triglyceride concentration and ischemic heart disease: an eight-year follow-up in the Copenhagen male study. Circulation. 1998;97(11):1029–36.

28. Sarwar N, Danesh J, Eiriksdottir G, Sigurdsson G, Wareham N, Bingham S, et al. Triglycerides and the risk of coronary heart disease: 10,158 incident cases among 262,525 participants in 29 western prospective studies. Circulation. 2007;115(4):450–8.

29. Nordestgaard BG, Benn M, Schnohr P, Tybjaerg-Hansen A. Nonfasting triglycerides and risk of myocardial infarction, ischemic heart disease, and death in men and women. JAMA. 2007;298(3):299–308.

30. Perk J, De Backer G, Gohlke H, Graham I, Reiner Z, Verschuren M, et al. European guidelines on cardiovascular disease prevention in clinical practice (version 2012): the fifth joint Task Force of the European Society of Cardiology and Other Societies on cardiovascular disease prevention in clinical practice (constituted by representatives of nine societies and by invited experts). Eur Heart J. 2012;33:1635–701.

31. Langlois MR, Delanghe JR, De Buyzere M, Rietzschel E, De Bacquer D. Unanswered questions in including HDL-cholesterol in the cardiovascular risk estimation. Is time still on our side? Atherosclerosis. 2013;226(1):296–8.

32. McLaughlin T, Abbasi F, Cheal K, Chu J, Lamendola C, Reaven G. Use of metabolic markers to identify overweight individuals who are insulin resistant. Ann Intern Med. 2003;139(10):802–9.

12

Associations between risk factors in childhood (12–13 years) and adulthood (48–49 years) and subclinical atherosclerosis

Indre Ceponiene[1*], Jurate Klumbiene[2], Egle Tamuleviciute-Prasciene[1], Justina Motiejunaite[1], Edita Sakyte[2], Jonas Ceponis[3], Rimvydas Slapikas[1] and Janina Petkeviciene[2]

Abstract

Background: The data on the childhood determinants of adult cardiovascular disease (CVD) are lacking in populations of Eastern Europe that are characterised by substantially high CVD mortality. From a public health perspective, it is important to identify high-risk individuals as early as possible in order to have the greatest benefit of preventive interventions. The aim of this study was to evaluate the associations of childhood and adulthood traditional risk factors with subclinical atherosclerosis and arterial stiffness in a Lithuanian cohort followed up for 35 years.

Methods: The study cohort consisted of 380 adults aged 48–49 from Kaunas Cardiovascular Risk Cohort study, who were followed up since childhood (12–13 years). The baseline survey (1977) included blood pressure (BP) and anthropometric measurements and sexual maturity scale. In the follow-up survey (2012), BP, anthropometric and lipids measurements, interview about smoking, measurement of carotid intima-media thickness (IMT) and determination of pulse wave velocity (PWV) were performed. Two types of general linear models were applied to test the associations of childhood and adulthood risk factors with IMT and PWV. Model 1 included only childhood variables. In model 2, adulthood variables were added to childhood variables.

Results: In linear regression model with childhood variables childhood systolic BP ($\beta = 0.014$; $p = 0.016$) and BMI ($\beta = 0.006$; $p = 0.003$) were directly associated with IMT only in women. When adulthood variables were included into regression model, the association between childhood systolic BP and IMT remained significant ($\beta = 0.013$; $p = 0.021$), while childhood BMI was not associated with IMT ($\beta = 0.003$; $p = 0.143$). Additionally, association of adult smoking and IMT was found in women ($\beta = 0.033$; $p = 0.018$). IMT of men was directly related to adult systolic BP ($\beta = 0.022$; $p = 0.018$) and inversely to HDL cholesterol level ($\beta = -0.044$; $p = 0.021$). PWV was directly associated only with adult systolic BP in both genders ($\beta = 0.729$ for men and $\beta = 0.476$ for women; $p = 0.001$).

Conclusions: Sex differences in the associations between childhood and adulthood risk factors and subclinical atherosclerosis were found. The results of the study support efforts to reduce conventional risk factors both in childhood and adulthood for the primary prevention of atherosclerosis.

* Correspondence: indreva@gmail.com
[1]Department of Cardiology, Medical Academy, Lithuanian University of Health Sciences, Eiveniu 2, Kaunas LT-50009, Lithuania
Full list of author information is available at the end of the article

Background

Atherosclerotic diseases such as coronary heart disease, stroke and peripheral artery disease are great threats to public health in Lithuania which has one of the highest cardiovascular mortality in Europe [1]. The process of atherosclerosis begins early in childhood and typically remains asymptomatic until later in life. The cardiovascular risk factors induce changes in the arterial wall that lead to stiffening and atherosclerotic plaque formation. Carotid intima-media thickness (IMT) demonstrates structural changes in the arterial wall even in early subclinical stages of atherosclerosis. IMT is directly related to increased cardiovascular risk and can predict cardiovascular events, such as myocardial infarction or stroke in asymptomatic adults [2]. Prospective cohort studies have demonstrated that blood pressure, lipid levels, body mass index (BMI) and some health behaviours, identified in childhood, predict increased IMT in adulthood [3–6]. Childhood risk factors measured at or after the age of 9 showed the strongest associations with subclinical atherosclerosis in adulthood [7].

Arterial stiffness expressed as pulse wave velocity (PWV) is a strong predictor of future cardiovascular events [8–10]. PWV is associated with subclinical target organ damage in the coronary, peripheral arterial, cerebral, and renal arterial beds [11]. Previous observations concerning the relationship between risk factors in childhood and arterial stiffness have been controversial. In the Bogalusa Heart Study and in the Cardiovascular Risk in Young Finns Study, systolic BP in childhood was directly associated with PWV in adulthood, whereas in the Atherosclerosis Risk in Young Adults (ARYA) Study no association between childhood BP and adult PWV was found [12–14]. Controversy in the results from these studies might be due to differences in methodology of PWV measurement and different age of the participants during the last follow-up (27–30 years in the ARYA study, compared to 30–45 years in the Young Fins study and 24 to 44 years in the Bogalusa study).

Population-based data from prospective cohort studies linking childhood risk factors with adulthood risk factors and preclinical markers of cardiovascular health are of particular importance because they help to identify individuals at high CVD risk. Such data are lacking in populations of Eastern Europe that are characterised by considerably high CVD risk profile and mortality rates and one of the highest male–female differences in cardiovascular health in Europe [15]. From a public health perspective, high priority should be given for early prevention of CVD in those countries including Lithuania. Preventive interventions are more likely to be successful when aimed at individuals who have an increased risk of developing CVD.

The aim of this study was to determine the associations of childhood and adulthood traditional risk factors with subclinical atherosclerosis and arterial stiffness in a Lithuanian cohort followed up for 35 years.

Methods

Study design and sample

This study used data from the Kaunas Cardiovascular Risk Cohort study, a prospective study with the baseline data collected in 1977 on a random sample of 1082 Kaunas schoolchildren aged 12–13 years [16, 17]. Over the period of follow-up, 8.4 % (n = 91) individuals died, 9.5 % (n = 103) emigrated from Lithuania, 0.4 % (n = 4) were severely ill and the addresses of 8.3 % (n = 90) subjects were not available in the National Population Register. In 2012, 507 participants (63.9 % of eligible sample) aged 48–49 were surveyed; however, only individuals who had both vascular ultrasound and pulse wave measurements performed were included in the analysis (n = 380).

The study protocol was approved by the Lithuanian Bioethics Committee (permission No. BE-2-30). Written consent on behalf of the children enrolled in the first survey (1977) was obtained from parents or guardians. Written informed consent for the participation in the follow-up survey (2012) was obtained from all participants.

Measurements in childhood

BP measurements were performed with a standard mercury sphygmomanometer in the sitting position after 5 minutes of rest. BP was measured to the nearest 2 mmHg on the right arm. The first Korotkoff phase was used to determine systolic BP, and the fifth phase was used to determine diastolic BP. Three consecutive BP measurements were taken. The average of these three measurements was used in the analysis.

The height of participants, without shoes, was measured to the nearest centimetre with a stadiometer. The body weight of participants, wearing light indoor clothing and no shoes, was measured to the nearest 0.1 kg with standardised medical scales. BMI was calculated as weight divided by height squared (kg/m²).

A modified Tanner scale (excluding examination of the testes) was used for evaluation of sexual maturity. The development of axillary hair and pubic hair for girls and boys, growth of moustache for boys, and the development of breast and menstruation for girls were assessed for calculation of sexual maturity score [16]. The sexual maturity scores could vary from 0 to 12 in boys and from 0 to 15 in girls (the higher numbers mean higher sexual maturity).

Measurements in adulthood

BP, height and weight were measured using the same methodology as in childhood. Blood samples for lipids measurements in adulthood were taken in the morning after fasting at least 12 hours. All measurements were performed in a certified laboratory on an automatic analyser

Cobas Integra 400 plus. Serum lipid levels were determined using conventional enzymatic methods.

Information on cigarette smoking was collected by a standard questionnaire. Participants were divided in daily smokers and others. Level of education was determined by the following question: 'What is your education?' Possible answer choices were: 1) incomplete secondary, 2) secondary, 3) vocational school, 4) college, 5) university. Participants were categorized into three educational groups: low education (incomplete secondary or secondary education), intermediate education (vocational school), and high education (college or university).

Carotid intima-media thickness measurement

Carotid ultrasonography to assess IMT of the common carotid artery was performed using high-resolution B-mode ultrasound 7 MHz vascular probe (Vivid 7®, GE). During the exam patient was in supine position; the patient's neck was positioned in hyperextension and slightly inclined at 45°. IMT measurement was carried out in the anterior and posterior wall of both common carotid arteries, at a distance of 1–1.5 cm from the carotid bifurcation. A 10-mm-long segment of the region of interest was placed manually for detection of the carotid intima–media [18]. Using a software package for semi-automated border detection loaded on the system (EchoPAC®, GE), mean carotid IMT values were obtained. Three measurements were taken on each carotid artery, and mean values of IMT were calculated for further analysis.

Measurement of pulse wave velocity

PWV measurements were performed using the technique of SphygmoCor System (AtCor Medical Pty Ltd., Head Office, West Ryde, Australia) [18, 19]. To ensure haemodynamic stability, the measurements were performed in the supine position after the participants had been resting in this position for a minimum of 10 minutes. All subjects were familiarised with the environment, the procedure, and the devices. After 10 min of rest in the supine position, the brachial artery BP was recorded twice consecutively with a 1 min interval between each measurement with a mercury sphygmomanometer using the auscultatory method. The PWA profile was obtained by placing tonometer over the radial artery.

PWV was measured estimating the delay in pulse wave at carotid and femoral level as compared to the electrocardiogram wave. The distance from the carotid site to the suprasternal notch (proximal distance) and the distance from the suprasternal notch to the femoral site (distal distance) were measured. The path length was calculated as the difference between the distal and proximal distances. The tonometer probe was placed at the right carotid and femoral arterial sites subsequently. PWV was calculated automatically as the carotid-femoral path length in meters divided by the carotid–femoral transit time in seconds using the intersecting tangent algorithm. To account for a distance measurement error, 'real' PWV was calculated by multiplying obtained PWV by 0.8 [20, 21].

Fifty measurements of IMT and PWV were assessed by a second investigator with between-observer coefficient of variation 4 % for IMT and 6 % for PWV.

Statistical analysis

All statistical analyses were performed using statistical software package IBM SPSS Statistics 20. Categorical variables were expressed as percentages and tested by the χ^2 test. The normality of distribution of continuous variables was tested by Kolmogorov-Smirnov test. Means and standard deviations (SD) were presented for the normally distributed continuous variables while median and interquartile range was calculated for the distributions that did not meet the criteria of normality. Student t test was used to compare the mean values of normally distributed variables and Mann–Whitney test was applied for the comparison of non-normal distributions.

General linear models (GLM) were applied to test the effect of childhood and adulthood risk factors on IMT and PWV. Two types of models were fitted. Model 1 included childhood systolic BP, BMI and sexual maturity score. Effect modification by sexual maturity score was examined by adding interaction terms of the score with systolic BP and BMI to the model. In model 2, adulthood variables (systolic BP, BMI, high-density lipoprotein (HDL) cholesterol, low-density lipoprotein (LDL) cholesterol, smoking, and educational level) were added to childhood variables.

All analyses were performed separately for men and women. P values of less than 0.05 were considered statistically significant.

Results

The characteristics of the study participants are presented in Table 1. In childhood, systolic BP and BMI were significantly higher in girls than in boys. The degree of sexual maturation differed between girls and boys. Girls were more sexually mature than boys. The proportion of girls who had reached menarche was 37.7 %. They had higher systolic BP (121.8 (13.8) mmHg) and BMI (21.1 (3.4 kg/m^2) then those who were less sexually mature (114.3 (11.0) mmHg and 18.3 (2.7) kg/m^2 respectively; p < 0.001).

Adult men had worse cardiovascular risk profile compared to women. Systolic and diastolic BP, also the prevalence of hypertension and smoking were higher, whereas levels of HDL cholesterol were lower in men than in women. Men had higher values of IMT and PWV.

The linear regression model with childhood variables (model 1) showed that childhood systolic BP and BMI were directly associated with IMT only in women (Table 2). No

Table 1 Characteristics of the study population in childhood and adulthood

Characteristic	Men	Women	P value
	n = 168	n = 212	
Childhood (12–13 years)			
Systolic BP, mm Hg (mean; SD)	112.3 (10.7)	116.6 (12.4)	0.001
Diastolic BP, mm Hg (mean; SD)	55.1 (10.2)	55.6 (11.1)	0.649
BMI, kg/m^2 (median; IQR)	17.9 (16.5;20.0)	18.6 (17.1;20.2)	0.021
Sexual maturity score (median; IQR)	0 (0;1)	6 (4;9)	<0.001
Adulthood (48–49 years)			
Systolic BP, mm Hg (median; IQR)	134.3 (123.5;150.0)	125.6 (116.2;138.7)	<0.001
Diastolic BP, mm Hg (median; IQR)	89.3 (82.0;96.0)	80.7 (74.8;88.0)	<0.001
LDL cholesterol, mmol/l (mean; SD)	4.0 (1.1)	3.8 (1.1)	0.106
HDL cholesterol, mmol/l (mean; SD)	1.4 (0.5)	1.8 (0.4)	<0.001
BMI, kg/m^2 (median; IQR)	26.7 (24.5;29.5)	25.7 (23.0;29.6)	0.145
Hypertension, N (%)	106 (63.1)	77 (36.3)	<0.001
Smoking, % N (%)	68 (40.5)	41 (19.3)	<0.001
Intima- media thickness, mm (mean; SD)	0.66 (0.11)	0.61 (0.08)	<0.001
Pulse wave velocity, m/s (mean; SD)	7.1 (2.1)	6.1 (1.7)	<0.001
Educational level, N (%)			
Low	54 (32.1)	47 (22.2)	0.058
Intermediate	53 (31.5)	67 (31.6)	
High	61 (36.3)	98 (46.2)	

Abbreviations: *BMI* body mass index; *BP* blood pressure; *HDL* high density lipoprotein; *IQR* interquartile range (25 percentile and 75 percentile values); *LDL* low density lipoprotein; *SD* standard deviation

Table 2 Associations between intima-media thickness and variables measured in childhood and adulthood

Variable	Men			Women		
	β	95 % CI	P value	β	95 % CI	P value
Model 1						
Childhood systolic BP, mm Hg (for a 1-SD change)	0.001	−0.001;0.003	0.357	0.014	0.003;0.025	0.016
Childhood BMI kg/m^2	−0.002	−0.008;0.004	0.514	0.006	0.002;0.010	0.003
Sexual maturity score	−0.004	−0.016;0.009	0.570	−0.003	−0.006;0.001	0.183
R^2	0.008			0.082		
Model 2						
Childhood systolic BP, mm Hg (for a 1-SD change)	0.002	−0.020;0.023	0.867	0.013	0.002;0.025	0.021
Childhood BMI kg/m^2	−0.003	−0.10;0.004	0.380	0.003	−0.001;0.008	0.143
Sexual maturity score	−0.001	−0.014;0.011	0.853	−0.003	−0.007;0.001	0.147
Adult systolic BP, mm Hg (for a 1-SD change)	0.022	0.004;0.041	0.018	0.006	−0.006;0.018	0.320
HDL cholesterol mmol/l	−0.044	−0.082;-0.007	0.021	0.011	−0.017;0.040	0.431
LDL cholesterol mmol/l	0.002	−0.014;0.017	0.844	0.004	−0.006;0.014	0.390
Adult BMI, kg/m^2	0.002	−0.002;0.006	0.363	0.002	−0.001;0.005	0.114
Daily smoking	0.006	−0.003;0.041	0.755	0.033	0.006;0.06	0.018
Education	0.001	−0.022;0.021	0.991	0.007	−0.006;0.021	0.292
R^2	0.104			0.133		

Reference group for daily smokers was nonsmokers and occasional smokers.
Abbreviations: *BMI* body mass index; *BP* blood pressure, *CI* confidence interval; *HDL* high-density lipoprotein; *LDL* low-density lipoprotein

interaction between female sexual maturity score and systolic BP (p-value of interaction term 0.231) or BMI (p-value of interaction term 0.833) on IMT was found. When adulthood variables were included into model 2, the association of childhood BMI with IMT of women was attenuated, while the contribution of childhood systolic BP remained significant ($\beta = 0.013$; $p = 0.021$). Interestingly, association of adult smoking and IMT was significant in women ($\beta = 0.033$; $p = 0.018$), but not in men. IMT of men was directly related to adult systolic BP ($\beta = 0.022$; $p = 0.018$) and inversely to HDL cholesterol level ($\beta = -0.044$; $p = 0.021$). No associations between adult BMI as well as LDL cholesterol level and IMT were found in both genders. Analysed childhood and adulthood variables explained 10 % of variation of IMT in men and 13 % in women.

Linear regression analyses (model 1) did not demonstrate any association of childhood BP and childhood BMI with PWV in men and women (Table 3). Adult systolic BP was significantly associated with PWV in both genders ($\beta = 0.729$ for men and $\beta = 0.476$ for women; $p = 0.001$) (model 2). PWV was not related to adult BMI, lipid levels, and smoking. Variables included into model 2 explained 12 % of variation of PWV in men and 13 % in women.

Discussion

Our study demonstrated a significant association of childhood systolic BP with adult carotid IMT in women. We did not find any relationship between childhood risk factors and IMT in men. High adult systolic BP and low HDL cholesterol were associated with increased IMT in

Table 3 Associations between pulse wave velocity and variables measured in childhood and adulthood

Variable	Men			Women		
	β	95 % CI	P value	β	95 % CI	P value
Model 1						
Childhood systolic BP, mm Hg (for a 1-SD change)	0.221	−0.190;0.631	0.290	−0.076	−0.318;0.166	0.537
Childhood BMI kg/m²	0.054	−0.070;0.177	0.391	0.028	−0.064;0.121	0.544
Sexual maturity score	0.079	−0.184;0.342	0.553	0.102	0.015;0.188	0.022
R²	0.024			0.046		
Model 2						
Childhood systolic BP, mm Hg (for a 1-SD change)	0.045	−0.372;0.462	0.832	−0.165	−0.409;0.079	0.184
Childhood BMI kg/m²	0.069	−0.067;0.206	0.319	−0.003	−0.111;0.105	0.953
Sexual maturity score	−0.001	−0.014;0.011	0.853	0.100	0.014;0.185	0.023
Adult systolic BP, mm Hg (for a 1-SD change)	0.726	0.328;1.123	<0.001	0.476	0.208;0.744	0.001
HDL cholesterol mmol/l	−0.215	−1.028;0.598	0.602	−0.102	−0.727;0.523	0.748
LDL cholesterol mmol/l	−0.049	−0.363;0.266	0.761	−0.033	−0.249;0.183	0.763
Adult BMI, kg/m²	0.005	−0.083;0.094	0.903	0.025	−0.036;0.086	0.412
Daily smoking	0.263	−0.440;0.966	0.460	−0.314	−0.918;0.291	0.307
Education	−0.016	−0.434;0.401	0.939	−0.012	−0.318;0.294	0.939
R²	0.117			0.133		

Reference group for daily smokers was nonsmokers and occasional smokers.
Abbreviations: *BMI* body mass index; *BP* blood pressure, *CI* confidence interval; *HDL* high density lipoprotein; *LDL* low-density lipoprotein

men. PWV was not related to childhood risk factors. The association between adult systolic BP and PWV was significant in both genders.

Previous cohort studies found that childhood BP was predictive of adulthood vascular changes as measured by carotid IMT [3–5]. The Cardiovascular Risk in Young Finns Study has shown that childhood BP is significantly related to thickness of carotid IMT in adulthood taking into account adult BP levels [3]. However, the pooled analyses of four prospective studies demonstrated that only persistently elevated BP from childhood to adulthood was associated with increased risk of subclinical atherosclerosis, while the individuals with high childhood BP and normal adult BP did not have significantly increased IMT [22]. Our study found that, after adjustment for adult BP, childhood systolic BP was positively associated with carotid IMT in women. This is in line with the observations from Bogalusa Heart Study in which childhood systolic BP was significant predictor of carotid IMT only in white women [23]. The causes of sex differences in the associations between childhood BP and carotid IMT are not studied extensively. Physiological mechanisms underlying the observed sex differences might be related with the influence of sex hormones and other female-specific factors [24]. In baseline survey of our cohort, girls were more sexually mature and had higher values of systolic BP than boys. Meanwhile, the increase in BP from childhood to adulthood was much more pronounced in men than in women. Possibly, in men tracking of BP from childhood to adulthood had greater influence on risk of subclinical atherosclerosis than childhood BP.

Several cohort studies demonstrated that childhood BMI is associated with carotid IMT in adulthood [25–27]. The British cohort study found associations of childhood BMI with IMT in men but not in women, however, the follow-up period was much longer than in our study (till 60–64 years) when men have increased atherosclerotic risk compared to women [27]. The findings of the Bogalusa Heart Study showed that childhood BMI was positively related to adult levels of carotid IMT; however, the association was reduced, after controlling for adult BMI [26]. High IMT levels were observed only among overweight children who became obese adults [28]. Finnish investigators also reported that the association between adolescent BMI and adult IMT became non-significant after adjustment for BMI measured in adulthood [29]. In systematic review on childhood obesity and adult cardiovascular disease risk, Lloyd LJ et al. found little evidence that childhood obesity is an independent risk factor for carotid IMT [30]. The authors argued that the associations might reflect the tracking of BMI from childhood to adulthood. The findings of our study revealed the association of childhood BMI with carotid IMT only in women when the data were not adjusted for adult

BMI. The differences in the association of BMI with IMT between genders might be driven by the fact that girls were more mature compared to boys. However, after adjustment, the association became non-significant which is in line with earlier reported data. We did not perform tracking of BMI categories from childhood to adulthood due to small number of study participants in some of the subgroups.

In our study, adult smoking increased IMT in women, but not in men. The recent review of sex differences in cardiovascular risk factors concluded that smoking is significantly more hazardous for CVD developing in women than in men [24]. The mechanisms of such differences are not sufficiently investigated.

Limited data are available regarding the effects of childhood risk factors on adult arterial stiffness. The prospective Cardiovascular Risk in Young Finns Study demonstrated that conventional risk factors in childhood predict PWV in adulthood [13]. Moreover, this study showed that the favourable change in ideal cardiovascular index was inversely related to PWV [31]. This association remained significant after adjustment for the baseline index suggesting that positive changes in lifestyle and risk factors could have favourable impact on the stiffening process of arteries. In our study, childhood BP and BMI were not predictive for PWV, whereas higher adult systolic BP was associated with higher PWV in both genders. Similarly, the recent data from Bogalusa Heart Study showed no association between childhood BP and adult PWV measured 27 years later after adjustment for adulthood BP, although previously this study reported the adverse influence of elevated childhood BP on arterial stiffening process [12, 32].

Summarising the results of most prospective studies, positive associations between childhood risk factors and adult subclinical atherosclerosis were generally attenuated after adjustment for adult CVD risk factors. Those findings do not mean that early CVD prevention and intervention measures during childhood might be irrelevant. Our previous studies confirmed that childhood BP was related with adult hypertension, also childhood BMI was associated with risk of adult obesity, metabolic syndrome, hyperglycaemia and diabetes [17, 33]. A substantial part of individuals with elevated childhood BP and increased childhood BMI had high CVD risk profile in adulthood. Those data emphasize that CVD risk factors should be prevented as early as possible with continuation of health promotion activities throughout the life course. Promotion of healthy nutrition and physical activity in childhood might help to avoid excessive weight gain and to prevent adult high BP. CVD prevention programmes should be targeted to children with higher levels of CVD risk factors to maximize benefit of preventive measures.

The strength of the present study is the use of population-based data from a randomly selected cohort prospectively followed up for 35 years. BP and anthropometric measurements were performed using the same methodology in the first and in the last survey. A further strength is the use of measurements that allow determining early subclinical stages of atherosclerosis strongly related with future cardiovascular events. As a limitation of our study, it should be noted that the relatively small sample size might contribute to the observed sex variations in the associations between childhood and adulthood risk factors and subclinical atherosclerosis. Moreover, the number of risk factors measured in childhood was quite limited. Finally, the loss of participants over 35 years of follow-up was quite substantial. One of the reasons for this was a high rate of emigration from Lithuania over the last decades. Although no differences between participants and non-participants were found in existing baseline measurements [17], the bias due to differential loss to follow-up was possible.

Conclusions

Sex differences in the associations between childhood and adulthood risk factors and subclinical atherosclerosis were found. In women, childhood BP was predictive of IMT later in life irrespectively of adult risk factors. Vascular health of men was related mainly to adult BP. These results support efforts to reduce conventional risk factors both in childhood and adulthood for the primary prevention of atherosclerosis.

Abbreviations

CVD: Cardiovascular disease; BMI: Body mass index; BP: Blood pressure, CI, Confidence interval; HDL: High density lipoprotein; IMT: Intima-media thickness; LDL: Low-density lipoprotein; PWV: Pulse wave velocity.

Competing interests

The authors declare that they have no competing interests.

Authors' contributions

IC participated in examination of participants, made substantial contributions to conception and design of the manuscript, made interpretation of the data, drafted the manuscript; JK, JP and RS made substantial contributions to the design of the study, revised the manuscript critically; ET-P, JM and JC participated in examination of participants, was involved in drafting of the manuscript; ES analysed the data. All authors read and approved the final version of manuscript.

Acknowledgements

The study was supported by a research grant from the Research Council of Lithuania for National Research Programme 'Chronic Noncommunicable Diseases' (LIG-12019).

Author details

[1]Department of Cardiology, Medical Academy, Lithuanian University of Health Sciences, Eiveniu 2, Kaunas LT-50009, Lithuania. [2]Faculty of Public Health, Medical Academy, Lithuanian University of Health Sciences, Siaures av. 57, Kaunas LT-49264, Lithuania. [3]Department of Endocrinology, Medical Academy, Lithuanian University of Health Sciences, Eiveniu 2, Kaunas LT-50009, Lithuania.

References

1. Nichols M, Townsend N, Scarborough P, Rayner M. Cardiovascular disease in Europe 2014: epidemiological update. Eur Heart J. 2014;35:2950–9.
2. Naqvi TZ, Lee MS. Carotid intima-media thickness and plaque in cardiovascular risk assessment. JACC Cardiovasc Imaging. 2014;7:1025–38.
3. Raitakari OT, Juonala M, Kahonen M, Taittonen L, Laitinen T, Maki-Torkko N, et al. Cardiovascular risk factors in childhood and carotid artery intima-media thickness in adulthood: the Cardiovascular Risk in Young Finns Study. JAMA. 2003;290:2277–83.
4. Juonala M, Viikari JS, Raitakari OT. Main findings from the prospective Cardiovascular Risk in Young Finns Study. Curr Opin Lipidol. 2013;24:57–64.
5. Li S, Chen W, Srinivasan SR, Bond MG, Tang R, Urbina EM, et al. Childhood cardiovascular risk factors and carotid vascular changes in adulthood: the Bogalusa Heart Study. JAMA. 2003;290:2271–6.
6. Davis PH, Dawson JD, Riley WA, Lauer RM. Carotid intimal-medial thickness is related to cardiovascular risk factors measured from childhood through middle age: The Muscatine Study. Circulation. 2001;104:2815–9.
7. Juonala M, Magnussen CG, Venn A, Dwyer T, Burns TL, Davis PH, et al. Influence of age on associations between childhood risk factors and carotid intima-media thickness in adulthood: the Cardiovascular Risk in Young Finns Study, the Childhood Determinants of Adult Health Study, the Bogalusa Heart Study, and the Muscatine Study for the International Childhood Cardiovascular Cohort (i3C) Consortium. Circulation. 2010;122:2514–20.
8. Sutton-Tyrrell K, Najjar SS, Boudreau RM, Venkitachalam L, Kupelian V, Simonsick EM, et al. Elevated aortic pulse wave velocity, a marker of arterial stiffness, predicts cardiovascular events in well-functioning older adults. Circulation. 2005;111:3384–90.
9. Vlachopoulos C, Aznaouridis K, O'Rourke MF, Safar ME, Baou K, Stefanadis C. Prediction of cardiovascular events and all-cause mortality with central haemodynamics: a systematic review and meta-analysis. Eur Heart J. 2010;31:1865–71.
10. Ben-Shlomo Y, Spears M, Boustred C, May M, Anderson SG, Benjamin EJ, et al. Aortic pulse wave velocity improves cardiovascular event prediction: an individual participant meta-analysis of prospective observational data from 17,635 subjects. J Am Coll Cardiol. 2014;63:636–46.
11. Coutinho T, Turner ST, Kullo IJ. Aortic pulse wave velocity is associated with measures of subclinical target organ damage. JACC Cardiovasc Imaging. 2011;4:754–61.
12. Li S, Chen W, Srinivasan SR, Berenson GS. Childhood blood pressure as a predictor of arterial stiffness in young adults: the Bogalusa Heart Study. Hypertension. 2004;43:541–6.
13. Aatola H, Hutri-Kahonen N, Juonala M, Viikari JS, Hulkkonen J, Laitinen T, et al. Lifetime risk factors and arterial pulse wave velocity in adulthood: the Cardiovascular Risk in Young Finns Study. Hypertension. 2010;55:806–11.
14. Oren A, Vos LE, Uiterwaal CS, Gorissen WH, Grobbee DE, Bots ML. Adolescent blood pressure does not predict aortic stiffness in healthy young adults. The Atherosclerosis Risk in Young Adults (ARYA) Study. J Hypertens. 2003;21:321–6.
15. European Health for All Database (HFA-DB). Available: http://www.euro.who.int/hfadb. Accessed 02 June 2015.
16. Torok E, Caukas M, Gyarfas I, editors. International Collaborative Study on Juvenile Hypertension. Budapest: Hungarian Institute of Cardiology; 1987.
17. Petkeviciene J, Klumbiene J, Simonyte S, Ceponiene I, Jureniene K, Kriaucioniene V, et al. Physical, behavioural and genetic predictors of adult hypertension: the findings of the Kaunas Cardiovascular Risk Cohort study. PLoS One. 2014;9(10):e109974.
18. Laurent S, Cockcroft J, Van Bortel L, Boutouyrie P, Giannattasio C, Hayoz D, et al. Expert consensus document on arterial stiffness: methodological issues and clinical applications. Eur Heart J. 2006;27:2588–605.
19. Van Bortel LM, Duprez D, Starmans-Kool MJ, Safar ME, Giannattasio C, Cockcroft J, et al. Clinical applications of arterial stiffness, Task Force III: recommendations for user procedures. Am J Hypertens. 2002;15:445–52.
20. Ring M, Eriksson MJ, Zierath JR, Caidahl K. Arterial stiffness estimation in healthy subjects: a validation of oscillometric (Arteriograph) and tonometric (SphygmoCor) techniques. Hypertens Res. 2014;37:999–1007.
21. Van Bortel LM, Laurent S, Boutouyrie P, Chowienczyk P, Cruickshank JK, De Backer T, et al. Expert consensus document on the measurement of aortic stiffness in daily practice using carotid-femoral pulse wave velocity. J Hypertens. 2012;30:445–8.

22. Juhola J, Magnussen CG, Berenson GS, Venn A, Burns TL, Sabin MA, et al. Combined effects of child and adult elevated blood pressure on subclinical atherosclerosis: the International Childhood Cardiovascular Cohort Consortium. Circulation. 2013;128:217–24.

23. Li S, Chen W, Srinivasan SR, Tang R, Bond MG, Berenson GS. Race (black-white) and gender divergences in the relationship of childhood cardiovascular risk factors to carotid artery intima-media thickness in adulthood: the Bogalusa Heart Study. Atherosclerosis. 2007;194:421–5.

24. Appelman Y, van Rijn BB, Ten Haaf ME, Boersma E, Peters SA. Sex differences in cardiovascular risk factors and disease prevention. Atherosclerosis. 2015;241:211–8.

25. Juonala M, Magnussen CG, Berenson GS, Venn A, Burns TL, Sabin MA, et al. Childhood adiposity, adult adiposity, and cardiovascular risk factors. N Engl J Med. 2011;365:1876–85.

26. Freedman DS, Patel DA, Srinivasan SR, Chen W, Tang R, Bond MG, et al. The contribution of childhood obesity to adult carotid intima-media thickness: the Bogalusa Heart Study. Int J Obes (Lond). 2008;32:749–56.

27. Johnson W, Kuh D, Tikhonoff V, Charakida M, Woodside J, Whincup P, et al. Body mass index and height from infancy to adulthood and carotid intima-media thickness at 60 to 64 years in the 1946 British Birth Cohort Study. Arterioscler, Thromb, Vasc Biol. 2014;34:654–60.

28. Freedman DS, Dietz WH, Tang R, Mensah GA, Bond MG, Urbina EM, et al. The relation of obesity throughout life to carotid intima-media thickness in adulthood: the Bogalusa Heart Study. Int J Obes Relat Metab Disord. 2004;28:159–66.

29. Juonala M, Raitakari M, SA Viikari J, Raitakari OT. Obesity in youth is not an independent predictor of carotid IMT in adulthood. The Cardiovascular Risk in Young Finns Study. Atherosclerosis. 2006;185:388–93.

30. Lloyd LJ, Langley-Evans SC, McMullen S. Childhood obesity and adult cardiovascular disease risk: a systematic review. Int J Obes (Lond). 2010;34:18–28.

31. Aatola H, Hutri-Kahonen N, Juonala M, Laitinen TT, Pahkala K, Mikkila V, et al. Prospective relationship of change in ideal cardiovascular health status and arterial stiffness: the Cardiovascular Risk in Young Finns Study. J Am Heart Assoc. 2014;3(2):e000532.

32. Yun M, Li S, Sun D, Ge S, Lai CC, Fernandez C, et al. Tobacco smoking strengthens the association of elevated blood pressure with arterial stiffness: the Bogalusa Heart Study. J Hypertens. 2015;33:266–74.

33. Petkeviciene J, Klumbiene J, Kriaucioniene V, Raskiliene A, Sakyte E, Ceponiene I. Anthropometric measurements in childhood and prediction of cardiovascular risk factors in adulthood: Kaunas cardiovascular risk cohort study. BMC Public Health. 2015;15:218.

13

Comparison of lower extremity atherosclerosis in diabetic and non-diabetic patients using multidetector computed tomography

Ci He[1†], Jin-gang Yang[1†], Yun-ming Li[2], Jian Rong[3], Fei-zhou Du[1], Zhi-gang Yang[4] and Ming Gu[1*]

Abstract

Background: Lower extremity atherosclerosis (LEA) is among the most serious diabetic complications and leads to non-traumatic amputations. The recently developed dual-source CT (DSCT) and 320- multidetector computed tomography (MDCT) may help to detect plaques more precisely. The aim of our study was to evaluate the differences in LEA between diabetic and non-diabetic patients using MDCT angiography.

Methods: DSCT and 320-MDCT angiographies of the lower extremities were performed in 161 patients (60 diabetic and 101 non-diabetic). The plaque type, distribution, shape and obstructive natures were compared.

Results: Compared with non-diabetic patients, diabetic patients had higher peripheral neuropathy, history of cerebrovasuclar infarction and hypertension rates. A total of 2898 vascular segments were included in the analysis. Plaque and stenosis were detected in 681 segments in 60 diabetic patients (63.1%) and 854 segments in 101 non-diabetic patients (46.9%; p <0.05). Regarding these plaques, diabetic patients had a higher incidence of mixed plaques (34.2% vs. 27.1% for non-diabetic patients). An increased moderate stenosis rate and decreased occlusion rate were observed in diabetic patients relative to non-diabetic patients (35.8% vs. 28.3%; and 6.6% vs. 11.4%; respectively). In diabetic patients, 362 (53.2%) plaques were detected in the distal lower leg segments, whereas in non-diabetic patients, 551 (64.5%) plaques were found in the proximal upper leg segments. The type IV plaque shape, in which the full lumen was involved, was detected more frequently in diabetic patients than in non-diabetic patients (13.1% vs. 8.2%).

Conclusion: Diabetes is associated with a higher incidence of plaque, increased incidence of mixed plaques, moderate stenosis and localisation primarily in the distal lower leg segments. The advanced and non-invasive MDCT could be used for routine preoperative evaluations of LEA.

Keywords: Diabetes mellitus, Lower extremity, Atherosclerosis, Computed tomography, Angiography

Background

According to statistics from the International Diabetes Federation [1], the global diabetes prevalence reached 246 million in 2007, more than double the rate from the previous decade. It has been predicted that by 2025, the global diabetic patient population will reach 380 million [2]. Lower extremity atherosclerosis (LEA) is among the

most serious diabetic complications and leads to non-traumatic amputations [3]. The risk of amputation is 15–46-fold higher among diabetic patients than among non-diabetic patients [4]. Meanwhile, diabetes is complicated by cerebral vascular disease and coronary heart disease (CHD); therefore, the mortality of diabetic patients is significantly increased [5].

LEA is always insidious, and it is very important to conduct early and accurate imaging evaluations in diabetic patients to improve patient outcomes, reduce the amputation rates and amputation planes and reduce the treatment costs [6]. Digital subtraction angiography (DSA) is currently considered the 'gold standard' for vascular disease

* Correspondence: guming18@sina.com
†Equal contributors
[1]Department of Radiology, Chengdu Military General Hospital, Chengdu, Sichuan 610083, China
Full list of author information is available at the end of the article

diagnosis, and can offer interventional treatments at the same time; however, this technique is invasive, expensive, requires highly trained surgical staff and is potentially dangerous [7]. Regarding the development of imaging technologies, multidetector computed tomography (MDCT) has been widely used for non-invasive vascular imaging evaluations [8-10]. The recently introduced dual-source CT (DSCT) and 320-MDCT has been widely used to evaluate cardiovascular and head and neck vascular lesions [11-13]; however, few reports have described their usefulness for LEA lesions. The purposes of this study were to explore the application of MDCT angiography for LEA and evaluate the differences in LEA plaque prevalence and morphology between diabetic and non-diabetic patients.

Methods

Study patients

From November 2011 to November 2013, we retrospectively observed a total of 60 consecutive diabetic patients (13 women; mean age, 69.42 ± 11.04 years) and 101 non-diabetic patients (23 women; mean age, 68.50 ± 13.59 years) who underwent DSCT and 320-MDCT angiography of the arteries in both legs. The exclusion criteria included an allergy to the iodine contrast agent, liver, kidney or heart failure (Creatinine level ≥ 120 mol/L), pregnancy and leg amputation. The vascular exclusion criteria included vascular malformations, poor imaging and a lumen diameter <1.5 mm.

Baseline demographics and medical history were provided, such as age, gender, history of diabetes mellitus, hypertension, CHD, cerebrovasuclar infarction (CI) and laboratory tests. All subjects provided informed consent, and the study was approved by the ethics committees of West China Hospital and Military General Hospital of Chengdu PLA.

MDCT scanning

Examinations were performed with DSCT (Somatom Definition; Siemens Medical Solutions, Forchheim, Germany) (n = 136, from November 2011 to June 2013) at West China Hospital, and 320-MDCT (Aquilion one, Toshiba Medical Systems, Tokyo, Japan) (n = 25, from May 2013 to November 2013) at Military General Hospital of Chengdu PLA. The scan parameters of DSCT were as follows: tube voltages, 120 KV and 80 KV; tube currents, 55 mAs and 230 mAs; collimation, $2 \times 64 \times 0.6$ mm; pitch, 0.65; reconstruction thickness, 0.75 mm and interlayer spacing, 0.4 mm. CT data were acquired in the craniocaudal direction from the common iliac artery to the plantar plane. The delay between contrast injection and CT acquisition was determined using bolus tracking software. A circular region of interest (ROI) for attenuation measurement was placed in the common iliac artery; data acquisition was initiated as soon as the signal intensity in this ROI reached a threshold of 100 Hounsfield units (HU). A non-ionic contrast medium (80–100 mL of iopamidol, 370 mg iodine/mL; Bracco Sine Pharmaceutical Corp. Ltd., Shanghai, China) was immediately administered, followed by 40 mL of a saline chaser solution through an 18-gauge intravenous antecubital catheter with a dual-head power injector (Stellant; Medrad, Indianola, PA, USA) at a flow rate of 6 mL/s. 320-MDCT examination was obtained following standard protocols similar to DSCT.

Image reconstruction

The images were simultaneously transferred to 3D post-processing workstation 1 (Syngo-Imaging; Siemens Medical Solutions, Forchheim, Germany) and workstation 2 (Aquilion one, Toshiba Medical Systems, Tokyo, Japan). Post-processing reconstruction was performed on the workstation and incorporated multi-planar reconstruction (MPR), maximum intensity projection (MIP), volume rendering (VR) and curved planar reformation (CPR).

Image analysis

The bilateral lower extremity arteries were divided into 18 segments, or 9 per leg; these were the common iliac artery, internal iliac artery, external iliac artery, femoral artery, popliteal artery, anterior tibial artery, posterior tibial artery, peroneal artery and dorsalis pedis artery. These segments were also divided into 2 categories to include the upper leg arteries (common iliac artery, internal iliac artery, external iliac artery and femoral artery) and lower leg arteries (popliteal artery, anterior tibial artery, posterior tibial artery, peroneal artery and dorsalis pedis artery). The plaques were classified as non-calcified (<50 HU), mixed (60–100 HU) or calcified (>130 HU) according to the average HU value [14]. Luminal narrowing values were automatically calculated by the software. The artery stenosis grade was classified as mild stenosis (luminal narrowing, <50%), moderate stenosis (luminal narrowing, 50%–74%), severe stenosis (luminal narrowing, $\geq 75\%$) and occlusion (luminal narrowing, 100%) [15]. The atherosclerosis artery axial plane was divided into 4 quadrants, and the plaque shapes were described as type I, <25%; type II, 25–50%; type III, 50–75% and type IV, 75–100% (Figure 1).

Two experienced radiologists blinded to the diagnostic indices and each other's decisions evaluated the reconstructed images for plaque distribution and properties. Only in cases of disagreement did the 2 radiologists discuss a case to reach a decision.

Statistical methods

The clinical information, clinical symptoms, laboratory tests, number of diseased segments, types and shapes of plaques and grades of luminal narrowing were analysed

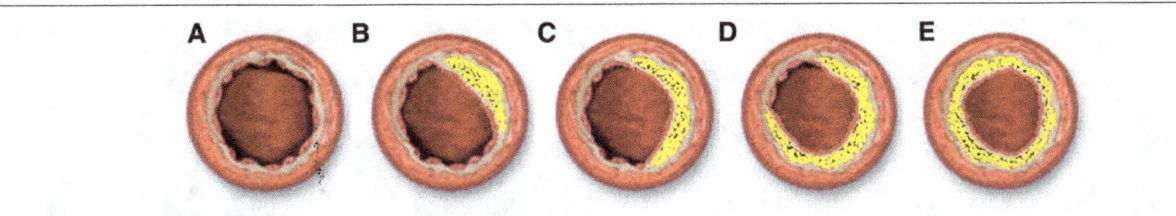

Figure 1 Plaque shapes. A. Normal lumen. **B**. Type I, <25%; **C**. Type II, 25–50%; **D**. Type III, 50–75%; **E**. Type IV, 75–100%.

statistically in each patient. Kolmogorov–Smirnov test was used to test the normality of the distribution. Continuous data are given as means ± standard deviations. Continuous variables such as laboratory tests were expressed as means ± standard deviations and were compared using Student's t-test for unpaired data or the Mann–Whitney two-sample statistic,as appropriate. Categorical variables such as the types and shapes of plaques were presented as numbers (percentages) and were compared using the χ^2 test. All data were analysed using the SPSS 16.0 statistical software package for Windows XP (SPSS Inc., Chicago, IL, USA). A p-value of <0.05 was considered statistically significant.

Results
General information
All examinations were successfully completed in all patients without the occurrence of any complications, and all examinations were of diagnostic image quality with good to excellent vessel visibility.

Compared with non-diabetic patients, diabetic patients had higher peripheral neuropathy, hypertension and history of CI incidence rates ($p < 0.05$). The remaining clinical data and laboratory test results are shown in Table 1.

Plaque type and stenosis degree
A total of 2898 vascular segments were included in the analysis. Plaque and stenosis were detected in 681 (63.1%) vessel segments in 60 diabetic patients and 854 (46.9%) vessel segments in 101 non-diabetic patients ($p < 0.001$). There was a statistical difference in plaque type between diabetic and non-diabetic patients ($p < 0.05$), and diabetic patients had a higher incidence of mixed plaques (Figure 2, Table 2).

Statistical difference was observed in the degree of stenosis between the 2 groups ($p < 0.05$). Compared with non-diabetic patients, diabetic patients had a higher incidence of moderate stenosis (35.8% vs. 28.3%) and a lower incidence of occlusion (6.6% vs. 11.4%), as shown in Table 2, Figure 3.

Plaque distribution and shape
Regarding plaque distribution, 362 (53.2%) plaques were detected in the distal lower leg segments of diabetic patients, and there was an increased involvement in the distal lower leg segments, particularly in the popliteal

artery, anterior tibial artery and posterior tibial artery. In non-diabetic patients, 551 (64.5%) plaques were found in the proximal upper leg segments. The increased distal segment involvement in diabetic patients and increased proximal segment involvement in non-diabetic patients represented significant differences ($p = 0.001$; Figure 4).

Extensive plaques were observed in both diabetic and non-diabetic patients; the plaque shapes were primarily classified as type II and type III, although the incidence of type IV, in which the full lumen is involved, was higher among diabetic patients than among non-diabetic patients and this difference was statistically significant (Table 2).

Discussion
LEA is a common complication of diabetes [16,17]. Dormandy et al. [16] reported that the prevalence of LEA among type 2 diabetic patients was as high as 23.5%. In our study, there were no significant differences with respect to age, sex, smoking status, and uric acid between

Table 1 Characteristics of study population

Characteristic	Non diabetic (n = 101)	Diabetic (n = 60)	P
Age (years)	68.50 ± 13.59	69.42 ± 11.04	>0.05
Gender (female)	23 (22.8%)	13 (21.7%)	>0.05
Smoking	43 (42.6%)	26 (43.3%)	>0.05
BMI	21.28 ± 2.9	22.34 ± 4.11	>0.05
Blood glucose (mmol/L)	5.92 ± 1.54	7.98 ± 1.42	0.001
Cholesterol (mmol/L)	3.94 ± 1.09	4.39 ± 1.18	0.017
Triglyceride (mmol/L)	1.33 ± 0.74	1.57 ± 0.74	0.042
HDL-C (mmol/L)	1.14 ± 0.31	1.12 ± 0.24	>0.05
LDL-C (mmol/L)	2.27 ± 0.86	2.52 ± 0.90	>0.05
Creatinine (mmol/L)	83.04 ± 25.53	82.39 ± 31.19	>0.05
Uric acid	311.57 ± 100.07	331.48 ± 105.26	>0.05
Hypertension	53 (52.5%)	42 (70.0%)	0.029
Peripheral neuropathy	22 (21.8%)	25 (41.7%)	0.007
History of CHD	29 (28.7%)	22 (36.7%)	>0.05
History of CI	72 (33.7%)	36 (60.0%)	0.001

Note: Data were expressed as n (%) or mean ± S.D.
BMI: body mass index; HDL-C: high density lipoprotein cholesterol; LDL-C: low density lipoprotein cholesterol. CHD: coronary heart disease; CI: cerebrovasuclar infarction.

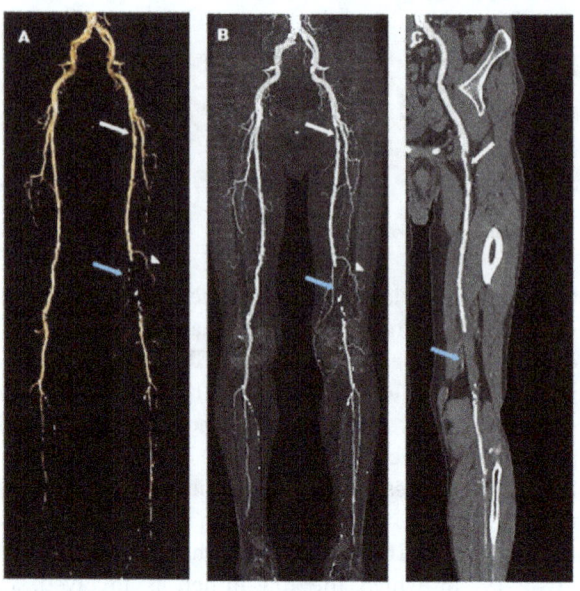

Figure 2 DSCT images of a 56-year-old man with diabetes for 15 years, 1 year of cold feet, show diffuse plaques and stenoses in both lower extremities. **A**, Volume-rendered reconstruction (VRT) after dual energy bone removal displays overview of both lower extremities with a mild stenosis (white arrow), an occlusion (blue arrow) and a compensatory artery (white triangle) in the right femoral artery. **B**, Maximum intensity projection (MIP) depicts the overview of plaques and stenosis. **C**, Both the mild stenosis (white arrow) and occlusion (blue arrow) are caused by non-calcified plaque as evidenced using curved planar reformation (CPR).

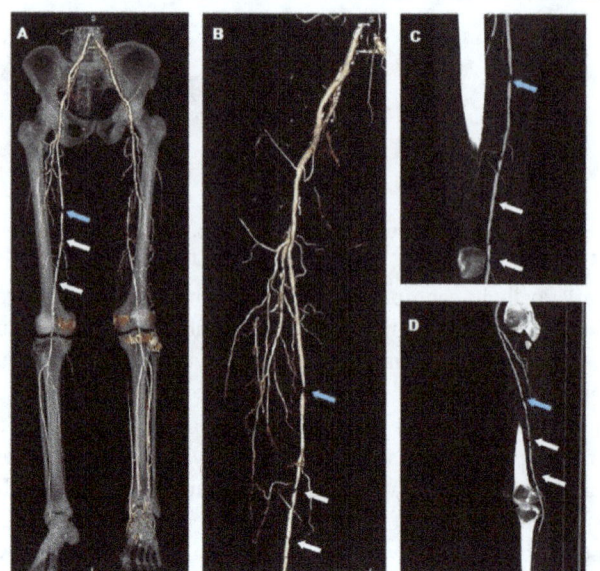

Figure 3 320-MDCT images of a 62-year-old man with diabetes for 10 years, intermittent claudication of both lower extremities for 6 months. **A**, VRT reflects overview artery tree of lower extremities with bone remaining, showing diffused stenoses in right femoral artery. **B**, VRT image after bone removal depicts a severe (blue arrow) and diffused mild to moderate stenosis (white arrows) in right femoral artery. **C**, All the stenoses are caused by non-calcified plaques as evidenced using coronal MIP. **D**, Sagital MIP displays the severe stenosis (blue arrow), mild to moderate stenoses (white arrows) in right femoral artery caused by non-calcified plaques.

diabetic and non-diabetic patients. Blood glucose levels, history of CI and peripheral neuropathy and hypertension incidence rates were significantly higher among diabetic patients, indicating that blood sugar and blood pressure statuses correlated closely with atherosclerosis development. These statuses also explained the more severe atherosclerotic lesions observed among diabetic patients relative to non-diabetic patients, a finding that corroborated relevant reports [18-20].

Our study found that the incidence of LEA was significantly higher among diabetic patients than among non-diabetic patients. In our study, a higher incidence of mixed plaques was observed in the diabetic group, a finding that was consistent with previous MDCT-based studies [21,22]. Rosamond et al. [22] reported that type 2 diabetes often led to the development of multiple atherosclerotic plaques, especially unstable mixed plaques. Unstable mixed plaques, which feature reduced calcification and increased fibrotic and lipid contents, are more vulnerable and more easily form ulcers and ruptures that lead to thrombosis, acute coronary heart syndrome and other serious and possibly life-threatening complications [23].

Artery stenoses were mainly mild to moderate in both groups. Compared with non-diabetic patients, diabetic

Table 2 Comparison of plaque and stenosis between diabetic and non-diabetic patients

Characteristics	Non-diabetic	Diabetic	P
N	854 (46.9%)	681 (63.1%)	<0.001
Plaque type			0.007
Non-calcified	217 (25.4%)	144 (21.2%)	
Mixed	231 (27.1%)	233 (34.2%)	
Calcified	406 (47.5%)	304 (44.6%)	
Grade of stenosis			<0.001
Mild (<50%)	363 (42.5%)	299 (43.9%)	
Moderate (≥50%)	242 (28.3%)	244 (35.8%)	
Severe (≥75%)	152 (17.8%)	93 (13.7%)	
Occlusion (=100%)	97 (11.4%)	45 (6.6%)	
Plaque shape			0.018
Type I < 25%	130 (15.2%)	91 (13.4%)	
Type II < 50%	377 (44.2%)	290 (42.6%)	
Type III < 75%	277 (32.4%)	211 (30.9%)	
Type IV ≤ 100%	70 (8.2%)	89 (13.1%)	

Note: Data were expressed as n (%).

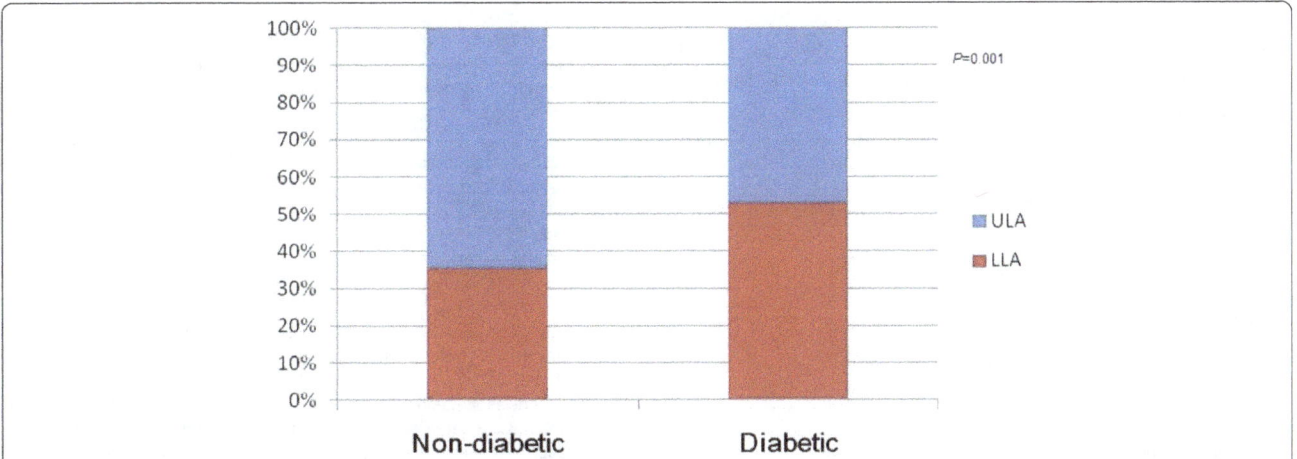

Figure 4 Bar graph demonstrates the main distribution of plaques between diabetic and non-diabetic patients, showing the increased distal segment involvement in diabetic patients (*P* = 0.01). ULA = Upper Leg arteries, LLA = Lower leg arteries.

patients had a higher incidence of moderate stenosis and a lower incidence of occlusion. Diabetes-induced atherosclerosis was primarily non-obstructive stenosis. Scholte et al. [2] evaluated the diabetes-related coronary atherosclerotic plaque and morphological statuses using 64-slice CT and found that approximately 82% of stenoses in diabetic patients were non-occlusive lesions, in accordance with our study. Other reports of ultrasound and CT studies [10,21] indicated that when compared with those in non-diabetic patients, atherosclerotic plaques in diabetic patients, which were mainly mixed plaques with reduced occlusion, were more unstable and thus more easily ruptured and thrombosed.

Our study found that the 2 groups differed significantly in terms of plaque distribution. Non-diabetic atherosclerosis primarily affected the proximal upper leg segments. In contrast, an increased involvement in the distal lower leg segments was observed in diabetic patients, particularly in the popliteal artery, anterior tibial artery and posterior tibial artery. Previous studies [24,25] have supported the finding that diabetes-induced atherosclerosis involved the distal segments; in particular, the distal segment atherosclerosis rate was as high as 58% among diabetic patients and was accompanied by more severe stenosis and an increased tendency toward vascular embolism. It was unclear why atherosclerosis distributions differed between diabetic and non-diabetic patients. We speculate that diabetes might alter the arterial remodelling process, thus resulting in diffusely narrowed arteries that lack compensatory enlargement, especially in distal segments.

In our study, we also found that plaque shapes in both groups were primarily type II and type III. The incidence of Type IV was higher among diabetic patients than among non-diabetic patients, indicating more widespread atherosclerosis among diabetic patients. Diabetic-induced atherosclerosis was usually multi-stage and widespread and beaded changes in the distal segments [16,18]. These characteristics might induce relatively more severe symptoms, a poorer prognosis and a higher amputation incidence. The more diffuse atherosclerotic burdens in diabetic patients were likely caused by the increased risk factors resulting from the metabolic disorders that have been described to cause atherosclerosis [26,27].

When considering non-invasive imaging, the magnetic resonance (MR) imaging and ultrasound results should also be compared. Following the developments in non-invasive imaging equipment and technology, ultrasound and MR are increasingly used in examinations of lower extremity arterial disease [28]. However, ultrasound analysis is operator-dependent. MR imaging, which features various imaging protocols and sequences, has a demonstrated ability to characterise morphological, structural and compositional features of atherosclerotic plaques in vivo [29]. However, this method is time-consuming and cannot be performed on some patients with pacemakers or stents. MDCT has undergone rapid development. In particular, dual-source CT and 320-MDCT have many advantages relative to conventional MDCT, such as higher temporal and spatial resolution, radiation dose reduction [30], and powerful post-processing capabilities.

This study has the following shortcomings. CT angiography has some limitations with respect to accurate determination of stenoses involving large plaques in distal small segments. Although the radiation dose provided by DSCT and 320-MDCT is significantly reduced, multiple inspections cannot be performed within a short time period.

Conclusion

The incidence of LEA was higher among diabetic patients than non-diabetic patients. Diabetic atherosclerosis, which featured a higher incidence of mixed plaque and moderate stenosis, was more extensive in the distal segments and primarily involved arteries in the lower leg. As an advanced non-invasive technique, MDCT could provide good evaluations of LEA plaque types, shapes, distributions and stenosis characteristics and could therefore be used for routine preoperative evaluations.

Competing interests

The authors declare that they have no competing interests.

Authors' contributions

All authors participated in the design and coordination of the study, reviewed the analysis and took part in writing the manuscript. They also read and approved the final manuscript.

Acknowledgments

This work was supported by Science Foundation of Military General Hospital of Chengdu PLA (NO. 2011YG-B38) and 12th Five-year Science Plan of Chengdu Military (NO.C12036).

Author details

[1]Department of Radiology, Chengdu Military General Hospital, Chengdu, Sichuan 610083, China. [2]Department of Neurosurgery, Chengdu Military General Hospital, Chengdu, Sichuan 610083, China. [3]Division of Geriatric Medicine, Department of Medicine, Chengdu Military General Hospital, Chengdu, Sichuan 610083, China. [4]Department of Radiology, West China Hospital, Sichuan University, Chengdu, Sichuan 610041, China.

References

1. Unwin N, Gan D, Whiting D: The IDF Diabetes Atlas: providing evidence, raising awareness and promoting action. Diabetes Res Clin Pract 2010, 87(1):2–3.

2. Scholte AJ, Schuijf JD, Kharagjitsingh AV, Jukema JW, Pundziute G, van der Wall EE, Bax JJ: Prevalence of coronary artery disease and plaque morphology assessed by multi-slice computed tomography coronary angiography and calcium scoring in asymptomatic patients with type 2 diabetes. Heart 2008, 94(3):290–295.

3. Ohnishi H, Sawayama Y, Furusyo N, Maeda S, Tokunaga S, Hayashi J: Risk factors for and the prevalence of peripheral arterial disease and its relationship to carotid atherosclerosis: the Kyushu and Okinawa Population Study (KOPS). J Atheroscler Thromb 2010, 17(7):751–758.

4. Nguyen LL, Hevelone N, Rogers SO, Bandyk DF, Clowes AW, Moneta GL, Lipsitz S, Conte MS: Disparity in outcomes of surgical revascularization for limb salvage: race and gender are synergistic determinants of vein graft failure and limb loss. Circulation 2009, 119(1):123–130.

5. Roper NA, Bilous RW, Kelly WF, Unwin NC, Connolly VM: Excess mortality in a population with diabetes and the impact of material deprivation: longitudinal, population based study. BMJ 2001, 322(7299):1389–1393.

6. Harrington C, Zagari MJ, Corea J, Klitenic J: A cost analysis of diabetic lower-extremity ulcers. Diabetes Care 2000, 23(9):1333–1338.

7. Willinsky RA, Taylor SM, TerBrugge K, Farb RI, Tomlinson G, Montanera W: Neurologic complications of cerebral angiography: prospective analysis of 2,899 procedures and review of the literature. Radiology 2003, 227(2):522–528.

8. Kock MC, Dijkshoorn ML, Pattynama PM, Myriam Hunink MG: Multi-detector row computed tomography angiography of peripheral arterial disease. Eur Radiol 2007, 17(12):3208–3222.

9. Mekle R, Hofmann E, Scheffler K, Bilecen D: A polymer-based MR-compatible guidewire: a study to explore new prospects for interventional peripheral magnetic resonance angiography (ipMRA). J Magn Reson Imaging 2006, 23(2):145–155.

10. Verim S, Tasci I: Doppler ultrasonography in lower extremity peripheral arterial disease. Turk Kardiyol Dern Ars 2013, 41(3):248–255.

11. Pflederer T, Marwan M, Renz A, Bachmann S, Ropers D, Kuettner A, Anders K, Bamberg F, Daniel WG, Achenbach S: Noninvasive assessment of coronary in-stent restenosis by dual-source computed tomography. Am J Cardiol 2009, 103(6):812–817.

12. He C, Yang ZG, Chu ZG, Dong ZH, Shao H, Deng W, Chen J, Peng LQ, Tang SS, Xiao JH: Carotid and cerebrovascular disease in symptomatic patients with type 2 diabetes: assessment of prevalence and plaque morphology by dual-source computed tomography angiography. Cardiovasc Diabetol 2010, 9:91.

13. He C, Yang ZG, Chu ZG, Dong ZH, Li YM, Shao H, Deng W: Comparison of carotid and cerebrovascular disease between diabetic and non-diabetic patients using dual-source CT. Eur J Radiol 2010, 80(3):e361–e365.

14. Ballotta E, Da Giau G, Renon L: Carotid plaque gross morphology and clinical presentation: a prospective study of 457 carotid artery specimens. J Surg Res 2000, 89(1):78–84.

15. North American Symptomatic Carotid Endarterectomy Trial Collaborators: Beneficial effect of carotid endarterectomy in symptomatic patients with high-grade carotid stenosis. N Engl J Med 1991, 325(7):445–453.

16. Dormandy JA, Betteridge DJ, Schernthaner G, Pirags V, Norgren L: Impact of peripheral arterial disease in patients with diabetes–results from PROactive (PROactive 11). Atherosclerosis 2009, 202(1):272–281.

17. Pomposelli F: Arterial imaging in patients with lower-extremity ischemia and diabetes mellitus. J Am Podiatr Med Assoc 2010, 100(5):412–423.

18. Federman DG, Kravetz JD: Peripheral arterial disease: diagnosis, treatment, and systemic implications. Clin Dermatol 2007, 25(1):93–100.

19. Cardoso CR, Leite NC, Freitas L, Dias SB, Muxfeld ES, Salles GF: Pattern of 24-hour ambulatory blood pressure monitoring in type 2 diabetic patients with cardiovascular dysautonomy. Hypertens Res 2008, 31(5):865–872.

20. Cacoub PP, Abola MT, Baumgartner I, Bhatt DL, Creager MA, Liau CS, Goto S, Rother J, Steg PG, Hirsch AT: Cardiovascular risk factor control and outcomes in peripheral artery disease patients in the Reduction of Atherothrombosis for Continued Health (REACH) Registry. Atherosclerosis 2009, 204(2):e86–e92.

21. Ibebuogu UN, Nasir K, Gopal A, Ahmadi N, Mao SS, Young E, Honoris L, Nuguri VK, Lee RS, Usman N, Rostami B, Pal R, Flores F, Budoff MJ: Comparison of atherosclerotic plaque burden and composition between diabetic and non diabetic patients by non invasive CT angiography. Int J Cardiovasc Imaging 2009, 25(7):717–723.

22. Rosamond W, Flegal K, Furie K, Go A, Greenlund K, Haase N, Hailpern SM, Ho M, Howard V, Kissela B, Kittner S, Lloyd-Jones D, McDermott M, Meigs J, Moy C, Nichol G, O'Donnell C, Roger V, Sorlie P, Steinberger J, Thom T, Wilson M, Hong Y: Heart disease and stroke statistics–2008 update: a report from the American Heart Association Statistics Committee and Stroke Statistics Subcommittee. Circulation 2008, 117(4):e25–e146.

23. Naghavi M, Libby P, Falk E, Casscells SW, Litovsky S, Rumberger J, Badimon JJ, Stefanadis C, Moreno P, Pasterkamp G, Fayad Z, Stone PH, Waxman S, Raggi P, Madjid M, Zarrabi A, Burke A, Yuan C, Fitzgerald PJ, Siscovick DS, de Korte CL, Aikawa M, Airaksinen KE, Assmann G, Becker CR, Chesebro JH, Farb A, Galis ZS, Jackson C, Jang IK, et al: From vulnerable plaque to vulnerable patient: a call for new definitions and risk assessment strategies: Part II. Circulation 2003, 108(15):1772–1778.

24. Carter A, Murphy MO, Turner NJ, Halka AT, Ghosh J, Serracino-Inglott F, Walker MG, Syed F: Intimal neovascularisation is a prominent feature of atherosclerotic plaques in diabetic patients with critical limb ischaemia. Eur J Vasc Endovasc Surg 2007, 33(3):319–324.

25. van der Feen C, Neijens FS, Kanters SD, Mali WP, Stolk RP, Banga JD: Angiographic distribution of lower extremity atherosclerosis in patients with and without diabetes. Diabet Med 2002, 19(5):366–370.

26. Wang TD, Goto S, Bhatt DL, Steg PG, Chan JC, Richard AJ, Liau CS: Ethnic differences in the relationships of anthropometric measures to metabolic risk factors in Asian patients at risk of atherothrombosis: results from the REduction of Atherothrombosis for Continued Health (REACH) Registry. Metabolism 2010, 59(3):400–408.

27. Escobedo J, Schargrodsky H, Champagne B, Silva H, Boissonnet CP, Vinueza R, Torres M, Hernandez R, Wilson E: Prevalence of the metabolic syndrome in Latin America and its association with sub-clinical carotid atherosclerosis: the CARMELA cross sectional study. Cardiovasc Diabetol 2009, 8:52.

28. Kreitner KF, Schmitt R: MultiHance-enhanced MR angiography of the peripheral run-off vessels in patients with diabetes. Eur Radiol 2007, 17(Suppl 6):F63–F68.

29. Lell M, Fellner C, Baum U, Hothorn T, Steiner R, Lang W, Bautz W, Fellner FA: Evaluation of carotid artery stenosis with multisection CT and MR imaging: influence of imaging modality and postprocessing. *AJNR Am J Neuroradiol* 2007, **28**(1):104–110.

30. Zhang LJ, Wu SY, Niu JB, Zhang ZL, Wang HZ, Zhao YE, Chai X, Zhou CS, Lu GM: Dual-energy CT angiography in the evaluation of intracranial aneurysms: image quality, radiation dose, and comparison with 3D rotational digital subtraction angiography. *AJR Am J Roentgenol* 2010, **194**(1):23–30.

14

Association between renin and atherosclerotic burden in subjects with and without type 2 diabetes

Isabel Gonçalves[1], Andreas Edsfeldt[1], Helen M. Colhoun[2], Angela C. Shore[3], Carlo Palombo[4], Andrea Natali[5], Gunilla Nordin Fredrikson[1], Harry Björkbacka[1], Maria Wigren[1], Eva Bengtsson[1], Gerd Östling[1], Kunihiko Aizawa[3], Francesco Casanova[3], Margaretha Persson[1], Kim Gooding[3], Phil Gates[3], Faisel Khan[2], Helen C. Looker[2], Fiona Adams[2], Jill Belch[2], Silvia Pinnola[5], Elena Venturi[5], Michaela Kozakova[5], Li-Ming Gan[6], Volker Schnecke[6], Jan Nilsson[1*], on behalf of the SUMMIT consortium

Abstract

Background: Activation of the renin-angiotensin-aldosterone-system (RAAS) has been proposed to contribute to development of vascular complications in type 2 diabetes (T2D). The aim of the present study was to determine if plasma renin levels are associated with the severity of vascular changes in subjects with and without T2D.

Methods: Renin was analyzed by the Proximity Extension Assay in subjects with ($n = 985$) and without ($n = 515$) T2D participating in the SUMMIT (SUrrogate markers for Micro- and Macro-vascular hard endpoints for Innovative diabetes Tools) study and in 205 carotid endarterectomy patients. Vascular changes were assessed by determining ankle-brachial pressure index (ABPI), carotid intima-media thickness (IMT), carotid plaque area, pulse wave velocity (PWV) and the reactivity hyperemia index (RHI).

Results: Plasma renin was elevated in subjects with T2D and demonstrated risk factor-independent association with prevalent cardiovascular disease both in subjects with and without T2D. Renin levels increased with age, body mass index, HbA1c and correlated inversely with HDL. Subjects with T2D had more severe carotid disease, increased arterial stiffness, and impaired endothelial function. Risk factor-independent associations between renin and APBI, bulb IMT, carotid plaque area were observed in both T2D and non-T2D subjects. These associations were independent of treatment with RAAS inhibitors. Only weak associations existed between plasma renin and the expression of pro-inflammatory and fibrous components in plaques from 205 endarterectomy patients.

Conclusions: Our findings provide clinical evidence for associations between systemic RAAS activation and atherosclerotic burden and suggest that this association is of particular importance in T2D.

Keywords: Renin, Type 2 diabetes, Atherosclerosis, Arterial stiffness, Endothelial dysfunction

Abbreviations: ABPI, Ankle-brachial pressure index; ACE, Angiotensin-converting enzyme; ARBs, Angiotensin receptor blockers; CVD, Cardiovascular disease; IMT, Carotid intima-media thickness; PWV, Pulse wave velocity; RAAS, Renin-angiotensin-aldosterone-system; RHI, Reactivity hyperemia index; SUMMIT, SUrrogate markers for Micro- and Macro-vascular hard endpoints for Innovative diabetes Tools; T2D, Type 2 diabetes

* Correspondence: jan.nilsson@med.lu.se
[1]Department of Clinical Sciences Malmö, Lund University, Malmö, Sweden
Full list of author information is available at the end of the article

Background

Activation of the renin-angiotensin-aldosterone-system (RAAS) has been implicated in the development of vascular complications in type 2 diabetes (T2D) [1, 2]. Approximately 75 % of subjects with T2D have hypertension [3]. Factors contributing to raising blood pressure in T2D include elevated production of angiotensinogen in abdominal fat and hyperinsulinemia-dependent activation of the sympathetic nervous system stimulating renin expression [4, 5]. Renin is the key activator of RAAS [6, 7]. It is primarily produced by the juxtaglomerular apparatus in the afferent arterioles of the kidney and functions by hydrolyzing angiotensinogen into angiotensin I. Angiotensin I is subsequently cleaved by angiotensin-converting enzyme (ACE) to generate angiotensin II, a powerful vasoconstrictor that increases blood pressure [7]. However, angiotensin II has also been reported to have several other biological effects including stimulation of smooth muscle cell proliferation and hypertrophy, oxidative stress, as well as the release of pro-inflammatory cytokines and pro-fibrotic factors that may contribute to the development of macrovascular complications in diabetes also in other ways beyond blood pressure [7–10]. Accordingly, blockade of angiotensin II receptors attenuates the development of atherosclerosis in apolipoprotein E knockout mice with streptozotocin-induced diabetes [11, 12]. However, stimulation of smooth muscle cell proliferation and extracellular matrix synthesis may also help stabilize vulnerable atherosclerotic plaques [13] suggesting that activation RAAS may have both detrimental and beneficial effects on cardiovascular disease in T2D. Intervention studies using ACE inhibitors or angiotensin receptor blockers (ARBs) in patients with diabetes have demonstrated a reduction of cardiovascular events [14–16], but it remains to be fully understood to what extent this involves effects on the vasculature that are unrelated to the effects of RAAS on the blood pressure.

To further explore the relation between activation of RAAS and vascular complications in diabetes we analyzed the association between plasma renin levels and markers of atherosclerosis, arterial stiffness and endothelial dysfunction in 1500 subjects with and without T2D matched for age, gender and prevalence of CVD participating in the SUMMIT (SUrrogate markers for Micro- and Macro-vascular hard endpoints for Innovative diabetes Tools) study. Furthermore to determine if plasma levels of renin were related with atherosclerotic plaque phenotype we analyzed their association with markers of inflammation and fibrous components in 205 carotid plaques obtained at endarterectomy.

Methods

Study populations

The SUrrogate markers for Micro- and Macro-vascular hard endpoints for Innovative diabetes Tools (SUMMIT) study cohort consisted of 4 groups; (1) subjects with T2D and clinically manifest CVD, (2) subjects with T2D but without clinical signs of CVD, (3) subjects with CVD but no diabetes and (4) subjects without both CVD and diabetes recruited from existing population cohorts and hospital registers at the university hospitals in Malmö (Sweden), Pisa (Italy), Dundee and Exeter (UK) between December 2010 and April 2013 [17]. Diabetes was defined by current or previous evidence of hyperglycemia (according to WHO 1998 criteria; fasting plasma glucose >7.0 mmol/l or 2-h plasma glucose >11.1 mmol/l, or both) or by current medication with insulin, sulphonylureas, metformin or other anti-diabetic drugs. A clinical history of CVD included a previous diagnosis in the clinical record of non-fatal acute myocardial infarction (MI), hospitalized unstable angina, resuscitated cardiac arrest, any coronary revascularization procedure, non-fatal stroke, transient ischemic attack confirmed by a specialist, lower extremities arterial disease defined as Ankle Brachial Pressure Index (ABPI) <0.9 with intermittent claudication or prior corrective surgery, angioplasty or above ankle amputation. T2D with and without CVD were matched at each center for gender, age (±5 years) and duration of diabetes (±5 years). Subjects without T2D were matched for gender and age (±5 years) at each center. Subjects with CVD with or without T2D were matched for CVD type. Exclusion criteria included renal replacement therapy, malignancy requiring active treatment, end-stage renal disease, any chronic inflammatory disease on therapy, previous bilateral carotid artery invasive interventions or age <40 years. Demographics, clinical characteristics including medication, physical and laboratory examinations were obtained according to a pre-defined study protocol at all 4 participating centers.

Carotid ultrasound, endothelial function, arterial stiffness and ankle brachial pressure index measurements

Carotid intima media thickness (IMT) was measured both in common carotid artery (CCA) and in the bulb as previously described [17]. To calculate carotid plaque area the proximal-distal boundaries of a plaque were set where the echo of the intima began to diverge from the adventitia echo forming a focal thickening of the intima-media-complex. The plaque area was assessed by outlining the contours of the plaque using the trace function on the ultrasound machine. The plaque area represents the sum of all plaques detected in the carotid artery and the values shown in this study represent the mean of the left and right carotid arteries.

Endothelial function was measured using EndoPat (Itamar Medical, Caesarea Ind. Park, Israel) to estimate the endothelium-dependent vasodilation following post-ischemic hyperemia [17].

The reactive hyperemia index (RHI) was calculated as a post-occlusion to pre-occlusion ratio of the signal amplitudes. Thirty-one subjects were excluded from the RHI analysis due to incomplete occlusion (brachial pulses from the occluded arm were visible during occlusion, despite an increase of the pressure of the cuff to the maximum level of 300 mmHg) or time of occlusion was > or < 5 mins.

Arterial stiffness was assessed by calculating pulse wave velocity (PWV) using a Sphygmocor device (Atcor Medical, Australia). The carotid and femoral pulses were captured. PWV (m/s) was automatically calculated as the measured distance divided by the differences in time between the R wave of the ECG to the foot of the carotid and femoral pulse curves as previously described [17].

The ankle brachial pressure index (ABPI) was calculated as the ratio between the highest systolic blood pressure values from each foot respectively and the blood pressure from the arm giving the highest value. Values given represent the mean of the left and right ABPI.

Carotid endarterectomy patients and analyses of plaque tissue

Two hundred and five human carotid plaques were collected at carotid endarterectomy. The indications for surgery were plaques associated with ipsilateral symptoms (transitory ischemic attack, stroke or amaurosis fugax) and stenosis >70 % or plaques not associated with symptoms and stenosis >80 %, measured by duplex. Patients were preoperatively assessed by a neurologist. Blood samples were collected one day before endarterectomy. Informed consent was given by each patient. The study was approved by the local ethical committee. Plaques were snap-frozen in liquid nitrogen immediately after surgical removal. Plaque homogenates were prepared as previously described [18]. One mm fragments, from the most stenotic region, were taken for histology. Stains for lipids (Oil Red O), vascular smooth muscle cells (α-actin) and macrophages (CD68) were performed as previously described [19]. Measurements of the area of plaque (% area) for the different stainings were quantified blindly using BiopixiQ 2.1.8 (Gothenburg, Sweden) after scanning with ScanScope Console Version 8.2 (LRI imaging AB, Vista CA, USA).

Finally aliquots of 50 μL of plaque homogenate were centrifuged at 13,000 g for 10 min. Twenty-five μL of the supernatant was removed and used for measuring different cytokines and growth factors. The procedure was performed according to the manufacturer's instructions (Human Cytokine/chemokine immunoassay, Millipore Corporation, MA, USA) and analyzed with Luminex 100 IS 2.3 (Austin, Texas, USA). Elastin and collagen in plaque homogenates were measured using the Fastin Elastin and Sircol soluble Collagen assays as previously described [19]. Renin levels in plaque homogenates were analyzed using the Proximity Extension Assay (see below).

Analysis of renin and IL-6 in plasma

Plasma levels of renin and IL-6 were analyzed by the Proximity Extension Assay (PEA) technique using the Proseek Multiplex CVD$^{96 \times 96}$ reagents kit (Olink Bioscience, Uppsala, Sweden) at the Clinical Biomarkers Facility, Science for Life Laboratory, Uppsala. Oligonucleotide-labeled antibody probe pairs were allowed to bind to their respective targets present in the plasma sample and addition of a DNA polymerase led to an extension and joining of the two oligonucleotides and formation of a PCR template. Universal primers were used to pre-amplify the DNA templates in parallel. Finally, the individual DNA sequences were detected and quantified using specific primers by microfluidic real-time quantitative PCR chip (96.96, Dynamic Array IFC, Fluidigm Biomark). The chip was run with a Biomark HD instrument. The mean coefficients of variance for intra-assay variation and inter-assay variation are 7 and 13 % for renin, and 8 and 10 % for IL-6, respectively. All samples were analyzed in the same run. Data analysis was performed by a preprocessing normalization procedure using Olink Wizard for GenEx (Multid Analyses, Sweden). All data are presented as arbitrary units (AU). General calibrator curves to calculate the approximate concentrations as well as technical information about the assays are available on the Olink homepage (http://www.olink.com).

Statistics

Statistical analyses were performed based on log2-transformed renin levels to approximate normal distribution. Assessment of association with other markers was done via Pearson correlation coefficient and linear regression models adjusted to study center and the individual factors from the Framingham risk score (age, gender, total cholesterol, HDL cholesterol, systolic blood pressure, and smoking). Statistical significance of the association in the linear regression model is judged by the p-value of the renin coefficient.

For assessing associations of renin levels with CVD risk logistic regression models were used, and adjustment for factors of the Framingham risk score and study center were done. Spearman correlations were used to determine associations between plasma renin levels and components of endarterectomy specimens. Statistical analyses of the SUMMIT study were done using the R version 3.1.1 and the IBM SPSS (version 22) software was used for the carotid endarterectomy study.

Results

Plasma renin levels are increased in both T2D and prevalent CVD

The design of the SUMMIT study has previously been reported [17]. Briefly, this cross-sectional cohort involves 985 T2D subjects and 515 subjects without T2D matched for age, gender and prevalence of CVD recruited at four different European academic health centers (Malmö, Dundee, Exeter and Pisa). The clinical characteristics of the study cohort are shown in Table 1. Plasma renin levels were significantly higher in subjects with T2D (median (IQR) 267 (157–458) versus 148 (98–260) AU in non-T2D). Subjects with prevalent CVD had increased levels of renin in both the T2D (333 (199–554) versus 214 (128–365) AU and non-T2D groups (214 (128–333) versus 119 (87–176) AU, Fig. 1). To determine if the renin association with CVD was independent of major cardiovascular risk factors we adjusted for the factors included in the Framingham risk score (e.g. age, gender, total cholesterol, HDL, systolic blood pressure and smoking) using logistic regression models. The results demonstrated that high levels of renin were independently associated with higher odds ratios for CVD in both the T2D and non-T2D groups. The associations with CVD remained significant when adjusting for renal function (estimated glomerular filtration rate; eGFR) and in the T2D also when adjusting for treatment with RAAS inhibitors (Table 2).

Association between plasma renin and risk factors

The levels of renin in plasma increased with age, body mass index (BMI), HbA1c and triglycerides, and showed inverse associations with LDL cholesterol, HDL cholesterol and renal function as assessed by the eGFR. Notably, these associations were at least as strong in non-T2D subjects as in the T2D group (Table 3). There was also a significant association with inflammation as assessed by plasma IL-6 levels in both groups. An inverse association between renin and systolic blood pressure was observed in the T2D group but not in the non-T2D group.

Association between plasma renin and measures of atherosclerosis, arterial stiffness and endothelial function

We next analyzed if renin levels were related to the severity of vascular changes. Peripheral artery disease was determined by the ankle-brachial pressure index (ABPI), carotid disease by the intima-media thickness (IMT) in the common carotid artery (CCA) and the carotid bulb as well as by carotid plaque area, arterial stiffness by measuring pulse wave velocity (PWV) and endothelial function by determining the Reactivity Hyperemia Index

Table 1 Clinical characteristics of the study cohort

	T2D with CVD	T2D without CVD	Non-T2D without CVD	Non-T2D with CVD
N	458	527	270	245
Male sex, n(%)	331 (72)	324 (61)	163 (60)	161 (66)
Age, years	69.3 (7.8)	66.2 (8.8)	66.4 (9.1)	67.9 (9.2)
T2D Duration, years	12.2 (8.8)	9.1 (6.9)	–	–
BMI, kg/m²	30.1 (4.9)	30.8 (5.5)	27.0 (4.0)	27.6 (4.1)
Medication				
Statin use, n(%)	401 (88)	321 (61)	97 (36)	171 (70)
Anti-hypertensive treatment use, n(%)	419 (92)	352 (67)	129 (48)	172 (70)
Blood pressure				
SBP, mmHg	138 (20.0)	136 (17.6)	132 (17.2)	134 (16.0)
DBP, mmHg	76 (10.3)	78 (9.8)	77 (9.4)	77 (9.2)
Pulse pressure, mmHg	62.6 (16.2)	58.2 (13.1)	54.5 (12.5)	57.2 (14.2)
Metabolic factors				
HbA1c, mmol/mol	58.8 (13.9)	56.6 (13.0)	38.4 (3.9)	39.8 (4.7)
%	8.0 (5.0)	7.9 (10.0)	5.8 (2.3)	5.8 (0.5)
Tot Cholesterol, mmol/l	3.92 (0.9)	4.38 (1.0)	5.03 (1.1)	4.47 (1.1)
HDL, mmol/l	1.19 (0.35)	1.32 (0.38)	1.51 (0.44)	1.42 (0.40)
LDL, mmol/l	2.06 (0.74)	2.42 (0.91)	3.01 (0.94)	2.52 (0.88)
Triglycerides, mmol/l	1.68 (0.94)	1.62 (0.92)	1.30 (0.65)	1.37 (0.70)
Renal function				
Creatinine, serum, µmol/l	93.4 (32.2)	80.0 (20.6)	81.3 (18.5)	83.3 (19.3)
ACR, mg/mmol	9.48 (37.4)	4.14 (16.5)	3.23 (22.7)	3.38 (15.3)
eGFR	60.8 (20.3)	71.3 (19.4)	69.6 (17.7)	66.9 (18.9)

Binary variables are reported as n(%) and quantitative data are reported as mean (SD)
BMI body mass index, *SBP* systolic blood pressure, *DBP* diastolic blood pressure, *HDL* high-density lipoprotein, *LDL* low-density lipoprotein, *ACR* albumin creatinine ratio, *eGFR* estimated glomerular filtration rate

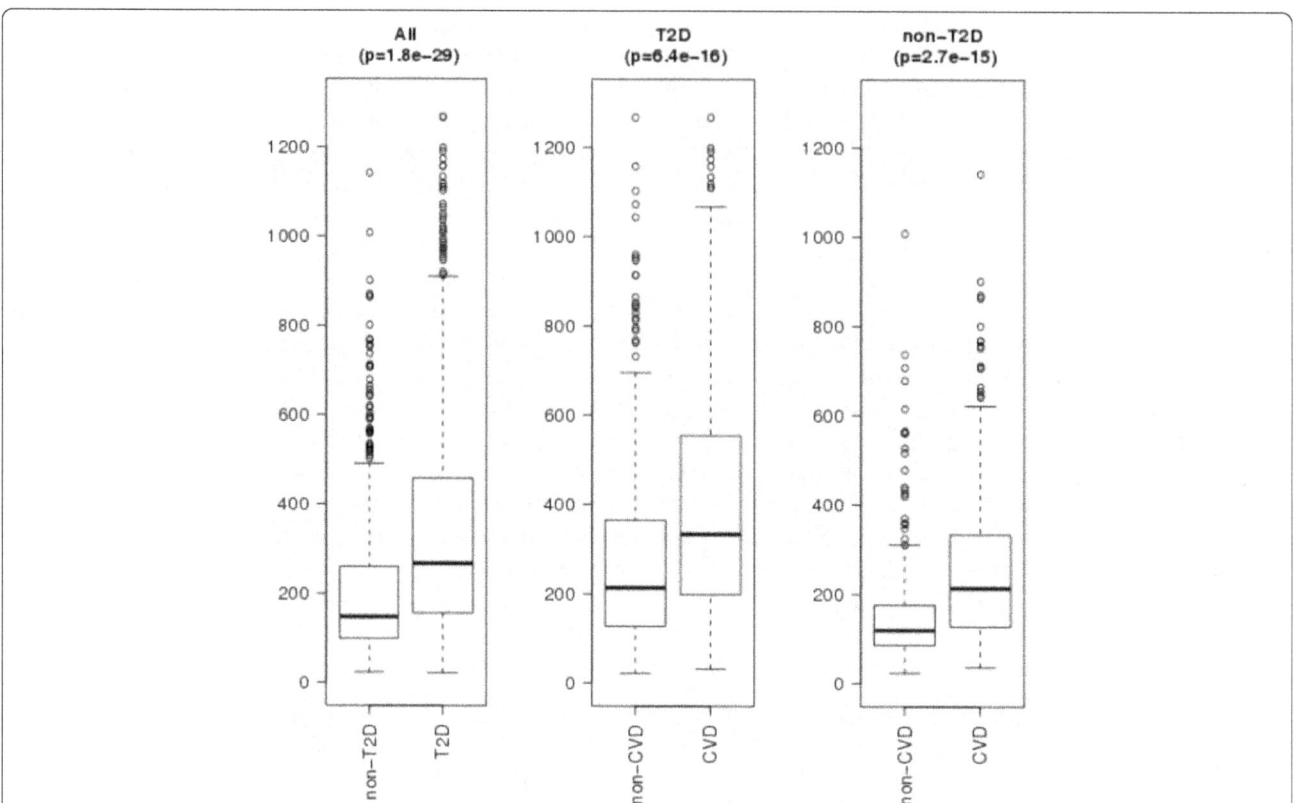

Fig. 1 Renin plasma levels in subjects with and without T2D and with and without CVD. Values are given as arbitrary units (linear scale). P-values were calculated using the Mann-Whitney U test

(RHI). Subjects with T2D had more severe carotid disease, increased arterial stiffness, and impaired endothelial function while there was no difference in ABPI between subjects with and without T2D (Table 4). Renin levels were significantly associated with the severity of atherosclerosis both in peripheral arteries and in the carotids. These associations were similar in subjects with and without T2D. Moreover, with the exception of the association between renin and CCA IMT in the non-T2D group they remained significant when adjusting for age, gender, total cholesterol, HDL, smoking and importantly also for systolic blood pressure (Table 5). There was a weak risk factor-independent relationship between high renin levels and a lower RHI among T2D subjects, but otherwise we found

no independent associations with arterial stiffness or endothelial dysfunction (Table 5).

Influence of RAAS inhibition

In an additional approach to explore the role of RAAS activation in vascular complications to T2D we analyzed if ongoing treatment with RAAS inhibitors (e.g. ACE inhibitors ARBs or renin inhibitors) was associated with any difference in markers of atherosclerosis, arterial stiffness and endothelial dysfunction. Subjects with or without prevalent CVD were analyzed separately since prevalent CVD has been shown to be associated with more severe vascular pathologies [17]. Seventy-seven percent of T2D subjects with prevalent CVD and 57 %

Table 2 Odds-ratios for CVD risk with increased plasma renin levels (log2 scale)

Covariates	All			T2D			Non-T2D		
	OR	(95 % CI)	p-value	OR	(95 % CI)	p-value	OR	(95 % CI)	p-value
Framingham (age, gender, total cholesterol, HDL, SBP, smoking)	1.37	(1.22–1.55)	9.5E-08	1.55	(1.34–1.80)	7.7E-09	1.45	(1.14–1.85)	3.0E-03
Framingham + eGFR	1.29	(1.14–1.45)	5.0E-05	1.42	(1.21–1.66)	1.2E-05	1.43	(1.12–1.83)	4.0E-03
Framingham + RAAS inhibitors	1.20	(1.06–1.36)	5.0E-03	1.41	(1.21–1.65)	1.3E-05	1.10	(0.84–1.44)	ns

P-values from separate logistic regression models adjusted for the individual components of the Framingham risk score and study center, and in addition for eGFR or RAAS inhibitors

SBP systolic blood pressure, *HDL* high-density lipoprotein, *eGFR* estimated glomerular filtration rate

Table 3 Pearson Correlations between plasma renin levels and factors related to CVD

	T2D		Non-T2D	
	r	p	r	p
Age	0.16 (0.10–0.23)	4.2E-07	0.26 (0.18–0.34)	2.5E-09
BMI	0.08 (0.01–0.14)	1.6E-02	0.19 (0.10–0.27)	2.0E-05
HbA1c	0.20 (0.14–0.26)	7.4E-10	0.25 (0.16–0.33)	3.3E-08
Systolic BP	−0.15 (−0.21–0.09)	4.0E-06	−0.04 (−0.13–0.05)	ns
HDL chol	−0.15 (−0.21–0.09)	4.8E-06	−0.21 (−0.29–0.12)	3.8E-06
LDL chol	−0.20 (−0.27–0.14)	8.4E-10	−0.28 (−0.36–0.19)	1.2E-09
Triglycerides	0.12 (0.06–0.19)	1.8E-04	0.09 (0.00–0.18)	5.0E-02
eGFR	−0.29 (−0.35–0.23)	<1.0E-16	−0.24 (−0.32–0.16)	6.9E-08
Plasma IL6	0.28 (0.22–0.33)	<1.0E-16	0.29 (0.21–0.37)	4.9E-11

BMI body mass index, *SBP* systolic blood pressure, *HDL* high-density lipoprotein, *LDL* low-density lipoprotein, *eGFR* estimated glomerular filtration rate

of the group with T2D subjects without prevalent CVD received treatment with any type of RAAS-inhibitor. Increased renin levels were observed in subjects treated with RAAS-inhibitors both in the CVD (median (IQR) 355 (231–584) versus 224 (151–377) AU) and non-CVD groups (271 (167–474) versus 167 (108–254) AU). No significant differences in ABPI, carotid IMT, carotid plaque area, PWV or RHI between T2D subjects with or without RAAS inhibitors (data not shown). In the non T2D subjects RAAS-inhibition was associated with increased plaque area in the CVD group and increased CCA IMT, carotid bulb IMT and PWV in the non-CVD group (Table 6).

To explore the possibility that the renin associations with CVD and atherosclerosis burden was explained by

Table 4 Differences in vascular changes between subjects with and without T2D

	T2D	Non-T2D	p-value
ABPI	1.16 (1.07, 1.25)	1.17 (1.08, 1.25)	ns
ABPI (right)	1.16 (1.07, 1.25)	1.17 (1.09, 1.25)	ns
ABPI (left)	1.16 (1.07, 1.25)	1.17 (1.08, 1.25)	ns
CCA IMT	0.91 (0.80, 1.04)	0.85 (0.75, 0.99)	5.1E-06
CCA IMT (right)	0.89 (0.77, 1.03)	0.84 (0.74, 0.97)	4.9E-05
CCA IMT (left)	0.91 (0.78, 1.06)	0.86 (0.74, 1.02)	5.9E-05
Bulb IMT	1.11 (0.93, 1.42)	1.05 (0.90, 1.30)	1.0E-03
Bulb IMT (right)	1.08 (0.90, 1.41)	1.01 (0.87, 1.30)	1.6E-03
Bulb IMT (left)	1.09 (0.92, 1.37)	1.05 (0.89, 1.28)	0.01
Plaque area	17.0 (10.7, 26.1)	15.6 (10.4, 22.6)	0.01
PWV	10.9 (9.3, 13.2)	9.6 (8.3, 11.4)	2.0E-16
RHI	2.01 (1.72, 2.48)	2.31 (1.90, 2.74)	4.1E-11

For each group the median is provided with the interquartile range, *p*-values from Mann-Whitney U-test

ns non significant, *ABPI* ankle brachial pressure index, *CCA* common carotid artery, *IMT* intima media thickness, *PWV* pulse wave velocity, *RHI* reactive hyperemia index

Table 5 Association between plasma renin levels and measures of atherosclerosis burden, arterial stiffness and endothelial function

		T2D	Non-T2D
ABPI	r	−0.19	−0.15
	95 % CI	(−0.26, −0.13)	(−0.23, −0.06)
	pCor	7.7E-09	0.001
	r2	0.14	0.20
	pReg	7.4E-09	0.006
CCA IMT	r	0.15	0.19
	95 % CI	(0.08, 0.21)	(0.10, 0.27)
	pCor	1.2E-05	4.7E-05
	r2	0.15	0.29
	pReg	0.015	ns
Bulb IMT	r	0.27	0.30
	95 % CI	(0.20, 0.33)	(0.21, 0.38)
	pCor	1.1E-14	1.8E-10
	r2	0.22	0.28
	pReg	8.7E-07	0.001
Plaque area	r	0.25	0.27
	95 % CI	(0.18, 0.32)	(0.17, 0.36)
	pCor	6.4E-12	1.4E-07
	r2	0.25	0.31
	pReg	3.3E-09	3.70E-05
PWV	r	0.08	0.18
	95 % CI	(0.01, 0.15)	(0.09, 0.27)
	pCor	0.029	1.2E-04
	r2	0.33	0.36
	pReg	ns	ns
RHI	r	−0.14	−0.14
	95 % CI	(−0.21, −0.08)	(−0.23, −0.05)
	pCor	1.8E-05	0.002
	r2	0.08	0.15
	pReg	0.025	ns

r Pearson correlation coefficient, *95 % CI* 95 % confidence interval for r, *pCor* p-value for correlation significance, *r2* proportion of variation explained by linear regression model adjusted for age, gender, total cholesterol, *HDL* systolic blood pressure, smoking, and study center, *pReg* p-value for significance of renin coefficient in this model; data of imaging variables has been log2-transformed to resemble normal distribution, *ABPI* ankle brachial pressure index, *CCA* common carotid artery, *IMT* intima media thickness, *PWV* pulse wave velocity, *RHI* reactive hyperemia index

a more frequent treatment with RAAS-inhibitors in subjects with more advanced disease we next analyzed subjects with and without RAAS-inhibitors separately. Subjects treated with renin inhibitors (n = 68) were excluded from these analyses as these do not have the same increasing effect on plasma renin as ACE inhibitors and ARBs. Moreover, since only 41 subjects in the non-CVD, non-T2D group were treated with ACE inhibitors

Table 6 Differences in vascular changes in non-T2D subjects without or without treatment with any type of RAAS inhibitor

Variable	No T2D with CVD					No T2D without CVD				
	Yes	No	MedianYes	MedianNo	p-value	Yes	No	MedianYes	MedianNo	p-value
ABPI	146	76	1.16 (1.08–1.25)	1.13 (1.02–1.23)	ns	49	196	1.17 (1.12–1.23)	1.17 (1.10–1.25)	ns
CCA IMT (mm)	147	73	0.88 (0.78–1.04)	0.88 (0.78–0.99)	ns	48	192	0.92 (0.82–1.03)	0.81 (0.72–0.96)	7.4E-04
Bulb IMT (mm)	132	66	1.20 (0.98–1.44)	1.07 (0.96–1.31)	ns	47	187	1.15 (0.99–1.38)	0.96 (0.84–1.15)	1.9E-04
Plaque area (mm^2)	128	67	18.5 (12.5–24.6)	13.58 (10.9–18.7)	0.004	40	134	15.8 (10.7–29.8)	13.2 (7.8–20.0)	ns
PWV (m/sec)	135	63	10.2 (8.3–11.8)	9.7 (8.5–11.8)	ns	46	189	9.8 (9.0–11.0)	9.2 (7.9–10.7)	0.025
RHI	158	77	2.2 (1.8–2.6)	2.3 (1.9–2.7)	ns	50	196	2.25 (1.88–2.48)	2.41 (2.00–2.81)	ns

Difference of imaging marker was assessed by Mann-Whitney U-test, medians are presented together with IQRs
ns not significant, ABPI ankle brachial pressure index, CCA common carotid artery, IMT intima media thickness, PWV pulse wave velocity, RHI reactive hyperemia index

and ARBs we restricted the analyses to the T2D group. In T2D subjects treated with RAAS inhibitors those with CVD ($n = 313$) had higher plasma renin than those without CVD ($n = 256$; 355 (231–584) versus 271 AU (167–465), $p = 9.2E-06$). Also in T2D subjects without RAAS inhibition higher renin levels was observed in the CVD group ($n = 150$) than in the non-CVD group ($n = 211$; 224 (151–377) versus 167 AU (108–253), $p = 3.3E-05$). The odds-ratio for CVD risk with increased plasma renin levels was 1.45 (95 % C.I. 1.19–1.76) for T2D subjects treated with RAAS inhibitors and 1.41 (95 % C.I. 1.04–1.93) for those not treated with RAAS inhibitors when controlling for age, gender, total cholesterol, HDL, systolic blood pressure, smoking and study center. The pattern of renin associations with measures of atherosclerosis burden, arterial stiffness and endothelial function were also similar in T2D subjects with or without treatment with RAAS inhibitors (Table 7). Taken together, these observations demonstrate that the renin associations with CVD and atherosclerosis burden observed in the present study is not due a more frequent treatment with RAAS-inhibitors in subjects with more advanced disease.

Plasma renin levels and atherosclerotic plaque structure
Since previous experimental data have shown that RAAS activation can stimulate inflammation, expression of fibrous proteins and smooth muscle cell growth we investigated if plasma levels of renin were related to atherosclerotic plaque content of these factors in a cohort of 205 carotid endarterectomy patients. The clinical characteristics of this cohort have been reported previously [19]. Weak but statistically significant associations were found between plasma renin levels and the plaque content of platelet-derived growth factor ($r = 0.14$, $p < 0.05$) and TNF-α ($r = -0.16$, $p < 0.05$), but there were no significant associations with plaque content of collagen, elastin, IL-6, monocyte chemotactic protein-1, vascular endothelial growth factor or immunostaining for macrophages or smooth muscle cells (data not shown). Renin levels in plaque homogenates were analyzed using the Proximity Extension Assay. There was a strong correlation between the levels of renin in plasma

and atherosclerotic plaque tissue ($r = 0.80$, $p = 1.0E-40$). However, with the exception of a trend for a correlation with the plaque content of platelet-derived growth factor ($r = 0.13$, $p = 0.07$) there were correlations between the plaque renin content and other plaque components.

Table 7 Associations between renin levels and measures of atherosclerosis burden, arterial stiffness and endothelial function

		T2D	
		RAASi	NoRAASi
ABPI	r	−0.19	−0.09
	pCor	1.6E-05	ns
	r2	0.14	0.16
	pReg	3.6E-04	ns
CCA IMT	r	0.14	0.13
	pCor	7.9E-04	0.021
	r2	0.15	0.20
	pReg	0.007	ns
Bulb IMT	r	0.26	0.29
	pCor	1.0E-08	9.40E-07
	r2	0.20	0.3
	pReg	3.3E-05	0.029
Plaque area	r	0.26	0.20
	pCor	7.7E-09	0.002
	r2	0.26	0.29
	pReg	3.2E-08	ns
PWV	r	0.02	0.09
	pCor	ns	ns
	r2	0.31	0.38
	pReg	ns	ns
RHI	r	−0.16	−0.15
	pCor	2.3E-04	0.007
	r2	0.09	0.11
	pReg	0.036	ns

r is Pearson correlation coefficient, and r2 is proportion of variation explained by a linear regression model adjusted for age, gender, total cholesterol HDL systolic BP, smoking, eGFR, IL6, and study center
RAASi RAAS inhibitor treatment

Discussion

There is evidence from clinical trials that treatment with RAAS inhibitors slows the onset of T2D and reduces the risk of renal complications in manifest T2D [20]. Moreover, experimental studies have shown that activation of RAAS stimulates processes known to be of importance for development of atherosclerosis including inflammation, oxidative stress, smooth muscle cell growth and fibrosis suggesting that it could play an important role also in the macrovascular complications associated with T2D [21]. The concept that RAAS promotes atherogenesis in diabetes has gained support from a few animal studies [11, 12], but evidence from randomized clinical trials of RAAS inhibitors with cardiovascular end points has been inconsistent [22]. Thus, the clinical importance of RAAS activation in the development of cardiovascular complications in T2D remains to be fully established. In the present study we investigated if RAAS activation, as assessed by circulating renin levels, was associated with the severity of vascular complications in T2D subjects with and without prevalent CVD. Our findings show that there is a significant association between circulating renin levels and atherosclerotic burden in the carotid and peripheral arteries in subjects with T2D and that these associations are independent of systolic blood pressure and other major cardiovascular risk factors. In accordance, T2D subjects with clinically manifest CVD were characterized by increased renin levels and this difference remained significant when adjusting for renal function, treatment with RAAS-inhibitors and cardiovascular risk factors including systolic blood pressure. Collectively these observations are well in line with the proposed role for RAAS activation in cardiovascular complications in T2D. Notably, plasma renin levels were elevated also in non-T2D subjects with prevalent CVD and demonstrated significant associations with markers of atherosclerosis also in this group. Moreover, renin levels were found to link with factors characteristic for T2D, such as HBA1c, BMI and low HDL, also among subjects without T2D. However, renin levels were lower in subjects without T2D and the vascular changes were less pronounced. These observations are in line with previous findings that insulin resistance stimulates the expression of renin and that this may contribute to a more severe progression of atherosclerosis in T2D [1, 2, 5].

In spite of the association between renin and markers of atherosclerotic burden we found no evidence for reduced atherosclerosis in subjects treated with RAAS-inhibitors. There are several possible explanations to this finding. First, it cannot be excluded that RAAS activation has no direct effect on atherosclerosis development in humans and that the association between renin and disease severity observed here is caused by association of renin with another atherogenic factor. However, the fact that renin remained significantly associated to atherosclerotic burden when adjusting for other cardiovascular risk factors, as well as renal function argues against this. Second, it could be that vascular changes caused by increased RAAS activation over many years are not easily reversible by providing RAAS inhibition in different time-frames. Third, it is possible that RAAS inhibition when given alone may be sufficient to reduce or inhibit the progression of disease but when co-administered with other potent anti-atherogenic drugs, such as statins, the effect of RAAS inhibition may become too small to be of clinical significance. In line with the latter possibility treatment with ACE-inhibition reduced myocardial events in the HOPE study in which only about 20 % received lipid-lowering therapy [14] while no significant effect of ACE-inhibition on major coronary events could be observed in the ADVANCE trial in which about 50 % received lipid-lowering therapy [23]. Unexpectedly, RAAS-inhibition was associated with more severe carotid atherosclerosis in non-T2D subjects. The reason for this association remains to be elucidated but it does not support the existence of an anti-atherogenic effect of RAAS inhibitors.

Experimental studies have shown that angiotensin II induces vascular oxidative stress leading to decreased endothelial relaxation and endothelial dysfunction [24]. In accordance with these findings we observed an inverse correlation between plasma renin and the RHI in the present study. However, no differences were observed in RHI between subjects with or without RAAS-inhibition. Angiotensin II has also been shown to affect processes involved in atherosclerotic plaque development and stability. Increased expression of adhesion molecules and pro-inflammatory cytokines including monocyte chemotactic protein-1 and IL-6 has been reported in monocytes, smooth muscle cells and endothelial cells exposed to angiotensin II [25–28]. Additionally, angiotensin II has been shown to stimulate smooth muscle cell growth and collagen production [10, 29, 30]. In the present study we found no or only weak associations between plasma renin and the expression of pro-inflammatory cytokines, fibrous proteins and smooth muscle cells in atherosclerotic plaques obtained from carotid endarterectomy patients. Taken together these findings suggest that RAAS activation does not significantly affect plaque composition and vulnerability. However, since the experimental data show that angiotensin II stimulates both inflammatory and repair processes it is possible that it may contribute to plaque development without affecting the balance between individual plaque components. It is also possible that local RAAS activation is of more importance for these processes than systemic RAAS activation.

There are some limitations of the present study that should be considered. Most importantly, the observational design of the study does not allow for conclusions regarding cause and effect relations. Thus, our findings do not provide clinical evidence for an atherogenic role of renin and RAAS activation. They are, however, well in line with experimental data suggesting that RAAS activation exuberate several biological processes involved in plaque development. The finding that treatment with RAAS-inhibitors does not affect atherosclerosis severity also needs to be interpreted with caution since this is an observational study and information regarding length of treatment is unfortunately lacking. Another important limitation is that RAAS activation was only assessed indirectly through analysis of renin levels.

Conclusions

Our findings provide clinical evidence for an association between RAAS activation and atherosclerotic burden both in subjects with and without T2D. Plasma renin and atherosclerosis are concomitantly increased in subjects with T2D as compared to age and sex-matched subjects without T2D suggesting that these associations may be of particular importance in vascular complication of diabetes. Importantly, the association between renin and atherosclerotic burden was independent of blood pressure and other major cardiovascular risk factors suggesting involvement of a direct effect of RAAS activation on the vascular wall. However, our findings also suggest that treatment with RAAS inhibitors may have limited effectiveness in counteracting the atherogenic effects of RAAS activation.

Acknowledgements
We are grateful to Ana Persson, Mihaela Nitulescu and Lena Sundius for expert technical assistance. The research was supported by the National Institute for Health Research (NIHR) Exeter Clinical Research Facility. The views expressed are those of the authors and not necessarily those of the NHS, the NIHR or the Department of Health, England.

Funding
Innovative Medicines Initiative (the SUMMIT consortium, IMI-2008/115006, the Swedish Heart-Lung Foundation, the Swedish Research Council and Marianne and Marcus Wallenberg Foundation).

Authors' contributions
IG and JN designed the study, analyzed data and wrote the first version of the manuscript. ACS, MHC, AN, CP, GÖ, LMG and MP contributed to the design of the study, developed technical protocols, performed analyses on patients and made critical revision of the manuscript. AE, GNF, HB, MW, EB, KA, CK, FC, KG, PG, FK, HCL, FA, JB, SP, EV and MK contributed to the development of the technical protocols, performed analyses on patients and made critical revision of the manuscript. VS performed the statistical analyses and made critical revision of the manuscript. All authors read and approved the final manuscript.

Competing interests
The authors declare that they have no competing interests.

Author details
[1]Department of Clinical Sciences Malmö, Lund University, Malmö, Sweden. [2]Medical Research Institute, University of Dundee, Dundee, UK. [3]Diabetes and Vascular Medicine, NIHR Exeter Clinical Research Facility and University of Exeter Medical School, Exeter, UK. [4]Department of Surgical, Medical, Molecular Pathology, and Critical Area Medicine, Pisa, Italy. [5]Department of Clinical and Experimental Medicine, University of Pisa, Pisa, Italy. [6]AstraZeneca, Cardiovascular and Metabolic Diseases, Mölndal, Sweden.

References
1. Gray SP, Jandeleit-Dahm K. The pathobiology of diabetic vascular complications–cardiovascular and kidney disease. J Mol Med. 2014;92(5):441–52.
2. Abuissa H, O'Keefe Jr J. The role of renin-angiotensin-aldosterone system-based therapy in diabetes prevention and cardiovascular and renal protection. Diabetes Obes Metab. 2008;10(12):1157–66.
3. Schutta MH. Diabetes and hypertension: epidemiology of the relationship and pathophysiology of factors associated with these comorbid conditions. J Cardiometab Syndr. 2007;2(2):124–30.
4. Frederich Jr RC, Kahn BB, Peach MJ, Flier JS. Tissue-specific nutritional regulation of angiotensinogen in adipose tissue. Hypertension. 1992;19(4):339–44.
5. Watanabe K, Sekiya M, Tsuruoka T, Funada J, Kameoka H, Miyagawa M, Kohara K. Relationship between insulin resistance and cardiac sympathetic nervous function in essential hypertension. J Hypertens. 1999;17(8):1161–8.
6. Batenburg WW, Danser AH. (Pro)renin and its receptors: pathophysiological implications. Clin Sci (Lond). 2012;123(3):121–33.
7. Te Riet L, van Esch JH, Roks AJ, van den Meiracker AH, Danser AH. Hypertension: renin-angiotensin-aldosterone system alterations. Circ Res. 2015;116(6):960–75.
8. Esteban V, Lorenzo O, Ruperez M, Suzuki Y, Mezzano S, Blanco J, Kretzler M, Sugaya T, Egido J, Ruiz-Ortega M. Angiotensin II, via AT1 and AT2 receptors and NF-kappaB pathway, regulates the inflammatory response in unilateral ureteral obstruction. J Am Soc Nephrol. 2004;15(6):1514–29.
9. Li XC, Zhuo JL. Intracellular ANG II directly induces in vitro transcription of TGF-beta1, MCP-1, and NHE-3 mRNAs in isolated rat renal cortical nuclei via activation of nuclear AT1a receptors. Am J Physiol Cell Physiol. 2008;294(4):C1034–45.
10. Gibbons GH, Pratt RE, Dzau VJ. Vascular smooth muscle cell hypertrophy vs. hyperplasia. Autocrine transforming growth factor-beta 1 expression determines growth response to angiotensin II. J Clin Invest. 1992;90(2):456–61.
11. Koitka A, Cao Z, Koh P, Watson AM, Sourris KC, Loufrani L, Soro-Paavonen A, Walther T, Woollard KJ, Jandeleit-Dahm KA, et al. Angiotensin II subtype 2 receptor blockade and deficiency attenuate the development of atherosclerosis in an apolipoprotein E-deficient mouse model of diabetes. Diabetologia. 2010;53(3):584–92.
12. Candido R, Jandeleit-Dahm KA, Cao Z, Nesteroff SP, Burns WC, Twigg SM, Dilley RJ, Cooper ME, Allen TJ. Prevention of accelerated atherosclerosis by angiotensin-converting enzyme inhibition in diabetic apolipoprotein E-deficient mice. Circulation. 2002;106(2):246–53.
13. Hansson GK. Inflammation, atherosclerosis, and coronary artery disease. N Engl J Med. 2005;352(16):1685–95.
14. Effects of ramipril on cardiovascular and microvascular outcomes in people with diabetes mellitus: results of the HOPE study and MICRO-HOPE substudy. Heart Outcomes Prevention Evaluation Study Investigators. Lancet. 2000; 355(9200):253–59.
15. Tatti P, Pahor M, Byington RP, Di Mauro P, Guarisco R, Strollo G, Strollo F. Outcome results of the Fosinopril Versus Amlodipine Cardiovascular Events Randomized Trial (FACET) in patients with hypertension and NIDDM. Diabetes Care. 1998;21(4):597–603.
16. Niskanen L, Hedner T, Hansson L, Lanke J, Niklason A, Group CS. Reduced cardiovascular morbidity and mortality in hypertensive diabetic patients on first-line therapy with an ACE inhibitor compared with a diuretic/beta-blocker-based treatment regimen: a subanalysis of the Captopril Prevention Project. Diabetes Care. 2001;24(12):2091–6.
17. Shore AC, Colhoun HM, Natali A, Palombo C, Ostling G, Aizawa K, Kennback C, Casanova F, Persson M, Gooding K, et al. Measures of atherosclerotic burden are associated with clinically manifest cardiovascular disease in type 2 diabetes: a European cross-sectional study. J Intern Med. 2015;278(3):291–302.

18. Goncalves I, Moses J, Dias N, Pedro LM, Fernandes e Fernandes J, Nilsson J, Ares MP. Changes related to age and cerebrovascular symptoms in the extracellular matrix of human carotid plaques. Stroke. 2003;34(3):616–22.

19. Edsfeldt A, Goncalves I, Grufman H, Nitulescu M, Duner P, Bengtsson E, Mollet IG, Persson A, Nilsson M, Orho-Melander M, et al. Impaired fibrous repair: a possible contributor to atherosclerotic plaque vulnerability in patients with type II diabetes. Arterioscler Thromb Vasc Biol. 2014;34(9):2143–50.

20. Abuissa H, Jones PG, Marso SP, O'Keefe Jr JH. Angiotensin-converting enzyme inhibitors or angiotensin receptor blockers for prevention of type 2 diabetes: a meta-analysis of randomized clinical trials. J Am Coll Cardiol. 2005;46(5):821–6.

21. Patel BM, Mehta AA. Aldosterone and angiotensin: role in diabetes and cardiovascular diseases. Eur J Pharmacol. 2012;697(1–3):1–12.

22. Hao G, Wang Z, Guo R, Chen Z, Wang X, Zhang L, Li W. Effects of ACEI/ARB in hypertensive patients with type 2 diabetes mellitus: a meta-analysis of randomized controlled studies. BMC Cardiovasc Disord. 2014;14:148.

23. Patel A, Group AC, MacMahon S, Chalmers J, Neal B, Woodward M, Billot L, Harrap S, Poulter N, Marre M, et al. Effects of a fixed combination of perindopril and indapamide on macrovascular and microvascular outcomes in patients with type 2 diabetes mellitus (the ADVANCE trial): a randomised controlled trial. Lancet. 2007;370(9590):829–40.

24. Rajagopalan S, Kurz S, Munzel T, Tarpey M, Freeman BA, Griendling KK, Harrison DG. Angiotensin II-mediated hypertension in the rat increases vascular superoxide production via membrane NADH/NADPH oxidase activation. Contribution to alterations of vasomotor tone. J Clin Invest. 1996;97(8):1916–23.

25. Ruiz-Ortega M, Lorenzo O, Ruperez M, Konig S, Wittig B, Egido J. Angiotensin II activates nuclear transcription factor kappaB through AT(1) and AT(2) in vascular smooth muscle cells: molecular mechanisms. Circ Res. 2000;86(12):1266–72.

26. Schieffer B, Schieffer E, Hilfiker-Kleiner D, Hilfiker A, Kovanen PT, Kaartinen M, Nussberger J, Harringer W, Drexler H. Expression of angiotensin II and interleukin 6 in human coronary atherosclerotic plaques: potential implications for inflammation and plaque instability. Circulation. 2000;101(12):1372–8.

27. Chen XL, Tummala PE, Olbrych MT, Alexander RW, Medford RM. Angiotensin II induces monocyte chemoattractant protein-1 gene expression in rat vascular smooth muscle cells. Circ Res. 1998;83(9):952–9.

28. Kranzhofer R, Schmidt J, Pfeiffer CA, Hagl S, Libby P, Kubler W. Angiotensin induces inflammatory activation of human vascular smooth muscle cells. Arterioscler Thromb Vasc Biol. 1999;19(7):1623–9.

29. Kim S, Izumi Y, Yano M, Hamaguchi A, Miura K, Yamanaka S, Miyazaki H, Iwao H. Angiotensin blockade inhibits activation of mitogen-activated protein kinases in rat balloon-injured artery. Circulation. 1998;97(17):1731–7.

30. Kato H, Suzuki H, Tajima S, Ogata Y, Tominaga T, Sato A, Saruta T. Angiotensin II stimulates collagen synthesis in cultured vascular smooth muscle cells. J Hypertens. 1991;9(1):17–22.

15

Association of Gestational Diabetes Mellitus (GDM) with subclinical atherosclerosis

Jing-Wei Li, Si-Yi He, Peng Liu, Lin Luo, Liang Zhao and Ying-Bin Xiao[*]

Abstract

Background: Gestational diabetes mellitus (GDM) is associated with an elevated risk of adverse health outcomes such as type 2 diabetes and cardiovascular diseases. Carotid intima-media thickness (cIMT) is increasingly used as a noninvasive marker for subclinical atherosclerosis. Whether there is a direct correlation between GDM and elevated cIMT is still controversial.

Methods: PubMed, Embase and reference lists of relevant papers were reviewed. Studies assessing the relationship between GDM and cIMT were included. Weighted Mean Difference (WMD) of cIMT was calculated using random-effect models.

Results: Fifteen studies with a total of 2247 subjects were included in our analysis, giving a pooled WMD of 0.05 (95% confidence interval [CI] 0.03 –0.07). Furthermore, meta regression and subgroup analysis found that the association between GDM and larger cIMT already existed during pregnancy, and this relation was stronger in obese GDM patients.

Conclusions: GDM in and after pregnancy is associated with subclinical atherosclerosis. Weight control may be helpful to prevent cardiovascular diseases for GDM patients.

Keywords: Gestational diabetes mellitus, Carotid intima-media thickness, Atherosclerosis

Background

Gestational diabetes mellitus (GDM) is one of the common complications during pregnancy, which incidence is approximately 5% (range from 1 to 14%) and this number is increasing due to increased prevalence of obesity [1]. GDM women have an increased risk for type 2 diabetes mellitus, cardiovascular disease and metabolic syndrome years after pregnancy, also offspring of GDM women have a higher risk for noncommunicable diseases and obesity rates [2].

Carotid intima-media thickness (cIMT) is measurement of the combined thickness of the intimal and medial layers of the carotid artery by B-mode ultrasound. cIMT is a noninvasive technique to dectect subclinical atheroscler-

osis [3], and is associated with multiple cardiovascular risk factors [4], cardiovascular events [5] and coronary artery diseases [6].

As GDM alone is independent predictors of obstructive coronary artery disease [7] and cardiovascular diseases. We suspect whether there is a direct correlation between GDM and elevated cIMT. However, studies focusing on this issue have been small and have reported conflicting results. Therefore, we conducted a meta-analysis to assess the correlation between GDM and cIMT.

Methods

Literature search

We searched the databases of EMBASE and PubMed and references lists of relevant papers to MAY 24, 2014. EMBASE search terms were 'pregnancy diabetes mellitus'/exp and 'arterial wall thickness'/exp. Similar search terms were used for PubMed. The search strategy

* Correspondence: xiaoyb@vip.sina.com
Institute of Cardiovascular Surgery, PLA, Xinqiao Hospital, Third Military Medical University, No. 183 Xinqiao Street, Chongqing 400037, PR China

(Additional file 1) has been put into the supplemental material. No language and time limitation was performed.

Study selection

We selected published trials that investigated the relationship between gestational diabetes and cIMT. Excluded were (1) studies published as conference articles; (2) cIMT was not measured in both gestational diabetes and control groups; and (3) reports having duplicate study population. All literature searches were independently reviewed by 2 authors (JW L and SY H) to identify relevant trials that met the inclusion criteria. Disparities were adjudicated by a third author (YB X). For each included article, study characteristics, including authors, publication year, country, ages, duration, BMI, mean and standard deviation of CIMT were extracted independently by two researchers (JW L and SY H). If the studies were studying the same population, we included the newer and completed ones in this meta-analysis.

Statistical analysis

The cIMT in both gestational diabetes and control groups were induced to our meta-analysis. Statistical heterogeneity between studies was tested by Cochran's test (P < 0.05). We used the random-effect model in this meta-analysis, which takes into account heterogeneity among studies, because the study design and measuring time were different across studies. The Cochrane Q test and I^2 was used to evaluate the presence of heterogeneity. If heterogeneity exists, subgroup analyses were conducted to evaluate effect modification by study-level characteristics including publish year, number of patients, ages at pregnancy, measuring time (in pregnancy or after pregnancy), BMI and duration. Publication bias was assessed with Egger's test. All statistical significance was set at a p value of 0.05, and CIs were calculated at the 95% level. Statistical analyses were performed with Stata software (version 11.0; Stata Corporation, College Station, TX).

Results

Search results and study characteristics

A total of 67 articles were identified in a combined search of PubMed and EMBASE. We also manually searched studies cited in previous reviews and of references list from retrieved articles. First 27 duplicates were removed, and then 18 articles were initially excluded through screening title and abstract. Among the 23 articles retrieved for further review of the full text, 6 were excluded for repeated reports, 1 for not reporting cIMT outcomes, and 1 study for conference reports. Akinci B and his colleagues investigated the association between GDM and CVD from different aspects and published five articles using the same population [1,8-11]. Mehmet Vural and his colleagues [12] studied the same population with Mehmet Ali Eren [13]. Eventually, 15 studies with a total of 2247 subjects were included in our meta-analysis (Figure 1) [11,13-26]. Study characteristics and exclusion criteria included in the analysis are shown in Table 1. Only the study of Gunderson [19] was evalauted at multivariate

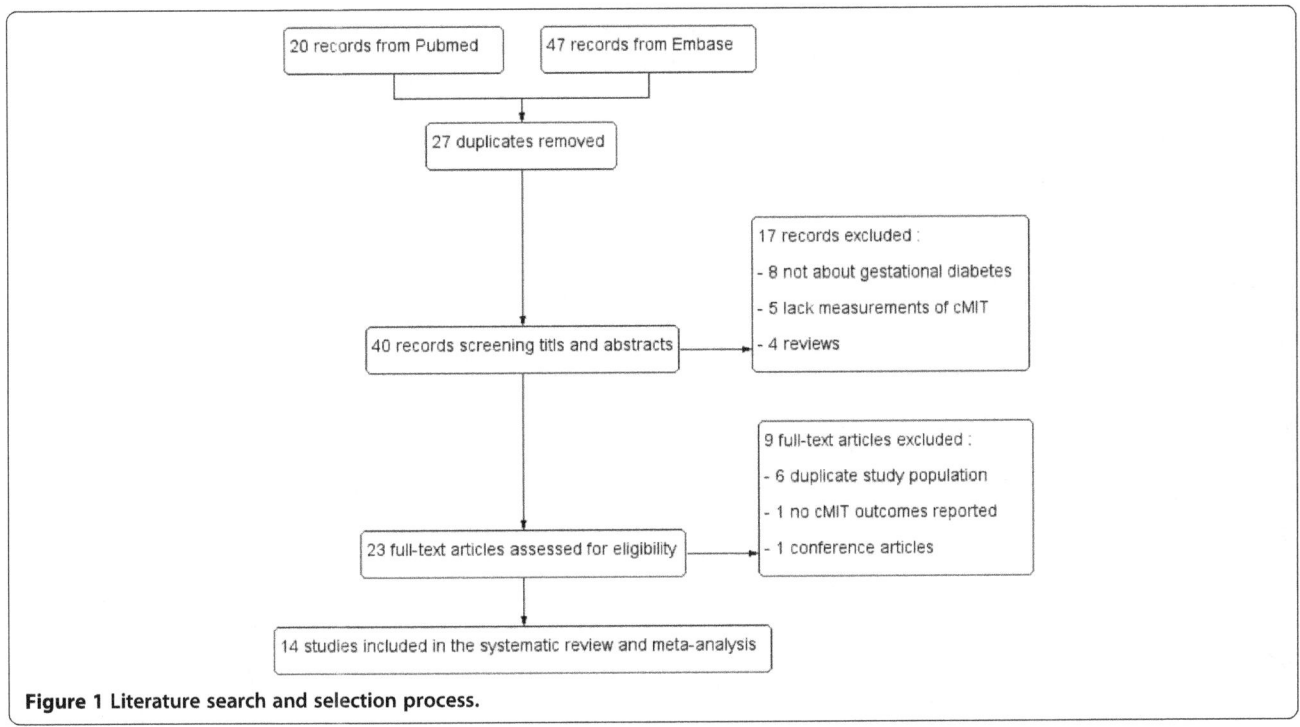

Figure 1 Literature search and selection process.

Table 1 Study characteristics of included studies

Author	Age	No. patient	Country	Duration(year)	BMI GDM	BMI CG	Waist GDM	Waist CG	Exclusion:
Baris Akinci [11]	35.1	190	Turkey	3.39	26.82 ± 4.25	26.5 ± 2.66	90.31 ± 11.68	87.45 ± 8.93	known cardiovascular disorders, type 1 or type 2 diabetes (diagnosed before the index pregnancy), familial hyperlipidemia, hypertension, acute infection, chronic inflammatory disease, coagulation disorders and other systemic diseases, on peri- or postmenopausal period at the time of sampling
A.E. Atay [14]	27.9	75	Turkey	2.29	32.2 ± 4.8	27.3 ± 4.2			receiving any medication during the last 3 months, with liver or renal dysfunction, hyperprolactinemia, or thyroid disease and smokers, with GDM and healthy pregnant women with a history of GDM in their previous pregnancies or glucose tolerance before the present pregnancy, healthy pregnant women with a family history of DM
S. Bo [15]	41.1	195	Italy	6.5	Group 1: 20.2 ± 2.2 Group 2: 23.6 ± 5.2	22.1 ± 3.1	Group 1: 73.6 ± 5.7 Group 2: 86.4 ± 13.5	79.9 ± 9.9	known pre-pregnancy conditions, such as diabetes mellitus, diseases affecting glucose metabolism, hypertension, chronic illness, and medical treatments (including hormonal preparations), presence of a positive OGCT, but an OGTT not diagnostic for GDM.
Mustafa Caliskan [16]	33.4	95	Turkey	6	26.9 ± 3.9	26.1 ± 2.7	85.0 ± 5.9	84.4 ± 4.9	presence of a valvular or congenital heart disease; cardiac rhythm other than sinus; previous myocardial infarction; hypo- or hyperthyroidism; chronic obstructive pulmonary disease or corulmonale; systemic diseases (etc. hemologic, hepatic, and renal diseases) or any disease that could impair coronaryflow reserve; hypertrophic cardiomyopathy; family history of coronary artery disease; excessive alcohol consumption (>120 g/day); previous lipid metabolism disorders; history of dyslipidemia; smoking; and diabetes mellitus.those with ST segment or T-wave changes specific for myocardial ischemia, Q-waves, and incidental left bundle branch block on ECG
Mehmet Ali Eren [13]	31	64	Turkey	0	31.8 ± 5.5	29.4 ± 5.4			smoking, alcohol abuse, preeclampsia, multiple pregnancies, pregestational diabetes for all study participants, and a family history of diabetes mellitus (for the control group only), pregnancies with GDM who had overt diabetes with 75-g standard OGTT in the 6-week after delivery
Hossein Fakhrzadeh [17]	33	40	Iran	4	27.63 ± 3.52	27.33 ± 5.64			current or previous smokers, patients who had pre-existing HTN, diabetes mellitus (DM), and women with symptomatic CVD
Claudia Maria Vilas Freire [18]	35.7	139	Brazil	2.7	29.01 ± 0.66	22.46 ± 0.42	92.09 ± 1.63	74.08 ± 1.14	any past condition afflicting them at previous pregnancies, other than GDM, was considered an exclusion criteria, especially those requiring hospital admission such as preeclampsia. alcoholism, drug addiction, uremia as well as those with liver, psychiatric, rheumatologic, and thyroid diseases or in use of corticosteroids

Table 1 Study characteristics of included studies (*Continued*)

Study			Country						Notes / Exclusion criteria
Erica P. Gunderson [19]	44.2	898	USA	20	24.8 (5.6)	23.3 (4.3)	74.4 (11.1)	71.7 (8.8)	heart disease or diabetes before pregnancies andthose without any post-baseline births,missing ccIMT measurements, and with history of heart disease,recently or currently pregnant, and with previous hysterectomy at baseline, with clinically relevant diabetes at baseline and those who developed diabetes before the first post-baseline birth
H Ijas [20]	52.2	116	Finland	19	27.1 ± 5.3	24.5 ± 4.2	94.4 ± 14.9	94.4 ± 14.2	GDM diagnosed in their subsequent pregnancy
Ufuk Ozuguz [22]	30.1	101	Turkey	0	29.95 ± 4.21	26.34 ± 4.08			previously knowndiagnosis of diabetes mellitus; the presence of an additional cardiovascular risk factor such as hypertension, hyperlipidemia or coronary artery disease; presence of other factors that may affect serum lipid profile and/or hsCRP level (acetylsalicylic acid, smoking, impaired liver and kidney functions, history of trauma, an acute infection within one month prior to presentation or a chronic infection); presence of an underlying chronic inflammatory condition such as collagen tissue and inflammatory bowel diseases.
E. TARIM [23]	29.4	70	Turkey	0	28.65 ± 4.75	27.17 ± 2.90			smokers, patients who had folic acid and vitamin B12 deficiency, hypertension, multiple pregnancy, fetal abnormalities, pre-existing hypertension and diabetes, thyroid disease or a history of significant severe diseases, family history of coronary heart disease and stroke
I Vastagh [24]	32.2	42	Hungary	0	28 ± 4	27 ± 4			have a history of diabetes mellitus or a previous GDM.
Gholamreza Yousefzadeh [26]	24.8	50	Iran	0	28.7 ± 4.5	26.5 ± 4.5			family history of cardiovascular disorders; history of hypertension; anti-hypertensive and cholesterol medication use; hyperlipidemia; overt diabetes or fasting plasma glucose (FPG) > 125 mg/dl;chronic renal or hepatic diseases; malignancies; recent hormonal medications; cigarette smoking; severe obesity (body mass index [BMI] >35 kg/m2); and history of infertility or polycystic ovarian disease, with the status of plaques/shadowing (> 1.0 mm) at any carotid site
Volpe, L. [25]	36.3	52	Italy	2	25.7 ± 8.9	23 ± 3.4	86.9 ± 9.7	79.6 ± 9.7	not mentioned
Yun Hyi Ku [21]	32.3	120	Korea	1	22.3 (20.4-24.2)	20.4 (19.5-23.1)	80.3 ± 7.7	74.5 ± 7.7	females who were diagnosed with gestational diabetes between the 24th and 28th week of pregnancy

analysis (adjusted for age, race, parity, pre-pregnancy BMI, HOMA-IR, weight gain, year 20-HOMA-IR + DBP, incident diabetes and metabolic syndrome), other studies used unadjusted data. Other characteristics of included studies have been put into the supplemental material (Additional file 2).

GDM is associated with cIMT

The cIMT from both GDM and control groups was pooled. The WMD was 0.05 (95% CI: 0.03–0.07, P < 0.001). The statistic value I^2 was 92.5%, P < 0.001 (Figure 2). No significant publication bias was found for WMD by Begg's test (P = 0.621) (Figure 3). We performed meta-regression analyses on cIMT to investigate the cause of heterogeneity, and found the BMI may be one of the main causes (P = 0.048, Table 2). Subgroup analysis was performed to distinguish the heterogeneity among these studies. Results showed that study object with higher BMI got larger cIMT (WMD: 0.07, 95% CI: 0.03–0.12 for those with BMI > 27.6 and WMD: 0.04, 95% CI: 0.02–0.06 for those with BMI < 27.6). Diagnostic criteria of GDM

might influence the results (WMD: 0.08, 95% CI: 0.05–0.11 for Carpenter and Coustan criteria, WMD: 0.03, 95% CI: –0.01–0.07 for NDDG criteria, WMD: 0.04, 95% CI: –0.01–0.09 for WHO criteria and WMD: 0.01, 95% CI: –0.06–0.07 for ADA 75 g criteria). There seemed no difference as to measuring time of cIMT with GDM (WMD: 0.07, 95% CI: 0.03–0.10 when measured in pregnancy and WMD: 0.05, 95% CI: 0.03–0.07 when measured years after pregnancy) and ages at pregnancy (WMD: 0.07, 95% CI: 0.03–0.11 for those with age < 31 and WMD: 0.04, 95% CI: 0.02–0.07 for those with age > =31). The GDM did not significantly increase cIMT as to publish year (WMD: 0.07, 95% CI: 0.03–0.10 for those published after 2013 and WMD: 0.05, 95% CI: 0.02–0.08 for those before 2013), number of patients (WMD: 0.06, 95% CI: 0.03–0.08 for number of patients above 90 and WMD: 0.05, 95% CI: 0.02–0.07 for number of patients below 90) and duration between the time of GDM diagnosed and cIMT measured (WMD: 0.05, 95% CI: 0.01–0.09 for duration > 4 and WMD: 0.05, 95% CI: 0.01–0.09 for duration between 0 and 4) (Table 3).

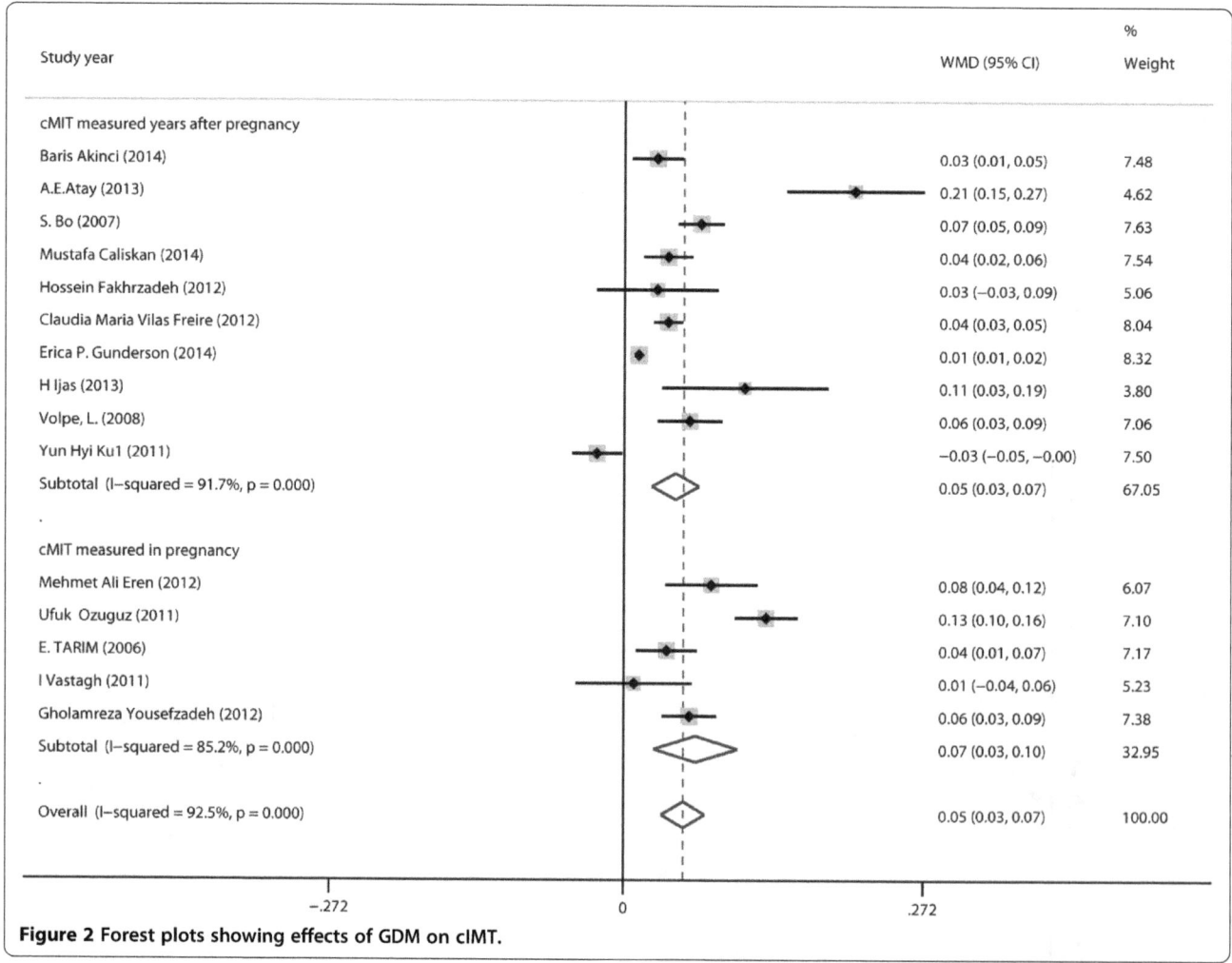

Figure 2 Forest plots showing effects of GDM on cIMT.

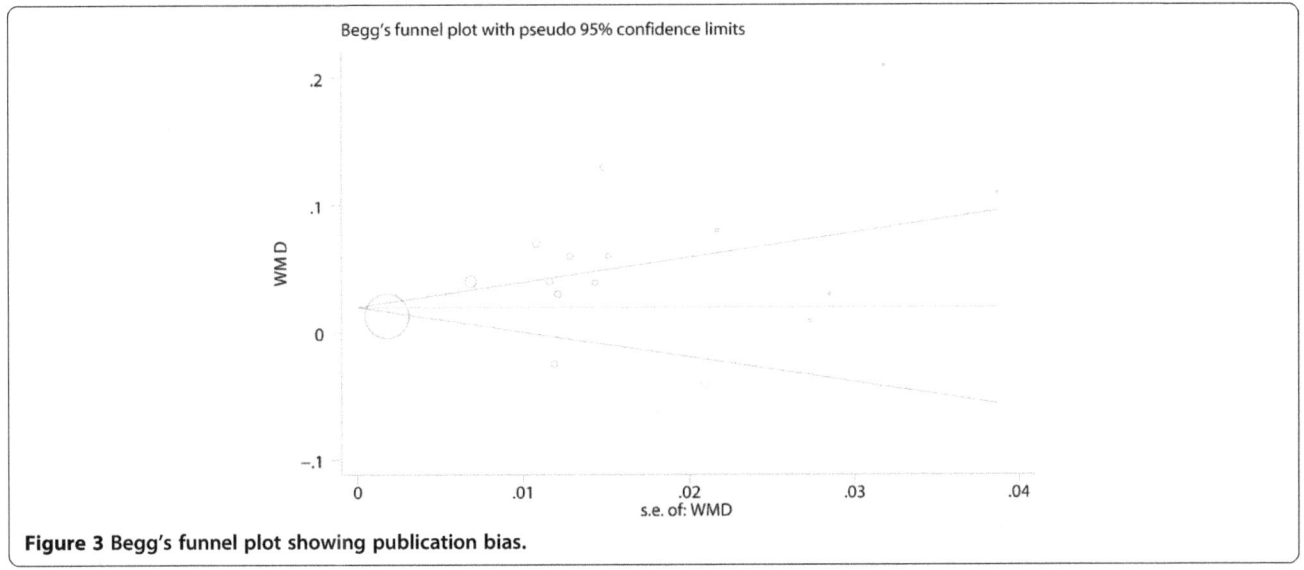

Figure 3 Begg's funnel plot showing publication bias.

Discussion

During pregnancy, insulin resistance increases. In healthy women compensatory insulin secretion counteracts this demand, while in GDM patients, not enough insulin is secreted to overcome the insulin demand. Compared with healthy ones, GDM patients are more likely to have type 2 diabetes and endothelial dysfunction, known conditions that leads to higher risk for cardiovascular diseases [27].

The results from our systematic review and meta-analyses indicate GDM was significantly associated with elevated cIMT, and this association already exists at the time of pregnancy. Fatty women with GDM seem to have larger cIMT.

Most of our included studies have found GDM is associated with larger cIMT. The study by A.E. Atay et al. [14] was the one finding the most significant difference of cIMT between GDM patients and control. The study population included in this study was fatter (BMI: 32.2 ± 4.8 for the GDM group vs 27.3 ± 4.2 for the control). Earlier study has found that obese patients with GDM

Table 2 Results of meta regression of GDM on cIMT

Item	Coef	P	95% CI	
Publish year	.0005284	0.930	-.0121875	.0132443
Age at pregnancy	-.0017171	0.704	-.0112528	.0078185
No. Patients	-.0000597	0.372	-.0001991	.0000797
BMI of GDM	.0100715	0.048	.0001263	.0200168
Measuring time	.013057	0.676	-.0529943	.0791082
Duration	-.0005414	0.823	-.0056708	.0045881
GDM Criteria	-.0234964	0.062	-.0484176	.0014249

Coef = regression coefficients.
CIs = confidence intervals.

had higher prevalence of chronic hypertension [28] and cardiovascular disease [29]. Our meta-regression and subgroup analyses confirms that the association between GDM and cIMT is influenced by BMI. The study of H Ijas et al. [20] showed that GDM patients with BMI > 25 had larger cIMT compared with those with BMI < 25 and controls. Also Gunderson and his colleagues [19] has found the association between GDM and cIMT changed from significance to insignificance after adjusting BMI. The study by Yun Hyi Ku [21] found there was no association between GDM and cIMT. As this study was conducted in Korea, the author compared their results with western ones and inferred it may be caused by culturally-based obesity. The author explained that as obesity was one of the major factor influencing cIMT, obesity is much less common in their country than in western ones (BMI of study objects were in normal range), which may lead to insignificance of their results. Contrary to these findings, the study of S. Bo et al. [15] found that GDM patients with BMI ≥ 25 had smaller cIMT that those with BMI < 25. This study regarded both BMI and metabolic syndrome as grouping criteria and BMI < 25 group also had no components of the metabolic syndrome. Metabolic syndrome may abolish this connection in this study.

We find that the diagnostic criteria of GDM may influence the impact of GDM on cIMT. Diagnosis of gestational diabetes significantly changed on the basis of the diagnostic criteria used, and influenced clinical outcomes [30,31]. However, too few studies included in NDDG, WHO, ADA 75 g subgroups. In fact the NDDG criteria indicate more severe GDM than Carpenter-Coustan one. But we got no statistically different result in NDDG subgroup analysis, while a statistically different one in Carpenter-Coustan subgroup. The heterogeneity

Table 3 Stratified analyses of GDM on cIMT

Item	Subgroup	No	WMD	95% CI		P. Het	I²	P. test
Publish year	>= 2013	5	0.07	0.03	0.10	<0.001	92.2	0.001
	<2013	10	0.05	0.02	0.08	<0.001	88.8	<0.001
No. pat	>= 90	8	0.05	0.02	0.07	<0.001	94.3	<0.001
	<90	7	0.07	0.03	0.10	<0.001	79.9	<0.001
Ages at pregnancy	>= 31	8	0.04	0.02	0.07	<0.001	85.4	0.001
	<31	7	0.07	0.03	0.11	<0.001	94.9	<0.001
Measuring time	In pregnancy	5	0.07	0.03	0.10	<0.001	91.7	<0.001
	After pregnancy	10	0.05	0.03	0.07	<0.001	85.2	0.001
Duration (years)	>4	4	0.05	0.01	0.09	<0.001	92.1	0.007
	>0, <4	6	0.05	0.01	0.09	<0.001	91.6	0.010
BMI	>= 27.6	7	0.07	0.03	0.12	<0.001	95.1	0.001
	<27.6	8	0.04	0.02	0.06	<0.001	83.8	0.001
GDM Criteria	Carpenter	7	0.08	0.05	0.11	<0.001	90.5	<0.001
	NDDG	3	0.03	<−0.01	0.07	0.001	85.2	0.072
	WHO	2	0.04	−0.01	0.09	0.102	62.6	0.114
	ADA-75 g	4	0.01	−0.06	0.07	<0.001	93.5	0.816

among different studies is relatively large, which may also cause this phenomenon.

The American Heart Association recommend to prevent heart disease in women with gestational diabetes, which was based on a higher risk of type 2 diabetes mellitus in these persons [32]. It is reported that cIMT adds predictive value to the Framingham risk score for cardiovascular events [5], is a level IIa recommendation for cardiovascular risk evaluation [33], cIMT has been confirmed to be able to predict incident coronary heart diseases [34]. Our finding that GDM is associated with early atherosclerosis even during pregnancy is important, because we can establish prevention strategy, such as weight control for GDM patients earlier in life.

Our research also finds increase of cIMT already exists at the time pregnancy. Another question raises our interests is that whether cIMT can predict GDM, as it's demonstrated that cIMT is elevated before the onset of clinical diabetes [35]. However, cIMT measured prior to the pregnancy fails to predict pregnancy outcome such as gestational diabetes [36]. Thus subclinical atherosclerosis may appear along with GDM, but is not a predictor of GDM. We find cIMT does not increase years after GDM has been diagnosed. A possible explanation is that these patients take certain drugs to delay the process of atherosclerotic formation, it's been reported that even subclinical atherosclerosis may be reduced by drugs [37]. As the medications of these patients were not fully reported in included studies, future researches are needed to study this issue.

The number of population in each study is limited; there was no study with number of GDM patients beyond 200. Prospective study of large samples is needed in the future.

Conclusion

In this meta-analysis we observed GDM is related to larger cIMT, the relation is stronger in obese GDM patients, and the association already exists at the time of pregnancy and remained significant years after pregnancy. Weight control may be helpful to prevent cardiovascular diseases for GDM patients.

Competing interests

The authors declare that they have no competing interests.

Authors' contributions

JL: Literature search, data extraction and manuscript writing; SH: Literature search and data extraction; PL: Statistical analysis; LL: Statistical analysis; LZ: Manuscript revision and experimental design. YBX is responsible for the overall content as the guarantor. All authors have read and approved the final manuscript.

Acknowledgments

This work has no one to acknowledge to.

References

1. Akinci B, Celtik A, Genc S, Yener S, Demir T, Secil M, Kebapcilar L, Yesil S: Evaluation of postpartum carbohydrate intolerance and cardiovascular risk factors in women with gestational diabetes. *Gynecol Endocrinol* 2011, 27(5):361–367.
2. Harreiter J, Dovjak G, Kautzky-Willer A: Gestational diabetes mellitus and cardiovascular risk after pregnancy. *Womens Health* 2014, 10(1):91–108.

3. Bauer M, Caviezel S, Teynor A, Erbel R, Mahabadi AA, Schmidt-Trucksäss A: Carotid intima-media thickness as a biomarker of subclinical atherosclerosis. Swiss Med Wkly 2012, 142:w13705.

4. Touboul PJ, Vicaut E, Labreuche J, Acevedo M, Torres V, Ramirez-Martinez J, Vinueza R, Silva H, Champagne B, Hernandez-Hernandez R, Wilson E, Schargrodsky H, CS Investigators: Common carotid artery intima-media thickness: the Cardiovascular Risk Factor Multiple Evaluation in Latin America (CARMELA) study results. Cerebrovasc Dis 2011, 31(1):43–50.

5. Polak JF, Pencina MJ, Pencina KM, O'Donnell CJ, Wolf PA, D'Agostino RB Sr: Carotid-wall intima-media thickness and cardiovascular events. N Engl J Med 2011, 365(3):213–221.

6. Zhang Y, Guallar E, Qiao Y, Wasserman BA: Is Carotid Intima-Media Thickness as Predictive as Other Noninvasive Techniques for the Detection of Coronary Artery Disease? Arterioscler Thromb Vasc Biol 2014, 37(7):1341–5. doi:10.1161/ATVBAHA.113.302075. Epub 2014 Apr 24.

7. Rademaker AA, Danad I, Groothuis JG, Heymans MW, Marcu CB, Knaapen P, Appelman YE: Comparison of different cardiac risk scores for coronary artery disease in symptomatic women: do female-specific risk factors matter? Eur J Prev Cardiol 2013, [Epub ahead of print].

8. Akinci B, Celtik A, Yener S, Genc S, Tunali S, Yuksel F, Ozcan MA, Secil M, Yesil S: Plasma thrombin-activatable fibrinolysis inhibitor levels are not associated with glucose intolerance and subclinical atherosclerosis in women with previous gestational diabetes. Clin Appl Thromb Hemost 2011, 17(6):E224–E230.

9. Akinci B, Celtik A, Yuksel F, Genc S, Yener S, Secil M, Ozcan MA, Yesil S: Increased osteoprotegerin levels in women with previous gestational diabetes developing metabolic syndrome. Diabetes Res Clin Pract 2011, 91(1):26–31.

10. Akinci B, Demir T, Celtik A, Baris M, Yener S, Ozcan MA, Yuksel F, Secil M, Yesil S: Serum osteoprotegerin is associated with carotid intima media thickness in women with previous gestational diabetes. Diabetes Res Clin Pract 2008, 82(2):172–178.

11. Akinci B, Celtik A, Tunali S, Genc S, Yuksel F, Secil M, Ozcan MA, Bayraktar F: Circulating apelin levels are associated with cardiometabolic risk factors in women with previous gestational diabetes. Arch Gynecol Obstet 2014, 289(4):787–793.

12. Vural M, Camuzcuoglu H, Toy H, Cece H, Aydin H, Eren MA, Kocyigit A, Aksoy N: Evaluation of the future atherosclerotic heart disease with oxidative stress and carotid artery intima media thickness in gestational diabetes mellitus. Endocr Res 2012, 37(3):145–153.

13. Eren MA, Vural M, Cece H, Camuzcuoglu H, Yildiz S, Toy H, Aksoy N: Association of serum amyloid A with subclinical atherosclerosis in women with gestational diabetes. Gynecol Endocrinol 2012, 28(12):1010–1013.

14. Atay AE, Simsek H, Demir B, Sakar MN, Kaya M, Pasa S, Demir S, Sit D: Noninvasive assessment of subclinical atherosclerosis in normotensive gravidae with gestational diabetes. Herz 2014, 39(5):627–632. Epub 2013 Jul 18.

15. Bo S, Valpreda S, Menato G, Bardelli C, Botto C, Gambino R, Rabbia C, Durazzo M, Cassader M, Massobrio M, Pagano G: Should we consider gestational diabetes a vascular risk factor? Atherosclerosis 2007, 194(2):e72–e79.

16. Caliskan M, Caklili OT, Caliskan Z, Duran C, Ciftci FC, Avci E, Gullu H, Kulaksizoglu M, Koca H, Muderrisoglu H: Does Gestational Diabetes History Increase Epicardial Fat and Carotid Intima Media Thickness? Echocardiography 2014, doi:10.1111/echo.12597. [Epub ahead of print].

17. Fakhrzadeh H, Alatab S, Sharifi F, Mirarefein M, Badamchizadeh Z, Ghaderpanahi M, Hashemi Taheri AP, Larijani B: Carotid intima media thickness, brachial flow mediated dilation and previous history of gestational diabetes mellitus. J Obstet Gynaecol Res 2012, 38(8):1057–1063.

18. Freire CM, Barbosa FB, De Almeida MC, Miranda PA, Barbosa MM, Nogueira AI, Guimaraes MM, Nunes Mdo C, Ribeiro-Oliveira A Jr: Previous gestational diabetes is independently associated with increased carotid intima-media thickness, similarly to metabolic syndrome - a case control study. Cardiovasc Diabetol 2012, 11:59.

19. Gunderson EP, Chiang V, Pletcher MJ, Jacobs DR, Quesenberry CP, Sidney S, Lewis CE: History of Gestational Diabetes Mellitus and Future Risk of Atherosclerosis in Mid-life: The Coronary Artery Risk Development in Young Adults Study. J Am Heart Assoc 2014, 3(2):e000490.

20. Ijas H, Morin-Papunen L, Keranen AK, Bloigu R, Ruokonen A, Puukka K, Ebeling T, Raudaskoski T, Vaarasmaki M: Pre-pregnancy overweight overtakes gestational diabetes as a risk factor for subsequent metabolic syndrome. Eur J Endocrinol 2013, 169(5):605–611.

21. Ku YH, Choi SH, Lim S, Cho YM, Park YJ, Park KS, Kim SY, Jang HC: Carotid intimal-medial thickness is not increased in women with previous gestational diabetes mellitus. Diab Metab J 2011, 35(5):497–503.

22. Ozuguz U, Isik S, Berker D, Arduc A, Tutuncu Y, Akbaba G, Gokay F, Guler S: Gestational diabetes and subclinical inflammation: evaluation of first year postpartum outcomes. Diabetes Res Clin Pract 2011, 94(3):426–433.

23. Tarim E, Yigit F, Kilicdag E, Bagis T, Demircan S, Simsek E, Haydardedeoglu B, Yanik F: Early onset of subclinical atherosclerosis in women with gestational diabetes mellitus. Ultrasound Obstet Gynecol 2006, 27(2):177–182.

24. Vastagh I, Horvath T, Garamvolgyi Z, Rosta K, Folyovich A, Rigo J, Kollai M, Bereczki D, Somogyi A: Preserved structural and functional characteristics of common carotid artery in properly treated normoglycemic women with gestational diabetes mellitus. Acta Physiol Hung 2011, 98(3):294–304.

25. Volpe L, Cuccuru I, Lencioni C, Napoli V, Ghio A, Fotino C, Bertolotto A, Penno G, Benzi L, Del Prato S, Di Cianni G: Early subclinical atherosclerosis in women with previous gestational diabetes mellitus. Diabetes Care 2008, 31:e32.

26. Yousefzadeh G, Hojat H, Enhesari A, Shokoohi M, Eftekhari N, Sheikhvatan M: Increased carotid artery intima-media thickness in pregnant women with gestational diabetes mellitus. J Tehran Heart Cent 2012, 7(4):156–159.

27. Sullivan SD, Umans JG, Ratner R: Gestational diabetes: Implications for cardiovascular health. Curr Diab Rep 2012, 12(1):43–52.

28. Sugiyama T, Nagao K, Metoki H, Nishigori H, Saito M, Tokunaga H, Nagase S, Sugawara J, Watanabe Y, Yaegashi N, Sagawa N, Sanaka M, Akazawa S, Anazawa S, Waguri M, Sameshima H, Hiramatsu Y, Toyoda N: Pregnancy outcomes of gestational diabetes mellitus according to pre-gestational BMI in a retrospective multi-institutional study in Japan. Endocr J 2014, 61:373–380.

29. Fadl H, Magnuson A, Ostlund I, Montgomery S, Hanson U, Schwarcz E: Gestational diabetes mellitus and later cardiovascular disease: a Swedish population based case–control study. BJOG 2014, doi:10.1111/1471-0528.12754. [Epub ahead of print].

30. Berggren EK, Boggess KA, Stuebe AM, Jonsson Funk M: National Diabetes Data Group vs Carpenter-Coustan criteria to diagnose gestational diabetes. Am J Obstet Gynecol 2011, 205(3):253 e251–257.

31. Simmons D, McElduff A, McIntyre HD, Elrishi M: Gestational diabetes mellitus: NICE for the U.S.? A comparison of the American Diabetes Association and the American College of Obstetricians and Gynecologists guidelines with the U.K. National Institute for Health and Clinical Excellence guidelines. Diabetes Care 2010, 33(1):34–37.

32. Mosca L, Benjamin EJ, Berra K, Bezanson JL, Dolor RJ, Lloyd-Jones DM, Newby LK, Pina IL, Roger VL, Shaw LJ, Zhao D, Beckie TM, Bushnell C, D'Armiento J, Kris-Etherton PM, Fang J, Ganiats TG, Gomes AS, Gracia CR, Haan CK, Jackson EA, Judelson DR, Kelepouris E, Lavie CJ, Moore A, Nussmeier NA, Ofili E, Oparil S, Ouyang P, Pinn VW, et al. Effectiveness-based guidelines for the prevention of cardiovascular disease in women–2011 update: a guideline from the American Heart Association. J Am Coll Cardiol 2011, 57:1404–1423.

33. Greenland P, Alpert JS, Beller GA, Benjamin EJ, Budoff MJ, Fayad ZA, Foster E, Hlatky MA, Hodgson JM, Kushner FG, Lauer MS, Shaw LJ, Smith SC Jr, Taylor AJ, Weintraub WS, Wenger NK, Jacobs AK, G American College of Cardiology Foundation/American Heart Asscoiation Task Force on Practice: 2010 ACCF/AHA guideline for assessment of cardiovascular risk in asymptomatic adults: executive summary: a report of the American College of Cardiology Foundation/American Heart Association Task Force on Practice Guidelines. Circulation 2010, 122:2748–2764.

34. Chambless LE, Heiss G, Folsom AR, Rosamond W, Szklo M, Sharrett AR, Clegg LX: Association of coronary heart disease incidence with carotid arterial wall thickness and major risk factors: the Atherosclerosis Risk in Communities (ARIC) Study, 1987–1993. Am J Epidemiol 1997, 146(6):483–494.

35. Hunt KJ, Williams K, Rivera D, O'Leary DH, Haffner SM, Stern MP, Gonzalez Villalpando C: Elevated carotid artery intima-media thickness levels in individuals who subsequently develop type 2 diabetes. Arterioscler Thromb Vasc Biol 2003, 23(10):1845–1850.

37. D'Ascenzo F, Agostoni P, Abbate A, Castagno D, Lipinski MJ, Vetrovec GW, Frati G, Presutti DG, Quadri G, Moretti C, Gaita F, Zoccai GB: **Atherosclerotic coronary plaque regression and the risk of adverse cardiovascular events: a meta-regression of randomized clinical trials.** *Atherosclerosis* 2013, **226:**178–185.

Expression levels of atherosclerosis-associated miR-143 and miR-145 in the plasma of patients with hyperhomocysteinaemia

Kejian Liu[1,2†], Saiyare Xuekelati[3†], Yue Zhang[3], Yin Yin[2], Yue Li[2], Rui Chai[2], Xinwei Li[2], Yi Peng[2], Jiangdong Wu[3*] and Xiaomei Guo[1*] (ID)

Abstract

Background: An elevated level of homocysteine (Hcy) in the blood is designated hyperhomocysteinaemia (Hhcy) and is regarded as a strong risk factor for the development of atherosclerosis (ATH), although the association remains controversial. Considered to be essential gene expression regulators, micro-RNAs (miRNAs) modulate cardiovascular disease development and thus can be regarded as potential biomarkers and therapeutic targets in atherosclerosis. The aim of the current study is to investigate the expression levels of atherosclerosis-associated miR-143 and miR-145 in Hhcy patients and predict the progress of atherosclerosis in Hhcy patients.

Methods: A total of 100 participants were enrolled and included normal control subjects (NC = 20), hyperhomocysteinaemia alone subjects (Hhcy = 25), hyperhomocysteinaemia and carotid artery atherosclerosis combined subjects (Hhcy + ATH = 30) and patients with standalone carotid artery atherosclerosis (ATH = 25). Plasma Hcy, supplementary biochemical parameters and carotid artery ultrasonography (USG) were measured in all participants. MicroRNA expression levels in the peripheral blood were calculated by real-time reverse transcription-polymerase chain reaction (qRT-PCR). The correlations of miR-143 and miR-145 with Hcy, blood lipid parameters and carotid artery atherosclerotic plaques were evaluated using Pearson's correlation coefficients. Receiver operating characteristic (ROC) curve analyses were performed to evaluate the capacities of miR-143 and miR-145 for the detection of Hhcy and atherosclerosis patients.

Results: MiR-143 and miR-145 exhibited trends towards significance with stepwise decreases from the NC to Hhcy groups and then to the Hhcy + ATH and ATH groups. Similar results were observed in the carotid artery plaque group (Hhcy + ATH and ATH grups) compared with the no-plaque group (NC and Hhcy groups). The miR-143 expression level exhibited significant negative correlations with Hcy, total cholesterol (TC) and low-density lipoprotein cholesterol (LDL-c). The miR-145 expression level exhibited significant negative correlations with Hcy, TC, triglyceride (TG) and LDL-c. MiR-143 and miR-145 exhibited the greatest area under the curves (AUCs) (0.775 and 0.681, respectively) for the detection of every Hhcy patient, including those in the Hhcy and Hhcy + ATH groups, from among all subjects.

(Continued on next page)

* Correspondence: 1556874645@qq.com; guoxiaomei6639@163.com
†Equal contributors
[3]The Key Laboratory of Xinjiang Endemic and Ethnic Diseases, Shihezi University, Shihezi, Xinjiang 832000, China
[1]Department of Cardiology, Tongji Hospital, Tongji Medical College, Huazhong University of Science and Technology, Wuhan 430030, China
Full list of author information is available at the end of the article

(Continued from previous page)

Conclusion: The results indicated that the levels of atherosclerosis-associated circulating miR-143 and miR-145 are linked to Hhcy. MiR-143 may be used as a potential non-invasive biomarkers of Hhcy and thus may be helpful in predicting the progress of atherosclerosis in Hhcy patients.

Keywords: miR-143, miR-145, Hyperhomocysteinaemia, Atherosclerosis, Correlation

Background

Homocysteine (Hcy) is an intermediate substance that is formed in the metabolic pathway of cysteine and methionine. Hyperhomocysteinaemia (Hhcy) is regarded as an emerging risk factor for the development of atherosclerosis and a variety of other cardiovascular diseases, such as coronary artery disease (CAD), hypertension, stroke, etc. [1–3]. Recent studies have demonstrated that homocysteine initiates an inflammatory response in vascular smooth muscle cells (VSMCs) and triggers the proliferation and migration of VSMCs [4, 5]. Moreover, it is well established that VSMC proliferation and migration play fundamental roles in the development of atherosclerosis [6, 7]. We hypothesize that Hhcy may induce the process of atherosclerosis. Although several studies have implicated Hhcy in atherosclerosis, the exact mechanism is not entirely understood.

MicroRNAs (miRNAs) are single-stranded noncoding RNA molecules of 22 nucleotides. miRNAs inhibit mRNA translation by interacting with the 3′ untranslated region (UTR) [8–10]. To determine the ability of atherosclerosis-associated microRNAs to predict the presence of atherosclerosis in Hhcy patients, miRNA databases (i.e., the TargetScan database, http://www.targetscan.org/ and miRBase, http: //http://www.mirbase.org/) [11] and other relevant literature were searched. MiR-143 and miR-145 were confirmed to be critical factors in the development of atherosclerosis [12]. Circulating miR-143 is critical for the regulation of VSMC phenotypes because it promotes differentiation and prevents the proliferation of VSMCs [13, 14]. Because miR-145 is the most abundant miRNA in the vascular wall, it plays a crucial role in differentiation of VSMCs and inhibits their proliferation [15, 16].

There is accumulating evidence demonstrating that miRNAs are a key factor in the development of atherosclerosis [9, 13, 17, 18] and other cardiovascular diseases. Down-regulation of miR-143/–145 has been predominantly expressed in VSMCs and play a role in several cardiovascular diseases, such as hypertension and coronary artery disease (CAD). Recent clinical fndings have demonstrated that the expression levels of miR-143/–145 were decreased in essential hypertension patients compared with healthy subjects [19, 20]. MiR-145 contributes to the pathogenesis of hypertension, as it mediates stretch-induced differentiation of VSMCs [21, 22]. These findings highlight the importance of miR-143/–145 as potential biomarkers for cardiovascular diseases. Vascular smooth muscle cells play an important role in plaque stabilization, particularly in the progression of atherosclerosis [23]. Gain and loss of function of VSMC-enriched miR-143/–145 in vivo results in reduced proliferation, which consequently limits neointima formation in vascular injury models. This leads to the assumption that the miR-143/–145 are inevitable for the pro-proliferative response of VSMCs to injury [24, 25]. This suggests that downregulation of miR-143/–145 may contribute to atherogenesis. MiR-143/–145 are relatively specific for VSMCs and thus are closely correlated with cardiovascular diseases such as atherosclerosis, hypertension and CAD.

However, the exact correlates of the expressions of atherosclerosis-associated microRNAs in Hhcy patients have yet to be fully elucidated. To determine whether these two miRNAs are related to hyperhomocysteinaemia and thus to the development of atherosclerosis, a study was conducted that involved a comparison of their expression levels in the plasma of hyperhomocysteinaemia alone patients and patients with both hyperhomocysteinaemia and carotid atherosclerosis and to further examine whether miRs-143/145 are related directly to hyperhomocysteinaemia and the development of carotid atherosclerotic plaques in humans, the associations with hyperhomocysteinaemia and atherosclerosis were re-analysed from a different perspective.

Methods

Research subjects

For this study, hyperhomocysteinaemia was defined as a plasma Hcy level above 15 μm/L [26]. Carotid artery atherosclerosis was determined by carotid artery ultrasonography (USG), which was used to determine the presence of plaque formation, which in turn was used to categorize the subjects into plaque and no-plaque groups. Approximately 310 newly diagnosed Hhcy patients were screened in the Department of Cardiovascular Diseases of the First Affiliated Hospital of Shihezi University Medical College from January 2014 to December 2015. Patients with histories of hypertension, ischaemic heart disease, diabetes mellitus, chronic liver diseases, chronic renal diseases and excessive drinking plus smoking were excluded. Ultimately, only 167 Hhcy patients were included. Of these, 30 Hhcy + ATH patients and 25 Hcy standalone patients were selected. The two groups were matched for age, sex, body mass index (BMI). Additionally, 25 ATH and 20 NC subjects were selected and were matched to the Hhcy + ATH group for age, sex and BMI. These subjects were extracted from 800 individuals who were already receiving health check-ups at the physical examination centre of the First Affiliated Hospital of Shihezi University Medical College during the same period.

Carotid artery ultrasonography to determine plaque formation

All patients underwent carotid artery ultrasonography (USG) to determine plaque formation. The patients were asked to lie down one by one in a semi-dark room in the supine position with their neck slightly extended and rotated away from the imaging transducer. Both the right and left carotid arteries and the bifurcation were visualized by an experienced radiologist via an ultrasonography device (Hitachi) using a 9-MHz linear probe. According to the study criteria, the absence of atherosclerotic plaque was considered "normal", and positive results were indicative of atherosclerotic plaque [27].

Biochemical assays

Whole blood samples were collected in Ethylene Diamine Tetraacetic Acid (EDTA) tubes from each subject in the morning after an 8-h fast. Plasma Hcy, TG, TC, high-density lipoprotein cholesterol (HDL-c), LDL-c, apolipoprotein A (ApoA), apolipoprotein B (ApoB), apolipoprotein A/B (Apo(A/B)), fasting blood glucose (FBG), alanine aminotransferase (ALT), aspartate aminotransferase (AST) and uric acid (UA) and serum creatinine (Cre) were measured using a Hitachi 7600 automated biochemistry analyser at the First Affiliated Hospital of Shihezi University Medical College.

RNA isolation and microRNA calculation

Whole blood samples were collected in tubes containing EDTA in the morning after 8 hs of fasting. The samples were immediately centrifuged at 3000 rpm for 10 mins at room temperature. After the separation phase, the plasma was collected, divided into two aliquots and frozen at −80 °C for later RNA isolation.

Total RNA, containing small RNA, was extracted from plasma using Trizol -Reagent (Tiangen, Biotech, Beijing, China), according to the manufacturer's protocol. For miRNA qPCR, prior RT was performed using miRNA FastKing RT Kit (Tiangen Biotech Co, Ltd., Beijing,

China, no. KR160815). For RT, 1 μg of RNA containing miRNA was polyadenylated by poly (A) polymerase and then reverse transcribed to cDNA. The cDNA (2 μl) then served as the template and was added to 1 μl primers for SYBR Green real-time PCR using miRcute Plus miRNA qPCR Detection Kit (Tiangen Biotech Co, Ltd., Beijing, China, no. FP160303). The sequence of the miR-143 specific forward primer was 5′-TGAGAT-GAAGCACTGTAGCTC-3′and the reverse primer was 5′-GCTGTCAACATACGCTACGTAACG-3′. The sequence of the miR-145 specific forward primer was 5′-GTCCAGTTTTCCCAGGAATCCCT-3′and the reverse primer was 5′-GCTGTCAACATACGCTACGTAACG-3′. Following the illustration in previous studies, measurements of microRNA levels were performed by quantitative RT-qPCR using cel-miR-54 as normalization control [28, 29]. The sequence of the cel-miR-54 forward primer was 5′-CCGCCCTACCCGTAATCTTCATAA-3′ and the reverse primer was 5′-GTGCAGGGTCC-GAGGT-3′. The RT reaction was performed at first at 37 °C for 30 min, followed by at 42 °C for 30 min and finally at 75 °C for another 5 min. The PCR reaction was performed initially at 95 °C for 3 min, followed by repeated 40 cycles at 95 °C for 10s and latter at 60 °C for 30s. The comparative Ct method (ΔCt) was exploited to calculate the relative expression level of miR. The relative expression of each miRNA after normalization to cel-miR-54 is displayed as $2^{-(Ct\ [miRNA]\ -Ct[cel-miR-54])}$ [30].

Statistical analysis

SPSS software (SPSS, Inc., Chicago, USA) for Windows version 20.0, STATA statistics software (Version 12.0, Stata corporation, College Station, Texas 77, 845 USA) and GraphPad Prism 5.0 software (GraphPad Software, Inc., La Jolla, CA, USA) were used for the statistical analysis. All data were subjected to a normality test (Kolmogorov-Smirnov). For the baseline characteristics of the patients and controls, the continuous variables were summarized as the means ± the SDs, and the discrete variables were summarized as counts and proportions. For the normally distributed data, one-way analysis of variance (ANOVA) and multiple comparison (LSD) tests were applied. The Kruskal-Wallis test was performed to compare the data that were not normally distributed. The significance of the microRNA level differences between the carotid artery plaque group and the no-plaque group were assessed with independent sample Student's t-tests. The χ [2] test was used to compare the gender distributions. Pearson correlations were used to explore the relationships of the miRNAs with Hcy, the lipid parameters, and the carotid atherosclerotic plaque value. Receiver operating characteristic (ROC) curve analyses were performed to evaluate the capacities of miR-143 and miR-145 to detect Hhcy and atherosclerosis patients. Combined diagnostic accuracy of circulating miRNAs both in the all Hhcy patients and all atherosclerosis patients by using STATA statistics software. $P < 0.05$ was regarded as statistically significant.

Results

Significant differences in the clinical features of the four groups

The basic characteristics and clinical features of the studied groups are provided in Table 1. Hcy, TG, TC and LDL-c exhibited differences between the groups ($P < 0.001$). No significant differences were found in the other clinical factors, which included the gender distribution, BMI, age, HDL-c, etc. (Table 1). LSD post hoc multiple comparison tests revealed that the serum TC and LDL-c levels in the Hhcy and Hhcy + ATH groups were significantly higher than that in the NC group. Additionally, the serum TC levels in the Hhcy + ATH group were higher than those in the Hhcy and ATH groups, whereas no differences in serum LDL-c levels were found between the Hhcy + ATH, Hhcy, and ATH subjects. The TG level in the Hhcy group was higher than those in the Hhcy + ATH and NC groups (Fig. 1).

MiR-143 and miR-145 were easily detected in the serum samples of all subjects

Before using $\Delta\Delta Ct$ for relative gene expression, we checked the efficiency of target genes and reference gene and amplification efficiency is consistent. MiR-143 and miR-145 were

stably measured in the serum samples of all subjects. No significant differences were discovered in the total RNA concentrations between the four groups (NC = 11.22 ± 2.14 ng/µl; Hhcy = 10.78 ± 1.41 ng/µl; Hhcy + ATH = 11.32 ± 1.23 ng/µl, and ATH = 11.15 ± 1.61 ng/µl) (Fig. 2a).

As displayed in Fig. 2b and c, both miR-143 and miR-145 exhibited significant trends towards stepwise decreases from the NC (3.99 ± 1.71 and 26.47 ± 8.47, respectively) to the Hhcy (2.89 ± 1.52 and 10.67 ± 5.26, respectively) to the Hhcy + ATH (1.96 ± 1.44 and 8.31 ± 7.21, respectively) and to the ATH (1.97 ± 1.35 and 8.35 ± 6.64, respectively) groups. No significant difference was found between the Hhcy and Hhcy + ATH subjects.

Expression levels of miR-143/145 in the carotid plaque group versus the no plaque group

To better understand the pathophysiology of the atherosclerotic process, we compared the expressions of the candidate miRNAs in the atherosclerotic plaque and normal arteries. Among all subjects, 55 patients had carotid artery plaques (35 men and 20 women; mean age = 48.15 ± 5.36 years), and 45 patients had no plaques (24 men and 21 women, mean age = 47.53 ± 5.02 years). Lower levels of the expressions of miR-143 and miR-145 (1.97 ± 1.39 vs 3.38 ± 1.69 and 8.33 ± 6.90 vs 17.69 ± 10.45; $P < 0.001$) were observed in the carotid artery plaque group compared with the no-plaque group (Fig. 3).

Table 1 Significant differences in clinical features among the four groups

	NC	Hhcy	Hhcy + ATH	ATH	P-value
Males/females	10/10	14/11	20/10	15/10	0.682
Age (years)	48.00 ± 4.44	47.16 ± 5.50	49.00 ± 5.47	46.92 ± 5.20	0.445
BMI (kg/m2)	24.13 ± 2.84	23.47 ± 2.30	25.03 ± 3.58	23.13 ± 2.68	0.080
TC (mmol/l)	3.94 ± 0.79	4.60 ± 0.99	5.56 ± 1.26	4.34 ± 1.04	<0.001**
TG (mmol/l)	1.12 ± 0.07	1.37 ± 0.04	1.45 ± 0.09	1.41 ± 0.11	0.001**
HDL-c (mmol/l)	1.43 ± 0.55	1.58 ± 0.63	1.59 ± 0.57	1.82 ± 0.66	0.176
LDL-c (mmol/l)	2.74 ± 0.91	3.46 ± 0.88	3.36 ± 0.93	3.18 ± 0.81	0.043*
ApoA(g/l)	1.32 ± 0.22	1.39 ± 0.27	1.39 ± 0.41	1.47 ± 0.31	0.480
ApoA/B	1.51 ± 0.42	1.57 ± 0.5	1.42 ± 0.45	1.53 ± 0.43	0.671
ApoB(g/l)	0.96 ± 0.25	0.93 ± 0.19	1.01 ± 0.28	1.01 ± 0.31	0.580
FBG (mmol/l)	5.06 ± 0.74	4.93 ± 0.55	5.07 ± 0.5	4.93 ± 0.59	0.722
ALT (U/l)	22.8 ± 13.02	19.8 ± 10.17	27.0 ± 12.8	20.48 ± 10.86	0.100
AST (U/l)	20.25 ± 10.17	20.84 ± 10.02	20.57 ± 12.36	21.2 ± 10.73	0.993
UA (umol/l)	255.65 ± 63.2	302.96 ± 105.9	258.9 ± 114.2	224.12 ± 106.1	0.795
Cre (umol/l)	73.68 ± 22.12	75.72 ± 24.12	71.3 ± 16.16	69.88 ± 19.84	0.754
Hcy (umol/l)	9.53 ± 2.99	19.07 ± 2.85	21.90 ± 4.69	11.16 ± 2.43	< 0.001**

Continuous and categorical variables data were expressed as mean ± SEM. The statistical P value was generated by the one-way ANOVA test or Kruskal-Wallis test. χ^2 test was employed to compare gender distribution. *P < 0.05 or **P < 0.001 was considered significant

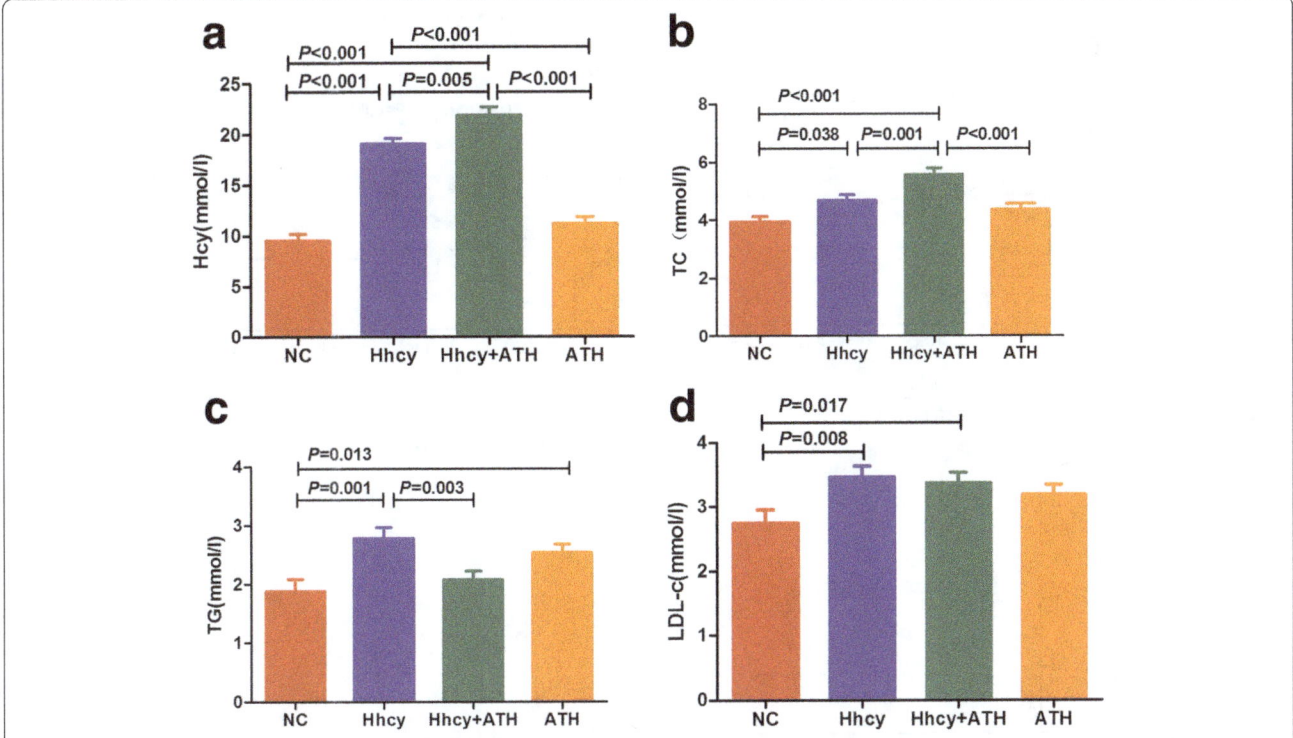

Fig. 1 Multiple comparisons of baseline characteristics (Hcy, TC, TG and LDL-c) among NC, Hhcy, Hhcy + ATH and ATH subjects. Data are shown as the mean ± SD. *P* values were generated by one-way ANOVA test followed by the LSD post hoc multiple comparisons test. *P* < 0.05 or *P* < 0.001 was considered significant

Correlations of miR-143 and miR 145 with Hcy and the lipid parameters

Baseline data about the correlations of miR-143/miR-145 with Hcy and the lipid parameters are presented in Table 2 and the Additional files (Additional file 1: Figure S1, Additional file 2: Figure S2, and Additional file 3: Figure S3). Pearson's correlation analyses demonstrated that Hcy was positively correlated with TC (r = 0.299, P = 0.003) and LDL-c (r = 0.279, P = 0.005). The miR-143 expression level exhibited negative correlations with Hcy (r = −0.214, P = 0.032), TC (r = −0.390, P < 0.001) and LDL-c (r = −0.608, P < 0.001). The miR-145 expression level also exhibited negative correlations with Hcy (r = −0.347, P < 0.001), TC (r = −0.468, P < 0.001), TG (r = −0.594, P < 0.001) and LDL-c (r = −0.219, P = 0.028). However, no correlation was found between miR-143 and TG. Similarly, no correlation of miR-143/miR-145 with ApoA, ApoB, ApoA/B, age, BMI and no association of miR-143/miR-145 with gender, were found (P > 0.05).

ROC curves for miR-143/145 for the definite detection of Hhcy and ATH patients

To further evaluate the predictive power of atherosclerosis-associated miR-143 and miR-145 for Hhcy. All those subjects were divided into hyperhomocysteinaemia patient (34 men and 21 women; mean age 48.16 ± 5.51 years) and atherosclerosis patient (35 men and 20 women; mean age 48.15 ± 5.36 years) groups, and ROCcurves were constructed to estimate the sensitivities and specificities of miR-143/miR-145 levels for the detection of Hhcy and ATH patients. As shown in Fig. 4a and b, ROC curve analysis of miR-143 or miR-145 exhibited strong differentiation power between Hhcy patients and other groups (NC and ATH). The AUC of miR-143 or miR-145 in Hhcy patients was 0.775 (P < 0.001), 0.681 (P < 0.001). Interestingly, the combination of the two miRNAs resulted in a little lower AUC value of 0.773 (P < 0.001) than the AUC of miR-143 or miR-145 (Fig. 2a–c). These data suggested that the combination of circulating miR-143 and miR-145, which were equal to the sensitivity and specificity of miR-143 alone for diagnosing Hhcy. In contrast, the miR-143 and miR-145 levels did not significantly aid the detection of between ATH patients and other groups (NC and Hhcy) (Fig. 5a–c).

Discussion

The present study is the only study to demonstrate the link between atherosclerosis-associated miR-143 and miR145 and hyperhomocysteinaemia in humans. In this

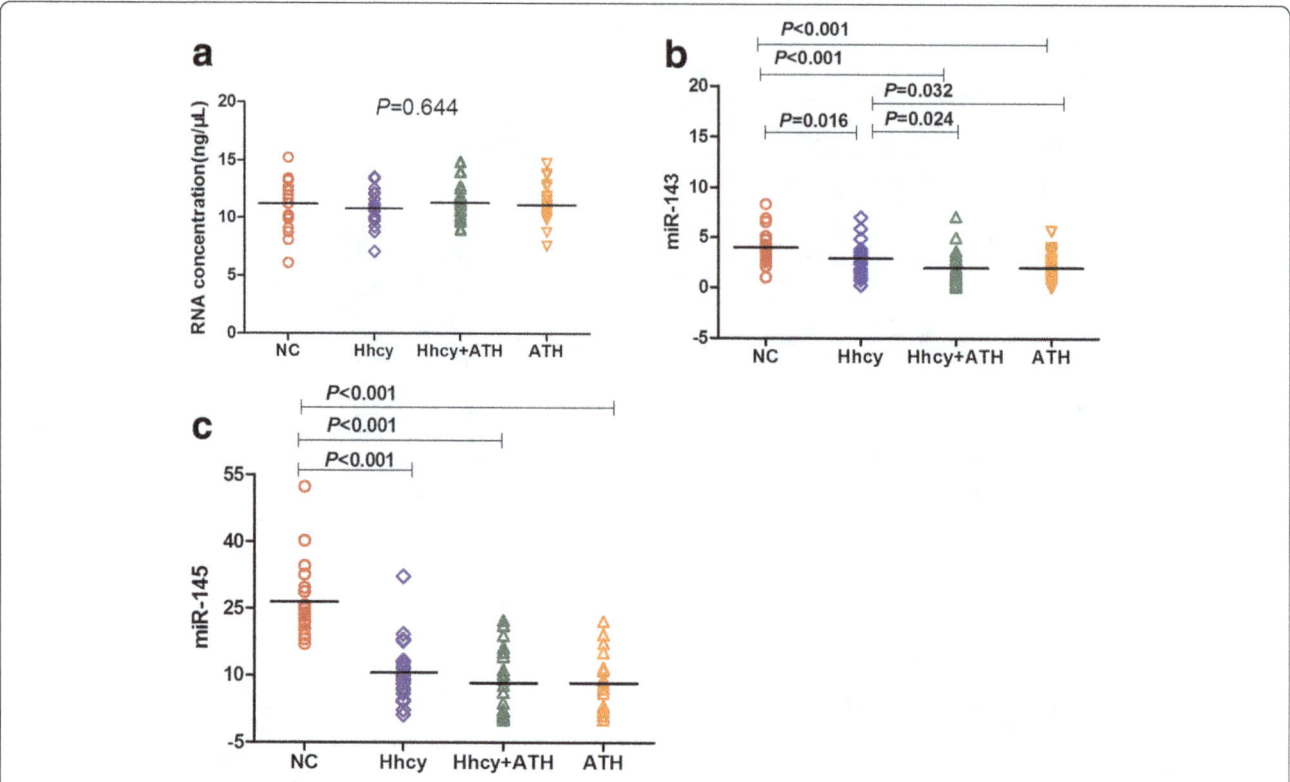

Fig. 2 a Concentration of all RNA samples has no significance difference among four groups. **b**, **c** The relative expression levels of miR-143 and miR-145 in the NC, Hhcy, Hhcy + ATH and ATH groups. The *horizontal lines* indicate the mean. *P* values were generated by one-way ANOVA test followed by the LSD post hoc multiple comparisons test. *P* < 0.05 or *P* < 0.001 was considered significant

study, all the subjects involved were freshly diagnosed with Hhcy and had never undergone any intervention whatsoever. Our study identified miR-143 and miR-145 as potential non-invasive biomarkers for Hhcy, which may be helpful in predicting the progress of atherosclerosis in Hhcy patients.

In this study, Hcy was positively correlated with TC and LDL-c, which indicates that elevated serum homocysteine might be closely related to dyslipidaemia and aggravate atherosclerosis. Meanwhile, qRT-PCR

results showed that plasma miR-143 and miR-145 were visibly down-regulated in Hhcy + ATH patients. Pearson's correlations revealed that the miR-143/−145 expression levels were negatively correlated with Hcy, TC, LDL-c or TG. The ROC analyses showed that the miR-143 might be suitable diagnostic markers for the detection of all Hhcy patients, including Hhcy and Hhcy + ATH patients.

Several studies have demonstrated that miR-143/−145 are molecular keys that determine VSMC phenotypic

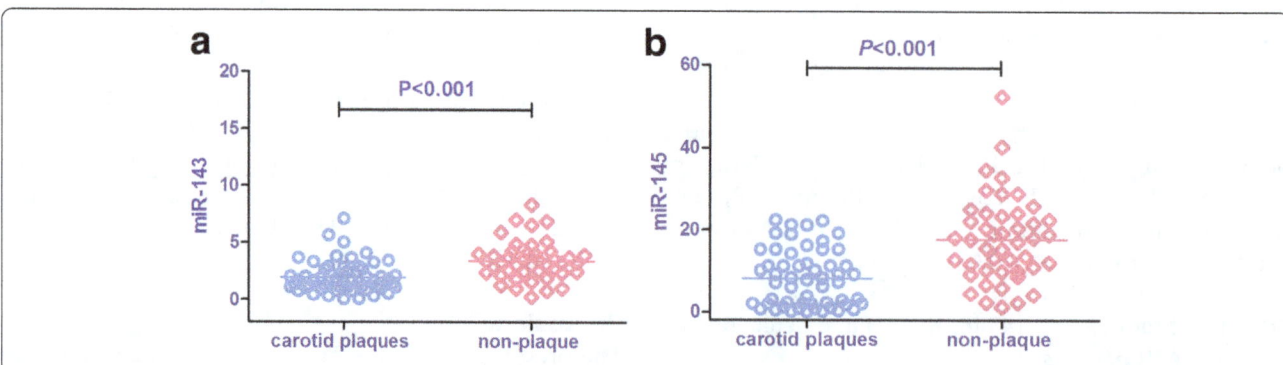

Fig. 3 MiR-143 and miR-145 levels in carotid plaques group and non-plaque group. *P* < 0.001 was considered significant. Carotid plaques, all objects with carotid plaque (Hhcy + ATH and ATH group); Non-plaque, all objects without carotid plaque (NC and Hhcy group)

Table 2 Correlations between miRNAs and Hcy, lipid profiles in all groups

		TC	LDL-c	TG	miR-143	miR-145
Hcy	r	0.299	0.279	0.053	−0.214	−0.347
	P	0.003*	0.005*	0.604	0.032*	<0.001**
TC	r		0.337	0.080	−0.390	−0.468
	P		0.001*	0.429	<0.001**	<0.001**
LDL-c	r			0.066	−0.608	−0.594
	P			0.513	<0.001**	<0.001**
TG	r				−0.123	−0.219
	P				0.223	0.028*
miR-143	r					0.690
	P					<0.001**

Pearson's correlation correlations were presented as correlation coefficients (r) and significance (P), *$P < 0.05$ or **$P < 0.001$ was considered significant

switching and are essential for VSMC differentiation [12], which is known to contribute to atherogenesis [31–33]. We found that that high level of LDL-c and Hcy are most important risk factor for atherosclerosis. And our data shows that miR-143/−145 expression level was negatively correlated with Hcy and LDL-c. Our data support the notion that Hcy was positively correlated with LDL-c. Several studies have demonstrated that elevated Hcy makes the correlation with LDL-c [34, 35]. This study demonstrated that elevated homocysteine levels may increase the risk of atherosclerosis.

The role of homocysteine in vascular plaque formation is multifactorial and includes smooth muscle proliferation, endothelial dysfunction and inflammation [36]. Previous studies have also confirmed the connection between Hhcy and dyslipidaemia, which is consistent with the results of present study [37]. The downregulations of miR-145 and miR-143 in injured or atherosclerotic vessels are associated with proliferating, less differentiated smooth muscle cells [38]. Interestingly, miR-143/−145 are significantly down-regulated in clinical atherosclerotic plaque arteries compared with

healthy arteries, which suggests that increasing miR-143 and miR-145 levels might contribute to the prevention of atherosclerotic plaque formation.

Because miR-143 and miR-145 are expressed in VSMCs, endothelial cells and inflammatory cells, it is not surprising that several animal and clinical studies have already demonstrated that miR-143 and miR-145 contribute to the pathogenesis of atherosclerosis [33, 39, 40]. MiR-145 has been found to be down-regulated in the proliferative VSMCs of atherosclerotic arteries in ApoE-knockout mice [41]. This finding implies that the down-regulation of miR-145 may contribute to atherogenesis. Hai Gao et al. [41] demonstrated that the plasma level of miR-145 is significantly lower in CAD patients compared to healthysubjects. This finding reveals that circulating miR-145 has been demonstrated to be regulated during coronary atherosclerosis. These studies indicate that miR-145 is involved in vascular injury and the migratory activity of VSMCs. In our study, the expressions of miR-143 and miR-145 were found to be down-regulated in individuals with carotid artery plaques. The athero-protective roles of miR-143 and miR-145 may be attributed to their abilities to promote the contractile VSMC phenotype and inhibit the synthetic VSMC phenotype, the latter of which is associated with atherosclerosis [6, 14].

MiRNA-based therapy has been regarded as a promising method for clinical applications in the treatment of cardiovascular diseases [42, 43]. Targeting miR-143/−145 may be a promising therapy for these cardiovascular diseases. However, to date, no miRNAbased therapy has been developed to treat cardiovascular diseases in human clinical trials. Several animal studies have demonstrated that targeting miR-143/−145 may be a promising therapy for vascular diseases. Our data just indicate that miR-143/−145 may be potential non-invasive markers of atherosclerosis in Hhcy patients, and our results may be impetus for these circulating miRNAs as prognostic biomarkers before long and possibly as therapeutic targets of atheroscleorsis in Hhcy patients.

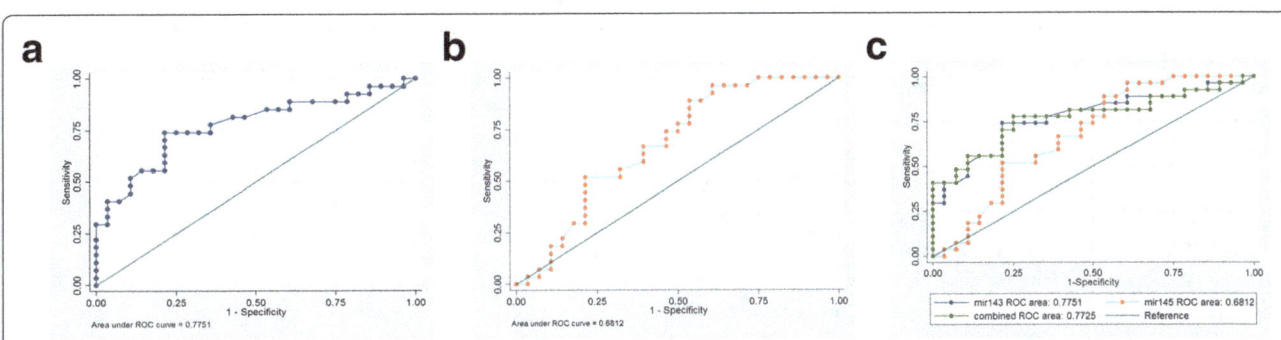

Fig. 4 ROC curve for plasma (**a**) miR-143, (**b**) miR-145, and (**c**) the combination of the two miRNAs were able to distinguish all Hhcy patients (Hhcy + ATH and Hhcy) from the (NC and ATH) cases

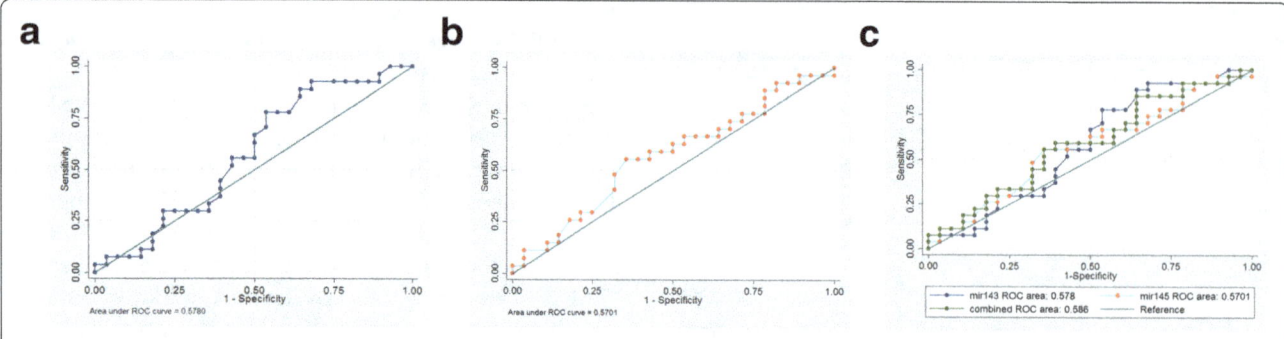

Fig. 5 ROC curve for plasma (**a**) miR-143, (**b**) miR-145, and (**c**) the combination of the two miRNAs were able to distinguish all atherosclerosis patients (Hhcy + ATH and ATH) from the (NC and Hhcy) cases

Remarkably, the plasma microRNA levels were not affected by a wide range of clinical confounders, including age, sex, body mass index, kidney function, hepatic function and fasting blood glucose level.

The current study not only corroborated previous animal studies of the effect of hyperhomocysteinaemia on atherosclerosis but also linked atherosclerosis-associated microRNAs and hyperhomocysteinaemia in humans. This relationship provides novel insight into the pathophysiology of atherosclerosis. Ourstudy has some limitations. First, the mechanisms of miR-143/−145 in regulating atherosclerosis are still not entirely clear in Hhcy human and unexplored in this study, while the underlying mechanisms postulated were based on previous studies. Further experimental studies are needed to explore unknown functions of miR-143/−145 that was expressed in Hhcy patients. Carotid intima-media thickness (CIMT) could not be applied as an evaluation index for atherosclerosis due to a lack of equipment in the hospital. Another potential limitation of our study is the small number of patients available due to the low prevalence of hyperhomocysteinaemia.

Conclusion
In conclusion, we demonstrated that atherosclerosis-related circulating miR-143/miR-145 have significantly variable expressions between NC, Hhcy, Hhcy + ATH and ATH individuals and between carotid plaque and no-plaque individuals. This study revealed that the miR-143/−145 expression levels were positively associated with Hcy and lipidaemia. Moreover, this study indicated that miR143may be regarded as a potential non-invasive biomarkers of atherosclerosis in patients with hyperhomocysteinaemia. However, prospective large-scale studies are required to determine the potential value of circulating miRNAs for the determination of atherosclerosis in patients with hyperhomocysteinaemia.

Additional files

Additional file 1: Figure S1. Pearson's correlation was used to explore the relationships between Hcy with TC and LDL. $P < 0.05$ or $P < 0.001$ was considered significant. (TIFF 57 kb)

Additional file 2: Figure S2. Pearson's correlation was used to explore the relationships between miR-143 with Hcy, TC and LDL-c. $P < 0.05$ or $P < 0.001$ was considered significant. (TIFF 79 kb)

Additional file 3: Figure S3. Pearson's correlation was used to explore the relationships between miR-145 with Hcy, TC, LDL and TG. $P < 0.05$ or $P < 0.001$ was considered significant. (TIFF 94 kb)

Abbreviations
ALT: Alanine aminotransferase; ApoA: Apolipoprotein A; Apo A/B, apolipoprotein A/B; ApoB: Apolipoprotein B; AST: Aspartate aminotransferase; ATH: Carotid artery atherosclerosis alone subjects; BMI: Body mass index; Cre: Serum creatinine; FBG: Fasting blood glucose; Hcy: Homocysteine; HDL-c: High-density lipoprotein cholesterol; Hhcy: Hyperhomocysteinaemia alone subjects; Hhcy + ATH: Hyperhomocysteinaemia and carotid artery atherosclerosis combined subjects; LDL-c: Low-density lipoprotein cholesterol; NC: Normal control subjects; TC: Total cholesterol; TG: Triglyceride; UA: Uric acid

Acknowledgements
We thank Inayat Azeem from Pakistan for assistance in language review.

Funding
This work was supported by National Natural Science Foundation of China (Grant nos. 81,270,353, 81,160,001).

Authors' contributions
KJ L, SX and JD W performed the data analysis and drafted the manuscript. JD W, KJ L and SX designed the study. KJ L, YY and YZ made the graphics. YL, RC, YP and XW L collected the clinical data, and the collection was supervised by JD W and. KJ L, YP, XW L, YY and YZ performed the laboratory experiments, which were supervised and analysed by JD W and XM G. All authors have read and approved the final manuscript.

Competing interests
The authors declare that they have no competing interests.

Author details

[1]Department of Cardiology, Tongji Hospital, Tongji Medical College, Huazhong University of Science and Technology, Wuhan 430030, China. [2]Department of Cardiology, the First Affiliated Hospital, Shihezi University School of Medicine, Shihezi, Xinjiang, China. [3]The Key Laboratory of Xinjiang Endemic and Ethnic Diseases, Shihezi University, Shihezi, Xinjiang 832000, China.

References

1. Li F, Chen Q, Song X, Zhou L, Zhang J. MiR-30b is involved in the Homocysteine-induced apoptosis in human coronary artery endothelial cells by regulating the expression of Caspase 3. Int J Mol Sci. 2015;16(8):17682–95.
2. Schaffer A, et al. Relationship between homocysteine and coronary artery disease. Results from a large prospective cohort study. Thromb Res. 2014;134(2):288–93.
3. Alpert MA. Homocyst(e)ine, atherosclerosis, and thrombosis. South Med J. 1999;92(9):858–65.
4. Jeon SB, Kang DW, Kim JS, Kwon SU. Homocysteine, small-vessel disease, and atherosclerosis: an MRI study of 825 stroke patients. Neurol. 2014;83(8):695–701.
5. Meng L, et al. Polyphenols and polypeptides in Chinese Rice wine inhibit Homocysteine-induced proliferation and migration of vascular smooth muscle cells. J Cardiovasc Pharmacol. 2016;67(6):482–90.
6. Rudijanto A. The role of vascular smooth muscle cells on the pathogenesis of atherosclerosis. Acta medica Indonesiana. 2007;39(2):86–93.
7. Dubland JA, Francis GA. So much cholesterol: the unrecognized importance of smooth muscle cells in atherosclerotic foam cell formation. Curr Opin Lipidol. 2016;27(2):155–61.
8. Deddens JC, et al. Circulating MicroRNAs as novel biomarkers for the early diagnosis of acute coronary syndrome. J Cardiovasc Transl Res. 2013;6(6):884–98.
9. Gao Y, et al. Functional regulatory roles of microRNAs in atherosclerosis. Clin Chim Acta. 2016;460:164–71.
10. Maegdefessel L. The emerging role of microRNAs in cardiovascular disease. J Intern Med. 2014;276(6):633–44.
11. Duan H, et al. MicroRNA-217 suppresses homocysteine-induced proliferation and migration of vascular smooth muscle cells via N-methyl-D-aspartic acid receptor inhibition. Clin Exp Pharmacol Physiol. 2016;43(10):967–75.
12. Cordes K, Sheehy R. N.T, white M.P. et al. MiR-145 and miR-143 regulate smooth muscle cell fate and plasticity. Nat. 2009;460(7256):705–10.
13. Zhang HP, et al. A regulatory circuit involving miR-143 and DNMT3a mediates vascular smooth muscle cell proliferation induced by homocysteine. Mol Med Rep. 2016;13(1):483–90.
14. Boettger T, et al. Acquisition of the contractile phenotype by murine arterial smooth muscle cells depends on the Mir143/145 gene cluster. J Clin Investig. 2009;119(9):2634–47.
15. Guo X, et al. MiRNA-145 inhibits VSMC proliferation by targeting CD40. Sci Rep. 2016;6:35302.
16. Shimizu C, et al. Differential expression of miR-145 in children with Kawasaki disease. PLoS One. 2013;8(3):1–12.
17. Urbich C, Kuehbacher A, Dimmeler S. Role of microRNAs in vascular diseases, inflammation, and angiogenesis. Cardiovasc Res. 2008;79(4):581–8.
18. Baldan A, Fernandez-Hernando C. Truths and controversies concerning the role of miRNAs in atherosclerosis and lipid metabolism. Curr Opin Lipidol. 2016;27(6):623–9.
19. Kontaraki JE, Marketou ME, Zacharis EA, et al. Differential expression of vascular smooth muscle-modulating microRNAs in human peripheral blood mononuclear cells: novel targets in essential hypertension. J Hum Hypertens. 2014;28(8):510–6.
20. Fu X, Guo L, Jiang ZM, et al. An miR-143 promoter variant associated with essential hypertension. Int J Clin Exp Med. 2014;7(7):1813–7.
21. Hu B, Song JT, Qu HY, et al. Mechanical stretch suppresses microRNA-145 expression by activating extracellular signalregulated kinase 1/2 and upregulating angiotensin-converting enzyme to alter vascular smooth muscle cell phenotype. PLoS One. 2014;9(5):e96338.
22. Turczynska KM, Sadegh MK, Hellstrand P, et al. MicroRNAs are essential for stretch-induced vascular smooth muscle contractile differentiation via microRNA (miR)-145-dependent expression of L-type calcium channels. J Biol Chem. 2012;287(23):19199–206.
23. Libby P, Ridker PM, Hansson GK. Progress and challenges in translating the biology of atherosclerosis. Nat. 2011;473:317–25.
24. Xin M, Small EM, Sutherland LB, et al. MicroRNAs miR-143 and miR-145 modulate cytoskeletal dynamics and responsiveness of smooth muscle cells to injury. Genes Dev. 2009;23:2166–78.
25. Cheng Y, Liu X, Yang J, et al. MicroRNA-145, a novel smooth muscle cell phenotypic marker and modulator, controls vascular neointimal lesion formation. Circ Res. 2009;105:158–66.
26. Kesherwani V, Nandi SS, Sharawat SK, Shahshahan HR, Mishra PK. Hydrogen sulfide mitigates homocysteine-mediated pathological remodeling by inducing miR-133a in cardiomyocytes. Mol Cell Biochem. 2015;404(1–2):241–50.
27. Arslan A, et al. The relationship between serum paraoxonase levels and carotid atherosclerotic plaque formation in Alzheimer's patients. Neurol Neurochir Pol. 2016;50(6):403–9.
28. Kuhlmann JD, et al. Circulating U2 small nuclear RNA fragments as a novel diagnostic tool for patients with epithelial ovarian cancer. Clin Chem. 2014;60(1):206–13.
29. Baraniskin A, et al. Circulating U2 small nuclear RNA fragments as a novel diagnostic biomarker for pancreatic and colorectal adenocarcinoma. Int J Cancer. 2013;132(2):E48–57.
30. Wang GK, et al. Circulating microRNA: a novel potential biomarker for early diagnosis of acute myocardial infarction in humans. Eur Heart J. 2010;31(6):659–66.
31. Lovren F, et al. MicroRNA-145 targeted therapy reduces atherosclerosis. Circ. 2012;126(11):S81–90.
32. Sala F, et al. MiR-143/145 deficiency attenuates the progression of atherosclerosis in Ldlr–/–mice. Thromb Haemost. 2014;112(4):796–802.
33. Rangrez AY, Massy ZA, Metzinger-Le Meuth V, Metzinger L. MiR-143 and miR-145: molecular keys to switch the phenotype of vascular smooth muscle cells. Circ Cardiovasc Genet. 2014;4(2):197–205.
34. Seo H, Oh H, Park H, et al. Contribution of dietary intakes of antioxidants to homocysteine-induced low density lipoprotein (LDL) oxidation in atherosclerotic patients. Yonsei Med J. 2010;51(4):526–33.
35. Chernyavskiy I, Veeranki S, Sen U, Tyagi SC. Atherogenesis: hyperhomocysteinemia interactions with LDL, macrophage function, paraoxonase 1, and exercise. Ann N Y Acad Sci. 2016;1363(1):138–54.
36. Ganguly P, Alam SF. Role of homocysteine in the development of cardiovascular disease. Nutr J. 2015;14:6.
37. Pang H, Han B, Fu Q, Zong Z. Association of High Homocysteine Levels with the risk stratification in hypertensive patients at risk of stroke. Clin Ther. 2016;38(5):1184–92.
38. Navickas R, et al. Identifying circulating microRNAs as biomarkers of cardiovascular disease: a systematic review. Cardiovasc Res. 2016;111(4):322–37.
39. Santovito D, et al. Overexpression of microRNA-145 in atherosclerotic plaques from hypertensive patients. Expert Opin Ther Targets. 2013;17(3):217–23.
40. Liu X, et al. Flank sequences of miR-145/143 and their aberrant expression in vascular disease: mechanism and therapeutic application. J Am Heart Assoc. 2013;2(6):e000407.
41. Gao H, et al. Plasma levels of microRNA-145 are associated with severity of coronary artery disease. PLoS One. 2015;10(5):e0123477.
42. van Rooij E, Olson EN. MicroRNA therapeutics for cardiovascular disease: opportunities and obstacles. Nat Rev Drug Discov. 2012;11(11):860–72.
43. Dangwal S, Tum T. MicroRNA therapeutics in cardiovascular disease models. Annu Rev Pharmacol Toxicol. 2014;54:185–203.

17

A potential protective element of myocardial bridge against severe obstructive atherosclerosis in the whole coronary system

Lisheng Jiang[1,3*†], Min Zhang[2,3†], Hong Zhang[4], Lan Shen[1,3], Qin Shao[3], Linghong Shen[1,3] and Ben He[1,3*] (iD)

Abstract

Background: Myocardial bridge (MB) is generally described as a congenital benign variation. Previous studies have suggested that MB prevents atherosclerotic plaques from accumulating within the bridge segment but promotes coronary stenosis in the proximal segment adjacent to MB. However, it is still not clear whether MB has positive or negative effects on severe obstructive atherosclerosis in the whole coronary artery system.

Methods: In this study, 6774 patients with symptoms of angina who were clinically diagnosed coronary artery disease (CAD) or suspected CAD underwent coronary angiography (CAG) in our center. The presence of MB was diagnosed, and a retrospective analysis was performed between MB and severe obstructive CAD requiring percutaneous coronary intervention (PCI) or coronary artery bypass grafting (CABG) in the whole coronary system.

Results: Among 6774 patients, 3583 (52.89%) were diagnosed with severe obstructive CAD (SOCAD) requiring a treatment of PCI or CABG and enrolled into the SOCAD group; and 3191 (47.11%) without SOCAD into the non-SOCAD group. Non-SOCAD and SOCAD groups had 512(16.05%) and 66(1.84%) patients with MB, respectively ($P < 0.0001$). The rate of SOCAD requiring PCI or CABG in patients with MB was much lower than that in patients without MB (11.42% vs. 56.76%, $P < 0.0001$). After adjusting for sex, age, diabetes mellitus, hypertension, and other risk factors, MB still had some positive role in preventing severe obstructive CAD (log-OR = − 2.134, p-value < 0.0001) through logistic regression.

Conclusions: Our results provided a clue that MB might act as a potential protective element against severe obstructive atherosclerosis in the whole coronary artery system.

Background

Myocardial bridge (MB) is referred to muscle overlying intramyocardial segment of an epicardial coronary artery, usually in the middle segment of the left anterior descending coronary artery (LAD) [1, 2]. Some studies reported anatomical properties of MB on atherosclerosis evolution in LAD. Location, length, and thickness are closely interrelated, and longer or thicker MBs are located significantly proximally in LAD [3]. Its charac-teristic compression of the tunneled coronary segment is clinically silent in many cases but is of interesting to clinical researchers due to its association with myocardial ischemia [4, 5].

The golden standard of MB diagnosis in angiography is defined as systolic milking effect produced by systolic compression by the intramyocardial segment [6]. MB is the most common congenital coronary variation, and the prevalence of MB varies from less than 5% [1, 6] under angiography, to 23% with intravascular ultrasound (IVUS) [6], to 55.6% under autopsy [7] due to the reason that short and thin bridges causing little systolic compression are easy to be ignored [8].

The presence of MB can be associated with various complications such as angina, acute myocardial infarction, arrhythmias, and even sudden death [4, 9–18]. MB

---

* Correspondence: jls1025@aliyun.com; drhe_renji@163.com
†Lisheng Jiang and Min Zhang contributed equally to this work.
¹Department of Cardiology, Shanghai Jiao Tong University Affiliated Chest Hospital, Shanghai, China
Full list of author information is available at the end of the article

can also be considered a benign variation of coronary arteries [19], or a double-edged sword [5]. The cause of angina is generally thought to be a distinct reduction of coronary artery flow due to muscular compression during systole [5, 20, 21]. Previous studies have suggested that in the intramyocardial segments, the vessel is protected from obstructive atherosclerosis, however, it is not clear whether MB has positive or negative effects on obstructive atherosclerosis in the whole coronary artery system. In the present study, we aimed at exploring a clinical relationship between MB and severe obstructive atherosclerosis requiring treatment with percutaneous coronary intervention (PCI) or coronary artery bypass grafting (CABG) in the whole coronary artery system.

Methods

Study oversight

This study is a retrospective observation based on hospital records from Renji Hospital, School of Medicine, Shanghai Jiaotong University, China. The authors assume responsibility for the accuracy and completeness of the data and data analyses.

Data collection

From December 2012 to February 2015, 6774 patients with symptoms of angina who were clinically diagnosed with coronary artery disease (CAD) or suspected CAD underwent 6848 coronary angiographies in Renji Hospital. We conducted a retrospective study on MB by retrieving these patients' hospital records, including sex, age, coronary risk factors, diagnoses of coronary angiography and invasive treatments. All clinical diagnoses follow the standard of ICD-10.

The presence of MB was recognized by the angiographic finding of transient reduction in the lumen of one epicardial coronary artery during systole as shown in Fig. 1. The severe obstructive coronary artery disease (SOCAD) requiring invasive treatment with PCI or CABG was defined as the presence of stenosis over 75% or occlusion in at least one major coronary artery, or stenosis less than 75% but over 50%, which was evaluated with an indication of PCI or CABG by coronary interventional cardiologist or cardiac surgeon. According to angiography results, patients with SOCAD underwent treatment with PCI or CABG and were enrolled into the SOCAD group; while patients without severe obstructive coronary artery lesion were enrolled into the non-SOCAD group.

The traditional risk factors including advanced age, hypertension, diabetes mellitus (DM) and impaired glucose tolerance (IGT), hyperlipidemia, chronic kidney disease (CKD), ischemic cerebrovascular disease (ICVD), etc. were documented to be linked with atherosclerosis. In the present study, both the incidence of MB and the risk factors as above were therefore recorded and analyzed.

Statistical analyses

Mean values with standard deviations and counts with percentages were used to describe baseline characteristics and the incidence of MB. Differences were calculated separately in different subgroups according to presence or absence of SOCAD or MB, and sex. The differences were evaluated using one-way analysis of variance for continuous variables and Fisher's exact test for categorical variables. The association between SOCAD and MB was further evaluated in the context of logistic

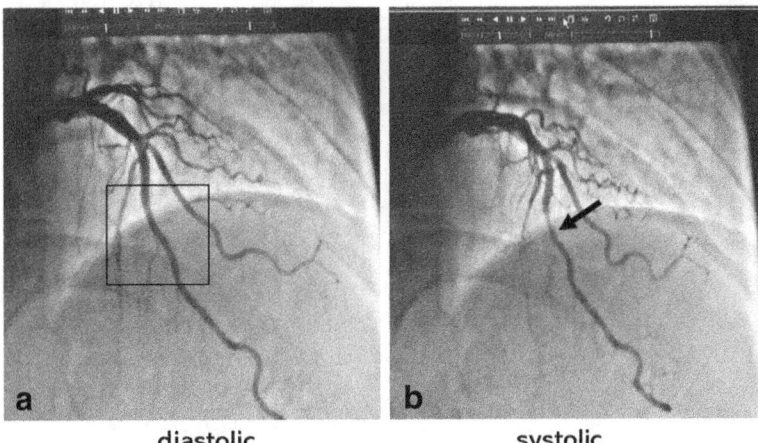

diastolic   systolic

Fig. 1 The typical characteristics of MB under angiography. The box in diagram **a** represents the segment of myocardial bridge free of compressing in left anterior descending artery during diastole; the arrow in diagram **b** represents the compressing segment of myocardial bridge in the same artery during systole

regression model with or without interaction terms by adjusting for some baseline risk factors and the widely used stepwise variable selection strategy based on Akaike's information criterion [22] was used to select those factors potentially associated with SOCAD.

All P values were two-sided, and a P value of < 0.05 was considered with statistical significances. The R program, version 3.4.0, was used to perform statistical analyses.

Results

Findings of myocardial bridge
As listed in Table 1, out of the 6774 patients underwent angiography, 578 (319 male and 259 female)were diagnosed with MB including 571 located in the left anterior descending artery (LAD), 4 in left circumflex (LCX) and 3 in right coronary artery (RCA).

Incidence of MB and risk factors between patients with or without SOCAD
There were significant differences when comparing the incidence of MB between patients with or without SOCAD. As listed in Table 2, the incidence of MB in the SOCAD group was much lower than the non-SOCAD group (proportions: 1.84% vs. 16.05%, respectively; $P < 0.0001$). Besides, in the SOCAD group, there were older age (mean [±SD], 65.08 ± 10.55 years vs. 63.34 ± 10.33 years; $P < 0.0001$), higher proportion of male (74.83% vs. 52.74%, $P < 0.0001$), and higher rates of risk factors including, hypertension, diabetes and/or impaired glucose tolerance, chronic kidney disease and ischemic cerebrovascular disease. However, the rate of hyperlipidemia in the SOCAD group was lower than that in the non-SOCAD group, which might be linked with the reason that patients in the SOCAD group were given an intensive lipid-lowering therapy even before admission (some of them had a long history of coronary heart disease).

Incidence of SOCAD and risk factors between patients with or without myocardial bridge
As shown in Table 3, in comparison with the non-MB group, patients in the MB group had much lower rate of SOCAD requiring PCI/CABG (11.42% vs. 56.76%, $P < 0.0001$), higher rate of female (44.81% vs. 34.72%, $P < 0.0001$), younger age (mean [±SD], 61.10 ± 9.93 vs. 64.56 ± 10.49, $P < 0.0001$), and lower rates of risk factors including hypertension (50.00% vs.61.54%, $P < 0.0001$), impaired glucose metabolism including DM and IGT (14.01% vs. 29.78%, $P < 0.0001$), ischemic cerebrovascular diseases (3.63% vs. 6.71%, $P = 0.0026$), and chronic kidney disease (1.21% vs.3.78%, $P = 0.0006$), but not for hyperlipidemia ($P = 0.934$).

Differences on incidence of MB and clinical characteristics between male and female
Compared with the male, the female patients had a higher proportion of MB (10.75% vs. 7.31%, $P < 0.0001$), much older age (66.09 ± 10.09 vs. 63.25 ± 10.56 years old, $P < 0.0001$), higher rate of hyperlipidemia (9.46% vs. 6.35%, $P < 0.0001$), but much lower SOCAD requiring PCI or CABG (37.43%% vs. 61.43%, $P < 0.0001$) (Table 4).

Logistic regression
Association intensities (log-ORs) between risk factors and severe obstructive atherosclerosis requiring PCI or CABG were reported in Table 4. There was a strong negative linear relationship between MB and severe obstructive atherosclerosis (log-OR = − 2.134, $P < 0.0001$), and other significant risk factors (including interaction terms) included old age ($P = 0.0025$), female sex ($P < 0.0001$), hypertension ($P < 0.0001$), impaired glucose metabolism ($P < 0.0001$), hyperlipidemia ($P = 0.0436$), interaction term between age and sex ($P < 0.0001$), interaction term between age and impaired glucose metabolism ($P = 0.0003$), and interaction term between sex and hypertension ($P = 0.0122$).

Table 1 Clinical characteristics in patients with myocardial bridge (MB)

Characteristics	Values
Incidence of MB, n/total (%)	578/6774 (8.53%)
Location of MB: LAD[a], n (%)	571(98.79%)
LCX[b], (%)	4 (0.69%)
RCA[c], (%)	3 (0.52%)
Age (years, mean ± SD)	61.10 ± 9.93
Sex	
Male, n (%)	319 (55.19%)
Female, n (%)	259 (44.81%)
Hypertension, n (%)	289 (50.00%)
DM[d], n (%)	59 (10.21%)
IGT[e], n (%)	22 (3.81%)
DM/IGT[f], n (%)	81 (14.01%)
Hyperlipidemia, n (%)	42 (7.27%)
Ischemic cerebrovascular disease, n (%)	21 (3.63%)
Chronic kidney disease, n (%)	7 (1.21%)
SOCAD[g], n (%)	66 (11.42%)

[a]LAD, left anterior descending artery
[b]LCX, left circumflex
[c]RCA, right coronary artery
[d]DM, diabetes mellitus
[e]IGT, impaired glucose tolerance
[f]DM/IGT, diabetes mellitus/impaired glucose tolerance
[g]SOCAD, severe obstructive coronary artery disease requiring treatment with percutaneous coronary intervention or coronary artery bypass grafting

Table 2 Comparisons on incidence of myocardial bridge and risk factors in patients with or without SOCAD[d]

Event	Non-SOCAD	SOCAD	P value
	N = 3191 (47.11%)	N = 3583 (52.89%)	
Age (years, mean ± SD)	63.34 ± 10.33	65.08 ± 10.55	< 0.0001
Sex			
Male, n (%)	1683(52.74%)	2681(74.83%)	< 0.0001
Female, n (%)	1508(47.26%)	902(25.17%)	
Myocardial bridge, n (%)	512(16.05%)	66(1.84%)	< 0.0001
Hypertension, n (%)	1725(54.06%)	2377(66.34%)	< 0.0001
DM[a], n (%)	527(16.52%)	1078(30.09%)	< 0.0001
IGT[b], n (%)	124(3.89%)	197(5.50%)	0.0078
DM/IGT[c], n (%)	651(20.40%)	1275(35.58%)	< 0.0001
Hyperlipidemia, n (%)	272(8.52%)	233(6.50%)	0.0016
Ischemic cerebrovascular disease, n (%)	178(5.58%)	259(7.23%)	0.0064
Chronic kidney disease, n (%)	83(2.60)	158(4.41%)	< 0.0001

[a]DM, diabetes mellitus
[b]IGT, impaired glucose tolerance
[c]DM/IGT, diabetes mellitus/impaired glucose tolerance
[d]SOCAD, severe obstructive coronary artery disease requiring treatment with percutaneous coronary intervention or coronary artery bypass grafting

A negative log-OR means a protective effect against severe obstructive atherosclerosis, and vice versa. Log-ORs of age, hypertension, impaired glucose metabolism, interaction term between age and sex, and interaction term between sex and hypertension were positive, while log-ORs of MB, female sex, hyperlipidemia, and interaction between age and glucose metabolism were negative. The log-OR of myocardial bridge was − 2.134, suggesting a potential protective element of MB against severe obstructive atherosclerosis requiring PCI or CABG (Table 5).

Discussion

Currently, many studies consider MB as a contributing factor in myocardial ischemia, angina, myocardial infarction and arrhythmia [4, 9–17]. However, less atherosclerotic lesions are found in bridge segments in contrast to non-bridged coronary arteries [18, 23–27]. Limited proof indicates that compression by contracting myocardial muscles may provide some potential anti-atherosclerotic mechanisms linked with the release of anticoagulant and growth factors [18]. However, the overall protective or

Table 3 Comparisons on incidence of SOCAD and risk factors in patients with or without myocardial bridge

Event	Without MB	With MB	P value
	N = 6196 (91.47%)	N = 578 (8.52%)	
Age (years, mean ± SD)	64.56 ± 10.49	61.10 ± 9.93	< 0.0001
Sex			
Male, n (%)	4045(65.28%)	319(55.19%)	< 0.0001
Female, n (%)	2151(34.72%)	259(44.81%)	
Hypertension, n (%)	3813(61.54%)	289(50.00%)	< 0.0001
DM[a], n (%)	1546(24.95%)	59(10.21%)	< 0.0001
IGT[b], n (%)	299(4.83%)	22(3.81%)	0.5441
DM/IGT[c], n (%)	1845(29.78%)	81(14.01%)	< 0.0001
Hyperlipidemia, n (%)	463(7.47%)	42(7.27%)	0.934
Ischemic cerebrovascular disease, n (%)	416(6.71%)	21(3.63%)	0.0026
Chronic kidney disease, n (%)	234(3.78%)	7(1.21%)	0.0006
SOCAD[d], n (%)	3517(56.76%)	66(11.42%)	< 0.0001

[a]DM, diabetes mellitus
[b]IGT, impaired glucose tolerance
[c]DM/IGT, diabetes mellitus/impaired glucose tolerance
[d]SOCAD, severe obstructive coronary artery disease requiring treatment with percutaneous coronary intervention or coronary artery bypass grafting

Table 4 Comparisons on incidence of myocardial bridge and clinical characteristics between male and female

Event	Male	Female	P value
	N = 4364 (64.42%)	N = 2410 (35.58%)	
Age (years, mean ± SD)	63.25 ± 10.56	66.09 ± 10.09	< 0.0001
Myocardial bridge, n (%)	319(7.31%)	259(10.75%)	< 0.0001
Hypertension, n (%)	2617(59.97%)	1485(61.62%)	0.1855
DM[a], n (%)	1010(23.14%)	595(24.69%)	0.1274
IGT[b], n (%)	221(5.06%)	100(4.15%)	0.2371
DM/IGT[c], n (%)	1231(28.21%)	695(28.84%)	0.8594
Hyperlipidemia, n (%)	277(6.35%)	228(9.46%)	< 0.0001
Ischemic cerebrovascular disease, n (%)	258(5.91%)	179(7.43%)	0.0174
Chronic kidney disease, n (%)	178(4.08%)	63(2.61%)	0.0016
SOCAD[d], n (%)	2681(61.43%)	902(37.43%)	< 0.0001

[a]DM, diabetes mellitus
[b]IGT, impaired glucose tolerance
[c]DM/IGT, diabetes mellitus/impaired glucose tolerance
[d]SOCAD, severe obstructive coronary artery disease requiring treatment with percutaneous coronary intervention or coronary artery bypass grafting

detrimental role of MB in the whole coronary system and knowledge on the mechanisms are still desired.

According to previous studies, formation of atherosclerotic plaque can frequently be found at segment proximal to the bridge, while the intramural segment is typically absent [18, 23], but not in all cases [26]. As supported by a morphological observation of cholesterol-fed rabbits, foam cells and modified smooth muscle cells have the same distribution on a cellar level with atheromatous plaques at proximal segments but not at intramural segments [25]. Also, endothelial cells proximal to MB were arranged in a pavement-like, polygonal and flat appearance because of a high sheer stress [27]. These pathologic changes in proximal segment may be due to the accumulation of ApoB, proliferating cell nuclear antigens (PCNA) in smooth muscle cells and increased endothelial cell permeability [25].

Diagnosis of MB under coronary angiography is based on the typical "milking effect" and a "step down-step up" phenomenon induced by muscle compression during

Table 5 Analysis of logistic regression (with interaction terms)

	log-OR[b]	Std. error	z value	P value
(Intercept)	−0.383	0.217	−1.762	0.0780
Age	0.010	0.003	3.019	0.0025
MB	−2.134	0.137	−15.545	< 0.0001
Female sex	−3.139	0.379	−8.285	< 0.0001
Hypertension	0.341	0.073	4.689	< 0.0001
Impaired glucose metabolism[a]	1.160	0.215	5.389	< 0.0001
Hyperlipidemia	−0.205	0.102	−2.018	0.0436
Ischemic cerebrovascular disease (ICVD)	−0.025	0.136	−0.183	0.8545
Chronic kidney disease (CKD)	0.254	0.146	1.735	0.0828
Age × Sex (female vs. male)	0.028	0.006	4.852	< 0.0001
Age × Impaired glucose metabolism[a]	−0.012	0.003	−3.628	0.0003
MB × ICVD	−12.698	179.070	−0.071	0.9435
Sex × Hypertension	0.301	0.120	2.507	0.0122
Sex × Impaired glucose metabolism[a]	0.118	0.067	1.770	0.0767
Hypertension × Impaired glucose metabolism[a]	−0.134	0.071	−1.881	0.0600
Impaired glucose metabolism × ICVD	0.175	0.124	1.416	0.1568

[a]Impaired glucose metabolism including diabetes mellitus and impaired glucose tolerance
[b]log-OR: log-odds ratio. A negative log-OR means a protective effect against severe obstructive coronary artery disease (SOCAD) requiring treatment with percutaneous coronary intervention or coronary artery bypass grafting on the premise that the presence of SOCAD was coded as 1 and non-SOCAD was coded as 0

systole [6]. Though coronary angiography is now the gold standard and is most widely used in diagnosing MB, it has some technical restrictions compared with other new imaging techniques, such as intravenous ultrasound (IVUS), intracoronary Doppler ultrasound, multi-detector computed tomography, and intracoronary pressure devices [1, 3, 7]. In other words, the percentage of MB varies with different diagnostic method and equipment. In this retrospective study, the overall incidence of MB was 8.53%, but the female had higher morbidity of MB than the male (10.75% vs. 7.31%, $P < 0.0001$). In the non-SOCAD group, the rate of MB was much higher than that in the SOCAD group (16.05% vs. 1.84%, $P < 0.0001$); whereas, in patients with MB, the rate of SOCAD requiring treatment with PCI or CABG was much lower than that in patients without MB (11.42% vs 56.76%, $P < 0.0001$). Take this in account, we speculated that MB might produce a potential positive role against severe obstructive atherosclerosis in the whole coronary artery system. Accordingly, we analyzed the relationship between MB and severe obstructive atherosclerosis by adjusting for age, sex, hypertension, impaired glucose metabolism, hyperlipidemia, ischemic cerebrovascular diseases, and chronic kidney diseases. Based on our results, there seemed to be a clue that MB might produce a potential protective element against severe obstructive atherosclerosis in the whole coronary artery system (log-OR = – 2.134; $P < 0.0001$).

Hyperlipidemia is a significant risk factor of CAD, which is a wide-accepted truth [28]. In the present study, however, we observed that the rate of hyperlipidemia in SOCAD group was lower than that in non-SOCAD group. We must mention that, it is not interpreted from our result that hyperlipidemia is negatively associated with severe obstructive CAD because of the reasons that patients without SOCAD didn't receive intensive lipid-lowering management, whereas patients with SOCAD (some of them had a long history of coronary heart disease) received an intensive lipid-lowering therapy even before admission according to the current guidelines.

Although the possible mechanisms of atherogenic protection of MB is unknown, there is still some supported evidence. Loukas et al. [18] found that the bridged segments demonstrated weaker proliferative activities of Ki-67 (a cellular marker for proliferation), and a decreased count of smooth muscle cells and macrophages. This phenomenon might be explained with that the MB-related contracting myocardium compression stimulates the release of anticoagulant and growth factors, which could produce a synergistic effect in preventing the endothelium from denudation, inflammation, and resultant atherosclerosis in vessels with MB and possibly in the whole coronary system. In addition, multi-slice

CT scanning showed that the presence of MB was associated with a lower Agatston Calcium Score in the bridged segments [29]. The presence of an MB may also influence arterial tissue through the alteration of hemodynamic forces. According to previous study [24], any atherosclerosis in the MB-segment is suppressed histopathologically and ultrastructurally. Abrupt changes of endothelial cell morphology in the intima beneath the bridge were observed with scanning electron microscopy, which indicates that the arterial tissue beneath the bridge is protected by hemodynamic factors. In cholesterol-fed rabbits, the intima in the MB segment covered by myocardial tissue was free of atherosclerotic lesions, and the endothelial cells were spindle-shaped and engorged [25], which also indicates that the protective element of MB against atherosclerosis might be linked with an alteration of endothelial permeability due to hemodynamic force changes tending towards a higher shear stress. Based on the documented studies as above, the role of myocardial bridges to suppress coronary atherosclerosis might be potential, but it still deserves further scientific research in biochemical and pathophysiological fronts.

Despite the presence of MB can be associated with various complications such as angina, acute myocardial infarction, arrhythmias, and even sudden death [4, 9–17], it can also be considered a benign variation of coronary arteries [19]. So, the treatment of MB is still uncertain due to the lack of convincing evidence. In clinical practice, beta-blockers are usually the first choice of treatment in symptomatic patients [30], other treatments including coronary stents and surgical interventions such as myotomy or bypass are also considered a second-line option. According to a recent systematic review and pooled analysis raised by Enrico Cerrato and colleagues [31], patients with symptomatic isolated MB generally have a good long-term prognosis; pharmacological treatment alone, especially with beta-blockers, can improve angina in most cases. In other words, their study clearly supports that MB is a benign variation of coronary arteries.

Limitations of this study

There are some limitations in our study, including its non-randomization because of retrospective nature and lack of standardization when MB was diagnosed with coronary angiography. Considering the unreliability of patient's subjective statement, smoking and family history for CAD, two major risk factors for CAD, were not included in the present study. Furthermore, it is also difficult for us to interpret the exact mechanisms of the potential of MB against severe obstructive atherosclerosis in the whole coronary artery system.

Conclusions

In conclusion, our results provided a clue that MB might be acted as a potential protective element against severe obstructive atherosclerosis in the whole coronary artery system by adjusting for sex, age, diabetes mellitus, hypertension, and other risk factors, but it still needs further scientific research due to lack of convincing evidence.

Abbreviations

CABG: Coronary artery bypass grafting; CAD: Coronary artery disease; CKD: Chronic kidney disease; DM: Diabetes mellitus; ICVD: Ischemic cerebrovascular disease; IGT: Impaired glucose tolerance; MB: Myocardial bridge; PCI: Percutaneous coronary intervention; SOCAD: Severe obstructive coronary artery disease

Authors' contributions

BH and LJ designed and supervised the study; LJ and MZ prepared the manuscript; LJ, MZ, LS, QS, and LHS performed this study; HZ and LS analyzed and interpreted data; BH and LJ performed critical revision of the article and approved the final version of the manuscript for publication. All authors read and approved the final version of the article, and all have given the necessary attention to ensure the accuracy and integrity of the work.

Competing interests

The authors declare that they have no competing interests.

Author details

Department of Cardiology, Shanghai Jiao Tong University Affiliated Chest Hospital, Shanghai, China. 2Department of Clinical Medicine, Shanghai Medical School, Fudan University, Shanghai, China. 3Department of Cardiology, Renji Hospital, School of Medicine, Shanghai Jiaotong University, Shanghai, China. 4Institution of Biostatistics, School of Life Science, Fudan University, Shanghai, China.

References

1. Möhlenkamp S, Hort W, Ge J, Erbel R. Update on myocardial bridging. Circulation. 2002;106:2616–22.
2. Alegria JR, Herrmann J, Holmes DR Jr, Lerman A, Rihal CS. Myocardial bridging. Eur Heart J. 2015;26:1159–68.
3. Ishikawa Y, Akasaka Y, Ito K, Akishima Y, Kimura M, et al. Significance of anatomical properties of myocardial bridge on atherosclerosis evolution in the left anterior descending coronary artery. Atherosclerosis. 2006;186:380–9.
4. Angelini P, Trivellato M, Donis J, Leachman RD. Myocardial bridges: a review. Prog Cardiovasc Dis. 1983;26:75–88.
5. Kunamneni PB, Rajdev S, Krishnan P, Moreno PR, Kim MC, et al. Outcome of intracoronary stenting after failed maximal medical therapy in patients with symptomatic myocardial bridge. Catheter Cardiovasc Interv. 2008;71:185–90.
6. Tsujita K, Maehara A, Mintz GS, Doi H, Kubo T, et al. Comparison of angiographic and intravascular ultrasonic detection of myocardial bridging of the left anterior descending coronary artery. Am J Cardiol. 2008;102:1608–13.
7. Ferreira AG Jr, Trotter SE, König B Jr, Décourt LV, Fox K, et al. Myocardial bridges: morphological and functional aspects. Br Heart J. 1991;66:364–7.
8. Raimund E, Hans-Jürgen R, Junbo G, Thomas G, Günter G, et al. Coronary artery shape and flow changes induced by myocardial bridging. Echocardiography. 1993;10:71–7.
9. Erdogan HI, Gul EE, Gok H. Relationship between myocardial bridges and arrhythmic complications. J Invasive Cardiol. 2012;24:E300–2.
10. Noble J, Bourassa MG, Petitclerc R, Dyrda I. Myocardial bridging and milking effect of the left anterior descending coronary artery: normal variant or obstruction? Am J Cardiol. 1976;37:993–9.
11. Faruqui AM, Maloy WC, Felner JM, Schlant RC, Logan WD, et al. Symptomatic myocardial bridging of coronary artery. Am J Cardiol. 1978;41:1305–10.
12. den Dulk K, Brugada P, Braat S, Heddle B, Wellens HJ. Myocardial bridging as a cause of paroxysmal atrioventricular block. J Am Coll Cardiol. 1983;1:965–9.
13. Morales AR, Romanelli R, Tate LG, Boucek RJ, de Marchena E. Intramural left anterior descending coronary artery: significance of the depth of the muscular tunnel. Hum Pathol. 1993;24:693–701.
14. Boktor M, Mansi IA, Troxclair S, Modi K. Association of myocardial bridge and Takotsubo cardiomyopathy: a case report and literature review. South Med J. 2009;102:957–60.
15. Nardi F, Verna E, Secco GG, Rognoni A, Sante Bongo A, et al. Variant angina associated with coronary artery endothelial dysfunction and myocardial bridge: a case report and review of the literature. Intern Med. 2011;50:2601–6.
16. Kracoff OH, Ovsyshcher I, Gueron M. Malignant course of a benign anomaly: myocardial bridging. Chest. 1987;92:1113–5.
17. Sunnassee A, Zhu S, Liang R, Liang L. Unexpected death of a young woman: is myocardial bridging significant? —a case report and review of literature. Forensic Sci Med Pathol. 2011;7:42–6.
18. Loukas M, Bhatnagar A, Arumugam S, Smith K, Matusz P, et al. Histologic and immunohistochemical analysis of the antiatherogenic effects of myocardial bridging in the adult human heart. Cardiovasc Pathol. 2014;23:198–203.
19. Kramer JR, Kitazume H, Proudfit WL, Sones FM Jr. Clinical signicance of isolated coronary bridges: benign and frequent condition involving the left anterior descending artery. Am Heart J. 1982;103:283–8.
20. Krawczyk JA, Dashkoff N, Mays A, Klocke FJ. Reduced coronary flow in a canine model of "muscle bridge" with inflow occlusion extending into diastole; possible role of downstream vascular closure. Trans Assoc Am Phys. 1980;93:100–9.
21. Yamada R, Schnittger I, Tremmel JA, Lin S, Yock PG, et al. Abstract 12745: is myocardial bridging truly benign? Impact of myocardial bridging induced arterial compression on atherosclerotic plaque formation. Circulation. 2012;126:A12745.
22. Akaike H. A new look at the statistical model identification. IEEE Trans Autom Control. 1974;19:716–23.
23. Duygu H, Zoghi M, Nalbantgil S, Kirilmaz B, Türk U, et al. Myocardial bridge: a bridge to atherosclerosis. Anadolu Kardiyol Derg. 2007;7:12–6.
24. Ishii T, Asuwa N, Masuda S, Ishikawa Y. The effects of a myocardial bridge on coronary atherosclerosis and ischemia. J Pathol. 1998;185:4–9.
25. Ishikawa Y, Ishii T, Asuwa N, Masuda S. Absence of atherosclerosis evolution in the coronary arterial segment covered by myocardial tissue in cholesterol-fed rabbits. Virchows Arch. 1997;430:163–71.
26. de Winter RJ, Kok WE, Piek JJ. Coronary atherosclerosis within a myocardial bridge, not a benign condition. Heart. 1998;80:91–3.
27. Ishii T, Asuwa N, Masuda S, Ishikawa Y, Kiguchi H, et al. Atherosclerosis suppression in the left anterior descending coronary artery by the presence of a myocardial bridge: an ultrastructuralstudy. Mod Pathol. 1991;4:424–31.
28. Imes CC, Austin MA. Low-density lipoprotein cholesterol, apolipoprotein B, and risk of coronary heart disease: from familial hyperlipidemia to genomics. Biol Res Nurs. 2013;15:292–308.
29. Verhagen SN, Rutten A, Meijs MF, Isgum I, Cramer MJ, et al. Relationship between myocardial bridges and reduced coronary atherosclerosis in patients with angina pectoris. Int J Cardiol. 2013;167:883–8.
30. Schwarz ER, Klues HG, vom Dahl J, Klein I, Krebs W, Hanrath P. Functional, angiographic and intracoronary Doppler flow characteristics in symptomatic patients with myocardial bridging: effect of short-term intravenous beta-blocker medication. J Am Coll Cardiol. 1996;27:1637–45.
31. Cerrato E, Barbero U, D'Ascenzo F, Taha S, Biondi-Zoccai G, Omedè P, et al. What is the optimal treatment for symptomatic patients with isolated coronary myocardial bridge? A systematic review and pooled analysis. J Cardiovasc Med (Hagerstown). 2017;18:758–70.

18

Predicted impact of lipid lowering therapy on cardiovascular and economic outcomes of Swedish atherosclerotic cardiovascular disease guideline

Gunilla Journath[1]*[iD], Kristina Hambraeus[2], Emil Hagström[3], Billie Pettersson[4] and Mickael Löthgren[5]

Abstract

Background: The effects on cardiovascular disease (CVD) by treatment recommendations on prevention of atherosclerotic CVD remain to be evaluated. The objectives were to assess treatment gap for low density lipoprotein cholesterol (LDL-C) according to guidelines, potential impact on CVD outcomes, and possible avoided economic costs, in post myocardial infarction (MI) patients, if target LDL-C levels of ≤1.8 mmol/L would be achieved.

Methods: All patients registered in the Swedish Secondary Prevention after Heart Intensive care Admission register, with one-year post-MI follow-up during 2013 were selected. The REACH risk prediction and a calibrated model for recurrent cardiovascular events and death were used to estimate unadjusted risk prediction based on the REACH equation henceforth called base case, and calibrated CVD outcomes based on gender-specific risk factors. The predicted impact of the LDL-C reduction on the risk of CVD was based on the Cholesterol Treatment Trialists' Collaboration findings.

Results: A sample of $n = 5904$ patients (74% men) with a mean age of 64 years were included. Around 70% did not reach LDL-C target ≤1.8 mmol/L. Over a 10-year period, 820–2262 events were predicted to occur in those who did not reach target corresponding to 20% – 55% risk of CVD events. To achieve LDL-C target, the mean LDL-C had to be reduced by 0.73 mmol/L (29%). If this LDL-C reduction was achieved, 195–544 life years, 132–343 CVD events, and 7.9–20.9 million Swedish crowns (MSEK) of direct costs, and 19.3¯51.0 MSEK of total costs would be avoided.

Conclusion: Lowering of LDL cholesterol to achieve target levels according to guidelines for post-MI patients may lead to fewer cardiovascular events and avoidance of event costs.

Keywords: Cardiovascular disease, Costs, Guidelines, Lipids, Myocardial infarction

Background

Ischemic heart disease (IHD) is the most common CVD, and the leading cause of death in large parts of the world [1] Reduction of low-density lipoprotein cholesterol (LDL-C) with lipid lowering therapy (LLT) has shown a reduction of the risk of cardiovascular events in both high and low risk individuals [2–4]. Meta-analysis of statin trials observed that further risk reductions were found in patients obtaining LDL-C levels below 1.8 mmol/L [5, 6].

European guidelines recommend treatment target levels of LDL-C depending on predicted risk for cardiovascular events, with lower target levels for patients at high risk (very high risk: <1.8 mmol /L; high risk <2.5 mmol/L; moderate risk <3 mmol /L) [7]. Guidelines from the US have another approach recommending fixed-dose strategies instead of targeted goals to lower blood cholesterol [8]. High intensity statin therapy was recommended for patients with high or very high risk, and a low dose statin therapy to those with moderate risk of cardiovascular disease [8].

The Medical Product Agency in Sweden published treatment recommendations on prevention of atherosclerotic

* Correspondence: gunilla.journath@ki.se
[1]Cardiology unit, Department of Medicine, Karolinska Institutet, Karolinska University Hospital, Stockholm, Sweden
Full list of author information is available at the end of the article

cardiovascular disease in 2014 [9], with a similar approach as European guidelines with recommended treatment target of LDL ≤1.8 mmol/L for high risk patients. Patients with established coronary artery disease were classified as high-risk patients in all CVD prevention guidelines. The risk of recurrent disease remained high despite modern treatment for myocardial infarction [10]. Treatment with lipid-lowering agents is cost-effective, especially in high-risk patients [11, 12]. To our knowledge the potential consequences the Swedish guideline have not been published.

The aims were to assess treatment gap for LDL-C according to guidelines, potential impact on CVD outcomes, and possible avoided economic costs, in a cohort of Swedish post myocardial infarction (MI) patients, if target LDL-C levels of ≤1.8 mmol/L would be achieved.

Methods

Setting, study design, and study population

SWEDEHEART is a Swedish national register in which patients with acute coronary syndrome are prospectively registered. Patient characteristic, hospital treatments, drug treatments at discharge, and outcome for patients consecutively included and treated at all Swedish coronary care units are collected in this register [13]. The Swedish Secondary Prevention after Heart intensive care Admission (SEPHIA) is a sub register within SWEDEHEART collecting data on secondary prevention and cardiac rehabilitation [14]. Follow-up data were registered by office visits or phone call, supplemented by blood samples collected at the patient's primary care centre, at six to ten weeks and at 12 to 14 months post MI. Around 80% of all Swedish MI patients below the age of 75 years are included in this register [14].

In this study, a cohort of 5904 patients (74% men) registered in the SEPHIA register and who had one year follow-up during 2013, were included. Data from the SWEDEHEART/SEPHIA national register was extracted in an aggregated form. In accordance with Swedish regulations, written informed consent is not necessary for national registers, however all patients were informed about their participation in the register, and their right to decline participation.

Prediction of cardiovascular disease risk

The Reduction of Atherothrombosis for Continued Health (REACH) risk function was used to predict 20-month risk of recurrent CVD [15]. This model provided estimates of recurrent non-fatal and fatal CVD events based on the following risk factors: age (years), gender (male/female), smoking, diabetes mellitus; body mass index (BMI) <20 kg/m², number of vascular beds with CVD-manifestations (1, 2, 3), congestive heart failure, atrial fibrillation, statin treatment, and acetylsalicylic acid treatment [15]. The predicted 20-month fatal and non-fatal CVD risk were derived from the "next event" REACH equation using the detailed Cox regression model covariate coefficient estimates provided in Wilson et al. 2012 Appendix [15]. CVD rates were predicted separately for males and females, before calculating a weighted average the overall cohort risk, accounting for gender variation in risk factors. CVD risk was estimated separately for each year in the prediction time period, accounting for the yearly increase in cohort age and the impact of increased age on CVD risk. The predicted 20-months risks were annualized for each year of prediction. The effect on CVD risk derived from the lowering of LDL-C was calculated based on the Cholesterol Treatment Trialists' Collaboration (CTTC) meta-analyses results, linking LDL-C lowering to CVD event risk reduction [6]. Different rate ratios of CVD event reductions per mmol/L LDL-C reduction were used based on CTTC: MI (0.71), ischemic stroke (IS) (0.69) and fatal CHD (0.80) [6]. For fatal stroke a rate ratio of one was used based on the non-significant difference reported by CTTC [6]. The proportion (%) of non-fatal (MI and stroke) vs. fatal CVD event post MI, was based on Jernberg et al. reported event distribution of up to 24 months post MI: 46.8% CVD death, 37.8% MI, 15.4% stroke [16]. In the age ranges 55–64 to 65–74 years of fatal CHD vs. fatal stroke occurred in 96% vs. 4% post-MI, indicating that fatal CHD is more common than fatal strokes in post MI patients [17]. The direct costs of non-fatal MI and stroke were based on Hallberg et al. 2015 [18] and were for MI: Swedish crowns (SEK) 76,657, and ischemic stroke: SEK 88,790. These event cost estimates were from Table 4 in Hallberg et al. 2016, and from the incremental cost year (day 0–365 days after new CVD event) for the CVD history cohort. The reported cost estimates were converted to SEK using the same exchange rate of 1 € = 8.71 SEK as reported by Hallberg et al. 2015, p. 3. Fatal CVD costs were estimated, and based on Ara et al. 2009 [19] and were for CHD death costs SEK 11,345 (14.8% of MI costs) and stroke death SEK 40,577 (45.7% of stroke costs). Total directs costs of CV events were estimated in a first analysis step. In a second step the total cost including costs of informal care by family and relatives, indirect costs of productivity loss due to premature death, and reduced work capacity ere estimated based on previous findings have shown that direct costs accounted for around 41% of total costs [20].

The REACH risk prediction model was based on participants from around the world with different prior CVD events, not only MI [19]. Results from the UK Clinical Practice Research Datalink (CPRD) calibration analyses indicated that the REACH risk prediction significantly underestimated the risk of CVD events in a post-acute coronary syndrome population [21]. Analyses of the REACH risk prediction were therefore, calibrated according to CPRD analyses. The CPRD study included heart failure (HF) in addition to MI, stroke and CVD mortality outcomes, and hence the reported calibration factor of 3.36 for a post- acute coronary syndrome (ACS) population had to be adjusted for the purpose of this study. Based on the post-ACS cohort, the adjusted calibration factor was 3.06 = 3.36*(1–0.089) in the CPRD cohort accounting for HF incidence in patients between 64 and 73 years old. In addition to the prediction of fatal and non-fatal CVD event using the REACH risk prediction, the predictions account for Swedish age- and gender specific non-CVD mortality life tables from Statistics Sweden were used (available at www.scb.se/hitta-statistik).

Statistical analyses

Demographics and other baseline characteristics were presented for the overall study population, as well as for the controlled cohort (LDL-C ≤ 1.8 mmol/L), the non-controlled (LDL-C > 1.8 mmol/L) cohort, and in men and women separately. The REACH risk function was used to predict the CVD risk [15], as well as the calibrated CVD risk prediction described above [19]. The possible avoided costs were based on cases at baseline in REACH (henceforth called base case), the calibrated (scenario) risk predictions, the corresponding population's CVD costs and potential cost reductions linked to LDL-C reduction according to guidelines. This was predicted by combining event prediction and estimation of health care costs associated with each type of event.

Results

Table 1 shows the characteristics of the study population (n = 5904, 74% men). Around 70% of the overall cohort did not reach the target of LDL-C ≤ 1.8 mmol/L (men 69% and women 75%). An average LDL-C reduction of 0.73 mmol/L (men 0.70 mmol/L, women 0.81 mmol/L) was required to achieve the LDL-C target corresponding to an average LDL-C reduction of 29% (men 28% and women 31%). There was a lower proportion of patients with diabetes, and statin-treated patients, in the non-controlled group than in the controlled group (Table 1). The base case and calibrated risk predictions ranged from 820 to 2262 total CVD events over a 10-year period in the non-controlled group, corresponding to a baseline CVD event risk of 20% -55% (Fig. 1). Over a ten-year period, the LDL-C reductions to reach target was predicted to lead to 195–544 gained life years, 132–343 fewer CVD events (fatal [39–97], non-fatal MI, and stroke [93–246]) (Fig. 2). The corresponding total direct health care costs were predicted to be reduced by 7.9–20.9 (million Swedish crowns) MSEK and total health care costs by 19.3–51.0 MSEK (Fig. 3).

Discussion

This study shows that around 70% of very high risk patients with prior MI did not have controlled LDL-C, 12 months post MI. We found that an average additional LDL-C reduction by 29% (0.73 mmol/L) would be needed to achieve target level of LDL-C 1.8 mmol/L. This LDL-C reduction was estimated to lead to a total of 132–343 fewer CVD events with corresponding health care costs reduced by in total 19.3–51.0 MSEK, accounting for 20.1% of the total predicted event costs. Over a ten-year period 805–2262 CVD events was predicted to occur in the non-controlled patients (n = 4145),

Table 1 Characteristics of the study population

Variable	Overall cohort			Controlled cohort (LDL-C ≤ 1.8 mmol/L)			Non-controlled Cohort (LDL-C > 1.8 mmol/L)		
	Total	Men	Women	Total	Men	Women	Total	Men	Women
n (%)	5904 (100)	4386 (74)	1518 (26)	1759 (100)	1377 (78)	382 (22)	4145 (100)	3009 (73)	1136 (27)
LDL-C, mean (SD) mmol/L	2.2 (0.9)	2.2 (0.8)	2.3 (0.9)	1.4 (0.3)	1.4 (0.3)	1.4 (0.3)	2.5 (0.8)	2.5 (0.8)	2.6 (0.8)
Risk factors for REACH risk predictions									
Age, mean (SD)	64 (9)	63 (8)	65 (9)	64 (9)	64 (9)	64 (9)	64 (8)	63 (8)	65 (8)
Smoking´(%)	13	12	15	13	12	15	13	12	15
Diabetes mellitus (%)	25	24	27	31	30	34	23	22	25
BMI < 20 kg/m² (%)	2	1	4	2	1	4	2	1	3
Number of vascular beds affected	1.1	1.1	1.1	1.1	1.0	1.1	1.1	1.1	1.1
One vascular bed affected (%)	95	95	95	95	96	94	95	95	95
Two vascular beds affected (%)	5	5	5	5	4	6	5	5	5
Congestive heart failure (%)	2	2	2	3	3	3	2	2	2
Atrial fibrillation (%)	3	3	3	4	4	4	3	3	2
Statin treatment (%)	92	93	88	99	99	99	89	91	85
Acetylsalicylic acid treatment (%)	92	93	90	93	93	94	92	93	89

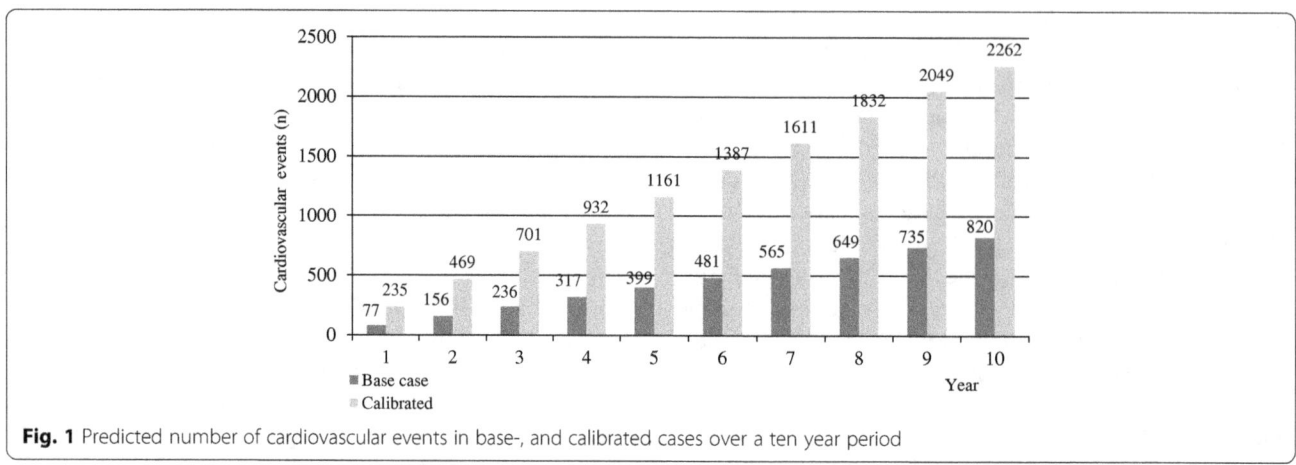

Fig. 1 Predicted number of cardiovascular events in base-, and calibrated cases over a ten year period

corresponding to a 20–55% ten-year risk of non-fatal MI, stroke and fatal CVD event. A total of 195–544 lives were predicted to be gained over ten years in the study population, if target LDL-levels were achieved.

In the western countries the incidence of MI has declined, and one-year post-MI survival has improved [22, 23]. However, patients who have survived a MI, are still at high risk and one in five was estimated to have a recurrent CVD event during a subsequent 10-year year period [16]. A large proportion of patients in this study received LLT but did not reach LDL-C target according to guidelines [9]. Treatment gaps between guidelines and real world results regarding risk factor control for CHD patients in Europe was reported in the EUROASPIRE-studies. Lipid control, defined as LDL <1.8 mmol/L increased from 6.1% in EUROASPIRE II (1999–2000) to 25.6% in EUROASPIRE IV (2012–2013), revealing a failure of current secondary prevention strategies to deliver best possible treatment to patients after a coronary

event [24]. Data from the Swedish quality registry SWEDEHEART showed that goal attainment for LDL-C improved, from 46% in 2014 to 51% in 2015 [25]. One explanation for the higher proportion of patients achieving LDL-C goal could be that access to high intensity statins increased, when prices for atorvastatin decreased following the patent expiration. Earlier changes in reimbursement schemes showed that around one fifth of the patients switched from low dose to higher doses of atorvastatin following a new reimbursement scheme, where higher doses of atorvastatin was covered while lower doses were not reimbursed in the new scheme [26]. Non-adherence to prescription may also be a reason for not achieving LDL-C target. Prior observational studies, in patients with IHD, have shown adherence to statin treatment in between 50% to 79% [27, 28]. Factors that may affect adherence could be demographic and socioeconomic factors, side effects, life-style, time since last provider visit and number of pills prescribed [29].

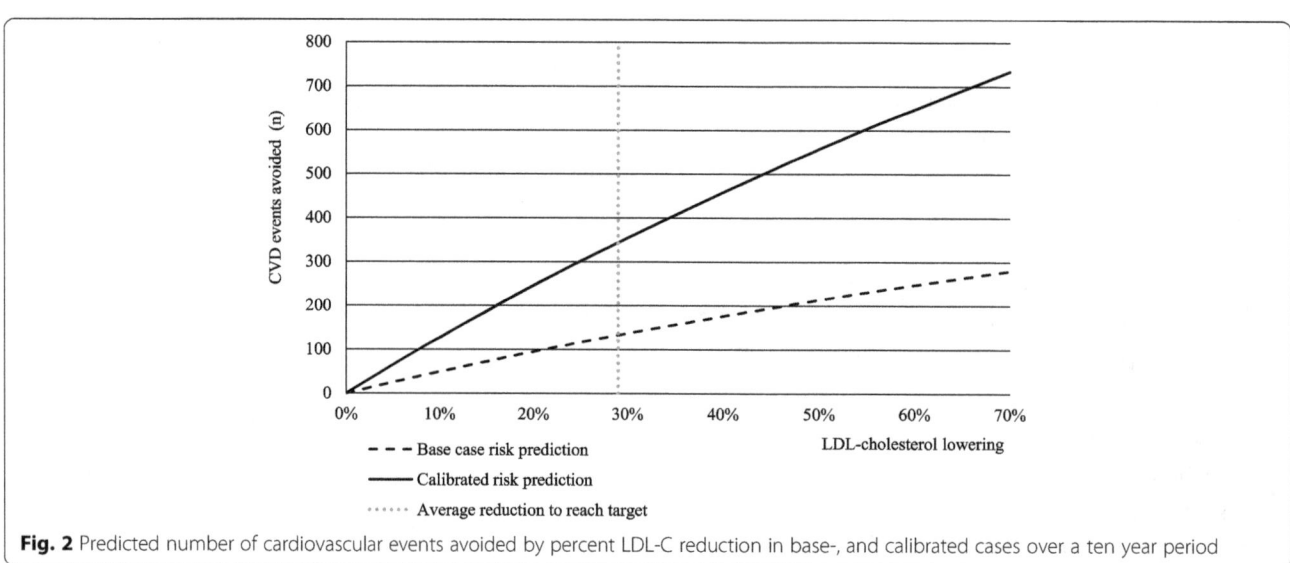

Fig. 2 Predicted number of cardiovascular events avoided by percent LDL-C reduction in base-, and calibrated cases over a ten year period

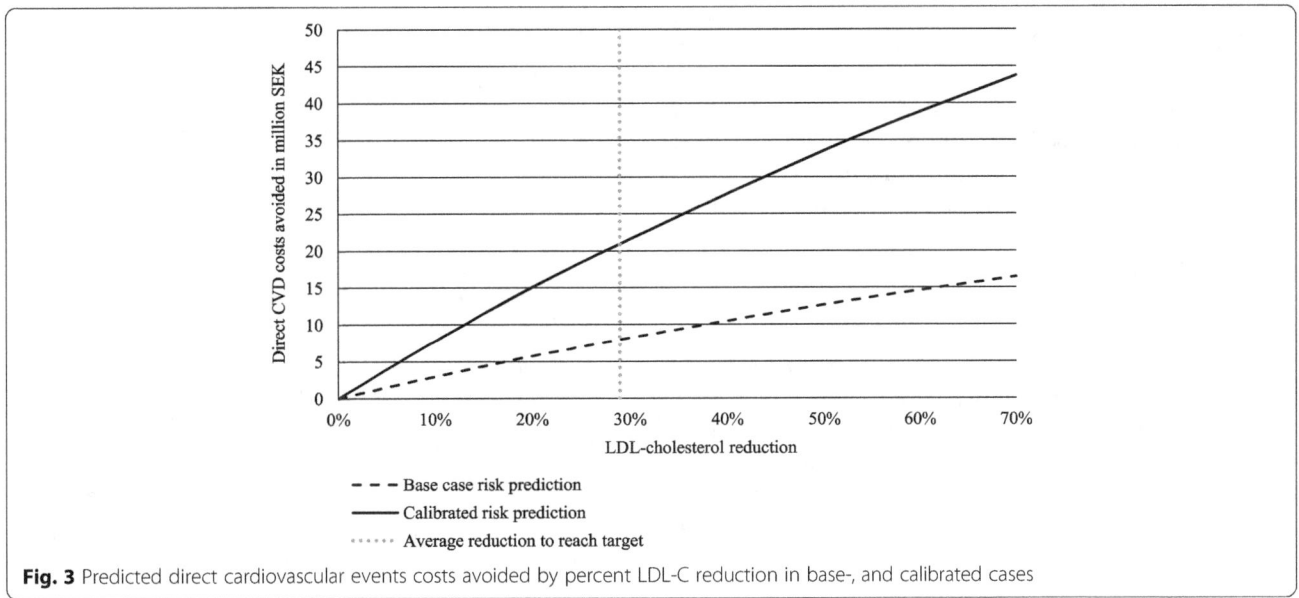

Fig. 3 Predicted direct cardiovascular events costs avoided by percent LDL-C reduction in base-, and calibrated cases

Strategies to improve adherence to secondary prevention medication need to be tailored to relevant patient- and community factors.

The results presented predicted CVD events and costs over a ten-year period for the analysed incident cohort. In order to assess the cost in a given year or over a period of years we needed to assess the CVD events and cost prediction for a prevalent population. This was done based on the available incident cohort and a life time prediction of CVD events and costs underestimated steady-state assumption (ie every year a cohort of same size and characteristics as the study cohorts were assumed to enter post MI). The cohort life-time predictions represented exactly the CVD events and costs expected to materialize in any given year. Under a life-time prediction horizon the base case and calibrated predictions indicated that 1396–2741 life years could be gained, 350–606 CVD events avoided and direct CVD costs reduced 21.4–39.2 MSEK if LDL-C levels were reduced on average 0.78 mmol/L. If willingness to pay for a life year gained is about 553,000 SEK [30, 31] then this would mean that the monetary value of the life years gained in our study would be 108–326 MSEK for the estimated 195–544 life-year gained in base case and risk calibrated scenario [30]. In a sensitivity analysis, using an LDL-C lowering up to 70%, up to 280 CVD events could potentially be avoided (vs case 132 events). Up to 19 M SEK due to CVD costs were estimated to be avoided over a 10-year period in the cohort. Ongoing outcomes studies with other non-statin therapies as PCSK9-inhibitors will add additional information on whether further lowering of LDL-C will prevent CVD events.

Limitations and strengths

The presented analyses and results focused on the assessment of the impact on CVD risk and costs if the current LDL-C target was reached in comparison with the current treatment patterns and practices. CVD risk and costs were predicted over a 10-year time horizon accounting for increased age and consequent increased CVD risk over time. However, the analysis was not accounting for any other risk factor changes over time, and is furthermore not accounting for possible future change of statin treatment goal and attainment rate which may change further with physicians' care or disease progression. The post-MI population in this study was younger, due to the age limit of the SEPHIA-register, more often revascularised, and had a higher proportion of men, also due to age inclusion criteria, compared with the MI population in general, which limited the generalizability. Since ICD-10 codes were used for morbidity data there was a possibility for coding errors. However, a validation of the Swedish in patient register showed that coding was concurrent in >98% of the cases [32]. The study was based on population averages, and not individual patient-level data. For the analysis of implementation of the guidelines focused on LDL-C this poses some challenges as the guidelines specifies that target LDL-C is ≤1.8 mmol/L, or if this cannot be achieved, a 50% reduction in LDL-C levels. Recently European Guidelines on CVD in clinical practice recommended an LDL-C goal <1.8 mmol/L, or a reduction of at least 50% if the baseline is between 1.8 and 3.5 mmol/L in very high risk patients [33]. The patients in this study represent around 80% of the total MI-population in Sweden in this age group and, potential selection bias was considered to be low. There is a risk of conservative bias, as patients with lower social, financial and health-related functioning may be less likely to attend follow-up visits. The study population should however provide a good estimate of treatment strategies and treatment goals attainment in usual care. Possible future research should compare these risk model based on predictions with actual real-world outcomes over a longer period in the SEPHIA register.

Conclusion

Despite the multitude of evidence of lowering the CVD risk by intensive secondary prevention there was a large treatment gap between guidelines and achievement of target LDL-C. Lowering of LDL cholesterol to achieve target levels according to guidelines for post-MI patients may lead to fewer cardiovascular events and avoidance of event costs.

Abbreviations

ACS: Acute coronary syndrome; CHD: Coronary heart disease; CPRD: The UK Clinical Practice Research Datalink; CTTC: The Cholesterol Treatment Trialists´ Collaboration; CVD: Cardiovascular disease; EUROASPIRE: European Society of Cardiology survey of secondary prevention of coronary heart disease; HF: Heart failure; IHD: Ichemic heart disease; LDL-C: Low density lipoprotein cholesterol; LLT: Lipid lowering theraphy; MI: Myocardial infarction; MSEK: Million Swedish crowns; REACH: The Reduction of Atherotrombosis for Continued Health; SEK: Swedish crowns; SEPHIA: The Swedish Secondary Prevention after Heart intensive care Admission Swedeheart: Swedish quality registers of coronary heart diseases; US: United States

Acknowledgements

We thank all participating centers in the SWEDEHEART register that collected the data, and Professor Johan Sundström, Uppsala Clinical Research Center, and Department of Medical Sciences, Uppsala University, Sweden, for valuable support during the planning of the study.

Funding

Amgen AB supported the study financially by paying the costs for extraction of data registers, and administration.

Authors' contributions

BP, GJ, KH, EH, and ML made substantial contributions to the conception, and design. KH, and EH contributed with acquisition of data. The manuscript was drafted by GJ and ML. ML and BP were responsible for the data analyses. All authors critically reviewed drafts of the manuscript, were responsible for the interpretation of the findings, and approved the final version of the manuscript.

Competing interests

Financial disclosures: GJ has received consultant fee from Amgen. KH has received lecture fees from Amgen, and Astra Zeneca, and an unrestricted grant from Gilead Inc. EH is an expert committee member, and have received lecture fees, and institutional research grant from Sanofi; institutional research grant and lecture fees from Amgen; institutional research grants from AstraZeneca; expert committee member for Ariad and MSD. BP and ML are employed by Amgen.

Author details

[1]Cardiology unit, Department of Medicine, Karolinska Institutet, Karolinska University Hospital, Stockholm, Sweden. [2]Department of Cardiology, Falun Hospital, Falun, Sweden. [3]Uppsala Clinical Research Center, and Department of Medical Sciences, Uppsala University, Uppsala, Sweden. [4]Amgen Inc, Thousand Oaks, California, USA. [5]Amgen (Europe) GmbH, Zug, Switzerland.

References

1. Mathers CD, Loncar D. Projections of global mortality, and burden of disease from 2002 to 2030. PLoS Med. 2006;3:e442.
2. Bjorck L, Rosengren A, Bennett K, Lappas G, Capewell S. Modelling the decreasing coronary heart disease mortality in Sweden between 1986 and 2002. Eur Heart J. 2009;30:1046–56.
3. Cholesterol Treatment Trialists CTT, Mihaylova B, Emberson J, et al. The effects of lowering LDL cholesterol with statin therapy in people at low risk of vascular disease: meta-analysis of individual data from 27 randomised trials. Lancet. 2012;380:581–90.
4. Zoungas S, Curtis AJ, McNeil JJ, Tonkin AM. Treatment of dyslipidemia and cardiovascular outcomes: the journey so far–is this the end for statins? Clin Pharmacol Ther. 2014;96:192–205.
5. Boekholdt SM, Arsenault BJ, Hovingh GK, et al. Levels and changes of HDL cholesterol and apolipoprotein A-I in relation to risk of cardiovascular events among statin-treated patients: a meta-analysis. Circulation. 2013;128:1504–12.
6. Cholesterol Treatment Trialists CTT, Baigent C, Blackwell L, et al. Efficacy and safety of more intensive lowering of LDL cholesterol: a meta-analysis of data from 170,000 participants in 26 randomised trials. Lancet. 2010;376:1670–81.
7. Perk J, De Backer G, Gohlke H, et al. European guidelines on cardiovascular disease prevention in clinical practice (version 2012): the fifth joint task force of the European Society of Cardiology and Other Societies on cardiovascular disease prevention in clinical practice (constituted by representatives of nine societies and by invited experts). Eur Heart J. 2012;33:1635–701.
8. Stone NJ, Robinson JG, Lichtenstein AH, et al. 2013 ACC/AHA guideline on the treatment of blood cholesterol to reduce atherosclerotic cardiovascular risk in adults: a report of the American College of Cardiology/American Heart Association task force on practice guidelines. Circulation. 2014;129:S1–45.
9. Medical product Agency. To prevent atherosclerotic cardiovascular disease with drugs- treatment recommendation. https://lakemedelsverket.se/upload/om-lakemedelsverket/publikationer/information-franlakemedelsverket/2014/Information_fran_lakemedelsverket_nr_5_2014_webb.pdf. Accessed 16 Oct 2016.
10. Fox KA, Carruthers KF, Dunbar DR, et al. Underestimated and under-recognized: the late consequences of acute coronary syndrome (GRACE UK-Belgian study). Eur Heart J. 2010;31:2755–64.
11. Lindgren P, Graff J, Olsson AG, Pedersen TJ, Jonsson B, Investigators IT. Cost-effectiveness of high-dose atorvastatin compared with regular dose simvastatin. Eur Heart J. 2007;28:1448–53.
12. Gandhi SK, Jensen MM, Fox KM, Smolen L, Olsson AG, Paulsson T. Cost-effectiveness of rosuvastatin in comparison with generic atorvastatin and simvastatin in a Swedish population at high risk of cardiovascular events. ClinicoEconomics and outcomes research : CEOR. 2012;4:1–11.
13. Jernberg T, Attebring MF, Hambraeus K, et al. The Swedish web-system for enhancement and development of evidence-based care in heart disease evaluated according to recommended therapies (SWEDEHEART). Heart. 2010;96:1617–21.
14. SWEDEHEART (2014). Annual report 2013. http://www.ucr.uu.se/swedeheart/. Accessed 16 Oct 2016.
15. Wilson PW, D'Agostino R Sr, Bhatt DL, et al. An international model to predict recurrent cardiovascular disease. Am J Med. 2012;125:695–703.
16. Jernberg T, Hasvold P, Henriksson M, Hjelm H, Thuresson M, Janzon M. Cardiovascular risk in post-myocardial infarction patients: nationwide real world data demonstrate the importance of a long-term perspective. Eur Heart J. 2015;36:1163–70.
17. Ara R, Tumur I, Pandor A, et al. Ezetimibe for the treatment of hypercholesterolaemia: a systematic review and economic evaluation. Health Technol Assess. 2008;12:21.
18. Hallberg S, Gandra SR, Fox KM, et al. Healthcare costs associated with cardiovascular events in patients with hyperlipidemia or prior cardiovascular events: estimates from Swedish population-based register data. Eur J Health Econ. 2015; doi:10.1007/s10198-015-0702-0.

Predicted impact of lipid lowering therapy on cardiovascular and economic outcomes of Swedish...

173

19. Ara R, Pandor A, Stevens J, Rees A, Rafia R. Early high-dose lipid-lowering therapy to avoid cardiac events: a systematic review and economic evaluation. Health Technol Assess. 2009;13:1–74. 5-118

20. Steen-Karlsson K, and Persson U. (2012) Kostnader för Hjärt-Kärlsjukdom år 2010 IHE Rapport Lund: Institutet för Hälso- och Sjukvårdsekonomi.

21. Danese M LM, Villa G, Lindgren P, van Hout B, and Taylor B. Differences between observed and predicted cardiovascular event rates using standard tools for risk prediction. The case of high-intensity statin users in the United Kingdom. Circulation 2015; 132: A18114 2015.

22. Nichols M, Townsend N, Scarborough P, Rayner M. Trends in age-specific coronary heart disease mortality in the European Union over three decades: 1980-2009. Eur Heart J. 2013;34:3017–27.

23. Nichols M, Townsend N, Scarborough P, Rayner M. Cardiovascular disease in Europe: epidemiological update. Eur Heart J. 2013;34:3028–34.

24. Kotseva K, Wood D, De Bacquer D, et al. EUROASPIRE IV: a European Society of Cardiology survey on the lifestyle, risk factor and therapeutic management of coronary patients from 24 European countries. Eur J Prev Cardiol. 2016;23:636–48.

25. SWEDEHEART (2017). Annual report 2016. http://www.ucr.uu.se/swedeheart/dokument-sh/arsrapporter. Accessed 2 March 2017.

26. Pettersson B, Hoffmann M, Wandell P, Levin LA. Utilization and costs of lipid modifying therapies following health technology assessment for the new reimbursement scheme in Sweden. Health policy. 2012;104:84–91.

27. Foody JM, Joyce AT, Rudolph AE, Liu LZ, Benner JS. Persistence of atorvastatin and simvastatin among patients with and without prior cardiovascular diseases: a US managed care study. Curr Med Res Opin. 2008;24:1987–2000.

28. Ho PM, Spertus JA, Masoudi FA, et al. Impact of medication therapy discontinuation on mortality after myocardial infarction. Arch Intern Med. 2006;166:1842–7.

29. Ho PM, Bryson CL, Rumsfeld JS. Medication adherence: its importance in cardiovascular outcomes. Circulation. 2009;119:3028–35.

30. Persson U, Norinder A, Hjalte K, Gralen K. The value of a statistical life in transport: findings from a new contingent valuation study in Sweden. J Risk Uncertainty. 2001;23:121–34.

31. Persson U, Hjelmgren J. Health services need knowledge of how the public values health. Lakartidningen. 2003;100(43):3436–7.

32. Ludvigsson JF, Andersson E, Ekbom A, et al. External review and validation of the Swedish national inpatient register. BMC Public Health. 2011;11:450.

33. Piepoli MF, Hoes AW, Agewall S, et al. 2016 European guidelines on cardiovascular disease prevention in clinical practice: the sixth joint task force of the European Society of Cardiology and Other Societies on cardiovascular disease prevention in clinical practice (constituted by representatives of 10 societies and by invited experts): developed with the special contribution of the European Association for Cardiovascular Prevention & rehabilitation (EACPR). Eur Heart J. 2016;37:2315–81.

34. SWEDEHEART. http://www.ucr.uu.se/swedeheart/. Accessed 3 August 2017.

19

Comparison of circulating dendritic cell and monocyte subsets at different stages of atherosclerosis: insights from optical coherence tomography

Jianhui Zhuang[1†], Yang Han[2†], Dachun Xu[1†], Guofu Zhu[1], Shekhar Singh[1], Luoman Chen[1], Mengyun Zhu[1], Wei Chen[1], Yawei Xu[1] and Xiankai Li[1,3*] ⓘ

Abstract

Background: While specific patterns of circulating dendritic cells (DCs) and monocytes are associated with the incidence of coronary artery disease, the characterization of circulating DC and monocyte subsets in patients with different stages of atherosclerosis remains unclear.

Methods: Forty-eight patients with unstable angina pectoris (UAP) diagnosed by angiography were enrolled. Likewise, 31 patients with ST-segment elevation myocardial infarction (STEMI) were enrolled and confirmed with the presence of thrombosis by angiography. Plaque features of 48 UAP patients were evaluated at the culprit lesions by OCT. Circulating myeloid DCs (mDCs), plasmacytoid DCs (pDCs) and monocyte subsets were analyzed using flow cytometry.

Results: The proportions and absolute counts of mDC2s, which specifically express CD141 and possess the ability to activate CD8+ T lymphocytes, significantly decreased in patients with UAP and STEMI when compared with controls ($0.08 \times 10^4 \pm 0.05 \times 104/ml$ and $0.08 \times 10^4 \pm 0.06 \times 104/ml$ vs. $0.11 \times 10^4 \pm 0.06 \times 104/ml$, $p = 0.027$). On the other hand, patients with UAP and STEMI had significantly higher proportions and counts of Mon2 subsets. In the OCT subgroup, patients with thin-cap fibroatheroma (TCFA) had higher proportions and absolute number of Mon2 ($11.96\% \pm 4.27\%$ vs. $9.42\% \pm 4.05\%$, $p = 0.034$; $5.17 \times 104/ml \pm 1.92 \times 104/ml$ vs. $3.53 \times 104/ml \pm 2.65 \times 104/ml$, $p = 0.045$) than those without TCFA. However, there was no remarkable difference in mDC2s between patients with and without TCFA.

Conclusions: Circulating Mon2 appears to be a promising marker for the severity of atherosclerotic plaque.

Keywords: Dendritic cells, Monocytes, Plaque vulnerability, Optical coherence tomography

Background

During the development of coronary atherosclerosis, atherosclerotic plaque enlargement accompanied with narrowing of arterial luminal results in a series of chronic ischemic manifestations. More seriously, plaque instability and ensuing rupture with superimposed thrombi eventually lead to myocardial infarction and sudden death [1]. Thin-cap fibroatheroma (TCFA) is the most common phenotype of vulnerable plaque and is the precursor of plaque rupture. Although a greater understanding of lesion dimensions favors the clinical detection of TCFA in coronary artery disease (CAD) patients, coronary angiography alone could not provide comprehensive information on plaque morphology beyond luminal narrowing. Current clinical studies have suggested that optical coherence tomography (OCT) is one of the most preferred invasive approaches that allow high-resolution (10 μm) tomographic intra-arterial imaging [2, 3].

* Correspondence: lixiankai@tongji.edu.cn

†Equal contributors

[1]Department of Cardiology, Shanghai Tenth People's Hospital, Tongji University School of Medicine, Shanghai, China

[3]Department of Cardiology, Shigatse People's Hospital, Shigatse, Tibet, China

Full list of author information is available at the end of the article

As professional antigen-presenting cells, monocytes and dendritic cells (DCs) possess the ability to recognize and present antigens to T cells [4]. Human circulating monocytes could be categorized into three subsets according to different expression of membrane receptors CD14 and CD16: a numerically dominant CD14++CD16- subset (Mon1), an intermediate CD14++CD16+ subset (Mon2), and a non-classical CD14 + CD16++ subset (Mon3) [5, 6]. Given the heterogeneity of circulating monocytes, the exact identity of atherosclerosis-related monocyte subsets deserves careful consideration. In this regard, some studies demonstrated that CD16 positive monocytes were associated with the incidence of myocardial infarction and in-stent restenosis [7, 8]. Furthermore, Rogacev et al. [9] observed that Mon2 subsets independently predicted the incidence of cardiovascular disease. Conversely, an earlier study by Shantsila et al. [10] did not find a marked correlation between monocyte subsets and the incidence of CAD. To our best knowledge, the relationship between monocyte subsets and atherosclerotic progress has not been examined.

Depending on the origin, location and function, DCs comprise two heterogeneous subpopulations. For human, plasmacytoid DCs (pDCs) express the surface marker blood dendritic cell antigen (BDCA)-2, while myeloid DCs (mDCs) could be categorized into mDC1 subsets with BDCA-1 and mDC2 subsets with BDCA-3 [11]. Recent reviews have helped solidify the knowledge of pDCs and mDCs in atherosclerosis [12]. Indeed, several clinical trials attempting to address whether circulating DC subsets correlate with the incidence and severity of CAD reached contradictory results [13, 14].

Toward this end, we sought to explore which subsets of DCs and monocytes are associated with the emergence, vulnerability and rupture of atherosclerotic plaques identified by coronary angiography and OCT.

Methods

Study population

Between April 2013 and July 2014, 112 subjects with acute chest pain as their first clinical manifestation undergoing coronary angiography and showing identifiable de novo culprit lesions in any native coronary artery were admitted at our hospital (Additional file 1: Figure S1). Among these individuals, 48 unstable angina pectoris (UAP) patients undergoing OCT were finally enrolled in the study. UAP was defined as angina at rest, accelerated angina or new-onset angina without elevation of cardiac markers [15]. Thirty-one ST-segment elevation myocardial infarction (STEMI) patients confirmed with the presence of acute thrombosis secondary to plaque rupture by angiography were also enrolled. The diagnosis of STEMI is clearly defined as ST-elevation in at least two contiguous leads >0.2 mV

(2 mm) in chest leads and/or >0.1 mV (1 mm) in limb leads, and elevation of serum cardiac troponin-T (cTnT) level with at least one value above the 99th percentile upper reference limit [16]. Thirty-three subjects with possible cardiac etiology but free of luminal diameter narrowing ≥50% at coronary angiography served as controls.

The study was approved by Ethics Committee of Shanghai Tenth People's Hospital and all individuals provided written informed concept before participation.

Angiography and optical coherence tomography analysis

The located vessel, minimum lumen area and percent diameter stenosis of culprit lesion were measured. Culprit lesions were identified from a combination of electrocardiographic changes, echocardiographic findings and angiographic lesion morphologies.

Frequency domain Optical coherence tomography (OCT) imaging (C7XR, St. Jude, USA) was performed before any intervention and after intracoronary administration of nitroglycerin (0.2 mg) in UAP patients with a TIMI flow grade of 3. OCT images were digitalized and analysed offline according to the principals of OCT imaging described elsewhere [2, 17]. Two independent experienced clinicians who were blinded to the angiographic and clinical data analyzed the OCT images using validated criteria for plaque characterization (Additional file 2: Figure S2). Lipid cores at culprit lesions were defined as diffusely bordered, signal-poor regions. A fibrous cap was identified as a signal-rich homogenous region overlying a lipid core, which was characterized by a diffusely bordered, signal-poor region on the OCT image. Fibrous cap thickness was measured at the thinnest point in culprit plaques for three different times and the average value was calculated. The thinnest fibrous cap thickness was defined as the distance from the arterial lumen to the inner border of the lipid pool where the fibrous cap thickness is considered minimal in non-ruptured lipid-rich plaques. TCFA was defined as a plaque presenting lipid content for >90 degrees, and with thinnest part of the fibrous cap measuring <65 μm [18]. In the current research, there is no case enrolled with TCFA in all 3 vessels at the same time as inner quality control.

Analysis of circulating DCs and monocytes by flow cytometry

Approximate 3–5 ml peripheral blood samples were taken at the day after admission from control group and UAP patients who had fasted overnight, while blood samples from STEMI patients were collected at the day of charge. It should be noted that all pheripheral blood samples from study population were obtained before coronary angiography. Peripheral leukocyte, polymorphonuclear granulocytes (PMNs), lymphocyte and monocyte counts were determined by Coulter Automated Hematology Analyzer (Beckman Coulter, USA). DC subsets from enrollments were analyzed using Blood Dendritic Cell Enumeration Kit (Miltenyi Biotec, Netherlands) [14]. Four-color flow cytometry (FACS Calibur, BD Biosciences, USA) was conducted using monoclonal antibodies against CD14, CD19, BDCA-1, BDCA-2 and BDCA-3 that were directly conjugated with fluorochromes. Dead cells, granulocytes, CD19+ B cells and CD14+ monocytes were excluded. The mDC1s were defined as cells positive for BDCA-1, while mDC2s were BDCA-3 immunopostive cells and pDCs were BDCA-2 immunopostive cells. To achieve the absolute mDC1, mDC2 and pDC count/ml, we set the above determined DC-proportions in relation to the total leucocyte count/ml. Monocyte subsets were analyzed in a whole-blood assay using 100 μl of whole blood as previously described [19]. FSC/SSC gate was positioned to exclude cell debris and granulocytes and monocytes were identified and gated in a CD45 (Miltenyi Biotec, Netherlands)/CD86 (BD Biosciences, USA) dot plots. Blood cells were simultaneously stained with anti-CD14-FITC (Miltenyi Biotec, Netherlands), anti-CD16-PE (Miltenyi Biotec, Netherlands) and anti-CCR2-APC (R&D Systems, UK) antibodies for 15 min at room temperature and analyzed by flow cytometry (Additional file 3: Figure S3). The flow cytometry for identifying DC and monocyte subsets was performed by one expert technician who was blind to the coronary angiography and OCT results.

Biochemical analysis

Plasma levels of fasting glucose, total cholesterol and triglyceride, low-density lipoprotein cholesterol (LDL-C), high-density lipoprotein cholesterol (HDL-C) and high sensitivity C-reactive protein (hs-CRP), and serum levels of cTnT and creatine kinase-MB (CK-MB) were measured by colorimetric enzymatic assay systems (Roche MODULAR P-800, Swiss Confederation). Plasma levels of fibrinogen (Diagnostic Stago, France) and MMP9 (R&D System, USA) were measure using enzyme-linked immunosorbent assay by an automatic microplate reader (SpectraMaxi3, Molecular Devices, USA).

Statistical anaylsis

Data were reported as mean ± standard deviation (SD) for continuous variables and as proportions for categorical variables. Student t test was undertaken to examine the differences between two groups. ANOVA test and Bonferroni correction were performed to compare the differences among controls, UAP patients and STEMI patients. The differences between categorical variables

were determined using χ [2] test. Correlations between circulating DC and monocyte subsets and plaque characteristics were tested using the Pearson's correlation test. A p value of <0.05 was considered statistically significant. Calculations were carried out using SPSS 14.0 software (SPSS Inc., USA).

Results
Baseline characteristics of patients

The baseline characteristics of enrollments are summarized in Additional file 4: Table S1. There was a male predominance in UAP and STEMI groups. The prevalence of smoking was higher in UAP and STEMI groups (35.4% and 51.6%, respectively) than in control group (12.1%). STEMI patients had higher levels of fasting glucose and triglyceride compared with healthy controls (fasting glucose: 7.4 ± 3.5 mmol/L vs. 5.5 ± 2.1 mmol/L; triglyceride: 3.0 ± 1.4 mmol/L vs. 1.7 ± 1.2 mmol/L). By definition, serum levels of cTnT and CK-MB were prominently higher in STEMI group as compared with control and UAP groups. Several established inflammatory markers such as hs-CRP, fibrinogen and MMP were markedly elevated in UAP and STEMI patients.

Comparison of circulating DC and monocyte subsets among control, UAP and STEMI groups

Compared with controls and UAP patients, percent PMNs and PMNs/lymphocytes ratio were significantly higher, while a relative lower percentage of lymphocytes was observed in STEMI patients (Table 1). Although the percentages of mDC1s, mDC2s and pDCs were markedly lower in UAP and STEMI patients, the total numbers of mDC1s, mDCs and pDCs were comparable among three groups because total leukocyte count was greatly higher in UAP and STEMI patients. In line with percent mDC2s, the absolute number of mDC2s was lower in UAP and STEMI patients when compared with healthy controls (0.08 × 10^4 ± 0.05 × 104/ml and 0.08 × 10^4 ± 0.06 × 104/ml vs. 0.11 × 10^4 ± 0.06 × 104/ml, p = 0.027). With regard to monocyte subsets, the percentage of total monocytes, as well as percent Mon1 subsets, was similar among three groups. The percentage of Monocyte 2 (Mon2) subsets was higher in UAP and STEMI patients than that in healthy controls (10.61% ± 4.17% and 13.38% ± 3.44% vs. 7.44% ± 2.40%, p < 0.001). In contrast, UAP and STEMI patients had lower percentages of Mon3 subsets as compared with healthy controls (6.97% ± 3.91% and 5.62% ± 4.96% vs. 10.29% ± 6.17%, p = 0.001). While the absolute number of Mon2 was markedly higher in UAP and STEMI patients (4.33 × 104/ml ± 2.39 × 104/ml vs. 7.22 × 104/ml ± 3.67 × 104/ml, p < 0.001), there was no significant difference in the absolute number of Mon3 among three groups (control, UAP and STEMI group: 4.43 × 104/

Table 1 Total counts and proportions of peripheral blood cells in three groups

	Control ($n = 33$)	UAP ($n = 48$)	STEMI ($n = 31$)	p value
WBC, $\times 10^6$/ml	6.47 ± 1.72	6.99 ± 1.97	8.88 ± 2.41	<0.001
PMN, % WBC	58.10 ± 8.81	60.74 ± 9.64	76.51 ± 10.59	<0.001
Lym, % WBC	32.48 ± 7.84	32.11 ± 9.43	16.65 ± 9.44	<0.001
PMN/Lym ratio	1.99 ± 0.96	2.26 ± 1.45	7.02 ± 5.66	<0.001
Mon, % WBC	6.60 ± 1.17	5.83 ± 1.33	6.18 ± 2.50	0.179
mDC1s, % WBC	0.29 ± 0.05	0.22 ± 0.05	0.19 ± 0.04	<0.001
mDC2s, % WBC	$1.69 \times 10^{-2} \pm 0.73 \times 10^{-2}$	$1.11 \times 10^{-2} \pm 0.42 \times 10^{-2}$	$0.81 \times 10^{-2} \pm 0.52 \times 10^{-2}$	<0.001
mDCs, % WBC	0.31 ± 0.05	0.23 ± 0.05	0.20 ± 0.04	<0.001
pDCs, % WBC	0.20 ± 0.05	0.16 ± 0.03	0.14 ± 0.02	<0.001
mDC1s, $\times 10^4$/ml	1.89 ± 0.66	1.60 ± 0.70	1.73 ± 0.58	0.151
mDC2s, $\times 10^4$/ml	0.11 ± 0.06	0.08 ± 0.05	0.08 ± 0.06	*0.027*
mDCs, $\times 10^4$/ml	2.00 ± 0.69	1.68 ± 0.73	1.81 ± 0.62	0.126
pDCs, $\times 10^4$/ml	1.19 ± 0.43	1.15 ± 0.37	1.20 ± 0.35	0.862
Mon1, % monocytes	82.37 ± 6.31	82.36 ± 5.54	81.03 ± 5.91	0.564
Mon2, % monocytes	7.44 ± 2.40	10.61 ± 4.17	13.38 ± 3.44	<0.001
Mon3, % monocytes	10.29 ± 6.17	6.97 ± 3.91	5.62 ± 4.96	*0.001*
Mon1, $\times 10^5$/ml	3.45 ± 0.95	3.42 ± 1.13	4.41 ± 1.97	*0.007*
Mon2, $\times 10^4$/ml	3.06 ± 1.13	4.33 ± 2.39	7.22 ± 3.67	<0.001
Mon3, $\times 10^4$/ml	4.43 ± 3.34	3.14 ± 2.20	3.32 ± 2.02	0.187

Values are mean ± SD

Abbreviations: *DC* dendritic cell, *Lym* lymphocyte, *mDC* myeloid dendritic cell, *Mon* monocyte, *pDC* plasmacytoid dendritic cell, *PMNs* polymorphonuclear granulocytes, *WBC* white blood cell. P-values of risk factors with significance are presented as italic form

ml ± 3.34 × 104/ml, 3.14 × 104/ml ± 2.20 × 104/ml and 3.32 × 104/ml ± 2.02 × 104/ml, $p = 0.187$) due to the gradually elevated number of circulating total monocytes.

Because of the significant differences in the history of smoking and the plasma levels of fasting glucose and triglyceride among three groups, we investigated whether circulating DC and monocyte subsets were associated with these established risk factors. There were no discrepancies in the percentage and count of DC and monocyte subsets among subjects with and without histories of smoking (Additional file 5: Table S2). Likewise, the percentage and count of DC and monocyte subsets were not correlated with the plasma levels of fasting glucose and triglyceride (Additional file 6: Table S3).

Considering the roles of DCs and monocytes in inflammation and myocardial infarction, we examined the correlation of circulating DC and monocytes subsets with inflammatory and myocardial necrotic markers. Hs-CRP was positively associated with the percentage and absolute number of Mon1 (Additional file 7: Table S4). Similarly, plasma levels of MMP9 were significantly associated with the percentage and absolute number of Mon1 and Mon2. Furthermore, Mon1, Mon2 and mDCs, especially mDC2s, were closely related to serum levels of cTnT and CK-MB, both of which reflected the severity of myocardial infarction.

Angiography and OCT findings

Of UAP patients, 20 (41.7%) were diagnosed as TCFA confirmed by OCT. The angiography and OCT data are shown in Table 2. Patients with TCFA had thinner fibrous cap (48.5 μm ± 10.9 μm vs. 119.6 μm ± 22.2 μm, $p < 0.001$) and larger lipid core (arc of lipid core, 252.0° ± 77.8° vs. 170.4° ± 67.7°, p < 0.001) compared with patients without TCFA. Plaque calcification was detected more frequently in patients with TCFA (45.0% vs. 17.9%, $p = 0.041$). No significant difference was found when comparing patients with and without TCFA in reference to the rate of multivessel disease, culprit lesion distribution, minimal lumen area and percentage of diameter stenosis.

Relation of circulating DCs and monocytes with plaque characteristics

In a subgroup analysis of 48 UAP patients with plaque morphologies determined by OCT, we found that patients with TCFA had higher proportions of Mon2 subsets (11.96% ± 4.27% vs. 9.43% ± 5.15%, $p = 0.035$) and lower proportions of Mon3 subsets (4.93% ± 3.22% vs. 8.43% ± 3.75%, $p = 0.001$) as compared with patients without TCFA (Table 3). In UAP patients with TCFA, the absolute number of Mon2 was significantly higher than those without TCFA (5.17 × 104/ml ± 1.92 × 104/

Table 2 Angiographic and OCT finding

	Patients with TCFA (n = 20)	Patients without TCFA (n = 28)	p value
Age, yrs	62.4 ± 7.7	60.8 ± 9.4	0.541
Male	14 (70.0)	25 (89.3)	0.091
Multivessel disease	6 (30.0)	7 (25.0)	0.701
Culprit vessel			
LAD	10 (50.0)	10 (35.7)	0.457
LCX	6 (30.0)	8 (28.6)	
RCA	4 (20.0)	10 (35.7)	
Fibrous cap thickness, μm	48.5 ± 10.9	119.6 ± 22.2	*<0.001*
Arc of lipid core, degrees	252.0 ± 77.8	170.4 ± 67.7	*<0.001*
Calcium	9 (45.0)	5 (17.9)	*0.041*
MLA, mm^2	4.5 ± 2.5	5.5 ± 2.7	0.215
Relative stenosis, %	56.8 ± 13.4	48.4 ± 16.2	*0.064*

Values are mean ± SD or n (%)

Abbreviations: *LAD* left anterior descending coronary artery, *LCX* left circumflex coronary artery, *MLA* minimum lumen area, *OCT* optical coherence tomography, *RCA* right coronary artery, *TCFA* thin-cap fibroatheroma. *P*-values of risk factors with significance are presented as italic form

ml vs. 3.53×10^4/ml ± 2.65×10^4/ml, $p = 0.045$), whereas the counts of Mon3 did not differ between two groups (2.23×10^4/ml ± 1.44×10^4/ml vs. 3.66×10^4/ml ± 2.16×10^4/ml, $p = 0.059$). There were no significant differences in the percent PMNs and lymphocytes, PMNs/lymphocytes ratio, the absolute and percent DC subsets, and the proportion of Mon1 subsets between patients with and without TCFA. The correlation between plaque characteristics determined by OCT and circulating DCs and monocytes is summarized in Additional file 8: Table S5. The percentage of Mon3 was positively correlated with fibrous cap thickness ($r = 0.409$, $p = 0.004$) and inversely correlated with arc of lipid core ($r = -0.353$, $p = 0.014$). The absolute number of Mon2 was inversely correlated

Table 3 Total counts and proportions of peripheral blood cells in patients with and without TCFA

	Patients with TCFA (n = 20)	Patients without TCFA (n = 28)	p value
WBC, ×10^6/ml	6.88 ± 1.98	7.12 ± 1.98	0.690
PMN, % WBC	59.83 ± 9.45	61.33 ± 9.88	0.613
Lym, % WBC	32.75 ± 8.94	31.70 ± 9.87	0.717
PMN/Lym ratio	2.22 ± 1.69	2.29 ± 1.31	0.883
Mon, % WBC	5.83 ± 1.25	5.82 ± 1.41	0.989
mDC1s, % WBC	0.24 ± 0.05	0.21 ± 0.04	0.134
mDC2s, % WBC	$1.08 \times 10^{-2} \pm 0.39 \times 10^{-2}$	$1.13 \times 10^{-2} \pm 0.44 \times 10^{-2}$	0.664
mDCs, % WBC	0.25 ± 0.05	0.23 ± 0.05	0.151
pDCs, % WBC	0.15 ± 0.03	0.16 ± 0.03	0.285
mDC1s, ×10^4/ml	1.63 ± 0.61	1.57 ± 0.76	0.791
mDC2s, ×10^4/ml	0.08 ± 0.04	0.08 ± 0.05	0.605
mDCs, ×10^4/ml	1.71 ± 0.64	1.66 ± 0.79	0.825
pDCs, ×10^4/ml	1.07 ± 0.30	1.22 ± 0.41	0.173
Mon1, % monocytes	82.84 ± 6.17	82.02 ± 5.15	0.754
Mon2, % monocytes	11.96 ± 4.27	9.43 ± 5.15	*0.035*
Mon3, % monocytes	4.93 ± 3.22	8.43 ± 3.75	*0.001*
Mon1, ×10^5/ml	3.25 ± 0.96	3.52 ± 1.22	0.470
Mon2, ×10^4/ml	5.17 ± 1.92	3.53 ± 2.65	*0.045*
Mon3, ×10^4/ml	2.23 ± 1.44	3.66 ± 2.16	0.059

Values are mean ± SD

Abbreviations as Table 1 and Table 2. *P*-values of risk factors with significance are presented as italic form

with fibrous cap thickness ($r = -0.383$, $p = 0.014$) and positively correlated with arc of lipid core ($r = 0.413$, $p = 0.001$). However, the percentages and numbers of circulating DCs and Mon1 did not differ in UAP patients with and without calcified plaques (Additional file 9: Table S6).

Furthermore, according to the initiation and progression of atherosclerosis, the enrollments were divided into four groups as follows: control, non-TCFA, TCFA and STEMI groups. In this context, Fig. 1 shows a gradual increase in the proportion and absolute number of Mon2 subsets and a gradual decrease in the proportion of Mon3 subsets as the atherosclerosis worsen.

Discussion

In the present study, we investigated the association of circulating inflammatory cells with morphological characteristics of atherosclerotic plaque observed by coronary angiography and OCT. The results herein demonstrated that elevated CD14++CD16+ Mon2 subsets were associated with plaque vulnerability and rupture determined by angiography and OCT.

There were a growing number of researches regarding the relationships among circulating DCs, inflammation and their effects on coronary plaque, whereas conflicting results were reported. While Yilmaz et al. [13] and Kretzschmar et al. [20] observed markedly decreases in circulating mDCs, pDCs and total DCs in stable CAD and STEMI patients, Wen et al. [21] found a reduction

in circulating mDCs, but not pDCs, in patients with unstable CAD. The disparate findings among published literatures may be explained as follow. Total DCs make up only approximate a 0.4 percentage of leukocytes in peripheral blood. It is thus conceivable that the absolute numbers of circulating DC subsets may fluctuate wildly because of changes in total leukocyte counts in different disease states and errors in operation. In our study, we observed that UAP and STEMI patients had a lower level of circulating mDC2s when compared with controls without coronary plaque. Human mDC2s share most features with murine CD8α + DCs, while mDC1s represent human counterpart of murine CD8α- DCs [22]. In response to viral infections and inflammatory stimuli, mDC1s activates CD4+ T lymphocytes and possess the capacity to promote Treg differetiation [23]. Conversely, mDC2s prime CD8+ T lymphocytes [24]. The mechanisms of decreased circulating mDC2s in CAD are unclear; however, the possible theories have been postulated. In former studies, decreased circulating DCs in CAD were shown to be accompanied with a resident DC increase in the inflamed plaques and infarct myocardium, inferring that circulating DC precursor recruitment to inflamed plaques was a part of the underlying disease process [20, 25]. Additionally, the pathological study showed a high density of resident DCs with frequent T lymphocyte contacts in unstable plaques, suggesting that tissue-resident DCs, at least in

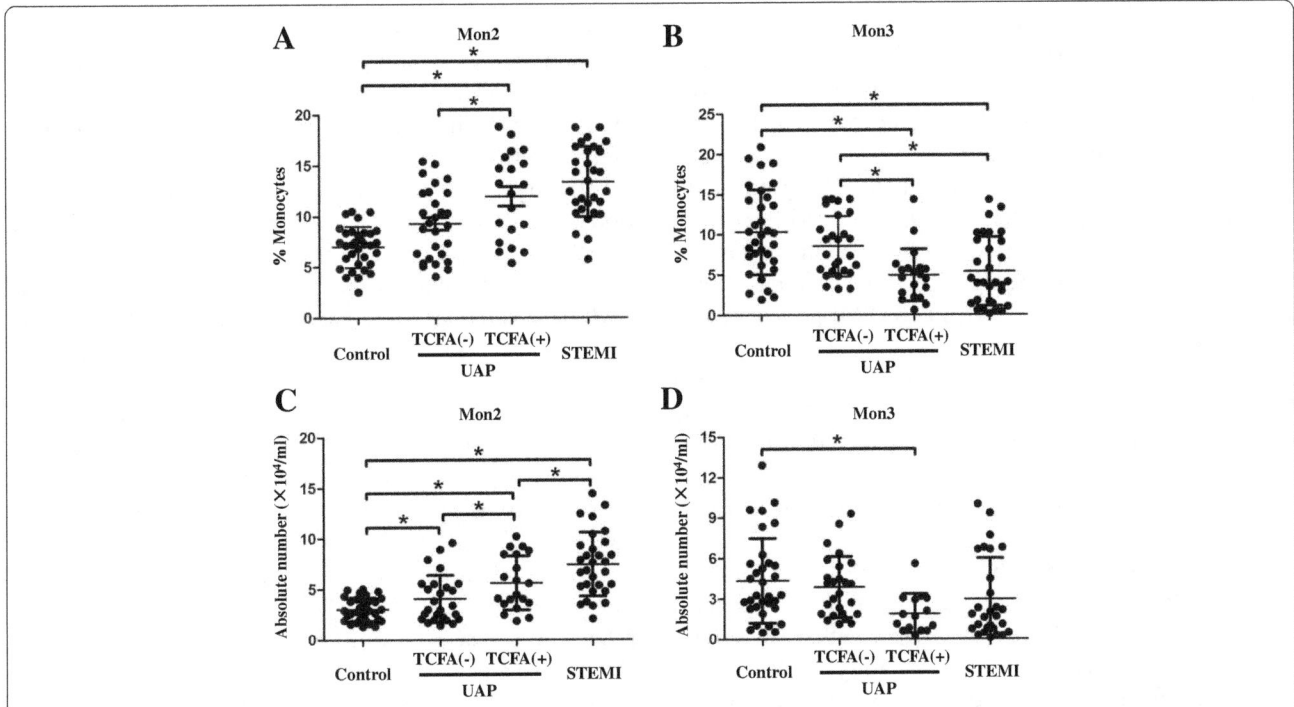

Fig. 1 Comparison of CD14++CD16+ Mon2 and CD14 + CD16++ Mon3 subsets at different stages of atherosclerosis. Comparison of the percentages of Mon2 (**a**) and Mon3 (**b**) subsets among four groups. Comparison of the absolute numbers of Mon2 (**c**) and Mon3 (**d**) among four groups. * $P < 0.05$

part, facilitated local T lymphocyte activation and aggravated atherosclerotic development [26, 27]. Collectively, it is likely that decreased circulating mDC2s in CAD patients are caused by their recruitment into inflamed lesions and infarct myocardium. Subsequently, mature mDC2s in response to inflammatory stimuli within vulnerable plaques promote CD8+ T lymphocyte activation and aggravate atherosclerotic development [27].

According to the severity of symptoms, some published studies grouped CAD patients into patients with stable angina pectoris (SAP) and with acute coronary syndrome (ACS). They reported that mDCs or pDCs were dramatically declined as CAD became more serious [13]. However, these subjects were not classified according to the plaque morphology in their coronary arteries. Although TCFA determined by OCT are found more prevalent in patients with ACS than in those with SAP, there are approximate 20% patients with SAP that have TCFA observed by OCT. [2] In agreement with the previous meta-analysis, the prevalence of TCFA is markedly higher in ACS group than that in SAP group [28]. TCFA harboring in patients with SAP seems to be neglected by clinical presentations but gradually evolve into plaque rupture [29]. Therefore, we applied OCT, which allows for the accurate assessment of plaque characteristics, to objectively identify the different stages of atherosclerosis. It should be noted that plaque rupture detected by OCT accounts for over 40% ACS, while the other ACS are caused by plaque erosion and calcified nodule [30]. As compared with plaque rupture, plaque erosion and calcified nodule are more prevalent in fibrous plaque than those in lipid plaque and TCFA [31]. Therefore, apart from vulnerable plaque characterized as TCFA, culprit plaque erosion and calcification pertain to fibrous plaque also contribute to the incidence of ACS. Additionally, TCFA alone is unable to correctly predict the adverse events in CAD patients. In contrast, TCFA combined with traditional risk factors is referred to be more feasible for evaluate the prognosis of CAD [28]. In patients undergoing coronary angiography, mDC2s were decreased in UAP and STEMI patients when compared with healthy controls, whereas the percentage and absolute number of mDC2s remained similar between UAP and STEMI patients. Moreover, as reported in the OCT subgroup, mDC2s were not significantly altered between patients with and without TCFA. Collectively, these results implied that decreased circulating mDC2s were associated with the presence of coronary plaque but not altered during plaque destabilization and rupture. Though CD11c + DCs were found to reside in vulnerable plaques in mice and humans, it was uncertain whether these resident DCs were derived from circulating common DC precursors or monocytes [25]. Moreover, the specific markers are needed to distinguish the different subsets of resident DCs in coronary plaques. [12]

Current studies unveil that monocyte subsets have different propensities to migrate the vascular wall and differentiate into particular subsets of DCs and macrophages located in plaques. [32, 33] This recognition prompted researchers to determine the association between distinct monocyte subsets and CAD. It is worth noting that some laboratories only referred to two monocyte subpopulations (CD14 + CD16- and CD14 + CD16+ monocytes). The consistent result of these studies was that the count of CD16 positive subsets was higher in patients with CAD and MI as compared with healthy controls.[34, 35] Rogacev et al. [9] found that the count of CD14++CD16+ Mon2 subsets was an independent predictor of adverse cardiovascular events. Tapp et al. [7] reported that circulating Mon2 subsets were prominently elevated in STEMI patients compared with patients with stable CAD and healthy volunteers. Our work extends the results of earlier studies on CAD patients diagnosed by coronary angiography. We showed that elevated CD14++CD16+ Mon2 subsets and reduced CD14 + CD16++ Mon3 subsets were associated with the presence and progression of coronary plaques determined by coronary angiography and OCT. In addition, we found that the proportion of circulating Mon3 subsets were positively correlated with fibrous cap thickness and negatively correlated with arc of lipid core, whereas none of monocyte subsets were significantly correlated with plaque volume. Considering that plaque composition, rather than plaque volume, plays an important role in the plaque disruption and subsequent thrombosis that leads to acute cardiovascular events [1], higher proportion and absolute number of Mon2 may provide important information to predict the presence of TCFA and the progression of atherosclerosis in coronary arteries.

Pathological studies have pushed forward the recognition of human monocyte heterogeneity and biological functions [5, 32]. Mechanistically, the intermediate Mon2 subsets expressing high levels of Tie-2 and CXCR4 possess pro-angiogenic properties [36, 37]. Recent studies uncovered that neovascularization of vasa vasorum within plaques facilitate macrophage infiltration and precipitate plaque vulnerability and rupture [38, 39]. Another important mechanism is that circulating monocytes eventually differentiate into resident DCs/macrophages in atheroma and myocardium, and continue to function during the development of atherosclerosis and myocardial infarction [40]. In this regard, our results revealed that Mon1 and Mon2 were highly related to the serological markers of plaque rupture and myocardial infarction. Murine counterparts of human circulating monocytes could be delineated as Ly-6C^{hi} and Ly-6C^{lo} monocytes. In murine experiments, Ly-6C^{hi} monocytes substantially increased in peripheral blood of

Apoe−/− mice fed a high-fat diet and differentiated into pro-inflammatory M1-type macrophages, while Ly-6C^{lo} monocytes differentiated more readily into anti-inflammatory M2-type macrophages [41]. Taken together, these phenomena suggest that both higher Mon2 counts may precipitate plaque destabilization and rupture.

Study limitations

There were some limitations associated with the present study. First, the study population was relatively small and the study design was cross-sectional in nature. Therefore, we were unable to distinguish whether or not the variation in circulating monocyte subsets is causative of atherosclerotic process. There is a need for prospective studies that investigate the predictive value of circulating DC and monocyte subsets for the development of coronary plaque. Additionally, currently, there was no standardization in the measurement of circulating DC and monocyte subsets.

Conclusions

Higher proportion and counts of Mon2 subsets are associated with atherosclerosis destabilization and rupture, which may be promising biomarkers for further clinic management.

Additional files

Additional file 1: Figure S1. Flow chart of the study. OCT = optical coherence tomography, STEMI = ST-segment elevation myocardial infarction, UAP = unstable angina pectoris. (TIFF 903 kb)

Additional file 2: Figure S2. Representative OCT images at culprit lesions. **A.** Fibrotic plaque. The thickness of fibrous cap was 130 μm. An arc delineates the lipid core. Arrows delineate the fibrous cap. **B.** Thin-cap fibroatheroma (TCFA). The thickness of fibrous cap was 60 μm. Arrows delineate the TCFA. **C.** Calcified plaque. (TIFF 8907 kb)

Additional file 3: Figure S3. Representative images showing the identification of circulating DC and monocyte subsets by flow cytometry. Upper panel, identification of DC subsets: mDC1s, mDC2s and pDCs were detected according to the markers. FSC/SSC dot plots were created to exclude debris and platelets. Gated on P1, CD14−/CD19−/SSC dot plots were generated. CD14+ monocytes, CD19+ B lymphocytes and CD14−/CD19−/SSC+ granulocytes were excluded. Gated on P2, CD1c + region was drawn to identify mDC1s and CD141+ region was drawn to define mDC2s. CD303+ region was circled to identify pDCs. Lower panel, identification of monocyte subsets: Mon1, Mon2 and Mon3 were detected according to the markers. Gated on P3 by FSC/SSC, CD45+/CD86 region was drawn to define total monocytes (P4 gate). Mon1, CD14++ CD16- monocytes; Mon2, CD14++CD16+ monocytes; Mon3, CD14+ CD16++ monocytes. FSC = Forward scatter, SSC = Side scatter. (TIFF 10999 kb)

Additional file 4: Table S1. Baseline characteristics of study population. (DOC 41 kb)

Additional file 5: Table S2. Total counts and proportions of DC and monocyte subsets in patients with and without smoking. (DOC 35 kb)

Additional file 6: Table S3. Correlation between glucose and triglyceride and circulating DC and monocyte subsets. (DOC 37 kb)

Additional file 7: Table S4. Correlation between inflammatory markers, myocardial necrotic markers and circulating DC and monocyte subsets. (DOC 45 kb)

Additional file 8: Table S5. Correlation between plaque characteristics and circulating DCs and monocytes. (DOC 40 kb)

Additional file 9: Table S6. Total counts and proportions of DC and monocyte subsets in patients with and without calcified plaque. (DOC 34 kb)

Abbreviations
CAD: Coronary artery disease; DC: Dendritic cell; Mon: monocyte; OCT: Optical coherence tomography; STEMI: ST-segment elevation myocardial infarction; TCFA: Thin-cap fibroatheroma; UAP: Unstable angina pectoris

Acknowledgments
We appreciate Fan Fan from Fudan University School of Medicine for her critical suggestions and comments on this manuscript.

Funding
This study was supported by Shanghai Municipal Commission of Health and Family Planning (No. 201440479) and National Natural Science Foundation of China (No. 81000113).

Authors' contributions
JZ performed the flow cytometry and wrote the paper. YH designed the study and performed the statistical analysis. DX participated in patient recruitment and biochemical analysis. GZ participated in patient recruitment. SS participated in biochemical analysis. LC performed the flow cytometry. MZ participated in patient recruitment and performed the statistical analysis. WC performed the coronary angiography and OCT analysis. YX performed the coronary angiography and OCT analysis. XL designed the study, performed the statistical analysis and wrote the paper. All authors read and approved the final manuscript.

Competing interests
The authors declare that they have no competing interests.

Author details
[1]Department of Cardiology, Shanghai Tenth People's Hospital, Tongji University School of Medicine, Shanghai, China. [2]Department of Pathology, Shanghai East Hospital, Tongji University School of Medicine, Shanghai, China. [3]Department of Cardiology, Shigatse People's Hospital, Shigatse, Tibet, China.

References
1. Finn AV, Nakano M, Narula J, Kolodgie FD, Virmani R. Concept of vulnerable/unstable plaque. Arterioscler Thromb Vasc Biol. 2010;30:1282–92.
2. Jang IK, Tearney GJ, MacNeill B, Takano M, Moselewski F, Iftima N, Shishkov M, Houser S, Aretz HT, Halpern EF, Bouma BE. In vivo characterization of coronary atherosclerotic plaque by use of optical coherence tomography. Circulation. 2005;111:1551–5.
3. Fujii K, Hao H, Shibuya M, Imanaka T, Fukunaga M, Miki K, Tamaru H, Sawada H, Naito Y, Ohyanagi M, Hirota S, Masuyama T. Accuracy of OCT, grayscale IVUS, and their combination for the diagnosis of coronary TCFA: an ex vivo validation study. JACC Cardiovasc Imaging. 2015;8:451–60.

4. Mann DL. The emerging role of innate immunity in the heart and vascular system: for whom the cell tolls. Circ Res. 2011;108:1133–45.

5. Wong KL, Tai JJ, Wong WC, Han H, Sem X, Yeap WH, Kourilsky P, Wong SC. Gene expression profiling reveals the defining features of the classical, intermediate, and nonclassical human monocyte subsets. Blood. 2011;118: e16–31.

6. Zawada AM, Rogacev KS, Rotter B, Winter P, Marell RR, Fliser D, Heine GH. SuperSAGE evidence for CD14++CD16+ monocytes as a third monocyte subset. Blood. 2011;118:e50–61.

7. Tapp LD, Shantsila E, Wrigley BJ, Pamukcu B, Lip GY. The CD14++CD16+ monocyte subset and monocyte-platelet interactions in patients with ST-elevation myocardial infarction. J Thromb Haemost. 2012;10:1231–41.

8. Liu Y, Imanishi T, Ikejima H, Tsujioka H, Ozaki Y, Kuroi A, Okochi K, Ishibashi K, Tanimoto T, Ino Y, Kitabata H, Akasaka T. Association between circulating monocyte subsets and in-stent restenosis after coronary stent implantation in patients with ST-elevation myocardial infarction. Circ J. 2010;74:2585–91.

9. Rogacev KS, Cremers B, Zawada AM, Seiler S, Binder N, Ege P, Grosse-Dunker G, Heisel I, Hornof F, Jeken J, Rebling NM, Ulrich C, Scheller B, Bohm M, Fliser D, Heine GH. CD14++CD16+ monocytes independently predict cardiovascular events: a cohort study of 951 patients referred for elective coronary angiography. J Am Coll Cardiol. 2012;60:1512–20.

10. Shantsila E, Tapp LD, Wrigley BJ, Pamukcu B, Apostolakis S, Montoro-Garcia S, Lip GY. Monocyte subsets in coronary artery disease and their associations with markers of inflammation and fibrinolysis. Atherosclerosis. 2014;234:4–10.

11. Mildner A, Jung S. Development and function of dendritic cell subsets. Immunity. 2014;40:642–56.

12. Zernecke A. Dendritic cells in atherosclerosis: evidence in mice and humans. Arterioscler Thromb Vasc Biol. 2015;35:763–70.

13. Yilmaz A, Schaller T, Cicha I, Altendorf R, Stumpf C, Klinghammer L, Ludwig J, Daniel WG, Garlichs CD. Predictive value of the decrease in circulating dendritic cell precursors in stable coronary artery disease. Clin Sci (Lond). 2009;116:353–63.

14. Fukunaga T, Soejima H, Irie A, Fukushima R, Oe Y, Kawano H, Sumida H, Kaikita K, Sugiyama S, Nishimura Y, Ogawa H. High ratio of myeloid dendritic cells to plasmacytoid dendritic cells in blood of patients with acute coronary syndrome. Circ J. 2009;73:1914–9.

15. Braunwald E. Unstable angina. A classification. Circulation. 1989;80:410–4.

16. Thygesen K, Alpert JS, Jaffe AS, Simoons ML, Chaitman BR, White HD, Katus HA, Lindahl B, Morrow DA, Clemmensen PM, Johanson P, Hod H, Underwood R, Bax JJ, Bonow RO, Pinto F, Gibbons RJ, Fox KA, Atar D, Newby LK, Galvani M, Hamm CW, Uretsky BF, Steg PG, Wijns W, Bassand JP, Menasche P, Ravkilde J, Ohman EM, Antman EM, Wallentin LC, Armstrong PW, Januzzi JL, Nieminen MS, Gheorghiade M, Filippatos G, Luepker RV, Fortmann SP, Rosamond WD, Levy D, Wood D, Smith SC, Hu D, Lopez-Sendon JL, Robertson RM, Weaver D, Tendera M, Bove AA, Parkhomenko AN, Vasilieva EJ, Mendis S. Third universal definition of myocardial infarction. Circulation. 2012;126:2020–35.

17. Prati F, Regar E, Mintz GS, Arbustini E, Di Mario C, Jang IK, Akasaka T, Costa M, Guagliumi G, Grube E, Ozaki Y, Pinto F, Serruys PW. Expert review document on methodology, terminology, and clinical applications of optical coherence tomography: physical principles, methodology of image acquisition, and clinical application for assessment of coronary arteries and atherosclerosis. Eur Heart J. 2010;31:401–15.

18. Tearney GJ, Regar E, Akasaka T, Adriaenssens T, Barlis P, Bezerra HG, Bouma B, Bruining N, Cho JM, Chowdhary S, Costa MA, de Silva R, Dijkstra J, Di Mario C, Dudek D, Falk E, Feldman MD, Fitzgerald P, Garcia-Garcia HM, Gonzalo N, Granada JF, Guagliumi G, Holm NR, Honda Y, Ikeno F, Kawasaki M, Kochman J, Koltowski L, Kubo T, Kume T, Kyono H, Lam CC, Lamouche G, Lee DP, Leon MB, Maehara A, Manfrini O, Mintz GS, Mizuno K, Morel MA, Nadkarni S, Okura H, Otake H, Pietrasik A, Prati F, Raber L, Radu MD, Rieber J, Riga M, Rollins A, Rosenberg M, Sirbu V, Serruys PW, Shimada K, Shinke T, Shite J, Siegel E, Sonoda S, Suter M, Takarada S, Tanaka A, Terashima M, Thim T, Uemura S, Ughi GJ, van Beusekom HM, van der Steen AF, van Es GA, van Soest G, Virmani R, Waxman S, Weissman NJ, Weisz G. Consensus standards for acquisition, measurement, and reporting of intravascular optical coherence tomography studies: a report from the international working Group for Intravascular Optical Coherence Tomography Standardization and Validation. J Am Coll Cardiol. 2012;59:1058–72.

19. Tapp LD, Shantsila E, Wrigley BJ, Montoro-Garcia S, Lip GY. TLR4 expression on monocyte subsets in myocardial infarction. J Intern Med. 2013;273:294–305.

20. Kretzschmar D, Betge S, Windisch A, Pistulli R, Rohm I, Fritzenwanger M, Jung C, Schubert K, Theis B, Petersen I, Drobnik S, Mall G, Figulla HR, Yilmaz A. Recruitment of circulating dendritic cell precursors into the infarcted myocardium and pro-inflammatory response in acute myocardial infarction. Clin Sci (Lond). 2012;123:387–98.

21. Wen J, Wen Y, Zhiliang L, Lingling C, Longxing C, Ming W, Qiang F. A decrease in the percentage of circulating mDC precursors in patients with coronary heart disease: a relation to the severity and extent of coronary artery lesions? Heart Vessel. 2013;28:135–42.

22. Geginat J, Nizzoli G, Paroni M, Maglie S, Larghi P, Pascolo S, Abrignani S. Immunity to pathogens taught by specialized human dendritic cell subsets. Front Immunol. 2015;6:527.

23. Layseca-Espinosa E, Korniotis S, Montandon R, Gras C, Bouillie M, Gonzalez-Amaro R, Dy M, Zavala F. CCL22-producing CD8alpha- myeloid dendritic cells mediate regulatory T cell recruitment in response to G-CSF treatment. J Immunol. 2013;191:2266–72.

24. Kang SJ. The bloodline of CD8alpha(+) dendritic cells. Mol Cells. 2012;34: 219–29.

25. Yilmaz A, Weber J, Cicha I, Stumpf C, Klein M, Raithel D, Daniel WG, Garlichs CD. Decrease in circulating myeloid dendritic cell precursors in coronary artery disease. J Am Coll Cardiol. 2006;48:70–80.

26. Yilmaz A, Lochno M, Traeg F, Cicha I, Reiss C, Stumpf C, Raaz D, Anger T, Amann K, Probst T, Ludwig J, Daniel WG, Garlichs CD. Emergence of dendritic cells in rupture-prone regions of vulnerable carotid plaques. Atherosclerosis. 2004;176:101–10.

27. Cochain C, Koch M, Chaudhari SM, Busch M, Pelisek J, Boon L, Zernecke A. CD8+ T cells regulate Monopoiesis and circulating Ly6C-high monocyte levels in atherosclerosis in mice. Circ Res. 2015;117:244–53.

28. Iannaccone M, Quadri G, Taha S, D'Ascenzo F, Montefusco A, Omede P, Jang IK, Niccoli G, Souteyrand G, Yundai C, Toutouzas K, Benedetto S, Barbero U, Annone U, Lonni E, Imori Y, Biondi-Zoccai G, Templin C, Moretti C, Luscher TF, Gaita F. Prevalence and predictors of culprit plaque rupture at OCT in patients with coronary artery disease: a meta-analysis. Eur Heart J Cardiovasc Imaging. 2016;17:1128–37.

29. Ahmadi A, Leipsic J, Blankstein R, Taylor C, Hecht H, Stone GW, Narula J. Do plaques rapidly progress prior to myocardial infarction? The interplay between plaque vulnerability and progression. Circ Res. 2015;117:99–104.

30. Jia H, Abtahian F, Aguirre AD, Lee S, Chia S, Lowe H, Kato K, Yonetsu T, Vergallo R, Hu S, Tian J, Lee H, Park SJ, Jang YS, Raffel OC, Mizuno K, Uemura S, Itoh T, Kakuta T, Choi SY, Dauerman HL, Prasad A, Toma C, McNulty I, Zhang S, Yu B, Fuster V, Narula J, Virmani R, Jang IK. In vivo diagnosis of plaque erosion and calcified nodule in patients with acute coronary syndrome by intravascular optical coherence tomography. J Am Coll Cardiol. 2013;62:1748–58.

31. Higuma T, Soeda T, Abe N, Yamada M, Yokoyama H, Shibutani S, Vergallo R, Minami Y, Ong DS, Lee H, Okumura K, Jang IK. A combined optical coherence tomography and intravascular ultrasound study on plaque rupture, plaque erosion, and calcified nodule in patients with ST-segment elevation myocardial infarction: incidence, morphologic characteristics, and outcomes after percutaneous coronary intervention. JACC Cardiovasc Interv. 2015;8:1166–76.

32. Woollard KJ, Geissmann F. Monocytes in atherosclerosis: subsets and functions. Nat Rev Cardiol. 2010;7:77–86.

33. Auffray C, Sieweke MH, Geissmann F. Blood monocytes: development, heterogeneity, and relationship with dendritic cells. Annu Rev Immunol. 2009;27:669–92.

34. Ozaki Y, Imanishi T, Taruya A, Aoki H, Masuno T, Shiono Y, Komukai K, Tanimoto T, Kitabata H, Akasaka T. Circulating CD14+CD16+ monocyte subsets as biomarkers of the severity of coronary artery disease in patients with stable angina pectoris. Circ J. 2012;76:2412–8.

35. Kashiwagi M, Imanishi T, Ozaki Y, Satogami K, Masuno T, Wada T, Nakatani Y, Ishibashi K, Komukai K, Tanimoto T, Ino Y, Kitabata H, Akasaka T. Differential expression of toll-like receptor 4 and human monocyte subsets in acute myocardial infarction. Atherosclerosis. 2012;221:249–53.

36. Matsubara T, Kanto T, Kuroda S, Yoshio S, Higashitani K, Kakita N, Miyazaki M, Sakakibara M, Hiramatsu N, Kasahara A, Tomimaru Y, Tomokuni A, Nagano H, Hayashi N, Takehara T. TIE2-expressing monocytes as a diagnostic marker for hepatocellular carcinoma correlates with angiogenesis. Hepatology. 2013;57:1416–25.

37. Ghattas A, Griffiths HR, Devitt A, Lip GY, Shantsila E. Monocytes in coronary artery disease and atherosclerosis: where are we now? J Am Coll Cardiol. 2013;62:1541–51.

38. Celletti FL, Waugh JM, Amabile PG, Brendolan A, Hilfiker PR, Dake MD. Vascular endothelial growth factor enhances atherosclerotic plaque progression. Nat Med. 2001;7:425–9.
39. Jaipersad AS, Lip GY, Silverman S, Shantsila E. The role of monocytes in angiogenesis and atherosclerosis. J Am Coll Cardiol. 2014;63:1–11.
40. Ley K, Miller YI, Hedrick CC. Monocyte and macrophage dynamics during atherogenesis. Arterioscler Thromb Vasc Biol. 2011;31:1506–16.
41. Swirski FK, Libby P, Aikawa E, Alcaide P, Luscinskas FW, Weissleder R, Pittet MJ. Ly-6Chi monocytes dominate hypercholesterolemia-associated monocytosis and give rise to macrophages in atheromata. J Clin Invest. 2007;117:195–205.

20

SHP2 inhibitor PHPS1 protects against atherosclerosis by inhibiting smooth muscle cell proliferation

Jia Chen[1], Zhiyong Cao[2] and Jingshu Guan[1]* (ID)

Abstract

Background: Smooth muscle cells play an important role in the development of atherosclerosis. SHP2 is known to regulate the proliferation and migration of smooth muscle cells. The purpose of this study was to determine whether the SHP2 inhibitor PHPS1 has a pro-atherosclerotic or an atheroprotective effect in vivo and in vitro.

Methods: After exposure to a high-cholesterol diet for 4 weeks, LDL receptor-deficient (Ldlr$^{-/-}$) mice were exposed to the SHP2 inhibitor PHPS1 or vehicle. Body weight, serum glucose and lipid levels were determined. The size and composition of atherosclerotic plaques were measured by en face analysis, Movat staining and immunohistochemistry. The phosphorylation of SHP2 and related signaling molecules was analyzed by Western blot. Mechanistic analyses were performed in oxLDL-stimulated cultured vascular smooth muscle cells (VSMCs) with or without 10 mM PHPS1 pretreatment. Protein phosphorylation levels were detected by Western blot, and VSMC proliferation was assessed by BrdU staining.

Results: PHPS1 decreased the number of atherosclerotic plaques without significantly affecting body weight, serum glucose levels or lipid metabolism. Plaque composition analysis showed a significant decrease in the number of VSMCs in atherosclerotic lesions of Ldlr$^{-/-}$ mice treated with PHPS1. Stimulation with oxLDL induced a dose-dependent increase in the number of VSMCs and in SHP2 and ERK phosphorylation levels, and these effects were blocked by PHPS1.

Conclusion: The SHP2 inhibitor PHPS1 exerts a protective effect against atherosclerosis by reducing VSMC proliferation via SHP2/ERK pathway activation.

Keywords: SHP2, PHPS1, Atherosclerosis, Smooth muscle cells, Proliferation, ERK

Background

Cardiovascular disease is a threat to human health and seriously impacts quality of life [1]. Atherosclerosis (AS) is a major pathological basis of cardiovascular and cerebrovascular diseases [2]. Although the mechanism underlying AS is complex, the basic pathology of AS is fibrous proliferation caused by the presence of progressive lipid deposits, accumulation of inflammatory cells and deposition of extracellular matrix [3, 4]. AS is not a separate patho-logical process; rather, it is regulated by a variety of cells and intracellular signaling pathways [5]. Smooth muscle cells (SMCs) play an important role in the development of AS [6, 7].

Protein tyrosine phosphorylation and dephosphorylation play significant roles in numerous intracellular signaling pathways and are influenced by several opposing kinases, such as protein tyrosine kinases (PTKs) and protein tyrosine phosphatases (PTPs) [8, 9]. PTKs catalyze tyrosine phosphorylation, whereas PTPs catalyze dephosphorylation [10]. Src homology 2 domain-containing protein tyrosine phosphatase 2 (SHP2), also known as protein tyrosine phosphatase N 11 (PTPN11), is an important PTP that acts downstream of various growth factors, cytokines and tyrosine kinases. It plays an integral role in multiple cellular

* Correspondence: guanjingshu@yeah.net
[1]Department of Cardiology, Shanghai Baoshan Hospital of Integrated Traditional Chinese and Western Medicine, Friendship Road 181, Baoshan District, Shanghai, China
Full list of author information is available at the end of the article

events that regulate various functions, including migration, differentiation, survival and metabolism [11–13]. Schramm found that pharmacological reduction of SHP2/FAK/Akt/mTOR signaling at all levels of the signaling cascade effectively prevents cardiomyocyte hypertrophy [14]. In recent years, SHP2 inhibitors have become available for research applications. A SHP2 inhibitor phenylhydrazono pyrazolone sulfonate 1 (PHPS1) is a potent and cell permeable inhibitor that is specific for SHP2 over the closely related tyrosine phosphatases SHP1 and PTP1B [15]. In neutrophils, inflammatory monocytes and pDCs, the level of SHP2 expression is much lower than SHP1 [16]. PTP1B is an enzyme that negatively regulates insulin signaling and is likely involved in the pathways leading to insulin resistance [17]. PHPS1 remarkably suppresses E2-induced gene transcription, rapid DNA synthesis and late effects on cell growth. The finding introduces a new mechanism for SHP2 oncogenic action and sheds new light on extranuclear ER-initiated actions in breast cancer [18]. SHP2 regulates the acute pulmonary inflammation induced by cigarette smoke through the ERK1/2 pathway. PHPS1 significantly inhibits ERK1/2 activation and attenuates the inflammatory response induced in mouse lungs [19].

The purpose of this study was to determine whether the SHP2 inhibitor PHPS1 has a pro-atherosclerotic or an atheroprotective effect in vivo and in vitro by evaluating the effect of phosphorylation or dephosphorylation on the development of AS in LDL receptor-deficient (Ldlr$^{-/-}$) mice.

Methods

Animal preparation

Ldlr$^{-/-}$ (005061) mice were purchased from Jackson Laboratory. All animal protocols were approved by the Ethics Committee for Animal Experimentation at the Second Military Medical University. Five mice were housed in a cage on a 12-h light/dark cycle with free access to water and food. The animals received a high-fat diet containing 1.25% cholesterol for 4 weeks. The SHP2 inhibitor PHPS1 was purchased from Sigma-Aldrich. PHPS1 was dissolved in saline with 0.5% DMSO. Thirty mice were randomly divided into three groups: an AS group, an AS+Vehicle group and an AS+PHPS1 group. Mice in the AS+PHPS1 group received an intraperitoneal (i.p.) injection of 3 mg/kg PHPS1 every day during the last week on the high-fat diet, and those in the AS +Vehicle group received an equal volume of saline with 0.5% DMSO on the same days.

Measurement of serum glucose and lipids

The mice were euthanized with an overdose of pentobarbital. Blood samples were collected in EP tubes containing 2 mM EDTA and centrifuged (13,000 g) for 15 min at 4 °C. Plasma aliquots were separated and stored at − 80 °C. The serum glucose level was determined using the glucose oxidase method (Beckman). Levels of triglycerides (TG), total cholesterol (TC), low-density lipoprotein cholesterol (LDL-C) and high-density lipoprotein cholesterol (HDL-C) were determined by high-performance liquid chromatography (HPLC).

AS quantification

Quantification of AS in the heart and aorta was performed by staining. Briefly, the heart and aorta were perfused with phosphate-buffered saline (PBS) from the left ventricle and dissected from the aortic arch to the iliac bifurcation. The adventitia was carefully cleaned from the surrounding material. The aorta was sliced into sections, fixed in 4% paraformaldehyde for 48 h, stained with Oil Red O, incubated for 30 min at 37 °C, and washed with PBS several times; the area of the atherosclerotic lesion was compared to the total area of the aorta using a dissection microscope and Adobe Photoshop software.

The heart was embedded in optimal cutting temperature (OCT) compound and frozen at − 80 °C. Serial sections (8 μm) were taken from the aortic sinus and valve region, and sections in which all three valve leaflets were visible were used for Movat staining.

Western blot analysis

Protein samples (30 μg) from cultured cells or aortic specimens were electrophoresed on a 12% polyacrylamide gel by SDS-PAGE and blotted onto a nitrocellulose membrane. After being blocked with 5% BSA for 2 h at room temperature, the membrane was incubated overnight at 4 °C with primary antibodies (PRS3901, M5670, SAB4500491, and SAB4502398; 1:1,000 dilution; Sigma-Aldrich), washed with TBST 3 times, incubated with anti-rabbit secondary antibody (1:5,000 dilution) for 1 h at room temperature and then washed with TBST 3 times.

Cell culture

Mouse aorta vascular smooth muscle cells (VSMCs) were purchased from ATCC. The cells were grown in 6-well culture plates in RPMI 1640 supplemented with 10% FBS, penicillin and streptomycin at 37 °C in a humidified atmosphere of 5% CO_2. The medium was changed daily, and the cells were passaged after treatment with 0.05% trypsin-0.02% EDTA solution. Cells at passage 5-8 were used in the subsequent experiments. Cells were confirmed as SMCs by their typical "hill-and-valley" morphological features and by the expression of smooth muscle α-actin by immunofluorescence. Cells were made quiescent by a 48-h incubation in RPMI 1640 medium containing 0.1% FBS.

Cytotoxicity assay

Cells were seeded in 96-well culture plates at a concentration of 5×10^5 cells/ml 24 h prior to experiments. The cultured cells were stimulated with 10 μM PHPS1 or an equal volume of DMSO for 30 min and then with 100 μg/ml oxLDL for 48 h. Then, cells were washed 3 times with PBS. To evaluate the cytotoxicity of PHPS1 and DMSO, the number of cells was determined using the thiazolyl blue (MTT) test. A 10-μl volume of 5 mg/ml MTT was added to each well, and the plates were incubated for 4 h at 37 °C. The medium was removed, and the formazan crystals inside the cells were dissolved in 200 μl of DMSO. The absorbance of each well was measured at 450 nm on a microplate reader.

BrdU incorporation assay

5-Bromo-2′-deoxyuridine (BrdU) uptake by VSMCs was measured using a kit obtained from Amersham International. Quiescent cells at 70% confluence in DMEM with 0.5% FBS were treated with different stimuli for 24 h. BrdU (1 μmol/L) was added and co-cultivated with the cells for the last 3 h of the 24-h stimulation period. BrdU incorporation into the cells was quantified using the BrdU cell proliferation assay kit (Roche Diagnostics, Indianapolis, IN, USA). The cells were counted under a microscope using a hemocytometer as previously described [20]. BrdU-labeled and unlabeled SMCs were counted in each section. The proliferation index was calculated by dividing the number of BrdU-labeled cells by the number of unlabeled cells.

Statistics

All data are presented as the mean ± SE. Differences between groups were assessed using Student's t-test or one-way analysis of variance for multiple comparisons. P values < 0.05 indicated statistical significance, and the significance levels are provided in the text.

Results

PHPS1 renders Ldlr$^{-/-}$ mice less susceptible to AS development

To determine the pro-atherosclerotic or anti-atherosclerotic role of PHPS1, we ascertained the effect of PHPS1 on the

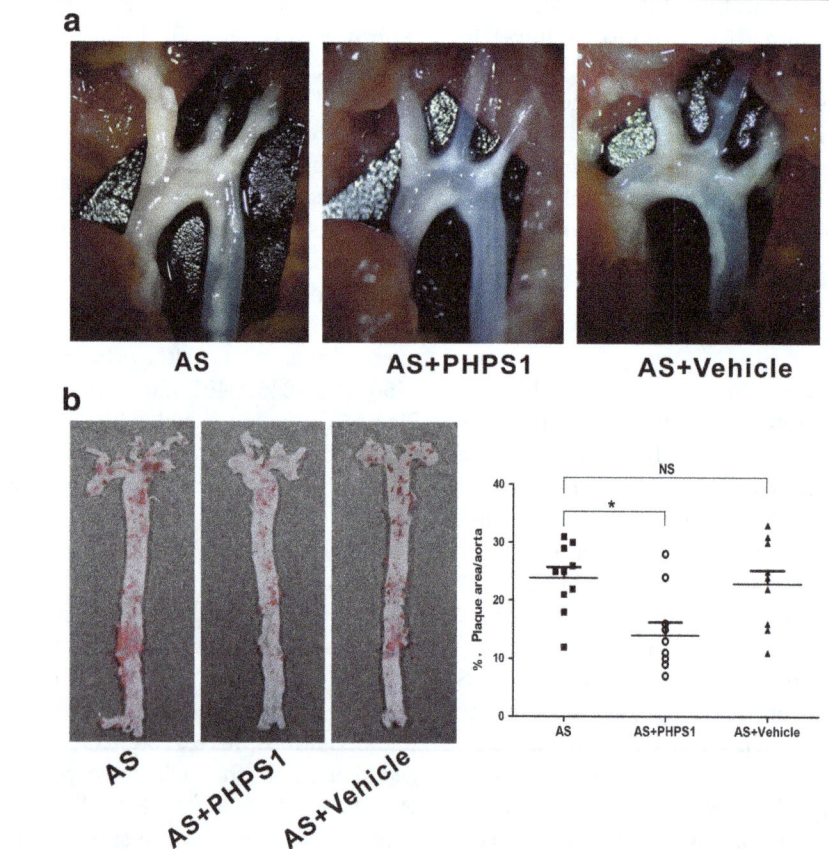

Fig. 1 The atherosclerotic plaque area was decreased in the AS+PHPS1 group. Ldlr$^{-/-}$ mice were fed a high-fat diet for 4 weeks. Mice in the AS+PHPS1 group were intraperitoneally injected with 3 mg/kg PHPS1 at the indicated time, and those in the AS+Vehicle group were injected with saline containing 0.5% DMSO. **a** Images of the aortic arch of Ldlr$^{-/-}$ mice in the AS, AS+PHPS1 and AS+Vehicle groups. **b** Left: representative en face images of the Oil Red O-stained whole aorta of Ldlr$^{-/-}$ mice. Right: quantification of the plaque area as a percentage of the aortic surface in Ldlr$^{-/-}$ mice. Data are presented as the mean ± SE ($n = 10$ per group). *$p < 0.05$ vs. the AS group

development and progression of AS in Ldlr$^{-/-}$ mice. No significant differences in body weight or the levels of serum glucose, TC, TG, HDL-C or LDL-C were observed among the three groups (Additional file 1: Figure S1). Remarkably, en face analysis of the aorta stained with Oil Red O revealed a significant decrease in atherosclerotic plaque size in the aorta of the AS+PHPS1 group compared with the other two groups (Fig. 1). The atherosclerotic plaque area at the aortic root was significantly decreased in Ldlr$^{-/-}$ mice treated with PHPS1. However, Movat staining showed no significant difference between the AS group and the Vehicle group. In the AS and AS+Vehicle groups, the intimal lesion was thicker, and both the vessel and lumen were narrowed. PHPS1 inhibited neointimal formation and SMC proliferation (Fig. 2).

PHPS1 treatment inhibits the phosphorylation of SHP2 and ERK

We analyzed the total and phosphorylated levels of JNK, p38^{MAPK} and ERK1/2 by Western blot. PHPS1 suppressed SHP2 and ERK phosphorylation without affecting JNK or p38^{MAPK} activation (Fig. 3), suggesting that PHPS1 might suppress P-SHP2 and P-ERK levels and consequently inhibit the progression of early lesions in Ldlr$^{-/-}$ mice.

Cytotoxic effects of PHPS1 on VSMCs in vitro

Because it was unknown whether PHPS1 is toxic to VSMCs, we treated cells with 10 µM PHPS1 or an equal volume of DMSO for 30 min. The doses of PHPS1 and DMSO used in the experiment were not toxic to the cells (Fig. 4).

OxLDL induces ERK phosphorylation and activation and promotes VSMC proliferation

VSMCs were incubated with 0, 25, 50 or 100 µg/ml oxLDL for 10 min. P-SHP2 and P-ERK levels were increased in the group treated with 25 µg/ml oxLDL compared with the control group and were highest in the 100 µg/ml group, revealing a concentration-dependent effect. The difference in total protein expression among groups was not statistically significant (Fig. 5a). The effect of oxLDL on VSMC proliferation was detected by the BrdU assay. As shown in Fig. 5b, stimulation with 100 µg/mL oxLDL for 24 h resulted in an approximate 50% increase in cell number, but that dose of oxLDL did not seem to affect VSMC proliferation to the same degree as 25 µg/mL oxLDL.

PHPS1 inhibits oxLDL-induced ERK phosphorylation and VSMC proliferation

Treatment of VSMCs with 100 µg/ml oxLDL increased the levels of phosphorylated SHP2 and ERK. PHPS1

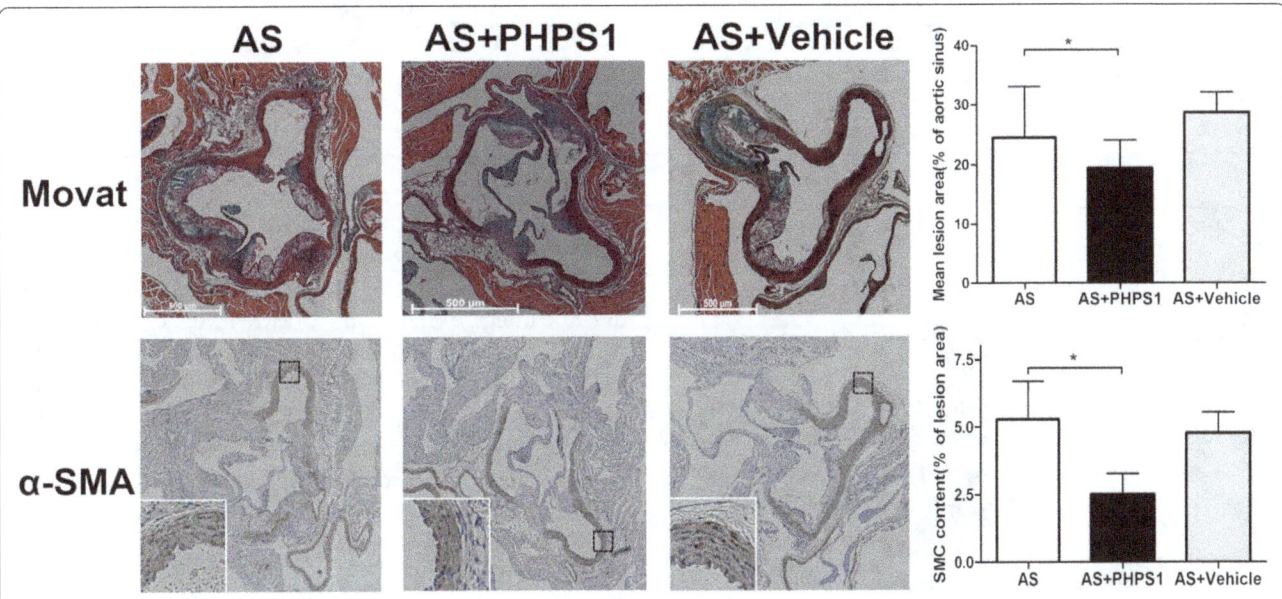

Fig. 2 Effect of PHPS1 on atherosclerotic lesion size in Ldlr$^{-/-}$ mice. The lesion volume/vessel volume ratio at the aortic root was analyzed by Movat staining. The number of smooth muscle cells in the plaques from the aortic root was determined by immunohistochemistry. PHPS1 treatment significantly reduced the atherosclerotic plaque area and inhibited the formation of atherosclerotic plaques. Compared with the intima in the other two groups, the intima was mildly thickened, the smooth muscle cells were arranged neatly, and smooth muscle cell proliferation was decreased in the AS+PHPS1 group. PHPS1 treatment inhibited the proliferation of vascular smooth muscle cells. Data are presented as the mean ± SE (n = 10 per group). *p < 0.05 vs. the AS group

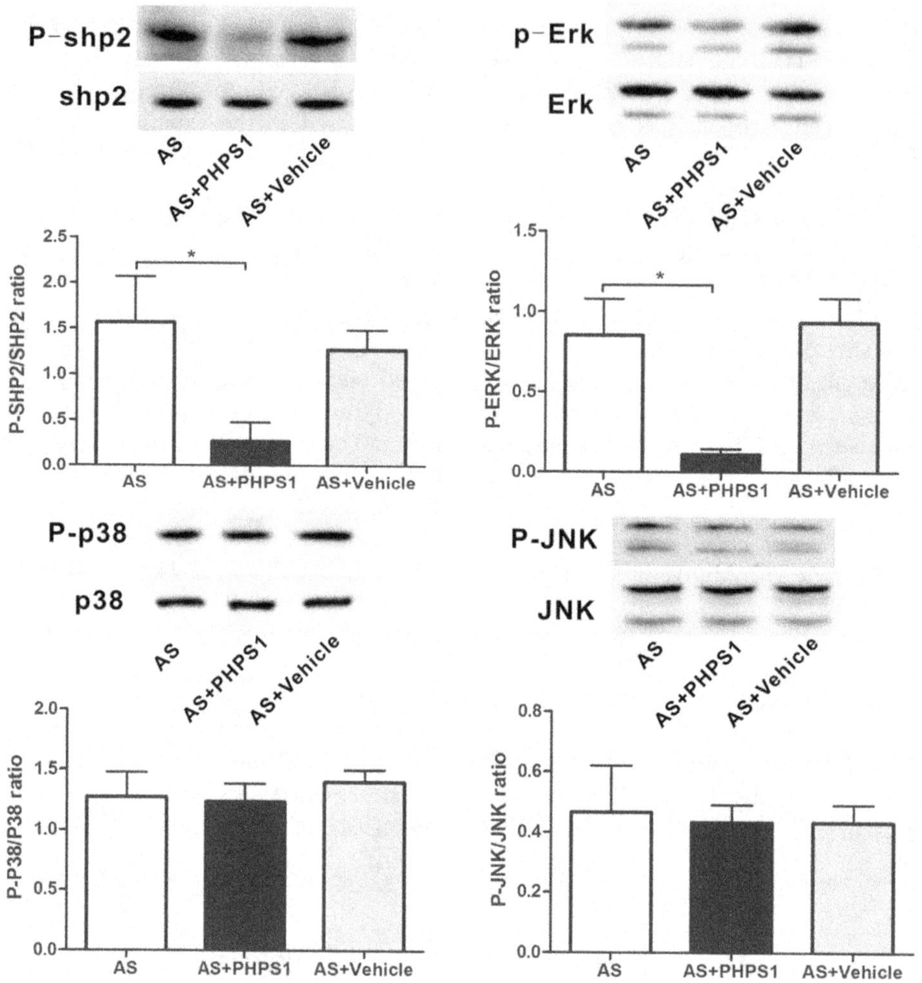

Fig. 3 The levels of total and phosphorylated SHP2, ERK, JNK and p38 were determined by Western blot analysis. There were no statistically significant differences in the total levels of SHP2, ERK, JNK or p38^{MAPK} among the three groups ($p > 0.05$). PHPS1 suppressed the levels of phosphorylated SHP2 and ERK. Data are presented as the mean ± SE. *$p < 0.05$ vs. the AS group

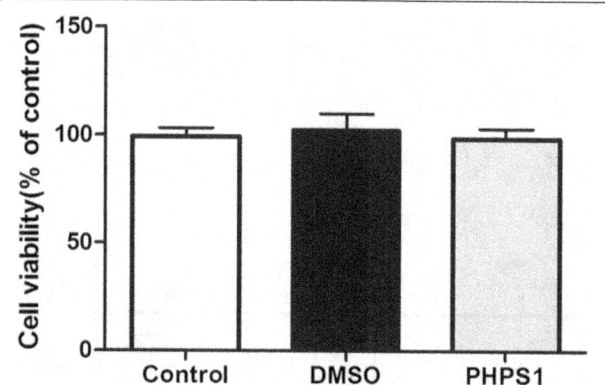

Fig. 4 Effects of DMSO and PHPS1 on the growth and viability of VSMCs. Cultured VSMCs were stimulated with 10 μM PHPS1 or an equal volume of DMSO for 30 min and then with 100 μg/ml oxLDL for 48 h. Cell number and viability were determined by the MTT assay. Data are presented as the mean ± SE. *$p < 0.05$ vs. the control group

attenuated P-SHP2 and P-ERK levels. In VSMCs, ERK phosphorylation was markedly inhibited after a 10-min treatment with 10 μM PHPS1. Treatment with DMSO did not affect P-SHP2 and P-ERK levels compared with control treatment (Fig. 6a). These results suggested that PHPS1 could inhibit oxLDL-induced SHP2-ERK signaling. As shown in Fig. 6b, VSMC proliferation was inhibited by PHPS1. Moreover, pretreatment with PHPS1 reversed the reinforcing effect of oxLDL on VSMC proliferation.

Discussion

This study showed that inhibiting the tyrosine phosphatase SHP2 with PHPS1 prevented the development of AS by inhibiting VSMC proliferation. This finding may provide a better understanding of the novel biological role of the SHP2 enzyme in the pathogenesis of AS.

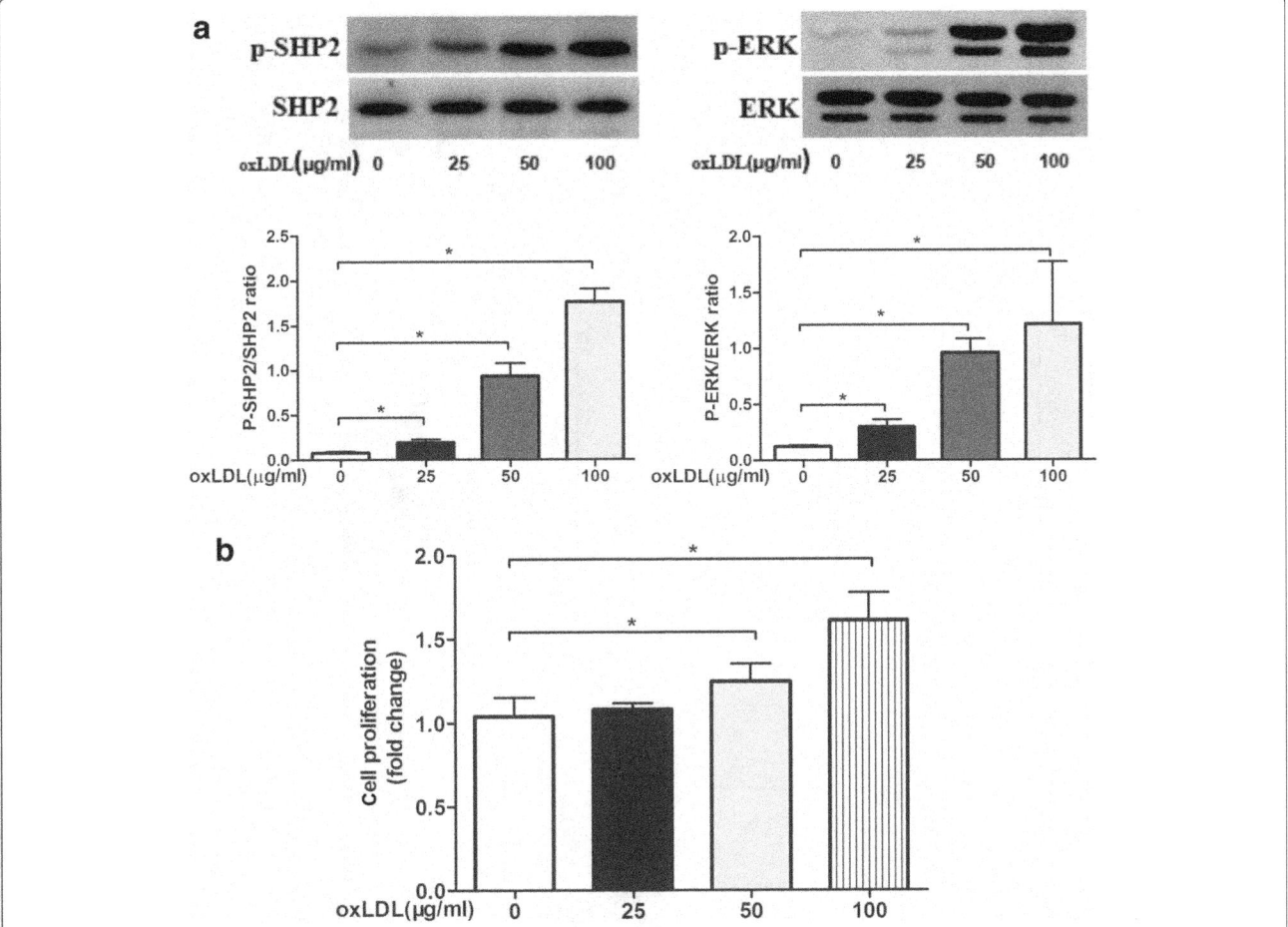

Fig. 5 a Quiescent cells were treated with different concentrations (0, 25, 50 or 100 µg/ml) of oxLDL for 10 min. Treatment was terminated by washing the cells with ice-cold PBS. Cells were lysed in 100 µl of lysis buffer containing protease and phosphatase inhibitor cocktails. Protein content in the samples was determined using the bicinchoninic acid assay, and the samples were heated at 100 °C in 5× protein loading dye for 5 min. Equal amounts of protein were separated by SDS-polyacrylamide gel electrophoresis, transferred to a polyvinylidene fluoride membrane and probed with monoclonal antibodies against total and phosphorylated SHP2 and ERK1/2. OxLDL activated SHP2 in a concentration-dependent manner. Total SHP2, phosphorylated SHP2, total ERK and phosphorylated ERK levels were examined by Western blot. Relative quantification of target proteins was performed by comparing band density levels among samples. The results are reported as the mean ± SE ($n = 3$ per group). $*p < 0.05$ vs. the no-oxLDL treatment group. **b** Effects of SHP2 on VSMC proliferation. Smooth muscle cells were exposed to different concentrations (0, 25, 50 or 100 µg/ml) of oxLDL for 24 h. BrdU (1 µmol/L) was added, and the cells were incubated for 3 h. BrdU incorporation was quantified using the BrdU cell proliferation assay kit. The percentage of BrdU-positive VSMCs was determined. Data are presented as the mean ± SE of three independent experiments. $*p < 0.05$ vs. the no-oxLDL treatment group

VSMCs participate in the development of AS [21]. Abnormal VSMC proliferation and migration contribute to atherosclerotic plaque formation, restenosis after percutaneous transluminal angioplasty and accelerated arteriopathy after cardiac transplantation [22, 23]. When chronic inflammation occurs in AS, arterial VSMCs become aberrantly regulated, leading to increased VSMC dedifferentiation and extracellular matrix formation in plaque areas [24]. Disturbances in hemodynamic forces could initiate a proinflammatory switch in the VSMC phenotype, even in the preclinical stages of AS [25]. Proinflammatory signals promote the further dedifferentiation of VSMCs in affected vessels and the propagation of pathological vascular remodeling [26, 27].

A number of studies have shown that SHP2 can promote VSMC proliferation and intimal hyperplasia [28, 29]. SHP2 was reported to be positively involved in the angiotensin II pathway, an important pathway involved in SMC proliferation [30]. SHP2 may act as an adaptor protein in the association of JAK2 with the AT_1 receptor, thus facilitating Ang II-induced JAK2 phosphorylation and activation [31]. By enhancing the phosphorylation levels of Syk and p38^{MAPK}, SHP2 facilitates the regulation of PDGF-BB-induced VSMC migration and neointima formation [32]. Induction by

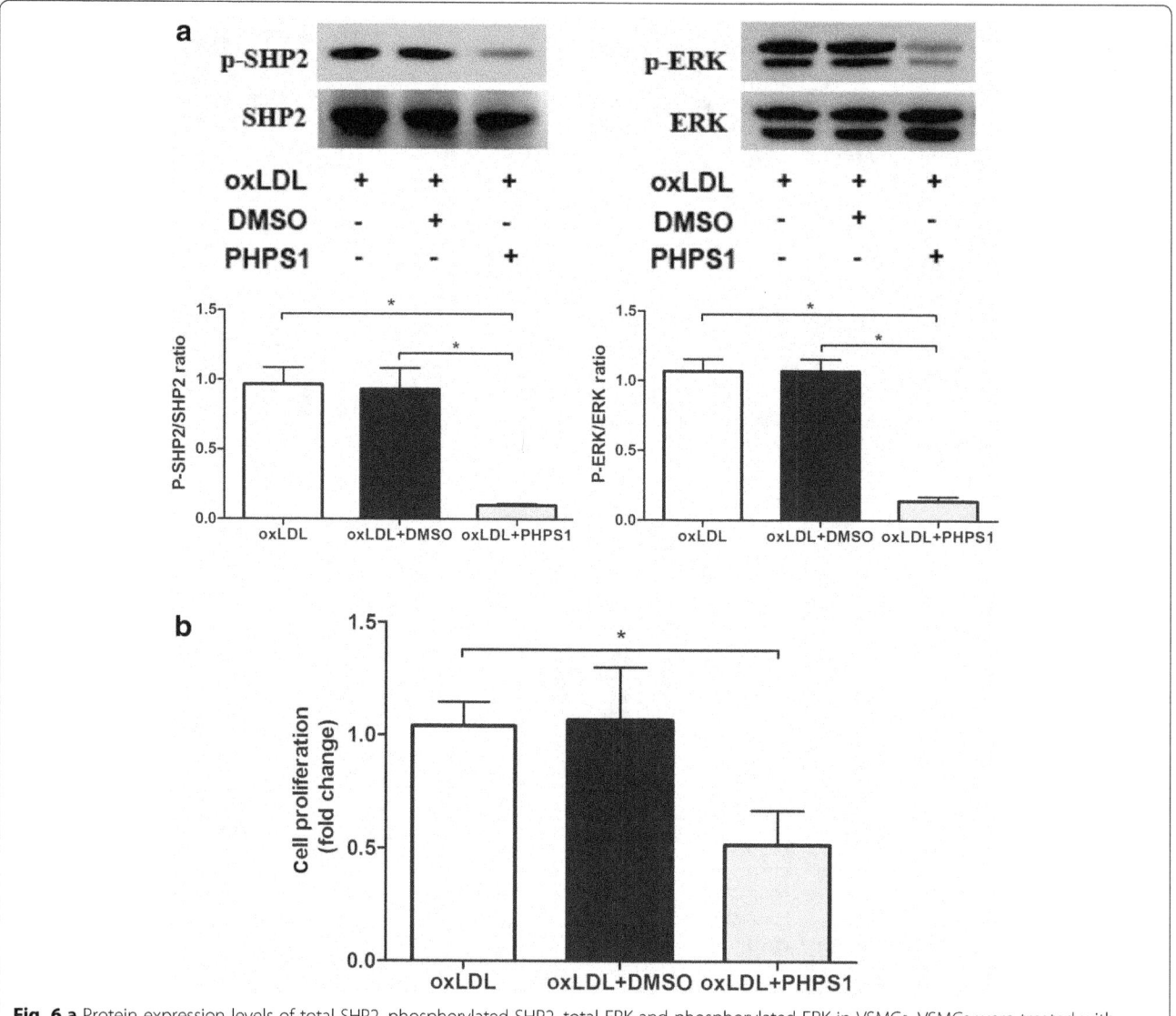

Fig. 6 a Protein expression levels of total SHP2, phosphorylated SHP2, total ERK and phosphorylated ERK in VSMCs. VSMCs were treated with PHPS1 or DMSO for 30 min and then with 100 µg/ml oxLDL for 10 min. Data are presented as the mean ± SE. *$p < 0.05$ vs. the oxLDL group. **b** Effects of SHP2 on VSMC proliferation. After preincubation in the presence or absence of 10 µM PHPS1 or an equal volume of DMSO for 30 min at 37 °C, cells were stimulated with oxLDL (100 µg/mL) for 24 h. BrdU (1 µmol/L) was added, and the cells were incubated for 3 h. BrdU incorporation was quantified using the BrdU cell proliferation assay kit. The percentage of BrdU-positive VSMCs was determined in the three groups. Compared with the other groups, the PHPS1 treatment group showed a decrease in the percentage of BrdU-positive VSMCs. *$p < 0.05$ vs. the oxLDL group

extracellular stimuli such as FBS, platelet-derived growth factor or insulin-like growth factor-1 enhances SHP2 levels and BrdU uptake in SMCs, suggesting that SHP2 may accelerate VSMC proliferation [28].

Our in vivo experiments showed that inhibition of SHP2 by PHPS1 had a protective effect on AS development by reducing VSMC proliferation. To evaluate the effect of SHP2 on AS, Ldlr$^{-/-}$ mice were fed a diet containing 1. 25% cholesterol for 4 weeks. As a result, early plaques formed in the aortic root. Subcutaneous injection of PHPS1 significantly inhibited VSMC proliferation and intimal thickening during the development of AS. Moreover, PHPS1

treatment significantly inhibited ERK phosphorylation in the aortic wall; ERK is a key regulator of cell proliferation [19], indicating that PHPS1 may attenuate VSMC proliferation by regulating the activation of ERK signaling cascade. Our in vitro experiment also verified the inhibitory effect of SHP2 on VSMC proliferation.

Our in vitro data showed that oxLDL increased SHP2 and ERK phosphorylation and simultaneously enhanced VSMC proliferation. However, these responses were suppressed by treatment with the SHP2 inhibitor PHPS1. These results implied that SHP2 positively regulated VSMC proliferation in response to oxLDL by regulating

ERK phosphorylation. SHP2 is reported to be involved in VSMC proliferation. OxLDL promotes the VSMC phenotypic switch from the contractile phenotype to the proinflammatory phenotype, which is associated with dedifferentiation and proliferation [33, 34]. In addition, OxLDL expedites the progression of AS through the accumulation of reactive oxygen species (ROS) and activation of the MAPK stress signaling cascade and stimulates the expression and secretion of ET-1 [35]. However, the relationship between SHP2 and oxLDL in VSMC proliferation remains unknown. This study showed that oxLDL stimulation further increased SHP2 phosphorylation, SHP2 activation by ERK phosphorylation promoted VSMC proliferation, and pretreatment with the SHP2 inhibitor PHPS1 inhibited the oxLDL-induced activation of SHP2 and VSMC proliferation. These results also indicated that SHP2 promoted VSMC proliferation via activation of the ERK signaling cascade.

Conclusion

The results of the present study suggest that the SHP2 inhibitor PHPS1 can inhibit VSMC proliferation by reducing the phosphorylation of ERK and suppressing activation of signaling cascade. PHPS1 is beneficial for delaying the development of AS, and it is a potential therapeutic target for cardiovascular diseases associated with vascular remodeling.

Abbreviations
AS: Atherosclerosis; BrdU: 5-bromo-2′-deoxyuridine; HDL-C: High-density lipoprotein cholesterol; LDL-C: Low-density lipoprotein cholesterol; OCT: Optimal cutting temperature; PBS: Phosphate-buffered saline; PHPS1: Phenylhydrazono pyrazolone sulfonate 1; PTK: Protein tyrosine kinase; PTP: Protein tyrosine phosphatase; PTPN11: Protein tyrosine phosphatase N 11; SHP2: Src homology 2 domain-containing protein tyrosine phosphatase 2; TC: Total cholesterol; TG: Triglyceride; VSMCs: Vascular smooth muscle cells

Acknowledgements
We would like to thank Yonghui He for his technical support. We gratefully acknowledge the support of the Pathology Department in our hospital.

Authors' contributions
JSG contributed to study conception and design and data acquisition, analysis, and interpretation and drafted the manuscript. JC designed the study, coordinated the blinding, performed the statistical analysis, and assisted with data collection and manuscript editing. ZYC conducted the experiments and analyzed the data. All authors have critically revised the manuscript and approved the final manuscript.

Competing interests
The authors declare that they have no competing interests.

Author details
[1]Department of Cardiology, Shanghai Baoshan Hospital of Integrated Traditional Chinese and Western Medicine, Friendship Road 181, Baoshan District, Shanghai, China. [2]Department of Cardiology, Shanghai Navy 411 Hospital, Shanghai, China.

References
1. Murray CJ, Barber RM, Foreman KJ, et al. Global, regional, and national disability-adjusted life years (DALYs) for 306 diseases and injuries and healthy life expectancy (HALE) for 188 countries, 1990-2013: quantifying the epidemiological transition. Lancet. 2015;386(10009):2145–91.
2. Ellulu MS, Patimah I, Khaza'ai H, et al. Atherosclerotic cardiovascular disease: a review of initiators and protective factors. Inflammopharmacology. 2016; 24(1):1–10.
3. Ley K, Miller YI, Hedrick CC. Monocyte and macrophage dynamics during atherogenesis. Arterioscler Thromb Vasc Biol. 2011;31(7):1506–16.
4. Galkina E, Ley K. Immune and inflammatory mechanisms of atherosclerosis (*). Annu Rev Immunol. 2009;27:165–97.
5. Osman I, Poulose N, Ganapathy V, et al. High fructose-mediated attenuation of insulin receptor signaling does not affect PDGF-induced proliferative signaling in vascular smooth muscle cells. Eur J Pharmacol. 2016;791:703–10.
6. Lim S, Park S. Role of vascular smooth muscle cell in the inflammation of atherosclerosis. BMB Rep. 2014;47(1):1–7.
7. Gray K, Kumar S, Figg N, et al. Effects of DNA damage in smooth muscle cells in atherosclerosis. Circ Res. 2015;116(5):816–26.
8. Patarca R. Protein phosphorylation and dephosphorylation in physiologic and oncologic processes. Crit Rev Oncog. 1996;7(5-6):343–432.
9. Paz C, Cornejo Maciel F, Gorostizaga A, et al. Role of protein phosphorylation and tyrosine phosphatases in the adrenal regulation of steroid synthesis and mitochondrial function. Front Endocrinol (Lausanne). 2016;7:60.
10. Fan G, Aleem S, Yang M, et al. Protein-tyrosine phosphatase and kinase specificity in regulation of SRC and breast tumor kinase. J Biol Chem. 2015; 290(26):15934–47.
11. Chong ZZ, Maiese K. The Src homology 2 domain tyrosine phosphatases SHP-1 and SHP-2: diversified control of cell growth, inflammation, and injury. Histol Histopathol. 2007;22(11):1251–67.
12. Mannell H, Krotz F. SHP-2 regulates growth factor dependent vascular signalling and function. Mini Rev Med Chem. 2014;14(6):471–83.
13. Kamiya N, Kim HK, King PD. Regulation of bone and skeletal development by the SHP-2 protein tyrosine phosphatase. Bone. 2014;69:55–60.
14. Schramm C, Edwards MA, Krenz M. New approaches to prevent LEOPARD syndrome-associated cardiac hypertrophy by specifically targeting Shp2-dependent signaling. J Biol Chem. 2013;288(25):18335–44.
15. Hellmuth K, Grosskopf S, Lum CT, et al. Specific inhibitors of the protein tyrosine phosphatase Shp2 identified by high-throughput docking. Proc Natl Acad Sci U S A. 2008;105(20):7275–80.
16. Abram CL, Lowell CA. Shp1 function in myeloid cells. J Leukoc Biol. 2017; 102(3):657–75.
17. Panzhinskiy E, Ren J, Nair S. Pharmacological inhibition of protein tyrosine phosphatase 1B: a promising strategy for the treatment of obesity and type 2 diabetes mellitus. Curr Med Chem. 2013;20(1875-533X (Electronic)):2609–25.
18. Li J, Kang Y, Wei L, et al. Tyrosine phosphatase Shp2 mediates the estrogen biological action in breast cancer via interaction with the estrogen extranuclear receptor. PLoS One. 2014;9(7):e102847.
19. Li FF, Shen J, Shen HJ, et al. Shp2 plays an important role in acute cigarette smoke-mediated lung inflammation. J Immunol. 2012;189(6):3159–67.
20. Matsuda M, Shimomura I, Sata M, et al. Role of adiponectin in preventing vascular stenosis. The missing link of adipo-vascular axis. J Biol Chem. 2002; 277(40):37487–91.
21. Zhang MJ, Zhou Y, Chen L, et al. SIRT1 improves VSMC functions in atherosclerosis. Prog Biophys Mol Biol. 2016;121(1):11–5.
22. Koga J, Aikawa M. Crosstalk between macrophages and smooth muscle cells in atherosclerotic vascular diseases. Vasc Pharmacol. 2012;57(1):24–8.
23. Johnson JL. Emerging regulators of vascular smooth muscle cell function in the development and progression of atherosclerosis. Cardiovasc Res. 2014; 103(4):452–60.
24. Yin YW, Liao SQ, Zhang MJ, et al. TLR4-mediated inflammation promotes foam cell formation of vascular smooth muscle cell by upregulating ACAT1

expression. Cell Death Dis. 2014;5:e1574.

25. Chistiakov DA, Orekhov AN, Bobryshev YV. Vascular smooth muscle cell in atherosclerosis. Acta Physiol (Oxf). 2015;214(1):33–50.

26. Kiyan Y, Tkachuk S, Hilfiker-Kleiner D, et al. oxLDL induces inflammatory responses in vascular smooth muscle cells via urokinase receptor association with CD36 and TLR4. J Mol Cell Cardiol. 2014;66:72–82.

27. Hakimi M, Peters A, Becker A, et al. Inflammation-related induction of absent in melanoma 2 (AIM2) in vascular cells and atherosclerotic lesions suggests a role in vascular pathogenesis. J Vasc Surg. 2014;59(3):794–803.

28. Seki N, Hashimoto N, Suzuki Y, et al. Role of SRC homology 2-containing tyrosine phosphatase 2 on proliferation of rat smooth muscle cells. Arterioscler Thromb Vasc Biol. 2002;22(7):1081–5.

29. Kandadi MR, Stratton MS, Ren J. The role of Src homology 2 containing protein tyrosine phosphatase 2 in vascular smooth muscle cell migration and proliferation. Acta Pharmacol Sin. 2010;31(10):1277–83.

30. Marrero MB, Venema VJ, Ju H, et al. Regulation of angiotensin II-induced JAK2 tyrosine phosphorylation: roles of SHP-1 and SHP-2. Am J Phys. 1998; 275(5 Pt 1):C1216–23.

31. Godeny MD, Sayyah J, VonDerLinden D, et al. The N-terminal SH2 domain of the tyrosine phosphatase, SHP-2, is essential for Jak2-dependent signaling via the angiotensin II type AT1 receptor. Cell Signal. 2007;19(3):600–9.

32. Won KJ, Lee HM, Lee CK, et al. Protein tyrosine phosphatase SHP-2 is positively involved in platelet-derived growth factor-signaling in vascular neointima formation via the reactive oxygen species-related pathway. J Pharmacol Sci. 2011;115(2):164–75.

33. Makino J, Asai R, Hashimoto M, et al. Suppression of EC-SOD by oxLDL during vascular smooth muscle cell proliferation. J Cell Biochem. 2016; 117(11):2496–505.

34. Hwang JS, Ham SA, Yoo T, et al. Sirtuin 1 mediates the actions of peroxisome proliferator-activated receptor delta on the oxidized low-density lipoprotein-triggered migration and proliferation of vascular smooth muscle cells. Mol Pharmacol. 2016;90(5):522–9.

35. Xu H, Duan J, Ren J, et al. alpha-Zearalanol attenuates oxLDL-induced ET-1 gene expression, ET-1 secretion and redox-sensitive intracellular signaling activation in human umbilical vein endothelial cells. Toxicol Lett. 2008; 179(3):163–8.

21

Association of Platelet to lymphocyte ratio with non-culprit atherosclerotic plaque vulnerability in patients with acute coronary syndrome: an optical coherence tomography study

Xuedong Wang[1,2], Zulong Xie[3], Xinxin Liu[1,2], Xingtao Huang[1,2], Jiale Lin[1,2], Dan Huang[1,2], Bo Yu[1,2] and Jingbo Hou[1,2]* (iD)

Abstract

Background: The platelet to lymphocyte ratio (PLR), an indirect inflammatory biomarker, has been recently demonstrated to be associated with severity of coronary artery disease. In the present study, we sought to investigate whether PLR is associated with vulnerable plaque characteristics of non-culprit lesions in patients with acute coronary syndrome (ACS).

Methods: The patients in our study were divided into two groups (high PLR group and low PLR group). A total of 119 non-culprit plaques from 71 patients with ACS were assessed by optical coherence tomography (OCT).

Results: The non-culprit plaques in high PLR group exhibited thinner fibrous cap thickness (FCT) (88.60 ± 44.70 vs. 119.28 ± 50.22 μm, $P = 0.001$), greater maximum lipid arc (271.73 ± 71.66 vs. 240.60 ± 76.69°, $P = 0.027$) and increased incidence of thin-cap fibroatheroma (TCFA) (34.0% vs. 15.9%, $P = 0.022$) compared with those in low PLR group. Meanwhile, PLR was negatively associated with FCT ($r = -0.329$, $P < 0.001$). Furthermore, multivariate regression analysis showed that PLR [OR: 1.023 (95% CI: 1.005–1.041), $P = 0.012$] and LDL-C [OR: 1.892 (95% CI: 1.106–3.239), $P = 0.020$] were significant predictors of TCFA.

Conclusions: High level of PLR may be associated with vulnerable plaque features of non-culprit lesions in patients with ACS. PLR, a cheap and easily available index, may surve as a useful inflammatory marker in reflecting plaque vulnerability.

Keywords: Platelet to lymphocyte ratio, Atherosclerosis, Plaque vulnerability, Optical coherence tomography

Background

Inflammation plays a vital role in the pathophysiological process of atherosclerotic disease [1]. At the instigation of atherogenic diet, endothelial cells became inflamed and proceeded with attracting leukocyte to the nascent atherosclerotic position. As the evolution of atherosclerotic lesions, leukocytes and other vascular wall cells secrete various proinflammatory mediators, which subsequently render the plaque vulnerable and prone to rupture. Vulnerable plaque, characterized by thin fibrous caps, large lipid core, macrophage infiltration and neovascularization, is closely related to inflammation [2–4]. The majority of acute coronary syndromes (ACS) can be attributed to plaque vulnerability [5].

Previous researches have demonstrated that elevated platelet counts or reduced lymphocyte counts were related to poor cardiovascular clinical outcomes [6–10]. Furthermore, platelet to lymphocyte ratio (PLR), initially served as a systemic inflammatory biomarker to predict the prognosis of neoplastic diseases [11–13], recently

* Correspondence: jingbohou@163.com
[1]Department of Cardiology, The Second Affiliated Hospital of Harbin Medical University, Harbin 150001, China
[2]Key Laboratory of Myocardial Ischemia, Ministry of Education, Harbin Medical University, Harbin 150001, China
Full list of author information is available at the end of the article

showed distinct predictive value on mortality or major adverse cardiovascular events [14, 15]. The severity of coronary artery disease was likewise shown to be associated with PLR [16, 17]. In spite of this, the relationship between PLR and atherosclerotic plaque vulnerability is still unclear.

Optical coherence tomography (OCT) has advantages in differentiating the vulnerable plaque including thin-cap fibroatheroma (TCFA) [18]. On account of high resolution, OCT made it possible to visualize the microstructure of vulnerable plaque in either culprit or non-culprit lesions in ACS [19]. Based on the above analyses, we aimed to evaluate whether high preoperative PLR was related to plaque vulnerability of non-culprit lesions in patients with ACS.

Methods

Study population

The present retrospective study included seventy-one patients who were diagnosed with ACS (non-ST segment elevated ACS and ST segment elevated myocardial infarction) and received percutaneous coronary intervention during admission between October 2012 and January 2014. Patients with chest pain that persisted for at least 30 min, ST-segment elevation > 1 mm in at least 2 contiguous leads or new-onset left bundle branch block on a 12-lead electrocardiogram, and elevated cardiac markers such as creatine kinase-myocardial band or troponin T/I were diagnosed with ST-segment elevated myocardial infarction (STEMI). The definition of non-ST segment elevated ACS included unstable angina pectoris (UAP) and non-ST segment elevated myocardial infarction (Non-STEMI). We defined non-STEMI as an acute myocardial infarction in the absence of elevated ST-segment on electrocardiogram. UAP was defined as new-onset angina, accelerated angina or angina at rest episodes but without cardiac markers elevation. In the present study, we defined non-culprit lesions as de novo atherosclerotic lesions with an angiographically intermediate diameter stenosis (50% to 75%) in the non-culprit/non-target locations. All of the patients had written informed consent prior to the enrollment. Our study was approved by the ethics committee at the Second Affiliated Hospital of Harbin Medical University (Harbin, China).

The exclusion criteria of this study comprised left main diseases, ostial lesions, severely calcified or tortuous lesions, left ventricular ejection fraction < 40%, cardiogenic shock, renal insufficiency (baseline serum creatinine > 2.0 mg/dl), or accompanied with malignant disease, peripheral arterial disease, chronic obstructive lung disease, hematologic disease, autoimmune disease, or other systemic inflammatory conditions.

Laboratory tests

For all patients, venous blood samples were drawn from antecubital vein immediately after admission. The parameters of differential leukocyte count and platelet count were determined. Glycosylated hemoglobin, lipid profiles, creatinine and high sensitivity C-reactive protein (hs-CRP) were also assessed. The PLR was calculated as the ratio of platelet count to lymphocyte count and the neutrophil-to-lymphocyte ratio (NLR) was calculated by dividing neutrophil count by lymphocyte count.

Angiographic analysis

The lesion distribution and plaque location of patients were recorded. Quantitative coronary angiography (QCA) was analyzed using the off-line software (CAAS 5.10.1, Pie Medical Imaging BV, Maastricht, the Netherlands). The reference vessel diameter (RVD), minimum lumen diameter (MLD) and diameter stenosis (DS) were analyzed.

OCT image acquisition and analysis

Intracoronary OCT examination was performed by using frequency-domain OCT system and the procedure was conducted as previously described [20]. Two independent observers, blinded to angiographic and laboratory characteristics, analyzed the OCT images according to the criteria for plaque measurement [21]. A signal-poor region with unclearly delineated borders was identified as a lipid core. The fibrous cap on OCT images appeared as signal-rich homogeneous regions overlying the lipid core. The fibrous cap thickness (FCT) was measured 3 times at the thinnest part of fibrous cap and the average was recorded. The maximum lipid arc was measured likewise on the cross-sectional images. When a lipid core took up at least two quadrants (maximum lipid core > 90°), it was defined as a lipid-rich plaque. Thin-cap fibroatheroma (TCFA) was defined as a lipid-rich plaque with the thinnest FCT < 65 μm (Fig. 1a). Calcification on OCT images appeared as a sharply delineated, heterogeneous region. Macrophage infiltration was defined as clusters of signal-rich spots in fibrous cap with backward shadowing (Fig. 1b). Cholesterol crystals were identified as linear regions with high signal intensity in the plaque. The presence of a tubular structure with the diameter of 50-300 μm on more than 3 consecutive cross sections was considered as a microchannel (Fig. 1c). Plaque rupture was defined as a plaque with the fibrous cap discontinuity and a cavity formation within the plaque (Fig. 1d). Plaque erosion was defined as formation of thrombus adjacent to the plaque surface without signs of overlying fibrous cap discontinuity. Thrombus on OCT images appeared as an irregular mass protruding into the lumen or attached to luminal surface.

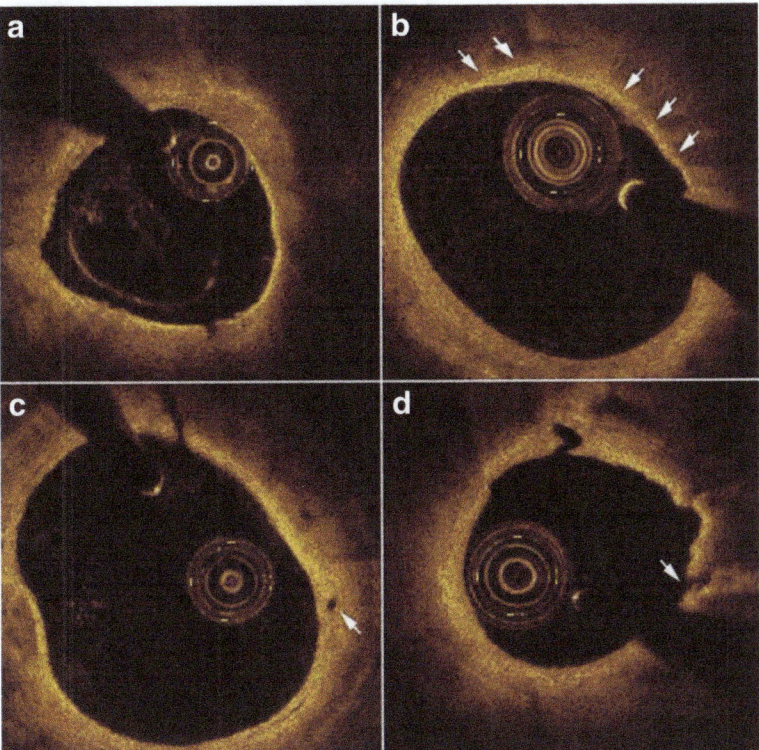

Fig. 1 Representative optical coherence tomography images. **a** Thin cap fibroatheroma (TCFA) was displayed as a lipid-rich plaque (maximum lipid core > 90°) with fibrou cap thickness < 65 μm. **b** Macrophage infiltration (*arrows*) was defined as clusters of bright spots with backward shadowing. **c** Microchannel (*arrow*) was shown as a black hole in the plaque. **d** Ruptured plaque (*arrow*) was observed as a plaque with the discontinuous fibrous cap and a communication between the lipid core and the lumen

Statistical analysis

Continuous variables are expressed as mean ± standard deviation (SD) or median (25th to 75th percentiles), according to the distribution type of variables. Categorical variables are expressed as number (percentages). Continuous values were compared by independent sample t-test or Mann-Whitney U test. Categorical data were analyzed by chi-square or Fisher exact test. Correlations between PLR and plaque characteristics were assessed using Pearson correlation test or Spearman correlation rank test. To determine the important factors which indicate the presence of TCFA, univariate and multivariate logistic regression analysis were performed. Parameters with $P < 0.05$ in the univariate analysis were entered into the multivariate analysis models. A 2-tailed P value < 0.05 was considered statistically significant. All of the statistical analyses were performed by IBM SPSS version 19.0 (IBM Corp., Armonk, NY, USA).

Results

Baseline characteristics

Seventy-one patients with 119 non-culprit plaques were enrolled in this study. According to the median of PLR (109), enrolled patients were divided into low PLR group (PLR < 109, 36 patients with 69 plaques) and high PLR group (PLR > 109, 35 patients with 50 plaques). The baseline clinical characteristics and laboratory parameters of the two groups are shown in Tables 1 and 2. The prevalence of dyslipidemia was higher in low PLR group (41.7% vs. 20.0%, $P = 0.048$), whereas the percentage of renin-angiotensin system (RAS) blocker usage was lower in low PLR group (19.4% vs. 45.7%, $P = 0.018$). No other differences were observed between the two groups.

As shown in Table 2, among laboratory parameters, the platelet number and NLR were significantly higher ($P = 0.01$ and $P = 0.007$, respectively), whereas the lymphocyte count was obviously lower ($P < 0.001$) in high PLR group. Meanwhile, the high PLR group presented with a mildly lower triglyceride level compared with the low PLR group ($P = 0.032$).

Angiographic fingdings

The qualitative and quantitative characteristics of angiographic fingdings are listed in Table 3. There was no difference in the lesion distribution between the two groups. Meanwhile, we found no difference in RVD,

Table 1 Baseline Characteristics

Parameters	Low PLR (*n* = 36)	High PLR (*n* = 35)	*P* Value
Age, years	57.97 ± 10.51	59.77 ± 8.88	0.439
Male, n (%)	28(77.8%)	26(74.3%)	0.73
Type of ACS, n (%)			
UAP	29(80.6%)	27(77.1%)	0.725
Non-STEMI	4(11.1%)	4(11.4%)	0.966
STEMI	3(8.3%)	4(11.4%)	0.662
Hypertension, n (%)	23(63.9%)	17(48.6%)	0.193
Diabetes mellitus, n (%)	13(36.1%)	13(37.1%)	0.928
Dyslipidemia, n (%)	15(41.7%)	7(20.0%)	0.048
Current smoker, n (%)	15(41.7%)	8(22.9%)	0.09
Previous MI, n (%)	12(33.3%)	11(31.4%)	0.864
LVEF, %	0.65 ± 0.08	0.62 ± 0.08	0.262
Medical therapy			
ASA, n (%)	36(100.0%)	35(100.0%)	1.000
P2Y12 receptor antagonist, n (%)	34(94.4%)	35(100.0%)	0.493
Statin, n (%)	36(100.0%)	35(100.0%)	1.000
RAS blocker, n (%)	7(19.4%)	16(45.7%)	0.018
β-blocker, n (%)	15(45.7%)	17(48.6%)	0.559
CCB, n (%)	16(44.4%)	11(31.4%)	0.259

Values are mean ± SD or n (%)

Abbreviations: *PLR* platelet to lymphocyte ratio, *ACS* acute coronary syndrome, *UAP* unstable angina pectoris, *STEMI* ST-segment elevation myocardial infarction, *MI* myocardial infarction, *LVEF* left ventricular ejection fraction, *ASA* acetylsalicylic acid, *RAS* renin-angiotensin system, *CCB* calcium channel blocker

Table 2 Laboratory Parameters

Parameters	Low PLR (*n* = 36)	High PLR (*n* = 35)	*P* Value
Lymphocyte, ×10^9/L	2.23 ± 0.45	1.66 ± 0.51	<0.001
Neutrophil, ×10^9/L	4.80 ± 1.34	4.85 ± 2.23	0.898
Platelets, ×10^9/L	202.75 ± 43.57	230.89 ± 45.47	0.01
NLR	2.21 ± 0.70	3.33 ± 2.31	0.007
RBC, ×10^{12}/L	4.67 ± 0.49	4.54 ± 0.47	0.252
Hemoglobin, g/L	145.89 ± 16.65	139.46 ± 13.86	0.082
RDW, %	12.81 ± 0.55	12.97 ± 0.79	0.329
hs-CRP, mg/L	2.93 ± 4.04	3.03 ± 4.93	0.924
Hemoglobin A1c, %	6.53 ± 1.24	6.43 ± 1.49	0.797
Total cholesterol, mg/dl	167.95 ± 46.49	161.20 ± 38.33	0.507
LDL-C, mg/dl	91.58 ± 30.68	89.35 ± 31.06	0.762
HDL-C, mg/dl	47.89 ± 9.48	50.41 ± 14.09	0.382
Triglycerides, mg/dl	176.99 ± 104.43	128.62 ± 79.55	0.032
apoA, mg/dl	127.20 ± 22.27	134.11 ± 27.99	0.257
apoB, mg/dl	87.46 ± 33.45	79.77 ± 24.40	0.276
Creatinine, mg/dl	0.97 ± 0.22	0.95 ± 0.16	0.739
Troponin I, μg/l	1.77 ± 7.15	2.26 ± 7.12	0.774

Values are mean ± SD

Abbreviations: *NLR* neutrophil-to-lymphocyte ratio, *RDW* red cell distribution width, *CRP* C-reactive protein, *HDL-C* high-density lipoprotein cholesterol, *LDL-C* low-density lipoprotein cholesterol

MLD and DS between the low PLR and the high PLR group.

OCT findings

Table 4 shows OCT findings of the two groups. Patients in the high PLR group presented more frequent occurrence of TCFA than those in the low PLR group (34.0% vs. 15.9%, *P* = 0.022). FCT in the high PLR group was strikingly thinner (88.60 ± 44.70 vs. 119.28 ± 50.22 μm, *P* = 0.001), in addition, the high PLR group showed greater maximum lipid arc than the low PLR group (271.73 ± 71.66 vs. 240.60 ± 76.69°, *P* = 0.027).

PLR and OCT findings

According to whether presenting with TCFA in non-culprit lesions, we divided study population into TCFA group (22 patients with 28 plaques) and non-TCFA group (49 patients with 91 plaques) and compared the PLR values between them. As presented in Fig. 2, the TCFA group showed significantly greater PLR than the non-TCFA group (*P* = 0.003). As shown in Fig. 3, there was a significant negative correlation between PLR and FCT (*r* = −0.329, *P* < 0.001).

We adopted univariate and multivariate logistic regression analysis to discuss which factors could predict the incidence of TCFA in non-culprit lesions

Table 3 Angiographic Findings

Parameters	Low PLR (n = 36)	High PLR (n = 35)	P Value
Total plaque number	69	50	
Vessel			0.159
LAD	26(37.7%)	18(36.0%)	
LCX	20(29.0%)	8(16.0%)	
RCA	23(33.3%)	24(48.0%)	
Lesion location			0.419
Proximal	26(37.7%)	15(30.0%)	
Mid	21(30.4%)	21(42.0%)	
Distal	22(31.9%)	14(28.0%)	
QCA data			
RVD, mm	3.36 ± 0.44	3.46 ± 0.51	0.253
MLD, mm	1.99 ± 0.58	2.10 ± 0.59	0.331
DS, %	41 ± 14	39 ± 15	0.576

Values are n (%) or mean ± SD

Abbreviations: *LAD* left anterior descending coronary artery, *LCX* left circumflex coronary artery, *RCA* right coronary artery, *QCA* quantitative coronary angiography, *RVD* reference vessel diameter, *MLD* minimum lumen diameter, *DS* diameter stenosis

of ACS (Table 5). Univariate regression analysis showed that LDL-C, PLR and NLR were possible predictors of the presence of TCFA. In multivariate regression analysis, LDL-C [odds ratio (OR): 1.892 (95% confidence interval (CI): 1.106–3.239), $P = 0.020$], PLR [OR: 1.023 (95% CI: 1.005–1.041), $P = 0.012$] remained independently predictable for TCFA.

Discussion

The main findings of this study are as follows: (i) non-culprit plaques in ACS patients with higher PLR values

Table 4 OCT Findings

Parameters	Low PLR (n = 36)	High PLR (n = 35)	P Value
Total plaque number	69	50	
Lesion length, mm	19.57 ± 7.94	20.88 ± 9.36	0.465
MLA, mm^2	3.41 ± 2.01	3.77 ± 2.03	0.342
Maximum lipid arc, °	240.60 ± 76.69	271.73 ± 71.66	0.027
FCT, μm	119.28 ± 50.22	88.60 ± 44.70	0.001
TCFA, %	11(15.9%)	17(34.0%)	0.022
Macrophage, %	38(55.1%)	23(46.0%)	0.328
Calcification, %	32(46.4%)	25(50.0%)	0.696
Cholesterol crystal, %	7(10.1%)	6(12.0%)	0.749
Microvessel, %	26(37.7%)	21(42.0%)	0.634
Plaque rupture, %	9(13.0%)	3(6.0%)	0.208
Plaque erosion, %	0	2(4.0%)	0.094
Thrombus, %	9(13.0%)	5(10.0%)	0.611

Values are mean ± SD or n (%)

Abbreviations: *FCT* fibrous cap thickness, *TCFA* thin-cap fibroatheroma, *MLA* minimum lumen area

exhibited more vulnerable characteristics (thinner FCT, greater maximum lipid arc and higher incidence of OCT-detected TCFA); (ii) PLR values were significantly and negatively correlated with FCT of non-culprit plaques; (iii) in multivariate regression analysis, PLR manifested as an independent indicator of TCFA in non-culprit leisons. To the best of our knowledge, this is the first study assessing the relation between PLR values and non-culprit plaque vulnerability using OCT in ACS patients.

TCFA has been postulated to be the precursor lesion of plaque rupture and subsequent luminal thrombosis which is the leading cause of ACS [5, 22, 23]. In ACS patients, besides of culprit lesions, the non-culprit lesions are often characterised by TCFA. A previous intravascular ultrasound (IVUS) sutdy demonstrated that ACS patients possessed more IVUS-derived TCFA in non-culprit lesions comparing with stable patients [24]. In another study, Kato et al. [25] evaluated the plaque characteristics of non-culprit leisons in patients with and without ACS by means of OCT, the results showed that TCFA was more frequent in the non-culprit lesions of ACS patients (64.7% versus 14.9%). However, in our present study, the OCT-detected TCFA in non-culprit lesions was fewer (31.0%). This discordance perhaps due to the relatively fewer incidence of plaque rupture (14.1%) in our study. Vergallo et al. [26] previously showed that patients with non-culprit rupture presented with higher frequency of TCFA.

PLR has recently been demonstrated to be correlated with various cardiovascular diseases [27–30]. In patients with acute myocardial infarction, PLR was also an independent predictor of short-term and long-term adverse clinical events [14, 15]. In addition, Kurtul et al. [16] demonstrated that higher PLR values (PLR ≥ 116) on admission were positively associated with the intermediate to high SYNTAX score in patients with ACS. Even so, the relationship between PLR and plaque characteristics has not been directly explored. By virtue of OCT which has advantages in identifying vulnerable plaques in vivo, our study provided the direct association of PLR and non-culprit plaques vulnerability in ACS patients. The mechanisms of the link between PLR and plaque vulnerability may be associated with immuno-inflammatory response which plays a crucial role in the plaque destabilization [31]. Previous studies demonstrated that PLR was positively associated with systemic inflammation markers such as CRP [16, 17]. Furthermore, higher platelet or lower lymphocyte counts per se can be regarded as the response to inflammatory stimuli [32, 33]. In ACS patients, platelet-derived chemokines, such as CXCL4 and CCL5, were elevated and played an important role in mediating the inflammatory response to plaque destabilization [34]. On the other hand, lymphocytopenia

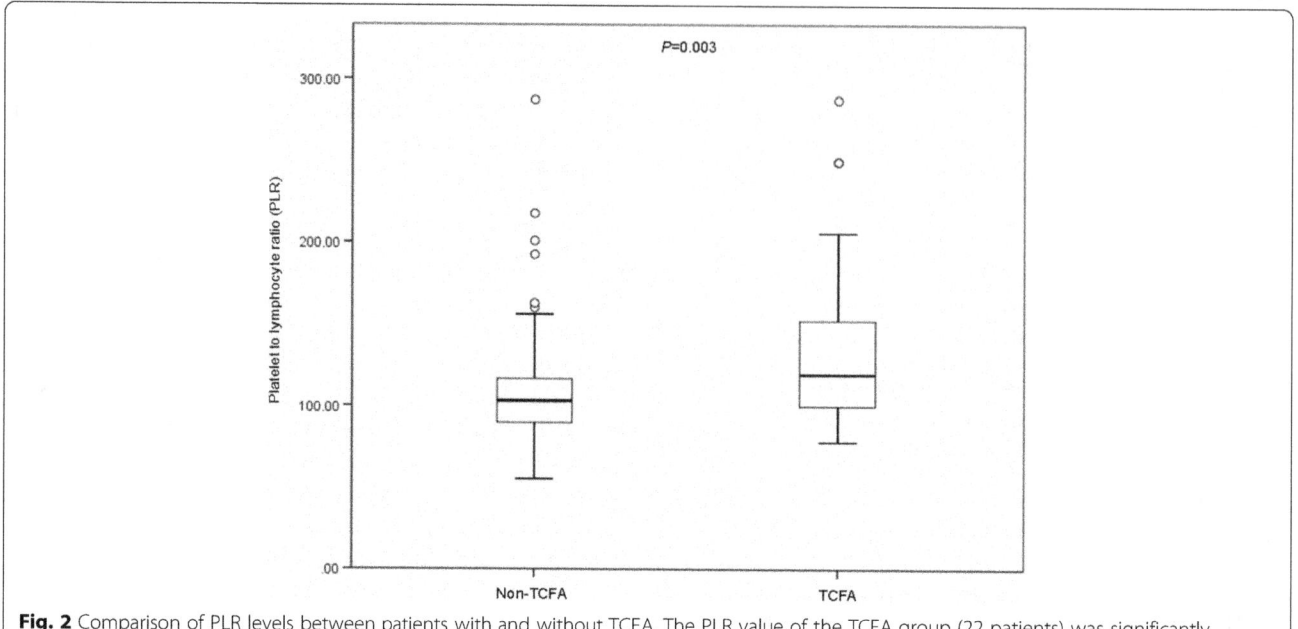

Fig. 2 Comparison of PLR levels between patients with and without TCFA. The PLR value of the TCFA group (22 patients) was significantly greater than the non-TCFA group (49 patients) (P = 0.003)

was also a pervasive phenomenon in the setting of ACS, which may be associated with lymphocytes apoptosis induced by inflammation [35].

In accordance with our findings, the ACS patients in the high PLR group possessed higher NLR values likewise (Table 2). Meanwhile, we found that the PLR was significantly correlated with NLR (r = 0.463, P < 0.001) which has been well-defined as a predictive marker for coronary artery disease severity. Arbel et al. [36] found

that higher NLR values (NLR > 3) were associated with more serious coronary artery disease and worse prognosis. Nilsson et al. [37] showed that NLR was significantly associated with non-calcified plaques detected by coronary computed tomographic angiography. The combined usefulness of PLR and NLR in predicting adverse clinical events in patients with CAD was also demonstrated by Cho et al. [38], their findings showed that higher preoperative PLR and NLR, alone or combined, were

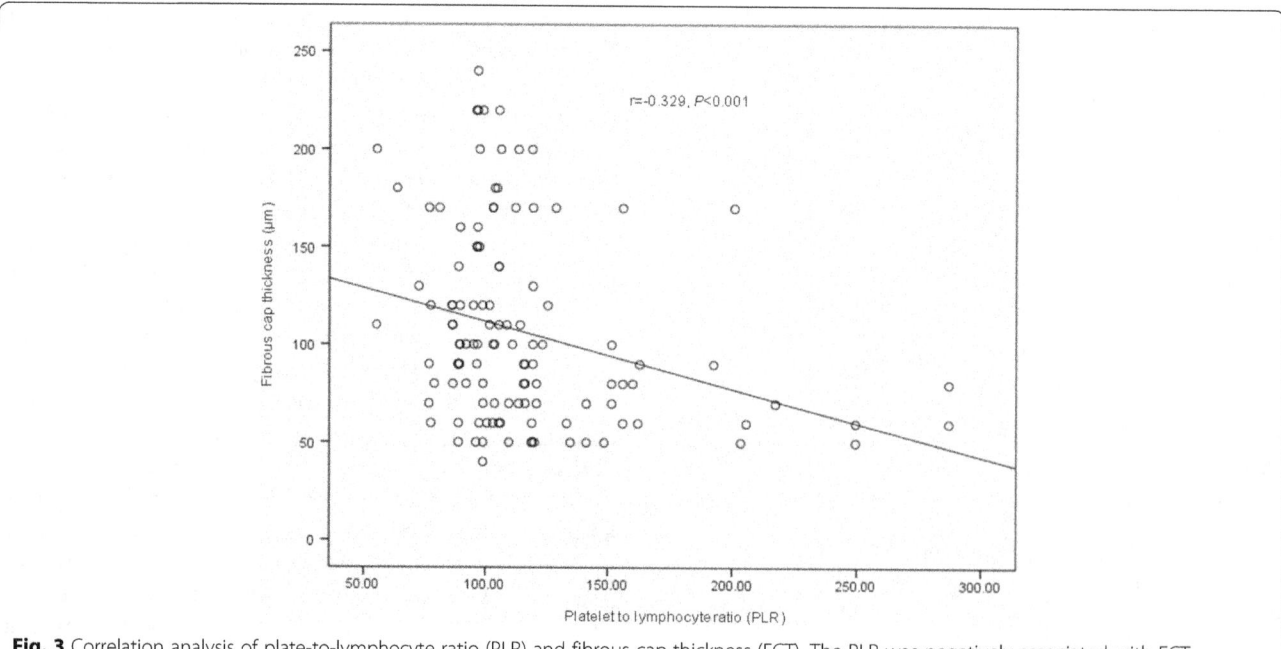

Fig. 3 Correlation analysis of plate-to-lymphocyte ratio (PLR) and fibrous cap thickness (FCT). The PLR was negatively associated with FCT (r = −0.329, P < 0.001)

Table 5 Logistic Regression Analysis of TCFA

Variables	Univariate		Multivariate	
	OR (95%CI)	P Value	OR (95%CI)	P Value
Age	1.004(0.962–1.047)	0.865		
Gender (male)	0.595(0.233–1.516)	0.276		
Diabetes mellitus	1.024(0.423–2.481)	0.958		
Current smoking	1.123(0.451–2.794)	0.803		
Prior MI	0.509(0.196–1.321)	0.165		
LDL-C	1.757(1.050–2.939)	0.032	1.892(1.106–3.239)	0.020
hs-CRP	0.996(0.906–1.095)	0.933		
PLR	1.015(1.005–1.025)	0.005	1.023(1.005–1.041)	0.012
NLR	1.242(1.001–1.539)	0.048	0.830(0.567–1.217)	0.341

significant predictors of long-term adverse clinical events. Further studies will be needed to identify the combined usefulness of PLR and NLR in predicting atherosclerotic plaque vulnerability.

It has been verified that the majority of ACS patients were at a high risk of recurrent cardiac events due to the lesions irrelevant to the initial ischemic events [39, 40]. According to the findings of PROSPECT study [41], non-culprit lesions and culprit lesions at baseline were equally contributed to the recurrence of major adverse cardiovascular events, furthermore, the non-culprit lesions associated with recurrent events were more likely to be IVUS-detected TCFA. In our study, the PLR presented as an independent indicator of OCT-detected TCFA in non-culprit lesions of ACS patients in multivariate regression analysis. We speculated that PLR, a simple and immediately obtained parameter, may be useful in identifying vulnerable plaques and patients with high risks. However, further studies are needed to verify all of our speculations.

Limitations
There are several limitations in the present study. Firstly, the sample size in the current study was small, so more well-designed studies are warranted to confirm our findings. Secondly, this is a retrospective, single-central, cross-sectional study with a specific patient cohort, therefore we should be cautious to generalize the results to all patients. Thirdly, instead of assessing dynamic changes, we just evaluated the spot value of PLR so that we cannot ensure whether it remains an indicator of TCFA subsequently. Finally, because of the limited penetration of OCT, we were not able to show additional characteristics related to plaque vulnerability (for example plaque burden).

Conclusions
The OCT-detected TCFA in non-culprit lesions is more frequent in ACS patients with higher levels of PLR.

Higher PLR levels show an important indicator of TCFA in non-culprit lesions. These findings reflect that PLR may serve as a useful indicator of atherosclerotic plaque vulnerability. Future prospective studies with large-scale samples are expected to validate the findings in our study.

Abbreviations
ACS: Acute coronary syndrome; DS: Diameter stenosis; FCT: Fibrous cap thickness; hs-CRP: High sensitivity C-reacitve protein; IVUS: Intravascular ultrasound; MLD: Minimum lumen diameter; NLR: Neutrophil-to-lymphocyte ratio; OCT: Optical coherence tomography; PLR: Platelet to lymphocyte ratio; QCA: Quantitative coronary angiography; RVD: Reference vessel diameter; STEMI: ST-segment elevated myocardial infarction; TCFA: Thin-cap fibroatheroma; UAP: Unstable angina pectoris.

Acknowledgements
Not applicable.

Funding
This study was supported by the National Natural Science Foundation of China (Grant No. 81271675).

Authors' contributions
XW contributed to the study design, participated in the interpretation of data and drafted the manuscript. JH contributed to the conception and design of the study and final revision of the manuscript. ZX, XL and XH participated in the study design and contributed to the data collection. JL and DH performed the statistical analysis and participated in drafting the manuscript. BY participated in the study design and data interpretation. All authors read and approved the final manuscript.

Competing interests
The authors declare that they have no competing interests.

Author details
[1]Department of Cardiology, The Second Affiliated Hospital of Harbin Medical University, Harbin 150001, China. [2]Key Laboratory of Myocardial Ischemia, Ministry of Education, Harbin Medical University, Harbin 150001, China. [3]Department of Cardiology, The Second Affiliated Hospital of Chongqing Medical University, Chongqing 400010, China.

References

1. Libby P. Inflammation in atherosclerosis. Nature. 2002;420:868–74.

2. Hansson GK, Libby P, Tabas I. Inflammation and plaque vulnerability. J Intern Med. 2015;278:483–93.

3. Newby AC, George SJ, Ismail Y, Johnson JL, Sala-Newby GB, Thomas AC. Vulnerable atherosclerotic plaque metalloproteinases and foam cell phenotypes. Thromb Haemost. 2009;101:1006–11.

4. Yamada S, Ding Y, Tanimoto A, Wang KY, Guo X, Li Z, et al. Apoptosis signal-regulating kinase 1 deficiency accelerates hyperlipidemia-induced atheromatous plaques via suppression of macrophage apoptosis. Arterioscler Thromb Vasc Biol. 2011;31:1555–64.

5. Virmani R, Kolodgie FD, Burke AP, Farb A, Schwartz SM. Lessons from sudden coronary death: a comprehensive morphological classification scheme for atherosclerotic lesions. Arterioscler Thromb Vasc Biol. 2000; 20:1262–75.

6. Thaulow E, Erikssen J, Sandvik L, Stormorken H, Cohn PF. Blood platelet count and function are related to total and cardiovascular death in apparently healthy men. Circulation. 1991;84:613–7.

7. Ly HQ, Kirtane AJ, Murphy SA, Buros J, Cannon CP, Braunwald E, et al. Association of platelet counts on presentation and clinical outcomes in ST-elevation myocardial infarction (from the TIMI trials). Am J Cardiol. 2006;98:1–5.

8. Iijima R, Ndrepepa G, Mehilli J, Bruskina O, Schulz S, Schömig A, et al. Relationship between platelet count and 30-day clinical outcomes after percutaneous coronary interventions: pooled analysis of four ISAR trials. Thromb Haemost. 2007;98:852–7.

9. Ommen SR, Hodge DO, Rodeheffer RJ, McGregor CG, Thomson SP, Gibbons RJ. Predictive power of the relative lymphocyte concentration in patients with advanced heart failure. Circulation. 1998;97:19–22.

10. Zouridakis EG, Garcia-Moll X, Kaski JC. Usefulness of the blood lymphocyte count in predicting recurrent instability and death in patients with unstable angina pectoris. Am J Cardiol. 2000;86:449–51.

11. Krenn-Pilko S, Langsenlehner U, Thurner EM, Stojakovic T, Pichler M, Gerger A, et al. The elevated preoperative platelet-to-lymphocyte ratio predicts poor prognosis in breast cancer patients. Br J Cancer. 2014;110:2524–30.

12. Zhang H, Gao L, Zhang B, Zhang L, Wang C. Prognostic value of platelet to lymphocyte ratio in non-small cell lung cancer: a systematic review and meta-analysis. Sci Rep. 2016;6:22618.

13. J. Y, GQ. Z, L. X. Preoperative platelet to lymphocyte ratio is a valuable prognostic biomarker in patients with colorectal cancer. Oncotarget. 2016;7:25516–27.

14. Ozcan Cetin EH, Cetin MS, Aras D, Topaloglu S, Temizhan A, Kisacik HL, et al. Platelet to lymphocyte ratio as a prognostic marker of in-Hospital and long-term major adverse cardiovascular events in ST-segment elevation myocardial infarction. Angiology. 2016;67:336–45.

15. Azab B, Shah N, Akerman M, McGinn JT Jr. Value of platelet/lymphocyte ratio as a predictor of all-cause mortality after non-ST-elevation myocardial infarction. J Thromb Thrombolysis. 2012;34:326–34.

16. Kurtul A, Murat SN, Yarlioglues M, Duran M, Ergun G, Acikgoz SK, et al. Association of platelet-to-lymphocyte ratio with severity and complexity of coronary artery disease in patients with acute coronary syndromes. Am J Cardiol. 2014;114:972–8.

17. Akboga MK, Canpolat U, Yayla C, Ozcan F, Ozeke O, Topaloglu S, et al. Association of Platelet to lymphocyte ratio with inflammation and severity of coronary atherosclerosis in patients with stable coronary artery disease. Angiology. 2016;67:89–95.

18. Jang IK, Tearney GJ, MacNeill B, Takano M, Moselewski F, Iftima N, et al. In vivo characterization of coronary atherosclerotic plaque by use of optical coherence tomography. Circulation. 2005;111:1551–5.

19. Kubo T, Imanishi T, Kashiwagi M, Ikejima H, Tsujioka H, Kuroi A, et al. Multiple coronary lesion instability in patients with acute myocardial infarction as determined by optical coherence tomography. Am J Cardiol. 2010;105:318–22.

20. Jia H, Dai J, Hou J, Xing L, Ma L, Liu H, et al. Effective anti-thrombotic therapy without stenting: intravascular optical coherence tomography-based management in plaque erosion (the EROSION study). Eur Heart J. 2017;38:792–800.

21. Tearney GJ, Regar E, Akasaka T, Adriaenssens T, Barlis P, Bezerra HG, et al. Consensus standards for acquisition, measurement, and reporting of intravascular optical coherence tomography studies: a report from the international working Group for Intravascular Optical Coherence Tomography Standardization and Validation. J Am Coll Cardiol. 2012;59:1058–72.

22. Burke AP, Farb A, Malcom GT, Liang YH, Smialek J, Virmani R. Coronary risk factors and plaque morphology in men with coronary disease who died suddenly. N Engl J Med. 1997;336:1276–82.

23. Kolodgie FD, Burke AP, Farb A, Gold HK, Yuan J, Narula J, et al. The thin-cap fibroatheroma: a type of vulnerable plaque: the major precursor lesion to acute coronary syndromes. Curr Opin Cardiol. 2001;16:285–92.

24. Rodriguez-Granillo GA, Garcia-Garcia HM, Mc Fadden EP, Valgimigli M, Aoki J, de Feyter P, et al. In vivo intravascular ultrasound-derived thin-cap fibroatheroma detection using ultrasound radiofrequency data analysis. J Am Coll Cardiol. 2005;46:2038–42.

25. Kato K, Yonetsu T, Kim SJ, Xing L, Lee H, McNulty I, et al. Nonculprit plaques in patients with acute coronary syndromes have more vulnerable features compared with those with non-acute coronary syndromes: a 3-vessel optical coherence tomography study. Circ Cardiovasc Imaging. 2012;5:433–40.

26. Vergallo R, Uemura S, Soeda T, Minami Y, Cho JM, Ong DS, et al. Prevalence and predictors of multiple coronary plaque ruptures: in vivo 3-vessel optical coherence tomography Imaging study. Arterioscler Thromb Vasc Biol. 2016; 36:2229–38.

27. Gary T, Pichler M, Belaj K, Hafner F, Gerger A, Froehlich H, et al. Platelet-to-lymphocyte ratio: a novel marker for critical limb ischemia in peripheral arterial occlusive disease patients. PLoS One. 2013;8:e67688.

28. Sunbul M, Gerin F, Durmus E, Kivrak T, Sari I, Tigen K, et al. Neutrophil to lymphocyte and platelet to lymphocyte ratio in patients with dipper versus non-dipper hypertension. Clin Exp Hypertens. 2014;36:217–21.

29. Yayla C, Canpolat U, Akyel A, Yayla KG, Yilmaz S, Acikgoz SK, et al. Association between platelet to lymphocyte ratio and saphenous vein graft disease. Angiology. 2016;67:133–8.

30. Yayla C, Akboga MK, Canpolat U, Akyel A, Yayla KG, Dogan M, et al. Platelet to lymphocyte ratio can be a predictor of infarct-related artery patency in patients with ST-segment elevation myocardial infarction. Angiology. 2015;66:831–6.

31. Hansson GK. Inflammation, atherosclerosis, and coronary artery disease. N Engl J Med. 2005;352:1685–95.

32. Damas JK, Waehre T, Yndestad A, Otterdal K, Hognestad A, Solum NO, et al. Interleukin-7-mediated inflammation in unstable angina: possible role of chemokines and platelets. Circulation. 2003;107:2670–6.

33. Nunez J, Minana G, Bodi V, Nunez E, Sanchis J, Husser O, et al. Low lymphocyte count and cardiovascular diseases. Curr Med Chem. 2011;18: 3226–33.

34. Blanchet X, Cesarek K, Brandt J, Herwald H, Teupser D, Kuchenhoff H, et al. Inflammatory role and prognostic value of platelet chemokines in acute coronary syndrome. Thromb Haemost. 2014;112:1277–87.

35. Hotchkiss RS, Karl IE. The pathophysiology and treatment of sepsis. N Engl J Med. 2003;348:138–50.

36. Arbel Y, Finkelstein A, Halkin A, Birati EY, Revivo M, Zuzut M, et al. Neutrophil/lymphocyte ratio is related to the severity of coronary artery disease and clinical outcome in patients undergoing angiography. Atherosclerosis. 2012;225:456–60.

37. Nilsson L, Wieringa WG, Pundziute G, Gjerde M, Engvall J, Swahn E, et al. Neutrophil/lymphocyte ratio is associated with non-calcified plaque burden in patients with coronary artery disease. PLoS One. 2014;9: e108183.

38. Cho KI, Ann SH, Singh GB, Her AY, Shin ES. Combined usefulness of the platelet-to-lymphocyte ratio and the neutrophil-to-lymphocyte ratio in predicting the long-term adverse events in patients who have undergone percutaneous coronary intervention with a drug-eluting stent. PLoS One. 2015;10:e0133934.

39. Kubo T, Maehara A, Mintz GS, Doi H, Tsujita K, Choi SY, et al. The dynamic nature of coronary artery lesion morphology assessed by serial virtual histology intravascular ultrasound tissue characterization. J Am Coll Cardiol. 2010;55:1590–7.

40. Cheruvu PK, Finn AV, Gardner C, Caplan J, Goldstein J, Stone GW, et al. Frequency and distribution of thin-cap fibroatheroma and ruptured plaques in human coronary arteries: a pathologic study. J Am Coll Cardiol. 2007;50:940–9.

41. Stone GW, Maehara A, Lansky AJ, de Bruyne B, Cristea E, Mintz GS, et al. A prospective natural-history study of coronary atherosclerosis. N Engl J Med. 2011;364:226–35.

22

Association of lecithin-cholesterol acyltransferase activity and low-density lipoprotein heterogeneity with atherosclerotic cardiovascular disease risk

Katsuaki Yokoyama[1], Shigemasa Tani[2]* (iD), Rei Matsuo[1] and Naoya Matsumoto[1]

Abstract

Background: Lecithin-cholesterol acyltransferase (LCAT) is believed to be involved in reverse cholesterol transport, which is known to play a key role in suppression of atherosclerosis. However, recent investigations have demonstrated that higher LCAT activity, measured in terms of the serum cholesterol esterification rate by an endogenous substrate method, is associated with increased formation of triglyceride (TG)-rich lipoproteins (TRLs), leading to a decrease in the low-density lipoprotein (LDL) particle size. The purpose of this hospital-based longitudinal study was to clarify the causal relationship between changes in the LCAT activity and changes in the LDL-particle size.

Methods: The subjects were a total of 335 patients, derived from our previous study cohort, with one or more risk factors for atherosclerotic cardiovascular disease (ASCVD). For this study, we measured the LDL-particle size (relative LDL migration [LDL-Rm value]) by polyacrylamide gel electrophoresis in the subjects, along with the changes in the LCAT activity, at the end of a follow-up period of at least 1 year.

Results: The results revealed that the absolute change (Δ) in the LDL-particle size increased significantly as the quartile of Δ LCAT activity increased ($p = 0.01$). A multi-logistic regression adjusted-analysis revealed that Δ LCAT activity in the fourth quartile as compared to that in the first quartile was independently predictive of an increased LDL-particle size (odds ratio [95% confidence interval]: 2.03 [1.02/4.04], $p = 0.04$). Moreover, the Δ LCAT activity was also positively correlated with Δ TRL-related markers (i.e., TG, remnant particle-like cholesterol [RLP-C], apolipoprotein B, apolipoprotein C-2, and apolipoprotein C-3).

Conclusions: The results lend support to the hypothesis that increased LCAT activity may be associated with increased formation of TRLs, leading to a reduction in the LDL-particle size in patients at a high risk for ASCVD. To reduce the risk of ASCVD, it may be important to focus not only on the quantitative changes in the serum LDL-cholesterol levels, but also on the LCAT activity.

Keywords: LCAT, TRLs, LDL-particle size

* Correspondence: tani.shigemasa@nihon-u.ac.jp
[2]Department of Health Planning Center and Cardiology, Nihon University Hospital, 1-6 Kanda-Surugadai, Chiyoda-ku, Tokyo 101-8309, Japan
Full list of author information is available at the end of the article

Background

Lecithin cholesterol acyltransferase (LCAT) is reported to be closely involved in reverse cholesterol transport (RCT), which is an anti-atherogenic process by which excess cholesterol is removed from the cells by high-density lipoprotein (HDL) and delivered to the liver for excretion [1].

However, according to the results of evaluation of the LCAT activity using the currently available assay methods, including both the exogenous and endogenous substrate methods, it appears quite likely that an increased LCAT activity is associated with the progression of atherosclerosis. Furthermore, several investigations have also suggested the existence of a positive correlation between increase in the serum levels of triglyceride (TG)-rich lipoproteins (TRLs) and elevation of the LCAT activity [2–4].

Recently, we reported that increased LCAT activity, as measured in terms of the serum cholesterol esterification rate by the endogenous substrate method, might be associated with a decrease in the LDL-particle size via its association with an increase in the serum levels of TRL-related markers in patients at a high risk for progression of atherosclerosis [5]. However, because this aforementioned study was designed as a cross-sectional study, and not as a longitudinal study or an interventional study, it was difficult to arrive at any definitive conclusions about the causal relationships based on the results.

Therefore, we designed this longitudinal study in an attempt to verify the hypothesis that elevation of the LCAT activity is associated with an increase in the serum levels of TRL-related markers, involved in disordered TG metabolism (i.e., TG, remnant particle-like cholesterol [RLP-C], apolipoprotein (apo) B, apo C-2, and apo C-3) [6], and is thereby involved in a reduction of the LDL-particle size.

The present study, with a longitudinal study design, as mentioned above, was undertaken to analyze the relationships between changes in the LCAT activity and changes in the LDL-particle size, particularly between elevation of the LCAT activity and diminution in the LDL-particle size.

Methods

Study design and populations

This study was designed as a hospital-based longitudinal study to investigate the relationship between the changes in the LCAT activity and changes in the LDL-particle size in the subjects of our previous cross-sectional study [5] who were available for additional measurements 1 year after completion of the previous study. The subjects underwent follow-up hematologic and blood biochemical tests at this institution at least 1 year after their participation in the completion of our previous study [5]. The primary endpoint was to evaluate the association between the absolute changes (Δ) in the LCAT activity and the Δ LDL-particle size using a multi-logistic regression analysis with adjustments for confounding factors, and the secondary endpoint was to investigate the associations between the Δ LCAT activity and Δ TRL-related markers, which are closely associated with TG metabolism.

The criterion for patient registration was the presence of one or more risk factors for atherosclerotic cardiovascular disease (ASCVD). The diagnostic criteria for the ASCVD risk factors were as follows: hypertension: systolic pressure ≥ 140 mmHg, diastolic pressure ≥ 90 mmHg, and/or current treatment with antihypertensive medication; diabetes mellitus (DM): fasting plasma glucose concentration ≥ 126 mg/dL, HbA1c ≥6.5%, and/or current treatment with anti-diabetic agents; dyslipidemia: serum LDL cholesterol (LDL-C) ≥140 mg/dL, serum TG ≥150 mg/dL, serum high-density lipoprotein cholesterol (HDL-C) ≤40 mg/dL, and/or current treatment with lipid-lowering medication; hyperuricemia: serum uric acid level ≥ 7.0 mg/dL and/or patient taking medications for control of blood uric acid levels; CKD: eGFR < 60 mL/min/1.73 m^2, with the severity of chronic kidney disease (CKD) being determined based on the estimated glomerular filtration rate (eGFR) using the abbreviated Modification of Diet in Renal Disease (MDRD) Study equation, modified by a Japanese coefficient [7]; Obesity: body mass index (BMI) ≥25 kg/m^2.

Patients were not enrolled if they met any of the following exclusion criteria: hepatic dysfunction (serum alanine aminotransferase and aspartate aminotransferase ≥2 times the upper limit of normal), known malignant disease, refusal to provide consent for participation in the study, diagnosis of acute coronary syndrome within 3 months prior to the study, and/or serum TG ≥400 mg/dL. The design and purpose of the study were approved by the Nihon University Surugadai Hospital Ethics Committee.

Measurement of laboratory parameters

Fasting blood samples were collected in the early morning hours after the subjects had fasted overnight for 12 h. Serum LCAT activity was determined by a self-substrate method (SRL Co., Ltd., Tokyo, Japan), in which the serum free cholesterol is measured enzymatically after incubation of the serum with synthetic dipalmitoyl lecithin using a commercially available kit (Nescoat LCAT kit-S, Alfresa Pharma, Osaka, Japan) [8]. The LCAT activity measured by the present method showed good correlation with the values measured by the endogenous substrate method using gas-liquid chromatography [8], and the exogenous substrate method [9], and with the LCAT mass concentrations measured by enzyme-linked immunosorbent assay [10]. The serum total cholesterol (TC), HDL-C, and TG levels were measured using standard methods. Serum LDL-C levels were calculated using the Friedewald formula [11]. The serum RLP-C levels were measured using an immunoadsorption assay (SRL). The serum apo levels were determined using turbidimetric latex agglutination assays (Daiichi Pure Chemicals Co., Ltd., Tokyo, Japan). Serum high-sensitivity C-reactive protein (hs-CRP) levels were measured using a nephelometric assay (Behring Diagnostic Marburg, Germany).

Measurement of the LDL-Rm value

The relative LDL migration (LDL-Rm) value, an indicator of the LDL-particle size, was measured relative to the mobility value of LDL by polyacrylamide-gel electrophoresis (PAGE) using the LipoPhor system (Joko, Tokyo, Japan). The LDL-Rm value was calculated as the distance between the very LDL (VLDL) peak and the LDL peak divided by the distance between the VLDL peak and the HDL peak (Fig. 1). Several studies have reported that an LDL-Rm value of ≥0.40 suggests the presence of a large amount of small-dense (sd)-LDL in the LDL fraction [12]; a decrease of the LDL-Rm value indicates an increase in the LDL-particle size [13, 14].

In order to distinguish LDL-particle size phenotype A (large buoyant LDL) and phenotype B (sd-LDL), Hirano et al., established a cutoff value in LDL diameter of 25.5 nm as determined by PAGE, corresponding to an LDL-Rm value of 0.40. [13]. As described above, LDL-Rm value is often used for qualitative evaluation of the LDL-particle size in a clinical practice setting. Therefore, LDL-Rm value represents the average size of all

LDL particles, which are aggregates of heterogeneously sized particles, and not the absolute amount of sd-LDL. However, the present study used LDL-Rm value as a continuous variable, which is keeping with previous drug interventional evaluating LDL-particle size conducted until now [15, 16].

Statistical analysis

Data are expressed as the mean ± standard deviation for continuous variables and as percentages for discrete variables. For variables with a significantly skewed distribution, the data are expressed as interquartile ranges. In a subset analysis performed according to quartiles of the Δ LCAT activity, we used analysis of variance (ANOVA) followed by Bonferroni's adjustment for covariates if differences were detected. A multi-logistic regression analysis was performed to identify the variables associated with changes of the LDL-Rm value. Increase/decrease of the LDL-Rm value from the baseline was entered as the dependent variable, and the patient characteristics, risk factors for ASCVD, use/non-use of lipid-modifying drugs, and quartiles of Δ LCAT activity were entered as independent variables. Regression analysis was performed using linear regression, with estimation of the Spearman's and Pearson's correlation coefficients. All the statistical analyses were performed using the SPSS software program (SPSS Inc., Chicago, Illinois, USA) for Windows (version 12.0.1).

Results
Patients

The patient characteristics and laboratory profiles are shown in Tables 1 and 2. Among the subjects ($n = 538$) enrolled in our previous cross-sectional study [5], 335 subjects who were available for follow-up hematologic and blood biochemical tests at least 1 year after participation in completion of the previous study [5] were enrolled in the present study. Of these 335 patients, none had experienced any cardiovascular events during the 1-year interval from the previous study.

Comparison of the Δ LDL-Rm value according to the Δ LCAT activity (as classified into quartiles)

Among the subjects of this cross-sectional study [7], we investigated the association between the Δ LCAT activity, as classified into quartiles, and the Δ LDL-Rm values in the 335 patients who could be followed up for at least 1 year. The Δ LCAT activity was correlated positively with the Δ LDL-Rm value (Fig. 2a). Moreover, a positive correlation between Δ LCAT activity and Δ LDL-Rm value was also found in both patients receiving and not receiving lipid-modifying drug treatment (Fig. 2b). The Δ LCAT activity ranged from − 41.8 to 43.4 nmol/ml/hr/37 ° C (mean ± SD: − 1.7 ± 13.8 nmol/ml/hr/37 °C, median;

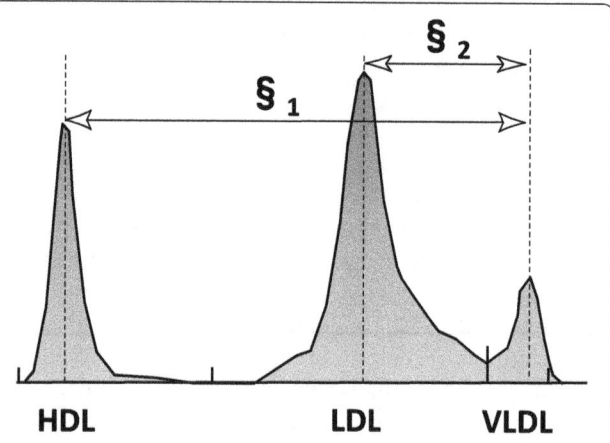

Fig. 1 Measurement of LDL-Rm value by lipoprotein polyacrylamide gel disc electrophoresis. LDL-Rm = relative LDL migration, LDL-Rm value calculated from densitometer analysis of polyacrylamide disc gel electrophoresis; HDL = high-density lipoprotein; LDL = low-density lipoprotein; VLDL = very LDL LDL-Rm value are expressed as §₂/§₁

Table 1 Patients characteristics

	$n = 335$
Male / Female, *n* (%)	233 (70) / 102 (30)
Age (years)	62 ± 11
BMI (kg/m2)	24.8 ± 3.8
Hypertension, *n* (%)	224 (67)
Diabetes mellitus, *n* (%)	92 (28)
HbA1c (%)	6.1 ± 0.9
Current smoking, *n* (%)	26 (7.8)
Dyslipidemia, *n* (%)	269 (80)
eGFR (ml/min/1.73 m2)	69 ± 17
CKD Stage 3≥, *n* (%)	89 (27)
Number of risk factors	4.0 ± 1.5
Cardiovascular disease, *n* (%)	100 (30)
Coronary artery disease	87 (26)
Cerebral infarction	12 (3.6)
Aortic dissection/aortic aneurysm	4 (1.2)
Peripheral arterial disease	3 (0.9)
Concomitant drug, *n* (%)	
Anti-platelets	101 (30)
ACEs/ARBs	191 (57)
β blockers	77 (23)
Calcium channel blockers	183(55)
Lipid-modifying drugs	201(60)
Statins	179 (53)
Fibrates	8 (2.4)
Ezetimibe	15 (4.5)

BMI body mass index, *Hb* hemoglobin, *e-GFR* estimated glomerular flow rate, *CKD* chronic kidney disease, *ACEI* angiotensin converting enzyme inhibitor, *ARB* angiotensin receptor blocker

Table 2 Laboratory profile

	$n = 335$
Lipids	
TC (mg/dL)	188 ± 32
LDL-C(kg/dL)	100 ± 26
HDL-C (mg/dL)	57 ± 15
LDL-C/HDL-C ratio	1.89 ± 0.72
non-HDL-C (mg/dL)	131 ± 31
TRLs-related markers	
TG (mg/dL)	103 (76/157)
RLP-C (mg/dL)	4.1 (3.1/5.7)
apo B (mg/dL)	91 ± 21
apo C-II (mg/dL)	4.9 ± 1.9
apo C-III (mg/dL)	10.5 ± 3.3
LCAT activity (nmol/ml/hr/37 °C)	95 ± 20
LDL-Rm value	0.37 ± 0.03

TC total cholesterol, *LDL* low-density lipoprotein, *HDL* high-density lipoprotein, *TG* triglyceride, *RLP* remnant-like particle, *apo* apolipoprotein, *LCAT* Lecithin-cholesterol acyltransferase, *LDL-Rm* relative LDL migration

for ASCVD, and history of use of lipid-modifying drugs revealed that Δ LCAT activity in the fourth quartile was an independent predictor of increased LDL-RM values, namely, smaller LDL-particle sizes (Table 3). However, no association between increased Δ LCAT activity and decreased Δ LDL-Rm value was found in the cases with serum LDL-C < 100 mg/dL, (1Q vs. 4Q, OR: 1.711; 95% CI: 0.649–4.510; $p = 0.277$).

Relationship between Δ LCAT activity and Δ TRL-related markers

Investigation of whether changes in the serum levels of TRL-related markers specifying the LDL-particle size might be correlated with changes in the LCAT activity was then pursued, inasmuch as the research hypothesis that elevation of LCAT activity was an independent predictor of diminution of the LDL-particle size had been verified. Figure 4 shows the simple correlations between the Δ LCAT activity and Δ serum TRLs-related markers. Positive correlations were noted between the Δ LCAT activity and all Δ TRL-related markers.

Discussion

This longitudinal study yielded the following findings. Elevation of LCAT activity, as measured in terms of the serum cholesterol esterification rate by the endogenous substrate method, was associated with a decrease in LDL-particle size, which exhibit potent atherogenic activity, and increased LCAT activity may be depend on increased serum levels of TRL-related markers in patients at high risk for ASCVD.

interquartile range in parentheses: − 1.5 (− 9.9/6.3 nmol/ml/hr/37 °C). The patients were divided into quartiles according to the Δ LCAT activity, as follows: first quartile, − 41.8 to − 10.0 nmol/ml/hr/37 °C (*n* = 83), second quartile, − 9.9 to − 1.7 nmol/ml/hr/37 °C (*n* = 83), third quartile, − 1.6 to 6.2 nmol/ml/hr/37 °C (*n* = 84), and fourth quartile, 6.3 to 43.4 nmol/ml/hr/37 °C (*n* = 85). The Δ LDL-Rm value increased with increasing quartile of Δ LCAT activity, the differences ($p = 0.023$) (Fig. 3) indicating that the higher the Δ LCAT activity, the smaller the Δ LDL-particle size.

Multi-logistic regression analysis to identify variables that were independently correlated with the changes of the LDL-Rm value, an estimate of the LDL-particle size

To investigate the relationships between elevation of the LCAT activity and diminution in the LDL-particle size, multiple logistic regression analysis in the 335 patients conducted with adjustments for age, gender, risk factors

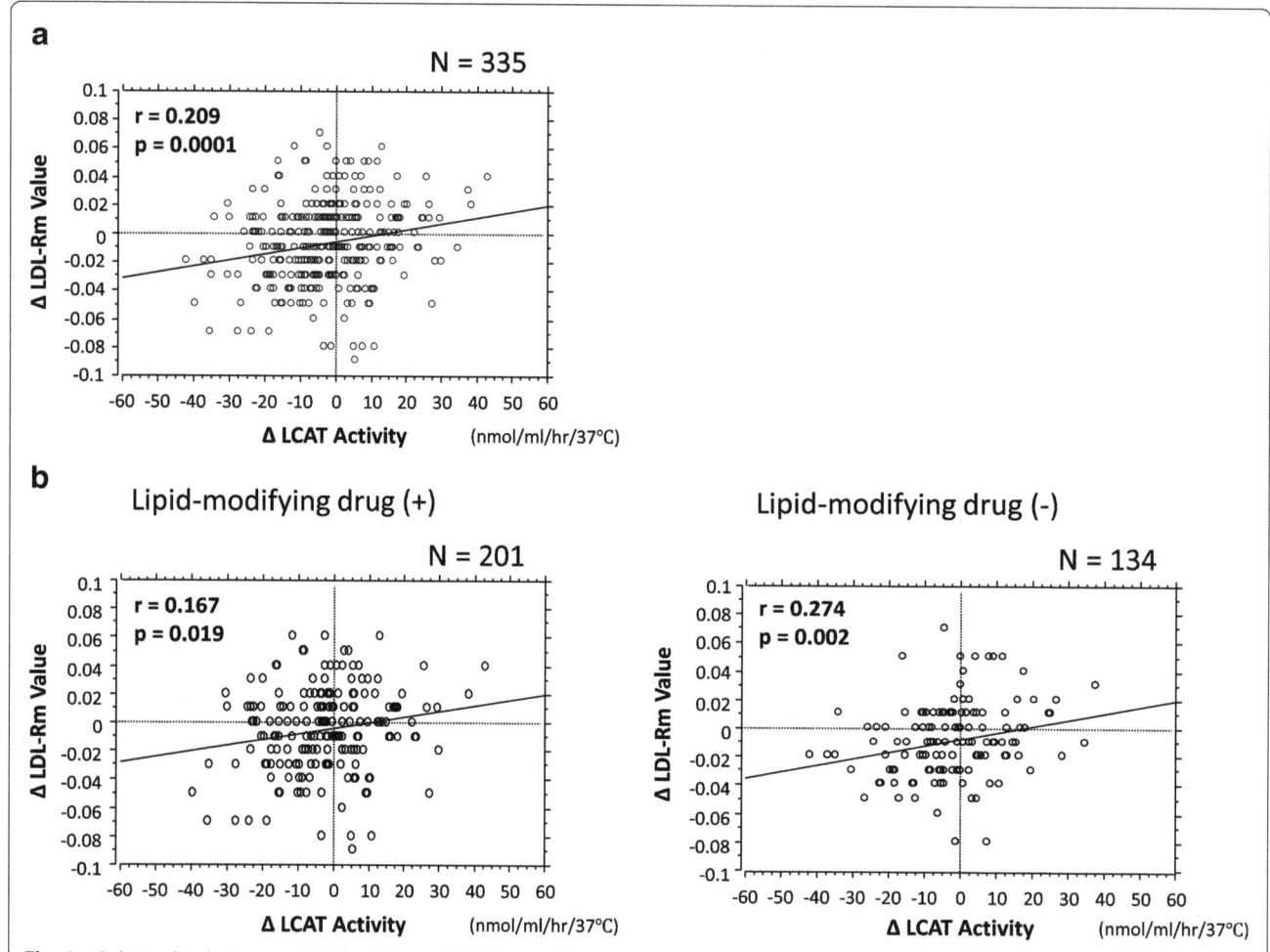

Fig. 2 a Relationship between Δ LCAT activity and Δ LDL-Rm value LCAT = lecithin-cholesterol acyltransferase, LDL-Rm = relative LDL migration, Regression analysis was performed using linear regression and Spearman's correlation coefficients. **b** LCAT = lecithin-cholesterol acyltransferase, LDL-Rm = relative LDL migration, Regression analysis was performed using linear regression and Spearman's correlation coefficients

The present longitudinal study on the correlations among LCAT activity, serum levels of TRL-related markers and the LDL-particle size was conducted in the same subject cohort as that in our previously reported cross-sectional study [5], and demonstrated that an increase in the LCAT activity may bring about elevations of the serum TRL-related markers, i.e., indicators of disordered triglyceride metabolism, and down-sizing of the LDL-particle size, and thereby possibly trigger an atherosclerogenic effect rather than exerting an anti-atherosclerogenic effect associated with activation of the RCT system. This is consistent with the findings reported heretofore [2–4].

Importantly, only cross-sectional study was unable to establish a causal relationship between the results, but the results of the two studies with different (cross-sectional [5] and longitudinal) designs taken together strongly suggests that an increase of the LCAT activity was associated with a decrease of the LDL-particle size.

It has been reported that the increased serum cholesterol esterification generated by the LCAT reaction may be the result of an increase in TRLs, and that it may, therefore, represent potentially decreased LDL-particle size through activities of cholesteryl ester transfer protein and hepatic lipase [3, 17, 18]. These reports provide support for what have been demonstrated in the present study, i.e., that elevation of LCAT activity constitutes a determinant of diminution of the LDL-particle size and that a positive correlation exists between absolute changes in LCAT activity and changes in the TRL-related markers from the baseline.

However, the RCT system represents a complicated network mediated not merely by the bioactivity of LCAT, but by the activities of many other enzymes as well, to exert an anti-atherosclerogenic effect of HDL in toto [19, 20]. We may have to interpret the present findings, solely focused upon the LCAT activity, TRL-related markers and LDL-particle size, as implying nothing

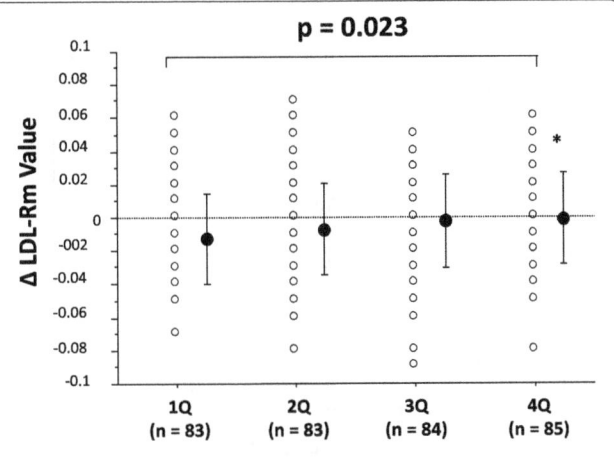

Fig. 3 Comparison of Δ LDL-Rm value according to Δ LCAT activity (as classified into quartile) Δ = absolute change from baseline, LDL-Rm = relative LDL migration, LCAT = lecithin-cholesterol acyltransferase. Error bar indicates mean ± standard deviation 1Q: −41.8–−10.0 nmol/ml/hr/37 °C, 2Q: −9.0–−1.7 nmol/ml/hr/37 °C, 3Q: 0–6.2 nmol/ml/hr/37 °C, 4Q: 6.3–43.4 nmol/ml/hr/37 °C. ANOVA and post hoc tests with Bonferroni correction were performed to test between-group differences. *$p < 0.01$ vs. 1Q

more than a demonstration of a causal relationship of these three factors with atherosclerogenic effect.

It has also been reported that the anti-atherosclerogenic effect of RCT is dependent on the state of lipid metabolism which has a profound bearing on progression of atherosclerosis. Several investigations suggest that in the presence of abnormal lipid metabolism that can cause ASCVD, RCT may be activated and LCAT may stimulate esterification of free

Table 3 Multi-logistic regression analysis to identify variables that were independently correlated with the changes of the LDL-Rm value, an estimate of the LDL-particle size

| Variable | OR | 95% CI | | $n = 335$ |
		Upper	Lower	p value
Age	0.973	0.951	0.995	0.018
Male gender	1.108	0.645	1.903	0.710
BMI	0.991	0.929	1.056	0.776
Current smoking	0.625	0.240	1.627	0.336
Diabetes mellitus	0.822	0.475	1.422	0.483
Hypertension	0.618	0.367	1.041	0.484
Dyslipidemia	1.704	0.768	3.781	0.190
Lipid-modifying drugs	1.368	0.734	2.552	0.324
ΔLCAT 1Q	Reference			
ΔLCAT 2Q	1.498	0.738	3.039	0.263
ΔLCAT 3Q	1.784	0.884	3.601	0.163
ΔLCAT 4Q	2.028	1.019	4.035	0.044

OR odds ratio, *CI* confidence interval, *BMI* body mass index, Δ absolute change from baseline, *LCAT* lecithin-cholesterol acyltransferase, *Q* quartile

cholesterol, possibly resulting in changes in the direction toward suppressed progression of atherosclerosis [20–22]. In support of these reported findings, a negative correlation between the plaque volume assessed by intravascular ultrasonography and the LCAT mass concentration has been documented in coronary artery disease patients in recent years, and the authors have suggested that LACT activity is up-regulated with a consequent facilitation of RCT, leading to a reduction in coronary artery plaques in patients with coronary artery disease [23].

There are few reports yet of large-scale prospective cohort studies investigating LCAT activity in relation to the prognosis of coronary artery disease. Most recently, in a prospective cohort study carried out in the general population in Japan, a positive correlation was observed between the LCAT activity, measured in terms of the serum cholesterol esterification rate assessed by the endogenous substrate method, and the serum levels of the TRLs, and the group with elevated LCAT activity showed a significantly higher incidence of sudden death and coronary artery disease [24]. This may provide evidence in support of our study results, although the cited study did not examine the relation between TRLs and the LDL-particle size.

Interestingly, what would deserve special mention here is that the coefficient of correlation between the Δ LCAT activity and Δ LDL-Rm was higher in the patient group receiving lipid-modifying drugs (mostly statins) as compared to that in the group that was not receiving lipid-modifying drugs (Fig. 2-2). Lipid-modifying drugs seem likely to suppress the downsizing of the LDL-particle size associated with elevation of the LCAT activity, although this may only be stated parenthetically in the presence of intergroup differences in sample size and patient background characteristics.

In the preceding investigation conducted as a cross-sectional study, a correlation was shown to exist between increase of LCAT activity and diminution of the LDL-particle size in patients with serum LDL-C levels of < 100 mg/dL. In this study, however, which was conducted using the data of patients at high risk for ASCVD, a multivariate logistic regression analysis indicated that in patients with serum LDL-C levels of < 100 mg/dL, who are assumed to have only a low tendency towards progression of atherosclerosis, increase of the LCAT activity had no impact on the LDL-particle size. This would be interpreted as being due to a decline in the statistical detection rate owing to the small case-sample size of this study. We propose to further verify the present research hypothesis through increasing the case-sample size. Figure 5 illustrated our hypothesis that increased LCAT activity might be associated with an increase in TRL-related markers and a reduction of LDL-particle size, possibly leading to the development of ASCVD.

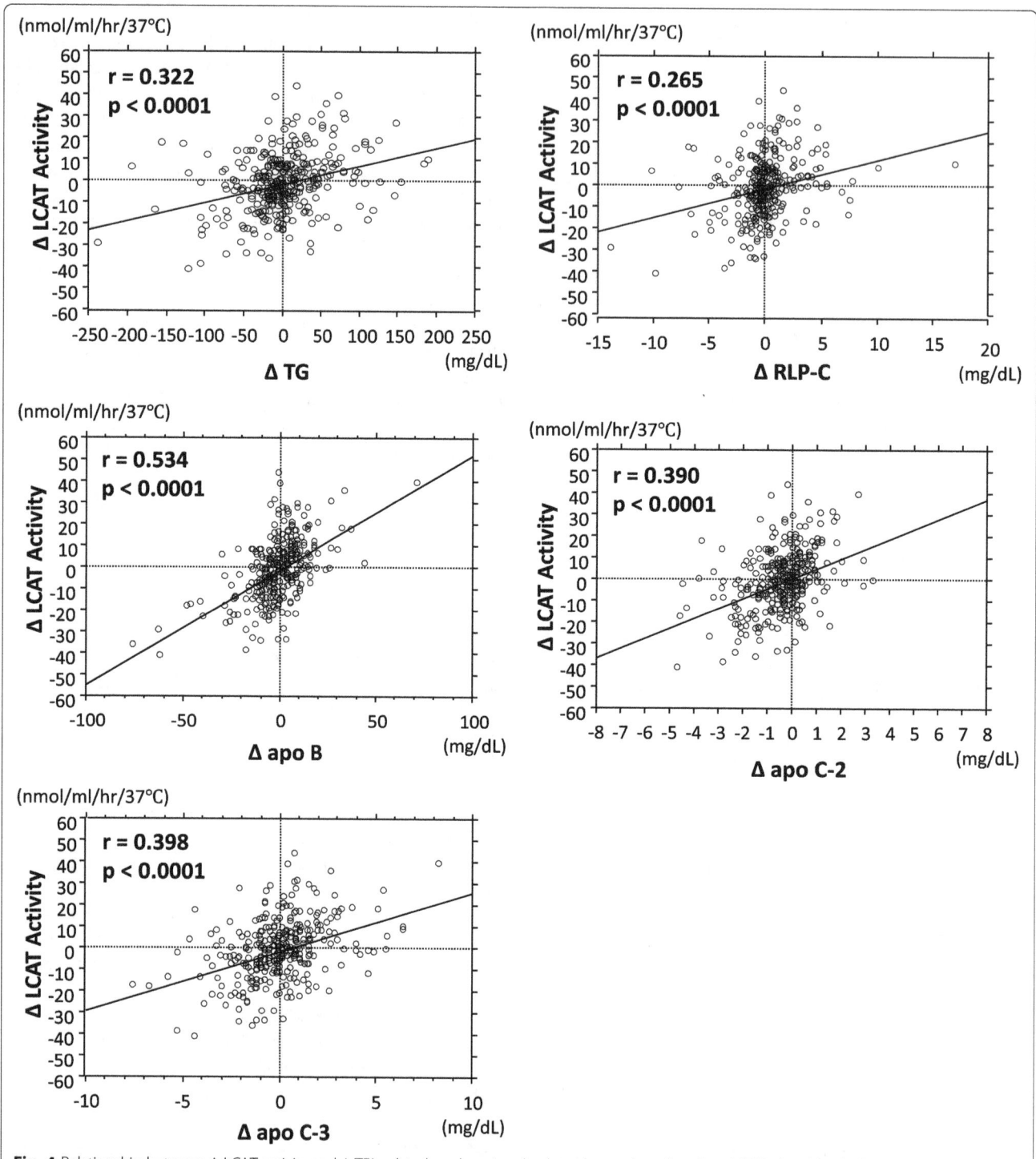

Fig. 4 Relationship between Δ LCAT activity and Δ TRL-related markers Δ = absolute change from baseline, LCAT = lecithin-cholesterol acyltransferase, TRL = triglyceride–rich lipoprotein. Regression analysis was performed using linear regression and Pearson's correlation coefficients

Study limitations and clinical implications

First, this study did not incorporate analysis of changes in the properties of the atherosclerotic lesions by diagnostic imaging [25]. Secondly, interventional studies using drugs which have the potential to modify LCAT activity (e.g., lipid-modifying drugs) may be useful for clarifying the relationship between LCAT activity and lipid metabolism [26]. It is expected that interventional studies with various drugs will be conducted in the future to examine the effect of LCAT on the progression of arteriosclerosis. We previously reported, in our original article, a patient with obesity who responded to prescribed dietary control with

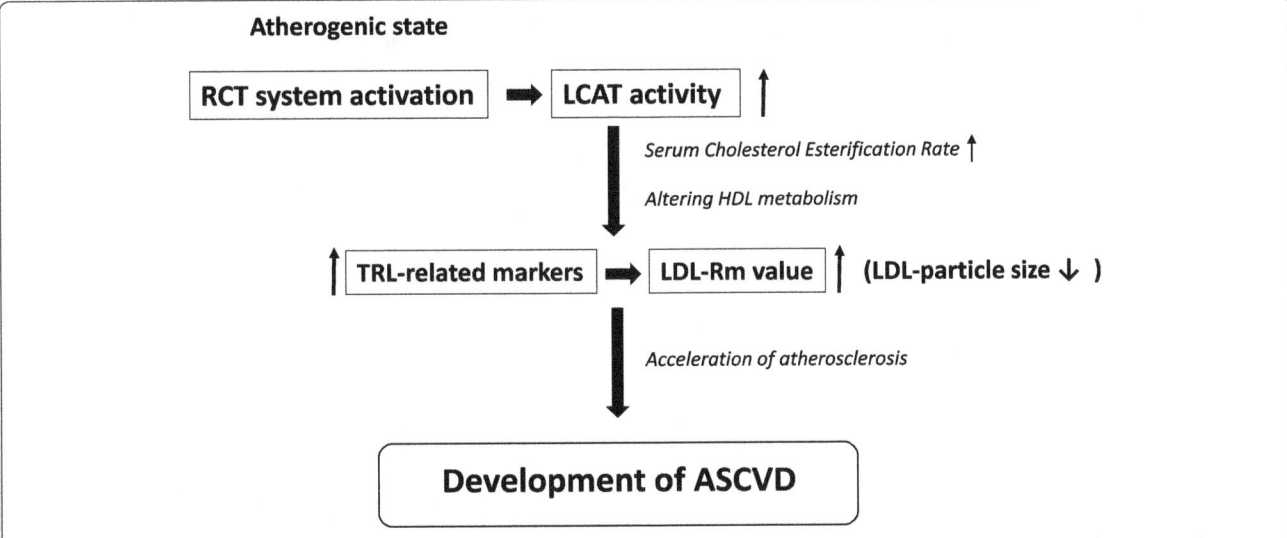

Fig. 5 A possible association of LCAT activity and LDL-Rm value, an indicator of LDL-particle size, with the development of ASCVD in this study. In an atherogenic state, RCT system might be activated. Accordingly, increased LCAT activity measured as a serum cholesterol esterification rate by the endogenous substrate method might be associated with altering HDL metabolism, resulting in an increase in the serum levels of TRL-related markers and a decrease in LDL-particle size (i.e. an increase in LDL-Rm value), leading to the development of ASCVD. However, further investigations are necessary for the elucidation of the precise mechanism involved in atherosclerosis associated with increased LCAT activity and decreased LDL particle size. LCAT = lecithin-cholesterol acyltransferase, LDL = low-density lipoprotein, LDL-Rm = relative LDL migration, ASCVD = atherosclerotic cardiovascular disease, RCT = reverse cholesterol transport, HDL = high-density lipoprotein, TRL = triglyceride–rich lipoprotein

weight reduction accompanied by lowering of the serum levels of TRLs and LCAT activity, and a decrease of the LDL-Rm value [27]. Similarly, there have been reports of lowering of the serum levels of TRLs and sd-LDL and LCAT activity associated with controlled weight reduction [28]. Thus, further evidence needs to be accumulated to establish the exact relation between the serum LCAT activity and LDL-heterogeneity. Thirdly, this study does not demonstrate the relationship between LCAT activity and clinical indices and/or outcomes, because it was only a pilot study. Finally, we have pursued the argument in this paper on the premise that LCAT activity represents an atherosclerosis-promoting factor; however, we may have to discuss with great deliberation whether LCAT facilitates, or in fact, suppresses atherosclerosis on the ground of evidence heretofore accumulated, by taking account of differences in LCAT assay procedure and characteristics of the study subjects (general population, high-risk cases of cardiovascular disease, gender) and of the expression profile of the LCAT gene in the pathophysiological state [29, 30]. In fact, no unified view has been obtained so far, based on carotid artery ultrasound study reports, as to the relation of the serum LCAT activity with progression/suppression of atherosclerosis [2, 31, 32].

In this study, we investigated the factors involved in the progression of atherosclerosis with our attention focused on the serum LCAT activity, TPL-related makers and LDL particle size. However, atherosclerosis pro-

gresses through a complex network also involving other elements than the above-mentioned factors alone [33]. Further verification of the results of this study will have to take into consideration these other factors as well.

Conclusions

In this longitudinal study, we confirmed that increased LCAT activity, measured in terms of the serum cholesterol esterification rate by the endogenous substrate method, might be associated with a decrease of the LDL-particle size through its association with an increase in the serum levels of TRL-related markers, which represents disordered TG metabolism. The causal relationship between increase of the LCAT activity and reduction of the LDL-particle size may be determined more clearly in our study due to its longitudinal study design. Thus, measurement of the LCAT activity may be useful for predicting ASCVD in patients at a high risk for progression of atherosclerosis.

Abbreviations
ANOVA: Analysis of variance; apo: apolipoprotein; ASCVD: Atherosclerotic cardiovascular disease; BMI: Body mass index; CAD: Coronary artery disease; CKD: Chronic kidney disease; DM: Diabetes mellitus; eGFR: estimated glomerular filtration rate; Hb: Hemoglobin; HDL: High-density lipoprotein; hs-CRP: high-sensitivity C-reactive protein; LCAT: Lecithin-cholesterol Acyltransferase; LDL-C: Low-density lipoprotein cholesterol; LDL-Rm: Relative LDL migration; MDRD: Modification of Diet in Renal Disease; RCT: Reverse cholesterol transport; RLP: remnant-like particle; sd: small-dense; SD: Standard deviation; TC: Total cholesterol; TG: Triglyceride; TRL: TG-rich lipoprotein; VLDL: Very-low density lipoprotein

Acknowledgements

The authors would like to thank International Medical Information Center (https://www.imic.or.jp/services/translation.html) for the English language review. The authors would also like to thank Mr. Gary Cooper for his help in editing the English manuscript.

Funding

No funding was obtained for this study.

Authors' contributions

ST has designed this study in whole and drafted this manuscript. KY, RM, and NM have contributed to collect data. ST has contributed to statistical analyses in this study. ST and KY have contributed to provide advice on interpretation of the results. ST revised this manuscript critically for important intellectual content and approved finally the manuscript submitted. All authors read and approved the final manuscript.

Competing interests

The authors declare that they have no competing interests.

Author details

[1]Department of Cardiology, Nihon University Hospital, 1-6 Kanda-Surugadai, Chiyoda-ku, Tokyo 101-8309, Japan. [2]Department of Health Planning Center and Cardiology, Nihon University Hospital, 1-6 Kanda-Surugadai, Chiyoda-ku, Tokyo 101-8309, Japan.

References

1. Glomset JA. The plasma lecithins:cholesterol acyltransferase reaction. J Lipid Res. 1968;9:155–67.
2. Dullaart RP, Perton F, Sluiter WJ, de Vries R, van Tol A. Plasma lecithin: cholesterol acyltransferase activity is elevated in metabolic syndrome and is an independent marker of increased carotid artery intima media thickness. J Clin Endocrinol Metab. 2008;93:4860–6.
3. Murakami T, Michelagnoli S, Longhi R, Gianfranceschi G, Pazzucconi F, Calabresi L, Sirtori CR, Franceschini G. Triglycerides are major determinants of cholesterol esterification/transfer and HDL remodeling in human plasma. Arterioscler Thromb Vasc Biol. 1995;15:1819–28.
4. Sutherland WH, Temple WA, Nye ER, Herbison PG. Lecithin:cholesterol acyltransferase activity, plasma and lipoprotein lipids and obesity in men and women. Atherosclerosis. 1979;34:319–27.
5. Tani S, Takahashi A, Nagao K, Hirayama A. Association of lecithin-cholesterol acyltransferase activity measured as a serum cholesterol esterification rate and low-density lipoprotein heterogeneity with cardiovascular risk: a cross-sectional study. Heart Vessel. 2016;31:831–40.
6. Miller M, Stone NJ, Ballantyne C, Bittner V, Criqui MH, Ginsberg HN, Goldberg AC, Howard WJ, Jacobson MS, Kris-Etherton PM, Lennie TA, Levi M, Mazzone T, Pennathur S, American Heart Association Clinical Lipidology, Thrombosis, and Prevention Committee of the Council on Nutrition, Physical Activity, and Metabolism; Council on Arteriosclerosis, Thrombosis and Vascular Biology, Council on Cardiovascular Nursing, Council on the Kidney in Cardiovascular Disease. Triglycerides and cardiovascular disease: a scientific statement from the American Heart Association. Circulation. 2011; 123:2292–333.
7. Imai E, Horio M, Nitta K, Yamagata K, Iseki K, Hara S, Ura N, Kiyohara Y, Hirakata H, Watanabe T, Moriyama T, Ando Y, Inaguma D, Narita I, Iso H, Wakai K, Yasuda Y, Tsukamoto Y, Ito S, Makino H, Hishida A, Matsuo S. Estimation of glomerular filtration rate by the MDRD study equation modified for Japanese patients with chronic kidney disease. Clin Exp Nephrol. 2007;11:41–50.
8. Nagasaki T, Akanuma Y. A new colorimetric method for the determination of plasma lecithin-cholesterol acyltransferase activity. Clin Chim Acta. 1997; 75:371–5.
9. Bartholome M, Niedmann D, Wieland H, Seidel D. An optimized method for measuring lecithin : cholesterol acyltransferase activity, independent of the concentration and quality of the physiological substrate. Biochim Biophys Acta. 1981;664:327–34.
10. Kobori K, Saito K, Ito S, Kotani K, Manabe M, Kanno T. A new enzyme-linked immunosorbent assay with two monoclonal antibodies to specific epitopes measure human lecithin-cholesterol acyltransferase. J Lipid Res. 2002;43:325–34.
11. DeLong DM, DeLong ER, Wood PD, Lippel K, Rifkind BM. A comparison of methods for the estimation of plasma low- and very low-density lipoprotein cholesterol. The Lipid Research Clinics Prevalence Study. JAMA. 1986;256: 2372–7.
12. Nakano T, Inoue I, Seo M, Takahashi S, Awata T, Komoda T, Katayama S. Rapid and simple profiling of lipoproteins by polyacrylamide-gel disc electrophoresis to determine the heterogeneity of low-density lipoproteins (LDLs) including small, dense LDL. Recent Pat Cardiovasc Drug Discov. 2009;4:31–6.
13. Hirano T, Ito Y, Yoshino G. Measurement of small dense low-density lipoprotein particles. J Atheroscler Thromb. 2005;12:67–72.
14. Tani S, Matsumoto M, Nagao K, Hirayama A. Association of triglyceride-rich lipoproteins-related markers and low-density lipoprotein heterogeneity with cardiovascular risk: effectiveness of polyacrylamide-gel electrophoresis as a method of determining low-density lipoprotein particle size. J Cardiol. 2014; 63:60–8.
15. Tani S, Takahashi A, Nagao K, Hirayama A. Effect of dipeptidyl peptidase-4 inhibitor, vildagliptin on plasminogen activator inhibitor-1 in patients with diabetes mellitus. Am J Cardiol. 2015;115:454–60.
16. Hiro T, Kimura T, Morimoto T, Miyauchi K, Nakagawa Y, Yamagishi M, Ozaki Y, Kimura K, Saito S, Yamaguchi T, Daida H, Matsuzaki M, JAPAN-ACS Investigators. Effect of intensive statin therapy on regression of coronary atherosclerosis in patients with acute coronary syndrome: a multicenter randomized trial evaluated by volumetric intravascular ultrasound using pitavastatin versus atorvastatin (JAPAN-ACS [Japan assessment of pitavastatin and atorvastatin in acute coronary syndrome] study). J Am Coll Cardiol. 2009;54:293–302.
17. Fielding CJ, Fielding PE. Regulation of human plasma lecithin: cholesterol acyltransferase activity by lipoprotein acceptor cholesteryl ester content. J Biol Chem. 1981;256:2102–4.
18. Chung BH, Segrest JP, Franklin F. In vitro production of beta-very low density lipoproteins and small, dense low density lipoproteins in mildly hypertriglyceridemic plasma: role of activities of lecithin:cholester acyltransferase, cholesterylester transfer proteins and lipoprotein lipase. Atherosclerosis. 1998;141:209–25.
19. Hutchins PM, Heinecke JW. Cholesterol efflux capacity, macrophage reverse cholesterol transport and cardioprotective HDL. Curr Opin Lipidol. 2015;26: 388–93.
20. Dobiásová M, Frohlich J. Understanding the mechanism of LCAT reaction may help explain the high predictive value of LDL/HDL cholesterol ratio. Physiol Res. 1998;47:387–97.
21. Dobiasova M, Stribrna J, Sparks DL, Pritchard PH, Frohlich JJ. Cholesterol esterification rates in very low density lipoprotein- and low density lipoprotein-depleted plasma. Relation to high density lipoprotein subspecies, sex, hyperlipidemia, and coronary artery disease. Arterioscler Thromb. 1991;11:64–70.
22. Tani S, Matsuo R, Kawauchi K, Yagi T, Atsumi W, Hirayama A. A cross-sectional and longitudinal study between association of n-3 polyunsaturated fatty acids derived from fish consumption and high-density lipoprotein heterogeneity. Heart Vessel. 2018;33:470–80.
23. Gebhard C, Rhainds D, He G, Rodés-Cabau J, Lavi S, Spence JD, Title L, Kouz S, L'Allier PL, Grégoire J, Ibrahim R, Cossette M, Guertin MC, Beanlands R, Rhéaume E, Tardif JC. Elevated level of lecithin:cholesterol acyltransferase (LCAT) is associated with reduced coronary atheroma burden. Atherosclerosis. 2018;276:131–9.
24. Tanaka S, Yasuda T, Ishida T, Fujioka Y, Tsujino T, Miki T, Hirata K. Increased serum cholesterol esterification rates predict coronary heart disease and sudden death in a general population. Arterioscler Thromb Vasc Biol. 2013; 33:1098–104.
25. Andrews JPM, Fayad ZA, Dweck MR. New methods to image unstable atherosclerotic plaques. Atherosclerosis. 2018;272:118–28.

26. Daniels JA, Mulligan C, McCance D, Woodside JV, Patterson C, Young IS, McEneny J. A randomised controlled trial of increasing fruit and vegetable intake and how this influences the carotenoid concentration and activities of PON-1 and LCAT in HDL from subjects with type 2 diabetes. Cardiovasc Diabetol. 2014;13:16.

27. Iida K, Tani S, Atsumi W, Yagi T, Kawauchi K, Matsumoto N, Hirayama A. Association of plasminogen activator inhibitor-1 and low-density lipoprotein heterogeneity as a risk factor of atherosclerotic cardiovascular disease with triglyceride metabolic disorder: a pilot cross-sectional study. Coron Artery Dis. 2017;28:577–87.

28. Asztalos BF, Swarbrick MM, Schaefer EJ, Dallal GE, Horvath KV, Ai M, Stanhope KL, Austrheim-Smith I, Wolfe BM, Ali M, Havel PJ. Effects of weight loss, induced by gastric bypass surgery, on HDL remodeling in obese women. J Lipid Res. 2010;51:2405–12.

29. Ossoli A, Simonelli S, Vitali C, Franceschini G, Calabresi L. Role of LCAT in atherosclerosis. J Atheroscler Thromb. 2016;23:119–27.

30. Calabresi L, Simonelli S, Gomaraschi M, Franceschini G. Genetic lecithin: cholesterol acyltransferase deficiency and cardiovascular disease. Atherosclerosis. 2012;222:299–306.

31. Calabresi L, Baldassarre D, Simonelli S, Gomaraschi M, Amato M, Castelnuovo S, Frigerio B, Ravani A, Sansaro D, Kauhanen J, Rauramaa R, de Faire U, Hamsten A, Smit AJ, Mannarino E, Humphries SE, Giral P, Veglia F, Sirtori CR, Franceschini G, Tremoli E. Plasma lecithin:cholesterol acyltransferase and carotid intima-media thickness in European individuals at high cardiovascular risk. J Lipid Res. 2011;52:1569–74.

32. Hovingh GK, Hutten BA, Holleboom AG, Petersen W, Rol P, Stalenhoef A, Zwinderman AH, de Groot E, Kastelein JJ, Kuivenhoven JA. Compromised LCAT function is associated with increased atherosclerosis. Circulation. 2005; 112:879–84.

33. Ross R. Atherosclerosis—an inflammatory disease. N Engl J Med. 1999;340: 115–26.

23

Long-term prognosis of patients with non-ST-segment elevation myocardial infarction according to coronary arteries atherosclerosis extent on coronary angiography

Karam Sadoon Alzuhairi[1*], Peter Søgaard[1,2], Jan Ravkilde[1], Aziza Azimi[3], Michael Mæng[4], Lisette Okkels Jensen[5] and Christian Torp-Pedersen[3]

Abstract

Background: Patients with non-ST-segment elevation myocardial infarction (NSTEMI) without obstructive coronary artery disease (CAD) are often managed differently than those with obstructive CAD, therefore we aimed in this study to examine the long-term prognosis of patients with NSTEMI according to the degree of CAD on coronary angiography (CAG).

Methods: We examined 8.889 consecutive patients admitted for first time NSTEMI during 2000–2011, to whom CAG was performed. Patients were classified by CAG into: 0-vessel disease (0VD), diffuse atherosclerosis (DA) (0% < stenosis <50%), 1-vessel disease (1VD), 2VD, and 3VD with stenosis ≥50%. Follow-up period: 13 years (median 4.5).

Results: One-year mortality for NSTEMI patients with 0VD was 3.7%, DA 5.7%, 1VD 2.5%, 2VD 4.8%, and 3VD 11. 5%. Non-diabetic 0VD patients had higher risk of mortality than 1VD patients (HR:1.59; 95% CI:1.21–2.02; $P < 0.001$), while those with diabetes mellitus (DM) had not significantly different risk. In addition 0VD group had higher risk of heart failure (HF) (HR 1.61; 95% CI: 1.39–1.88; $P < 0.001$), and lower risk of recurrent MI (HR:0.55; 95% CI:0.39–0. 77; $P < 0.001$) compared with 1VD. For patients with DA; mortality and HF risks were higher than 1VD and not different than 2VD, while recurrent MI risk was not different than 1VD and lower than 2VD.
Finally, the DA group had higher risk of mortality if they had DM, higher risk of recurrent MI, and not different risk of HF and stroke compared with the 0VD group patients.

Conclusion: Patients with NSTEMI and non-obstructive CAD (both normal coronaries and diffuse atherosclerosis) have a comparable prognosis to patients with one- or two-vessel disease. Patients with diffuse atherosclerosis have worse prognosis than those with angiographically normal coronary arteries.

Keywords: Acute coronary syndrome, Myocardial infarction, Prognosis, Non-obstructive coronary artery disease

* Correspondence: ksm.alzuhairi@gmail.com
[1]Department of Cardiology, Aalborg University Hospital, Hobrovej 18, –9000 Aalborg, DK, Denmark
Full list of author information is available at the end of the article

Background

Non-ST-segment elevation myocardial infarction (NSTEMI) with non-obstructive coronary arteries proven with coronary angiography is an important subgroup of patients with myocardial infarction (MI), because they are often managed differently, being less likely to receive recommended medical treatment after MI and more likely to discontinue double platelet inhibitors, than patients with NSTEMI with obstructive CAD [1, 2].

Studies investigating this subgroup reported a wide range of prevalence (4–13%) according to the definitions used, the type of MI, and the use of cardiac troponin (MI or acute coronary syndrome (ACS)) [3–5]. Previous studies suggested that factors predicting non-obstructive coronary arteries in MI patients are female, younger age, and lack of smoking and diabetes mellitus (DM) [2, 6, 7].

Previous studies showed that patients with NSTEMI with non-obstructive CAD had better prognosis compared with obstructive CAD [5, 6, 8–10]. Other studies reported a substantial risk in non-obstructive group with higher all-cause mortality [11] or similar risk of combined death, MI, admission for ACS, and non-fatal stroke compared with obstructive CAD group [2]. However, many of these studies were limited by a small sample size [1, 12] or a short duration of follow-up [6]. In addition, most of these prognostic studies compared patients with obstructive versus non-obstructive CAD, and studies dividing both these groups into subgroups according to coronary pathology are few [2, 10].

Therefore, the aim of this study was to assess the prognosis in a large number of NSTEMI patients divided into five groups according to their coronary artery atherosclerosis extent on the coronary angiography with a long-term follow-up.

Methods

Study design

This was a historical prospective study based on data collected from several Danish registries mentioned bellow. All citizens in Denmark have a unique identification number, which facilitates linkage between different registries on person-level.

The registries

Since 1977 the Danish National Patient Register has collected data including discharge diagnosis from all admissions to Danish hospitals [13]. MI diagnosis is with high sensitivity and specificity [14, 15].

The Western Denmark Heart Registry has collected patient and procedure data since 1999 for all interventions in the hospitals in western Denmark; and it is a validated research source [16].

Study population

We identified all patients discharged with first time NSTEMI or unspecific MI (ICD-10 codes: DI21.4 and DI21.9, respectively) in the Patient Register during the period January 1st, 2000 to August 31st, 2011, who underwent coronary angiography within 30 days. Patients discharged with unspecific MI diagnosis were included if NSTEMI diagnosis was confirmed from the Western Heart Registry, because this registry does not allow the use of (unspecific MI) diagnosis. From this registry clinical data and angiographic description of coronary arteries stenosis were obtained Patients were divided accordingly into five subgroups: zero-vessel disease (0VD) = angiographically normal coronary arteries; diffuse atherosclerosis (DA) = moderate focal or diffuse atherosclerosis either without stenosis ≥50%; one-vessel disease (1VD) with stenosis ≥50%; two-vessel disease (2VD) with stenosis ≥50%; or three-vessel disease (3VD) with stenosis ≥50%. Patients with left main stenosis ≥50% were included either in the 3VD group, if the right coronary was hypoplastic or with stenosis ≥50%, or in the 2VD group if the right coronary was without significant stenosis. From the Civil Registration System we obtained gender, age, and mortality status.

Study outcomes

Recurrent MI was identified from the Patient Register using ICD-10 code: DI21 (all types of MI). To avoid misclassification due to transfer between hospitals, we made a program to merge related admissions into one, and added 5 days after the discharge day, where no recurrent MI can be considered.

Moreover, we did a sensitivity analysis where no recurrent MI was considered within the first 30 days. Stroke event defined using ICD-10 code: DI61(intracerebral haemorrhage), DI62 (other non-traumatic intracranial haemorrhage), DI63 (cerebral infarction), or DI64 (stroke, not specified). Patients with stroke diagnosis before NSTEMI were not included in stroke outcome analysis. To identify heart failure (HF) event, we used either ICD-10 code: DI50.9 (heart failure, unspecified) or DI25.5 (ischemic cardiomyopathy).

Exclusion criteria

1- Missing data on coronary atherosclerosis description (628 (6%) of study population).
2- Previous MI.
3- Known with HF.
4- Prior revascularization treatment.

Follow up and end points

During a median follow up period of 4.5 years (1.3–13 years) the outcomes: mortality, recurrent MI, HF, and stroke were registered. Follow-up started on the day of admission with first NSTEMI and ended on the 31st December 2012, or the date of emigration or death.

Statistical analysis

Categorical variables are presented as numbers and percentages and compared using Chi-square test, while continuous variables presented as median with interquartile range, and compared using analysis of variance. Time to event curve was generated using Aalen-Nelson cumulative incidence estimator taking into account death as a competing risk.

Cox proportional hazard models were used to estimate hazard ratio with 95% confidence interval. The model was adjusted for: age, sex, DM, hypertension, current smoker status, renal insufficiency (defined as estimated glomerular filtration rate (eGFR) <60 ml/min/1.73m^2 using MDRD equation), and overweight (defined as body mass index ≥25). Left ventricular ejection fraction (EF) was not included in the primary analysis because only 45% of patients had available measurements; however, an additional analysis was done separately for this subgroup. Model assumptions for proportional hazard and linearity were found valid. Effect modification was tested using likelihood ratio test for clinically relevant variables: age, sex, hypertension, DM, renal insufficiency, and smoking. There was a significant and clinically important effect modification of DM (P 0.003) on mortality outcome; therefore we did the analysis with and without DM. No significant effect modification was found for DM on the other outcomes or for the other variables on all outcomes.

For more details in statistical analysis, please see online appendix A. All statistical analyses were performed using the SAS statistical software V.9.2 (SAS Institute Inc., Cary, North Carolina, USA), and R version 3.02 (R Development Core Team).

Results

Of 8889 first time NSTEMI patients who underwent coronary angiography, 1290 (14.5%) had non-obstructive coronary arteries. Of these 1290 patients, 988 (76.5%) had 0VD, and 302 (23.5%) had DA with no stenosis ≥50%. The proportion of patients with non-obstructive CAD increased throughout the study period reaching 18% in 2011.

Demographic data of the study population are showed in Table 1. Patients with 0VD had a comparable risk profile to those with 1VD except that the majority were females (59.9% vs. 29.6% $P < 0.001$), and they were less likely to be current smoker (32.4% vs. 42.7, $P < 0.001$) or overweight (57.7 vs. 67.3, $P < 0.001$). However, patients with 0VD were younger, more likely to be females, and less likely to have hypertension and DM than patients

with DA. The DA group had similar characteristics to the 2VD group, except it included more women (44.0% vs. 23.3%, $P < 0.001$) and less overweight (55.6% vs. 66.7, $P < 0.001$). Patients with all sub-groups of obstructive CAD were significantly more frequently treated with revascularization (either percutaneous coronary intervention or coronary by-pass grafting (Table 1), they were also more likely to receive double anti-platelet therapy than patients with 0VD or DA (Table 1).

Long-term prognosis of NSTEMI patients according to their coronary artery pathology
Mortality

Dividing NSTEMI patients according to coronary artery disease extent revealed that one-year mortality for patients with 0VD, DA, 1VD, 2VD, and 3VD were 36 (3.6%), 17(5.6%), 80(2.5%), 105(5.0%), and 251(11.5%), respectively (Table 2). 1VD had the lowest and 3VD had the highest unadjusted cumulative mortality rate (Fig. 1).

Patients with NSTEMI and without DM

After adjustment for covariates, mortality risk for the 0VD group was higher than the 1VD group (HR:1.59; 95% CI:1.21–2.02, $P < 0.001$) (Fig. 2, Additional file 1), and not significantly different from the DA (HR:0.82; 95% CI:0.54–1.26, $P = 0.37$), 2VD (HR:1.19; 95% CI:0.91–1.57, $P = 0.21$), and the 3VD groups (HR:0.83;95% CI:0.64–1.08, $P = 0.17$). On the other hand, patients with DA had higher risk of mortality compared with 1VD patients (HR:1.93; 95% CI:1.31–2.83, $P < 0.001$), nominally higher, but not statistically significant, compared with 2VD group (HR:1.44; 95% CI:0.97–2.13, $P = 0.06$), and not different than the 3VD group.

Patients with NSTEMI and DM

After multi-factorial adjustment, mortality risk for 0VD patients was not significantly lower than the 1VD group (Additional file 1), but significantly lower than the DA (HR:0.16; 95% CI:0.05–0.51, $P = 0.002$), 2VD (HR:0.26; 95% CI:0.09–0.72, $P = 0.01$), and the 3VD groups (HR:0.26; 95% CI:0.10–0.72, $P = 0.009$). For patients with DA and diabetes, mortality risk was higher than 1VD (HR: 2.5; 95% CI:1.28–4.90, $P = 0.007$), but not significantly different compared with both 2VD and 3VD.

Recurrent MI

One-year risk of recurrent MI was lowest in patients with non-obstructive CAD both the 0VD and the DA groups (Table 2). The 3VD group had the highest incidence of recurrent MI throughout the study period (Fig. 3).

Patients with 0VD had the lowest risk of recurrent MI in all groups after multi-factorial adjustment (Fig. 4), while patients with DA had a risk of recurrent MI that was higher than 0VD group (HR:1.7; 95% CI:1.05–

Table 1 Baseline characteristics of the study population

Variables	0VD (N = 988)	DA (N = 302)	1VD (N = 3295)	2VD (N = 2114)	3VD (N2190)	P values
Age (years)	62 {53, 72}	66 {56, 74}	63 {54, 71}	67 {59, 75}	71 {63, 78}	< 0.001
Female gender	585 (59.9)	131 (44.0)	966 (29.6)	489 (23.3)	587 (27.0)	< 0.001
Hypertension	368 (39.2)	143 (49.7)	1290 (41.6)	875 (44.4)	1088 (53.6)	< 0.001
Hyperlipidemia	427 (45.5)	144 (49.5)	1517 (48.9)	1060 (53.6)	1093 (53.9)	< 0.001
Diabetes mellitus	106 (11.0)	51 (17.2)	413 (12.9)	342 (16.6)	488 (23.0)	< 0.001
IHD in the family	347 (37.4)	113 (40.1)	1231 (40.5)	765 (39.3)	750 (37.9)	0.3072
Current smoker	293 (32.4)	100 (36.6)	1303 (42.7)	772 (39.4)	654 (33.0)	< 0.001
Overweight[a]	463 (57.7)	143 (55.6)	1764 (67.3)	1097 (66.7)	1059 (64.4)	< 0.001
Renal insufficiency[b]	107 (13.8)	39 (15.4)	353 (13.8)	310 (19.0)	457 (28.0)	< 0.001
EF < 50%	107 (22.1)	37 (25.2)	282 (19.5)	258 (28.7)	427 (42.3)	< 0.001
Previous stroke	36 (3.6)	15 (5.0)	113 (3.4)	111 (5.3)	189 (8.6)	< 0.001
Treatment						
Any revascularisation[c]	26 (2.6)	15 (5.0)	2764 (83.9)	1816 (85.9)	1688 (77.1)	< 0.001
PCI	21 (2.1)	11 (3.7)	2728 (82.8)	1588 (75.1)	769 (35.1)	< 0.001
CABG	5 (0.5)	4 (1.3)	36 (1.1)	228 (10.8)	919 (42.0)	< 0.001
Aspirin	883 (90.9)	288 (95.7)	3177 (96.6)	2039 (96.5)	2048 (93.8)	<0.001
P2Y12 receptor inhibitor	668 (67.7)	235 (78.1)	3097 (94.2)	1920 (90.9)	1642 (75.2)	<0.001
Beta blocker	758 (78.1)	263 (87.4)	2964 (90.1)	1892 (89.6)	1975 (90.5)	<0.001
ACE-inhibitor	428 (44.1)	147 (48.8)	1641 (49.9)	1175 (55.6)	1363 (62.4)	<0.001
Statin	808 (83.2)	277 (92.0)	3103 (94.3)	1968 (93.2)	1978 (90.6)	<0.001

Parameters presented as numbers (percentages from non-missing data) or median (25th, 75th percentile)
Abbreviations: *0VD* zero-vessel disease, *DA* diffuse atherosclerosis, *1VD* one-vessel disease, *2VD* two-vessel disease, *3VD* three-vessel disease, *IHD* ischemic heart disease, *EF* ejection fraction, *PCI* percutaneous coronary intervention, *CABG* coronary by-pass graft operation, *P2Y12-inhibitor* P2Y12 receptor inhibitor, *ACE* angiotensin-converting-enzyme
[a]Overweight defined as body mass index ≥25
[b]Renal insufficiency defined as estimated glomerular filtration rate < 60 ml/min/1.73m² using MDRD equation
[c]Revasculrisation defined as PCI within 30 days, and CABG within 60 days of non-ST-elevation myocardial infarction

2.89, $P = 0.03$), not significantly different from the 1VD (HR:0.91; 95% CI:0.60–1.39, $P = 0.66$), and lower than both the 2VD and 3VD groups. In patients with obstructive CAD, the risk of recurrent MI increased linearly with the severity of the disease.

Heart failure

One-year HF risk after first NSTEMI was substantial in patients with 0VD and DA (Table 2). Unadjusted cumulative incidence of HF was lowest in 1VD and highest in 3VD group (Fig. 5). After multi-factorial adjustment, the

Table 2 One-year and five-year prognosis of patients with NSTEMI according to their coronary artery atherosclerosis extent

Outcomes	0VD (N = 988)	DA (N = 302)	1VD (N = 3295)	2VD (N = 2114)	3VD (N = 2190)
1-year					
Death	36 (3.6%)	17 (5.6%)	80 (2.4%)	105 (5.0%)	251 (11.5%)
Recurrent MI	35 (3.5%)	19 (6.3%)	273 (8.3%)	285 (13.5%)	369 (16.8%)
Heart Failure	101 (10.2%)	40 (13.2%)	263 (8.0%)	249 (11.8%)	433 (19.8%)
Stroke	17 (1.7%)	4 (1.3%)	42 (1.3%)	37 (1.8%)	69 (3.2%)
5-years					
Death	120 (12.1%)	55 (18.2%)	327 (9.9%)	315 (14.9%)	609 (27.8%)
Recurrent MI	56 (5.7%)	29 (9.6%)	353 (10.7%)	360 (17.0%)	464 (21.2%)
Heart Failure	139 (14.1%)	45 (14.9%)	352 (10.7%)	367 (17.4%)	623 (28.4%)
Stroke	41 (4.1%)	16 (5.3%)	117 (3.6%)	94 (4.4%)	140 (6.4%)

The results presented in numbers (percent)
Abbreviations: *0VD* zero-vessel disease, *DA* diffuse atherosclerosis, *1VD* one-vessel disease, *2VD* two-vessel disease, *3VD* three-vessel disease

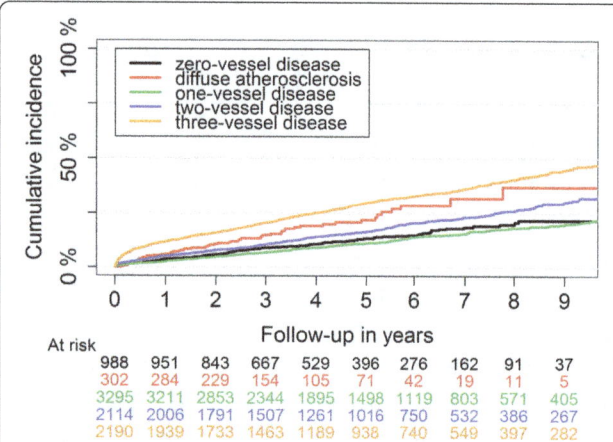

Fig. 1 Long-term mortality in patients with non-ST-segment elevation myocardial infarction according to their coronary artery atherosclerosis extent

risk of HF was not significantly different between 0VD and DA groups. Both groups had higher HF risk compared with 1VD (Fig. 4), not statistically different compared with 2VD, and lower risk compared with the 3VD group (HR:0.80; 95% CI: 0.69–0.93, $P = 0.004$; and HR: 0.60; 95% CI: 0.44–0.83, $P = 0.02$), respectively.

Stroke

One-year stroke risk was highest in patients with 3VD and comparable in the other 4 groups (Table 2). Incidence of

stroke was generally lower than other outcomes (Fig. 6). Adjusted risk of stroke in patients with 0VD compared with 1VD and 2VD were (HR:1.47; 95% CI: 0.98–2.20, $P = 0.06$) and (HR: 1.46; 95% CI: 0.95–2.23, $P = 0.09$), respectively. Stroke risk was similar in the 0VD compared with the DA and 3VD groups. Patients with DA had a similar stroke risk compared with all other groups.

Additional analyses
Cardiovascular mortality

Considering only cardiovascular (CV) mortality and not all-cause mortality: for patients without DM, the CV mortality for 0VD group was higher compared to 1VD (HR:1.52; 95% CI: 1.19–1.94, $P = <0.001$), not different compared to DA and 2VD groups, and lower than 3VD group (HR: 0.69; 95% CI:0.50–0.96, $P = 0.02$). While patients in the DA group had a CV mortality which was higher than both 1VD and 2VD groups (HR: 1.82; 95% CI: 1.27–2.60, $P = <0.001$), (HR: 1.76; 95% CI: 0.91–1.82, $P = 0.03$), respectively, and not different compared to 3VD.

For patients with NSTEMI and DM, whose in the 0VD group had CV mortality which was not significantly different compared to both 1VD, and 2VD groups, but lower than CV mortality of both 3VD, and DA groups (HR: 0.06; 95% CI:0.007–0.47, $P = 0.007$). While patients in the DA group had higher CV mortality than 1VD (HR:2.88; 95% CI:1.29–6.43, $P = 0.009$), and not different compared to 2VD, and 3VD groups.

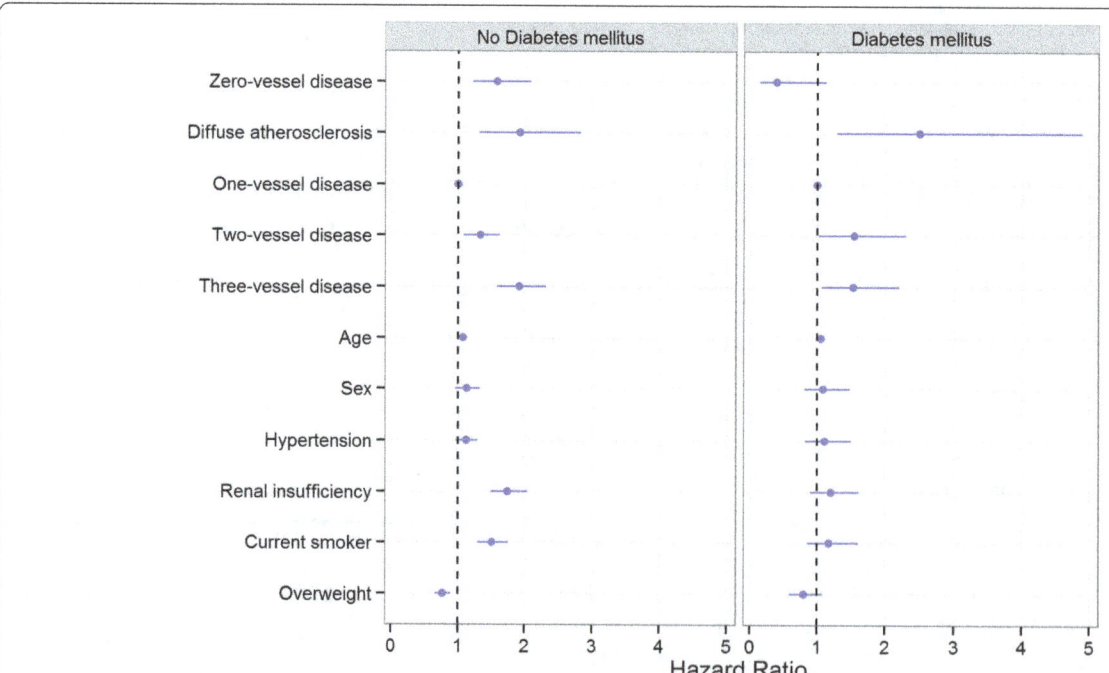

Fig. 2 Adjusted mortality hazard ratio for NSTEMI patients according to their coronary artery pathology. 1VD group was used as a reference group. The model was adjusted for age, sex, hypertension, renal insufficiency (eGFR < 60 ml/min/1.73m²), current smoker status, and overweight (BMI ≥ 25)

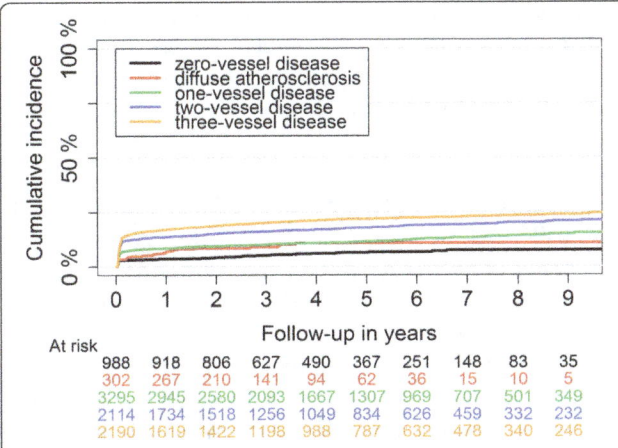

Fig. 3 Long-term recurrent myocardial infarction cumulative incidence in patients with first NSTEMI divided by their coronary artery atherosclerosis extent

Patients with available EF measurement

This subgroup analysis consisted of 3986 patients. Multifactorial adjustment including EF revealed that stroke hazard for 1VD group was significantly lower than all other groups. No other differences were observed for the other outcomes.

Sensitivity analysis considering recurrent MI only after 30 days

Recurrent MI risks from 30 to 365 days after NSTEMI were as follows: 0VD 0.7% (0.2–1.2%), DA 3.3% (1.3–

5.5%), 1VD 2.4% (1.8–2.8%), 2VD 4.4% (3.6–5.3%) and 3VD 7.4% (6.3–8.4%). After adjustment for risk factors, 0VD continued to have the lowest risk of recurrent MI among all groups. Patients with DA had a not significantly different risk compared with the 1VD, 2VD, and 3VD groups.

Discussion

Our study recruited 8889 patients with a follow-up duration of up to 13 years (median 4.5 years). It showed two important main findings: 1) NSTEMI patients with non-obstructive CAD (both 0VD and DA without significant stenosis) have a substantial risk of long-term adverse outcomes comparable to 1VD and 2VD patients; and 2) 0VD and DA groups are different in both risk profile and outcome.

This study showed that patients with 0VD were younger, mostly females, and had less co-morbidities than those with DA. This was also observed in another study [2]. An explanation of more females among both groups of non-obstructive CAD group could be that one half of females without significant stenosis have microvascular dysfunction [17].

The percentage of NSTEMI patients with non-obstructive coronary arteries increased gradually during the study to reach 18% in 2011, that might reflect the development of more sensitive troponin and the use of lower cut-off values in the definition of MI, and thus the

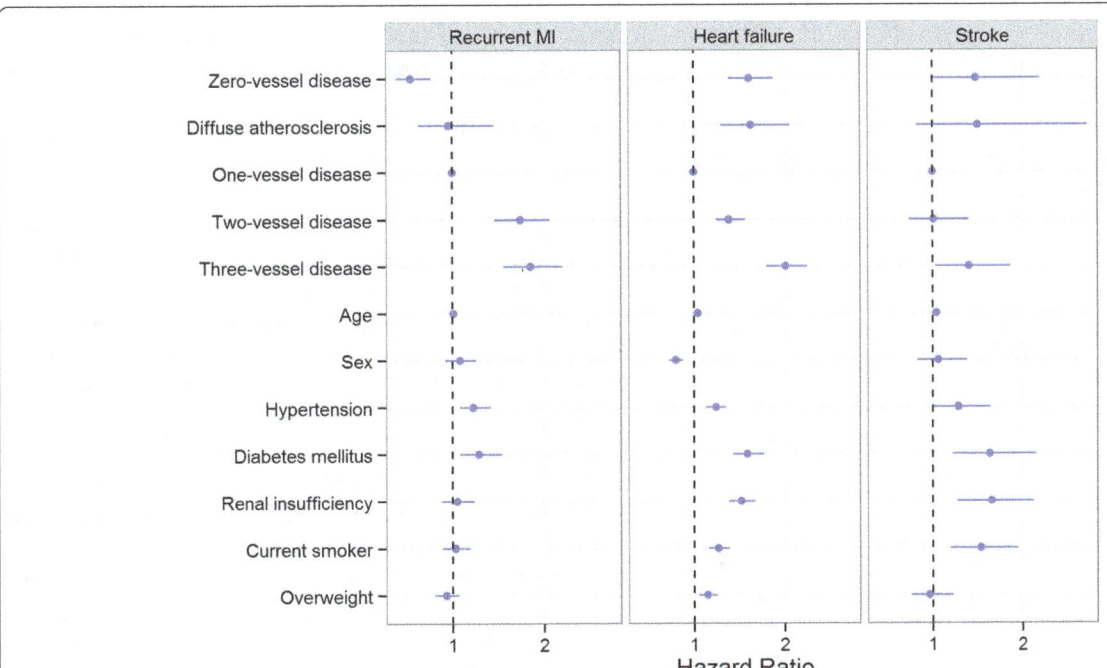

Fig. 4 Adjusted hazard ratio of long-term recurrent myocardial infarction, heart failure, and stroke in patients with NSTEMI according to their coronary artery disease. Hazard ratio was adjusted for age, sex, hypertension, diabetes mellitus, renal insufficiency (eGFR < 6060 ml/min/1.73m^2), current smoker status, and overweight (BMI ≥ 25)

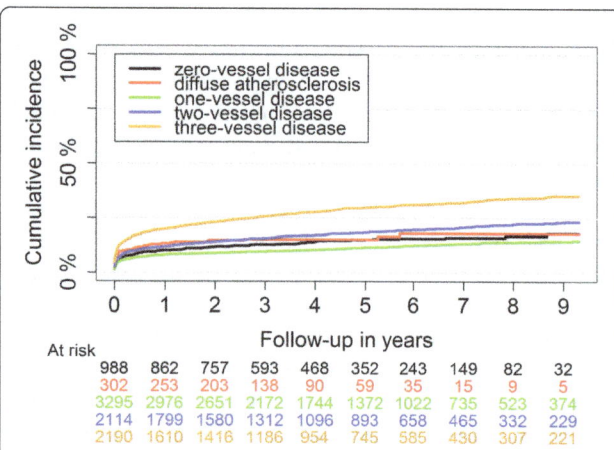

Fig. 5 Long-term heart failure cumulative incidence in patients with first NSTEMI divided by their coronary artery atherosclerosis extent

detection of smaller injuries to the myocardium [18]. This means also that we are dealing with growing subgroup of patients who need more attention in our management.

Mechanism of NSTEMI with non-obstructive CAD

There are several reported mechanisms of myocardial injury in these patients, like plaque disruption without significant stenosis on the angiogram proven with intra vascular ultrasound (IVUS) examination, [19] coronary artery spasm, [12, 20] microvascular disease, [21] or thrombophilias whether congenital or acquired [12]. Other possible non ischemic mechanisms including myocarditis which was observed in 7% of NSTEMI with non-obstructive CAD using cardiac MRI [3].

In our study 2.6% of 0VD and 5.0% of DA were treated with revascularization (either PCI or CABG). In the DA group, the explanation could be proven plaque rupture in non-obstructive lesion, and in the 0VD group, one of the explanations could be complications to the coronary

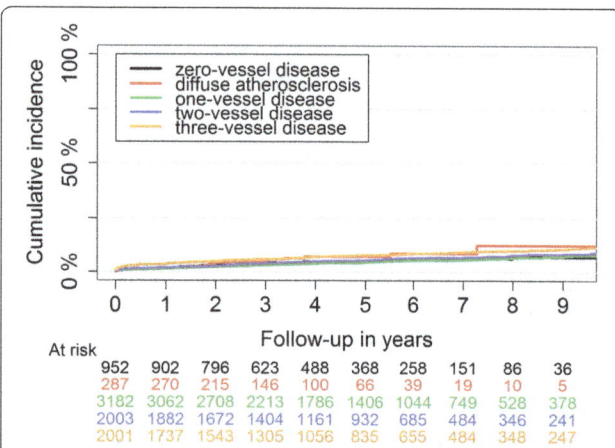

Fig. 6 Long-term stroke cumulative incidence in patients with first NSTEMI divided by their coronary artery atherosclerosis extent

angiography like perforation or dissection either with the diagnostic catheter or with optical coherence or IVUS wire. These complications might have led to revascularization in a patient without CAD.

Long-term mortality after first NSTEMI

Our study illustrated that non-diabetic NSTEMI patients with 0VD had higher mortality risk compared with 1VD group. On the other hand, patients with DA had a 2-fold higher mortality than those with 1VD and similar mortality to those with 2VD.

Another study concluded that NSTEMI with normal coronary arteries had the same mortality risk as both atherosclerosis and low risk anatomy obstructive CAD [10] while other studies showed no significant difference in mortality in patients with and without obstructive CAD after adjustment for risk factors for IHD [1, 7, 22]. A recent study reported higher risk of one-year mortality in NSTEMI patients with non-obstructive compared with obstructive CAD, mostly driven by non-cardiac death [11]. These studies, however, did not divide obstructive CAD into subgroups. A possible explanation for our findings could be that as our results showed that patients with NSTEMI with non-obstructive CAD were less likely to receive double anti-platelet therapy and other recommended medical treatment after MI according to ESC guidelines, [23]. This was also shown in another study, where these patients were also more likely to discontinue double platelet inhibitors if these were started [1, 2]. Another explanation might be that many of these patients, especially those with 0VD, might have suffered a type II MI, and comprises a heterogeneous group with different background pathology leading to myocardial injury without CAD. Mortality risk of type II MI was reported to be comparable or higher than type I MI [24, 25].

Recurrent MI

NSTEMI patients with 0VD had the lowest risk of recurrent MI among our five groups, and those with DA had the same risk as patients with 1VD. According to other studies, patients with non-obstructive CAD have lower risk of MI than obstructive CAD [2, 7]. However, these studies did not divide obstructive CAD into subgroups. Our findings might be explained by speculating that plaque burden might be comparable in the DA and 1VD groups; and both have higher plaque burden than the 0VD group. Previous studies using IVUS reported that plaque rupture is often not detected as significant stenosis by angiography, and is typically associated with eccentric and large plaque with positive remodeling [19, 26, 27]. A recent meta-analysis ([28] showed that shorter duration (<6 months) of double antiplatelet therapy, was associated with higher incidence of MI, less incidence of bleeding, and the same mortality and stent thrombosis rates. However, this study was in patients treated with PCI with second generation drug eluting stent, nevertheless, about 40% of patients were acute coronary syndrome patients. Although, our study population is different, but our results also indicated that a non-unreasonable anticipation is that some of the recurrent MI incidence in DA group is because of either not been given double anti-platelet therapy or shorter duration of treatment compared with obstructive CAD group.

Heart failure
NSTEMI patients with both 0VD and DA had a higher risk of HF than the 1VD, same risk as the 2VD, and lower risk than the 3VD group in this study. Another study showed that the risk of HF in ACS patients with or without obstructive CAD was similar, [22] but that study did not differentiate sub groups and included only patients ≥75 years.

One explanation of our findings could be that some of the patients were admitted with acute HF with symptoms, signs and troponin elevation that resembled MI. It is well known that HF can cause myocardial injury resembling MI [29]. However, we tried to restrict that possibility by excluding patients known with HF. Another explanation may be that especially patients with 0VD could have a myocardial disease in early stage which developed afterward to a manifest HF.

Stroke
Patients with NSTEMI with non-obstructive CAD had a similar risk of stroke compared with those with obstructive CAD. This confirms the findings of other studies [1, 2].

Study strength and limitations
The strengths include the large number of unselected patients with NSTEMI. Patients from both genders and all age groups were included, which helps generalization of our results.

However, our study has some limitations; patients with MI type II might have been included if the primary discharge diagnosis was NSTEMI, and it seems to be reasonable to assume that this was more applicable to 0VD and DA groups. These considerations, however, do not change that, according to our data, these two groups remain at high risk of adverse events. In angiography database the definitions of 0VD and DA were subject for inter- and intra-hospital different interpretations, thus some of the patients with DA might have been coded as 0VD. However, this misclassification would lead to minimize the differences between 0VD and DA groups, thus the real differences between these groups in outcome may be larger than that reported in our article. A core-lab for coronary angiography assessment was not used, thus inter-operator variation might exist. Lastly, only patients who underwent coronary angiography were included which make generalization of the results limited. The cut-off values and Troponin assays has been changed during the study years, which might led to that the MI size detected in the later years are smaller than that at the earlier years of the study.

Conclusion
Patients with NSTEMI with normal coronary arteries or atherosclerosis without significant stenosis have substantial risk of future cardiovascular events. Both patients with 0VD without diabetes and patients with DA have higher risk of mortality and heart failure compared with patients with 1VD; and patients with DA have a similar risk of recurrent MI compared with those with 1VD. Moreover, patients with 0VD have favorable risk profile, lower mortality (if patients were diabetic) and lower recurrent MI risk than patients with diffuse atherosclerosis. These findings call for considering these two subgroups of NSTEMI separately in future research and urge for further investigations to explore the best management and follow-up plans for each of these two subgroups.

Abbreviations
0VD: zero-vessel disease; 1VD: one-vessel disease; 2VD: two-vessel disease; 3VD: three-vessel disease; CAD: Coronary artery disease; DA: Diffuse atherosclerosis without significant stenosis; DM: Diabetes mellitus; HF: Heart failure; NSTEMI: Non-ST-segment elevation myocardial infarction

Acknowledgements
Not applicable.

Funding
None.

Authors' contributions
KSA designed the study, analyzed the data, and wrote the manuscript. PS, reviewed and corrected the manuscript, JR, MM, LOJ helped in collecting the data and correcting the manuscript. AA helped in data interpretation. CTP helped in study design, getting the permission for data access, supervising data analysis, and correcting the manuscript. All authors read and approved the final manuscript.

Competing interests
The authors declare that they have no competing interests.

Author details
[1]Department of Cardiology, Aalborg University Hospital, Hobrovej 18, –9000 Aalborg, DK, Denmark. [2]Department of Clinical Medicine, Aalborg University, Aalborg, Denmark. [3]Department of Health, Science and Technology, Aalborg University, Aalborg, Denmark. [4]Department of Cardiology, Aarhus University Hospital, Aarhus, Denmark. [5]Department of Cardiology, Odense University Hospital, Odense, Denmark.

References
1. Andre R, André RE. Prevalence, clinical profile and 3-year survival of acute myocardial infarction patients with and without obstructive coronary

lesions: the FAST-MI 2005 registry. Int J Cardiol. 2014;172:e247–49.

2. Rossini R, Capodanno D, Lettieri C, Musumeci G, Limbruno U, Molfese M, et al. Long-term outcomes of patients with acute coronary syndrome and nonobstructive coronary artery disease. Am J Cardiol. 2013;112:150–5.

3. Collste O, Sörensson P, Frick M, Agewall S, Daniel M, Henareh L, et al. Myocardial infarction with normal coronary arteries is common and associated with normal findings on cardiovascular magnetic resonance imaging: results from the Stockholm myocardial infarction with normal coronaries study. J Intern Med. 2013;273:189–96.

4. Agewall S, Daniel M, Eurenius L, Ekenbäck C, Skeppholm M, Malmqvist K, et al. Risk factors for myocardial infarction with normal coronary arteries and myocarditis compared with myocardial infarction with coronary artery stenosis. Angiology. 2012;63:500–3.

5. Cortell A, Sanchis J, Bodí V, Núñez J, Mainar L, Pellicer M, et al. Non-ST-elevation acute myocardial infarction with normal coronary arteries: predictors and prognosis. Rev española Cardiol. 2009;62:1260–6.

6. Patel MR, Chen AY, Peterson ED, Newby LK, Pollack CV, Brindis RG, et al. Prevalence, predictors, and outcomes of patients with non-ST-segment elevation myocardial infarction and insignificant coronary artery disease: results from the can rapid risk stratification of unstable angina patients suppress ADverse outcomes with early. Am Heart J. 2006;152:641–7.

7. Ohlow M-A, Wong V, Brunelli M, von Korn H, Farah A, Memisevic N, et al. Acute coronary syndrome without significant epicardial coronary disease: prevalence, characteristics, and outcome. Am J Emerg Med. 2015;33:150–4.

8. Zimmerman FH, Cameron A, Fisher LD, Ng G. Myocardial infarction in young adults: angiographic characterization, risk factors and prognosis (coronary artery surgery study registry). J Am Coll Cardiol. 1995;26:654–61.

9. Roe MT, Harrington RA, Prosper DM, Pieper KS, Bhatt DL, Lincoff AM, et al. Clinical and therapeutic profile of patients presenting with acute coronary syndromes who do not have significant coronary artery disease. Circulation. 2000;102:1101–6.

10. Larsen AI, Galbraith PD, Ghali WA, Norris CM, Graham MM, Knudtson ML. Characteristics and outcomes of patients with acute myocardial infarction and angiographically normal coronary arteries. Am J Cardiol. 2005;95:261–3.

11. Planer D, Mehran R, Ohman EM, White HD, Newman JD, Xu K, et al. Prognosis of patients with non-ST-segment-elevation myocardial infarction and nonobstructive coronary artery disease: propensity-matched analysis from the acute catheterization and urgent intervention triage strategy trial. Circ Cardiovasc Interv. 2014;7:285–93.

12. Da Costa A, Isaaz K, Faure E, Mourot S, Cerisier A, Lamaud M. Clinical characteristics, aetiological factors and long-term prognosis of myocardial infarction with an absolutely normal coronary angiogram; a 3-year follow-up study of 91 patients. Eur Heart J. 2001;22:1459–65.

13. Andersen TF, Madsen M, Jørgensen J, Mellemkjoer L, Olsen JH. The Danish National Hospital Register. A valuable source of data for modern health sciences. Dan Med Bull. 1999;46:263–8.

14. Madsen M, Davidsen M, Rasmussen S, Abildstrom SZ, Osler M. The validity of the diagnosis of acute myocardial infarction in routine statistics: a comparison of mortality and hospital discharge data with the Danish MONICA registry. J Clin Epidemiol. 2003;56:124–30.

15. Joensen AM, Jensen MK, Overvad K, Dethlefsen C, Schmidt E, Rasmussen L, et al. Predictive values of acute coronary syndrome discharge diagnoses differed in the Danish National Patient Registry. J Clin Epidemiol. 2009;62:188–94.

16. Schmidt M, Maeng M, Jakobsen C-J, Madsen M, Thuesen L, Nielsen PH, et al. Existing data sources for clinical epidemiology: the western Denmark heart registry. Clin Epidemiol. 2010;2:137–44.

17. Reis SE, Holubkov R, Conrad Smith AJ, Kelsey SF, Sharaf BL, Reichek N, et al. Coronary microvascular dysfunction is highly prevalent in women with chest pain in the absence of coronary artery disease: results from the NHLBI WISE study. Am Heart J. 2001;141:735–41.

18. Kostis WJ, Deng Y, Pantazopoulos JS, Moreyra AE, Kostis JB. Trends in mortality of acute myocardial infarction after discharge from the hospital. Circ Cardiovasc Qual Outcomes. 2010;3:581–9.

19. Reynolds HR, Srichai MB, Iqbal SN, Slater JN, Mancini GBJ, Feit F, et al. Mechanisms of myocardial infarction in women without angiographically obstructive coronary artery disease. Circulation. LIPPINCOTT WILLIAMS & WILKINS, 530 WALNUT ST, PHILADELPHIA, PA 19106–3621 USA. 2011;124: 1414–25.

20. Ong P, Athanasiadis A, Hill S, Vogelsberg H, Voehringer M, Sechtem U. Coronary artery spasm as a frequent cause of acute coronary syndrome: the CASPAR (coronary artery spasm in patients with acute coronary syndrome) study. J Am Coll Cardiol. 2008;52:523–7.

21. Yetkin E, Turhan H, Erbay AR, Aksoy Y, Senen K. Increased thrombolysis in myocardial infarction frame count in patients with myocardial infarction and normal coronary arteriogram: a possible link between slow coronary flow and myocardial infarction. Atherosclerosis. 2005;181:193–9.

22. Wong V, Farah A, von Korn H, Memisevic N, Richter S, Tukhiashvili K, et al. Patients ≥ 75 years with acute coronary syndrome but without critical epicardial coronary disease: prevalence, characteristics, and outcome. J Geriatr Cardiol. 2015;12:11–6.

23. Hamm CW, Bassand J-P, Agewall S, Bax J, Boersma E, Bueno H, et al. ESC guidelines for the management of acute coronary syndromes in patients presenting without persistent ST-segment elevation: the task force for the management of acute coronary syndromes (ACS) in patients presenting without persistent ST-segment elevatio. Eur Heart J. 2011;32:2999–3054.

24. Saaby L, Poulsen TS, Hosbond S, Larsen TB, Pyndt Diederichsen AC, Hallas J, et al. Classification of myocardial infarction: frequency and features of type 2 myocardial infarction. Am J Med Elsevier. 2013;126:789–97.

25. Nelson SE, Sandoval Y, Smith SW, Schulz KM, Murakami M, Pearce LA, et al. Role of delta cardiac troponin I to distinguish between type I NSTEMI and type ii myocardial infarction. J Am Coll Cardiol. 2013;61:E234.

26. Maehara A, Mintz GS, Bui AB, Walter OR, Castagna MT, Canos D, et al. Morphologic and angiographic features of coronary plaque rupture detected by intravascular ultrasound. J Am Coll Cardiol. 2002;40:904–10.

27. Stone GW, Maehara A, Lansky AJ, de Bruyne B, Cristea E, Mintz GS, et al. A prospective natural-history study of coronary atherosclerosis. N Engl J Med. 2011;364:226–35.

28. D'Ascenzo F, Moretti C, Bianco M, Bernardi A, Taha S, Cerrato E, et al. Meta-analysis of the duration of dual antiplatelet therapy in patients treated with second-generation drug-eluting stents. Am J Cardiol. 2016;117:1714–23.

29. Thygesen K, Alpert JS, Jaffe AS, Simoons ML, Chaitman BR, White HD, et al. Third universal definition of myocardial infarction. Eur Heart J. 2012;33:2551–67.

Permissions

All chapters in this book were first published in CD, by BioMed Central; hereby published with permission under the Creative Commons Attribution License or equivalent. Every chapter published in this book has been scrutinized by our experts. Their significance has been extensively debated. The topics covered herein carry significant findings which will fuel the growth of the discipline. They may even be implemented as practical applications or may be referred to as a beginning point for another development.

The contributors of this book come from diverse backgrounds, making this book a truly international effort. This book will bring forth new frontiers with its revolutionizing research information and detailed analysis of the nascent developments around the world.

We would like to thank all the contributing authors for lending their expertise to make the book truly unique. They have played a crucial role in the development of this book. Without their invaluable contributions this book wouldn't have been possible. They have made vital efforts to compile up to date information on the varied aspects of this subject to make this book a valuable addition to the collection of many professionals and students.

This book was conceptualized with the vision of imparting up-to-date information and advanced data in this field. To ensure the same, a matchless editorial board was set up. Every individual on the board went through rigorous rounds of assessment to prove their worth. After which they invested a large part of their time researching and compiling the most relevant data for our readers.

The editorial board has been involved in producing this book since its inception. They have spent rigorous hours researching and exploring the diverse topics which have resulted in the successful publishing of this book. They have passed on their knowledge of decades through this book. To expedite this challenging task, the publisher supported the team at every step. A small team of assistant editors was also appointed to further simplify the editing procedure and attain best results for the readers.

Apart from the editorial board, the designing team has also invested a significant amount of their time in understanding the subject and creating the most relevant covers. They scrutinized every image to scout for the most suitable representation of the subject and create an appropriate cover for the book.

The publishing team has been an ardent support to the editorial, designing and production team. Their endless efforts to recruit the best for this project, has resulted in the accomplishment of this book. They are a veteran in the field of academics and their pool of knowledge is as vast as their experience in printing. Their expertise and guidance has proved useful at every step. Their uncompromising quality standards have made this book an exceptional effort. Their encouragement from time to time has been an inspiration for everyone.

The publisher and the editorial board hope that this book will prove to be a valuable piece of knowledge for researchers, students, practitioners and scholars across the globe.

List of Contributors

Chan-Hee Jung, Kyu-Jin Kim, Bo-Yeon Kim, Chul-Hee Kim, Sung-Koo Kang and Ji-Oh Mok
Division of Endocrinology and Metabolism, Department of Internal Medicine, Soonchunhyang University College of Medicine, #170 Jomaruro, Wonmi-gu, Bucheon-si, Gyeonggi-do 420-767, South Korea

Sang-Hee Jung
Department of Obstetrics and Gynecology, Cha University School of Medicine, Bundang, Korea

Himanshu Gupta, Chun G. Schiros and Oleg F. Sharifov
Department of Medicine, Cardiovascular Disease, University of Alabama at Birmingham, 1808 7th Ave South, BDB 101, Birmingham, AL 35294, USA

Himanshu Gupta
VA Medical Center, Birmingham, AL, USA

Apurva Jain
School of Public Health, The University Of Texas Health Science Centre, Houston, TX, USA

Thomas S. Denney Jr
Department of Electrical and Computer Engineering, Auburn University, Auburn, AL, USA

Hui Ma
Department of Geriatrics, Zhong Shan Hospital, Fudan University, Shanghai 200032, China

Huandong Lin, Yu Hu, Xiaoming Li and Xin Gao
Department of Endocrinology and Metabolism, Zhong Shan Hospital, Fudan University, Shanghai 200032, China

Wanyuan He
Department of Ultrasonography, Zhongshan Hospital, Fudan University, Shanghai 200032, China

Xuejuan Jin
Clinical Epidemiology Center, Zhong Shan Hospital, Fudan University, Shanghai 200032, China

Jian Gao
Department of Clinical Nutrition, Zhong Shan Hospital, Fudan University, Shanghai 200032, China

Naiqing Zhao
Department of Biostatistics, College of Public Health, Fudan University, Shanghai 200032, China

Zhenqi Liu
Division of Endocrinology and Metabolism, Department of Medicine, University of Virginia Health System, Charlottesville, Virginia, USA

Valery S. Effoe, Haiying Chen, Alain G. Bertoni and Carlos J. Rodriguez
Division of Public Health Sciences, Wake Forest School of Medicine, Medical Center Blvd, Winston Salem, NC 27127, USA

Andrew Moran
Department of Medicine, Columbia University College of Physicians & Surgeons, New York, NY, USA

David A. Bluemke
National Institutes of Health/Clinical Center, Bethesda, MD, USA

Teresa Seeman
Division of Geriatrics, University of California at Los Angeles, Los Angeles, CA, USA

Christine Darwin
University of California at Los Angeles Research Center, Los Angeles, CA, USA

Karol E. Watson
Division of Cardiology, University of California at Los Angeles School of Medicine, Los Angeles, CA, USA

Teresa Auguet, Gemma Aragonès, Esther Guiu-Jurado, Alba Berlanga, Marta Curriu, Carmen Aguilar and Cristóbal Richart
Grup de Recerca GEMMAIR - Medicina Aplicada. Departament de Medicina I Cirurgia, Universitat Rovira i Virgili (URV), Institut Investigació Sanitària Pere Virgili (IISPV), 43007 Tarragona, Spain

Teresa Auguet, Ajla Alibalic and Cristóbal Richart
Servei Medicina Interna, Hospital Universitari Joan XXIII, 43007 Tarragona, Spain

Salomé Martinez
Servei Anatomia Patològica, Hospital Universitari Joan XXIII, 43007 Tarragona, Spain

Esteban Hernández and Vicente Martín-Paredero
Servei Angiologia I Cirurgia Vascular, Hospital Universitari Joan XXIII, 43007 Tarragona, Spain

María-Luisa Camara and Xavier Ruyra
Servei de Cirurgia Cardíaca, Hospital Germans Trias i Pujol, 08916 Badalona, Spain

Jina Choo and Jeong-Hyun Cho
College of Nursing, Korea University, Seoul, South Korea

Juneyoung Lee
Department of Biostatistics, College of Medicine, Korea University, Seoul, South Korea

Lora E Burke
School of Nursing and Epidemiology and Clinical and Translational Science Institute, University of Pittsburgh, Pennsylvania, USA

Akira Sekikawa
Department of Epidemiology, Graduate School of Public Health, University of Pittsburgh, Pennsylvania, USA

Sae Young Jae
College of Arts and Physical Education, University of Seoul, Seoul, South Korea

In-Kyung Jeong
Department of Endocrinology and Metabolism, Kyung Hee University School of Medicine, Kyung Hee University Hospital at Gangdong, Seoul, South Korea

Sin-Gon Kim
Korea University Anam Hospital, Seoul, South Korea

Dong Hyeok Cho
Chonnam National University Hospital, Gwangju, South Korea

Chong Hwa Kim
Sejong General Hospital, Gyeonggi-do, South Korea

Chul Sik Kim
Hallym University Sacred Heart Hospital, Gyeonggi-do, South Korea

Won-Young Lee
Kangbuk Samsung Hospital, Seoul, South Korea

Kyu-Chang Won
Yeungnam University Medical Center, Daegu, South Korea

Doo-Man Kim
Department of Internal Medicine, Kangdong Sacred Heart Hospital, Hallym University Medical Center, Gil-Dong, Gangdong-Gu, Seoul, South Korea

Lu Qian, Saroj Thapa, Lu-yuan Tao, Shao-Ze Wu, Lu-Ping Wang, Jiao-Ni Wang, Jie Wang, Ji Li, Ji-Fei Tang and Kang-Ting Ji
Department of Cardiology, the Second Affiliated Hospital, Wenzhou Medical University, Wenzhou, Zhejiang 325000, China

Xiao-Yan Wang and Gao-Jiang Luo
Department of Cardiology, Yiwu Central Hospital, Yiwu 322000, China

Yu-Feng Li, Quan-Zhou Feng, Ya Huang and Yun-Dai Chen
The Department of Cardiology, Chinese PLA General Hospital, Fuxing Road 28, Beijing 100853, China

Wen-Qian Gao
The First Department of Geriatric Cardiology, Chinese PLA General Hospital, Beijing 100853, China

Xiu-Jing Zhang
The First Clinics, Administrative and Supportive Bureau, Chinese PLA General Logistics Department, Jia 14, Fuxing Road 22, Beijing 100842, China

Wen-Qian Gao, Quan-Zhou Feng, Yu-Feng Li, Ya Huang, Yan-Ming Chen, Bo Yang and Cai-Yi Lu
The Department of Cardiology, Chinese PLA General Hospital, Beijing 100853, China

Wen-Qian Gao
The First Department of Geriatric Cardiology, Chinese PLA General Hospital, Beijing 100853, China

Yuan-Xin Li
Navy Wangshoulu Clinics, Xicui Road, Beijing 100036, China

Julian P. Halcox
Institute of Life Sciences 2, Swansea University College of Medicine, Singleton Park, Swansea SA2 8PP, UK

José R. Banegas
Department of Preventive Medicine and Public
Health, School of Medicine, Universidad Autónoma
de Madrid/IdiPaz and CIBER of Epidemiology
and Public Health (CIBERESP), Madrid, Spain

Carine Roy and David Hajage
INSERM CIC-EC 1425 and Département
d'Épidémiologie et Recherche Clinique, Assistance
Publique–Hôpitaux de Paris, Hôpital Bichat, Paris,
France

Jean Dallongeville
INSERM U 744, Institut Pasteur de Lille, Université
Lille-Nord de France, Lille, France

Guy De Backer
Department of Public Health, University of Ghent,
Ghent, Belgium

Eliseo Guallar
Departments of Epidemiology and Medicine and
Welch Center of Prevention, Epidemiology and
Clinical Research, Johns Hopkins Bloomberg School
of Public Health, Baltimore, MD, USA

Joep Perk
School of Health and Caring Sciences, Linnaeus
University, Kalmar, Sweden

Karin M. Henriksson
Department of Medical Sciences, Uppsala University,
Uppsala, Sweden

Claudio Borghi
Department of Internal Medicine, Ageing and
Clinical Nephrology, University of Bologna,
Bologna, Italy

**Indre Ceponiene, Egle Tamuleviciute-Prasciene,
Justina Motiejunaite and Rimvydas Slapikas**
Department of Cardiology, Medical Academy,
Lithuanian University of Health Sciences, Eiveniu
2, Kaunas LT-50009, Lithuania

**Jurate Klumbiene, Edita Sakyte and Janina
Petkeviciene**
Faculty of Public Health, Medical Academy,
Lithuanian University of Health Sciences, Siaures
av. 57, Kaunas LT-49264, Lithuania

Jonas Ceponis
Department of Endocrinology, Medical Academy,
Lithuanian University of Health Sciences, Eiveniu
2, Kaunas LT-50009, Lithuania

Ci He, Jin-gang Yang, Fei-zhou Du and Ming Gu
Department of Radiology, Chengdu Military
General Hospital, Chengdu, Sichuan 610083, China

Yun-ming Li
Department of Neurosurgery, Chengdu Military
General Hospital, Chengdu, Sichuan 610083, China

Jian Rong
Division of Geriatric Medicine, Department of
Medicine, Chengdu Military General Hospital,
Chengdu, Sichuan 610083, China

Zhi-gang Yang
Department of Radiology, West China Hospital,
Sichuan University, Chengdu, Sichuan 610041,
China

**Gunilla Nordin Fredrikson, Harry Björkbacka, Maria
Wigren, Eva Bengtsson, Gerd Östling, Margaretha
Persson and Jan Nilsson**
Department of Clinical Sciences Malmö, Lund
University, Malmö, Sweden

**Faisel Khan, Helen C. Looker, Fiona Adams and
Jill Belch**
Medical Research Institute, University of Dundee,
Dundee, UK

**Kunihiko Aizawa, Francesco Casanova, Kim
Gooding and Phil Gates**
Diabetes and Vascular Medicine, NIHR Exeter
Clinical Research Facility and University of Exeter
Medical School, Exeter, UK

Carlo Palombo
Department of Surgical, Medical, Molecular
Pathology, and Critical Area Medicine, Pisa, Italy

**Silvia Pinnola, Elena Venturi and Michaela
Kozakova**
Department of Clinical and Experimental Medicine,
University of Pisa, Pisa, Italy

Li-Ming Gan and Volker Schnecke
AstraZeneca, Cardiovascular and Metabolic
Diseases, Mölndal, Sweden

**Jing-Wei Li, Si-Yi He, Peng Liu, Lin Luo, Liang
Zhao and Ying-Bin Xiao**
Institute of Cardiovascular Surgery, PLA, Xinqiao
Hospital, Third Military Medical University, No.
183 Xinqiao Street, Chongqing 400037, PR China

Kejian Liu and Xiaomei Guo
Department of Cardiology, Tongji Hospital, Tongji Medical College, Huazhong University of Science and Technology, Wuhan 430030, China

Kejian Liu, Yin Yin, Yue Li, Rui Chai, Xinwei Li and Yi Peng
Department of Cardiology, the First Affiliated Hospital, Shihezi University School of Medicine, Shihezi, Xinjiang, China

Saiyare Xuekelati, Yue Zhang and Jiangdong Wu
The Key Laboratory of Xinjiang Endemic and Ethnic Diseases, Shihezi University, Shihezi, Xinjiang 832000, China

Lisheng Jiang, Lan Shen, Linghong Shen and Ben He
Department of Cardiology, Shanghai Jiao Tong University Affiliated Chest Hospital, Shanghai, China

Min Zhang
Department of Clinical Medicine, Shanghai Medical School, Fudan University, Shanghai, China

Lisheng Jiang, Min Zhang, Lan Shen, Qin Shao, Linghong Shen and Ben He
Department of Cardiology, Renji Hospital, School of Medicine, Shanghai Jiaotong University, Shanghai, China

Hong Zhang
Institution of Biostatistics, School of Life Science, Fudan University, Shanghai, China

Gunilla Journath
Cardiology unit, Department of Medicine, Karolinska Institutet, Karolinska University Hospital, Stockholm, Sweden

Kristina Hambraeus
Department of Cardiology, Falun Hospital, Falun, Sweden

Emil Hagström
Uppsala Clinical Research Center, and Department of Medical Sciences, Uppsala University, Uppsala, Sweden

Billie Pettersson
Amgen Inc, Thousand Oaks, California, USA

Mickael Löthgren
Amgen (Europe) GmbH, Zug, Switzerland

Jianhui Zhuang, Dachun Xu, Guofu Zhu, Shekhar Singh, Luoman Chen, Mengyun Zhu, Wei Chen, Yawei Xu and Xiankai Li
Department of Cardiology, Shanghai Tenth People's Hospital, Tongji University School of Medicine, Shanghai, China

Yang Han
Department of Pathology,Shanghai East Hospital, Tongji University School of Medicine, Shanghai, China

Xiankai Li
Department of Cardiology, Shigatse People's Hospital, Shigatse, Tibet, China

Jia Chen and Jingshu Guan
Department of Cardiology, Shanghai Baoshan Hospital of Integrated Traditional Chinese and Western Medicine, Friendship Road 181, Baoshan District, Shanghai, China

Zhiyong Cao
Department of Cardiology, Shanghai Navy 411 Hospital, Shanghai, China

Xuedong Wang, Xinxin Liu, Xingtao Huang, Jiale Lin, Dan Huang, Bo Yu and Jingbo Hou
Department of Cardiology, The Second Affiliated Hospital of Harbin Medical University, Harbin 150001, China

Xuedong Wang, Xinxin Liu, Xingtao Huang, Jiale Lin, Dan Huang, Bo Yu and Jingbo Hou
Key Laboratory of Myocardial Ischemia, Ministry of Education, Harbin Medical University, Harbin 150001, China

Zulong Xie
Department of Cardiology, The Second Affiliated Hospital of Chongqing Medical University, Chongqing 400010, China

Katsuaki Yokoyama, Rei Matsuo and Naoya Matsumoto
Department of Cardiology, Nihon University Hospital, 1-6 Kanda-Surugadai, Chiyoda-ku, Tokyo 101-8309, Japan

Shigemasa Tani
Department of Health Planning Center and Cardiology, Nihon University Hospital, 1-6 Kanda-Surugadai, Chiyoda-ku, Tokyo 101-8309, Japan

Karam Sadoon Alzuhairi, Peter Søgaard and Jan Ravkilde
Department of Cardiology, Aalborg University Hospital, Hobrovej 18, –9000 Aalborg, DK, Denmark

Peter Søgaard
Department of Clinical Medicine, Aalborg University, Aalborg, Denmark

Aziza Azimi and Christian Torp-Pedersen
Department of Health, Science and Technology, Aalborg University, Aalborg, Denmark

Michael Maeng
Department of Cardiology, Aarhus University Hospital, Aarhus, Denmark

Lisette Okkels Jensen
Department of Cardiology, Odense University Hospital, Odense, Denmark

Index

www.ingramcontent.com/pod-product-compliance
Lightning Source LLC
Chambersburg PA
CBHW080407190526
45161CB00003B/156